Occupational Therapy in Australia and Aotearoa New Zealand

This outstanding new edition offers a comprehensive introduction to occupational therapy in Australia and Aotearoa New Zealand, framing the profession's role within health systems as well as the breadth of its practice.

The book is divided into three sections: the first explores historical and contemporary contexts, including regulatory and professional frameworks; while the second addresses professional issues such as diverse client groups, collaborative partnerships, and core principles shaping practice. The final section focuses on practical issues, including assessment, assistive technology, primary health care, sustainability, health promotion, leadership, and practice management. Each chapter includes case studies, key concept explanations, and review questions, while an overarching theme is the building of respectful relationships with Aboriginal and Torres Strait Islander peoples and Pacific and Māori communities, guided by principles of truth, recognition, and reconciliation.

Including a companion site with adaptable PowerPoint slides for lecturers and educators who adopt the edited text for education purposes, this is the complete resource for students beginning their journey toward becoming occupational therapists in Australia or Aotearoa New Zealand.

Ted Brown, Professor of Occupational Therapy and Undergraduate Course Director, Monash University – Peninsula Campus, Frankston, Victoria, Australia

Helen Bourke-Taylor, Professor of Occupational Therapy and Undergraduate Research Honours Coordinator, Monash University – Peninsula Campus, Frankston, Victoria, Australia

Stephen Isbel, Professor, Discipline of Occupational Therapy, University of Canberra Hospital, Bruce, Australian Capital Territory, Australia

Louise Gustafsson, Professor, Discipline of Occupational Therapy, Griffith University, Nathan, Queensland, Australia

Yvonne Thomas, Professor and Research Coordinator, The School of Occupational Therapy/Te Kura Whakaora Ngangahau, Otago Polytechnic/Te Kura Matatini ki Otago, Dunedin, Aotearoa New Zealand

Ema Tokolahi, Associate Professor, The School of Occupational Therapy/Te Kura Whakaora Ngangahau, Otago Polytechnic/Te Kura Matatini ki Otago, Dunedin, Aotearoa New Zealand

Occupational Therapy in Australia and Aotearoa New Zealand

Professional and Practice Issues

Third Edition

*Edited by Ted Brown, Helen Bourke-Taylor,
Stephen Isbel, Louise Gustafsson,
Yvonne Thomas, and Ema Tokolahi*

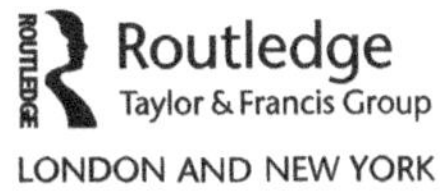

Routledge
Taylor & Francis Group

LONDON AND NEW YORK

Designed cover image: Getty Images

Third edition published 2027
by Routledge
4 Park Square, Milton Park, Abingdon, Oxon, OX14 4RN

and by Routledge
605 Third Avenue, New York, NY 10158

Routledge is an imprint of the Taylor & Francis Group, an informa business

For Product Safety Concerns and Information please contact our EU representative GPSR@taylorandfrancis.com. Taylor & Francis Verlag GmbH, Kaufingerstraße 24, 80331 München, Germany.

Trademark notice: Product or corporate names may be trademarks or registered trademarks, and are used only for identification and explanation without intent to infringe.

First edition published by Allen and Unwin 2017

Second edition published by Routledge 2021

British Library Cataloguing-in-Publication Data
A catalogue record for this book is available from the British Library

ISBN: 978-1-032-80141-4 (hbk)
ISBN: 978-1-032-80142-1 (pbk)
ISBN: 978-1-003-49566-6 (ebk)

DOI: 10.4324/9781003495666

Typeset in Sabon
by Apex CoVantage, LLC

Access the Support Material: www.routledge.com/9781032801421

Ted Brown

- David Stevens, life partner and constant source of support and patience for the time my academic pursuits take up.
- Archer and Oscar, our two Burmese cats who are constant sources of occupational engagement, intrigue, companionship, and playfulness.
- John Waugh and Colin Martin, dear friends who listened and laughed with me along the way.
- My academic colleagues in the Department of Occupational Therapy, Monash University – Peninsula Campus for their ongoing collegiality, collaboration, friendship, and support of my educational, research, professional, and personal endeavours over the years.
- Professor Sylvia Rodger, Professor Jane Case-Smith, Professor Jim Hinojosa, and Professor Gary Kielhofner, four occupational therapy scholars, educators, researchers, champions, and visionaries whose contributions to the profession were exceptional, enduring, and selfless.

Helen Bourke-Taylor

- I dedicate my work on this book to all my colleagues over the years who have joined me in expending energy and passion into growing the profession in Australia into the evidence-based health profession it is becoming today.
- I embrace ideas and actions which will contribute to aligning occupational therapy with culturally and ethically safe practice for individuals and collectives everywhere.
- I thank my family and friends for their love and for sharing the fun times in life.

Stephen Isbel

- I dedicate this book to all occupational therapists and
  occupational therapy students. I hope this book assists
  you in your work and study wherever it may be.

Louise Gustafsson

- This is dedicated to my occupational therapy colleagues (past
  and present) – thank you for your support and friendship, and
  for the promotion of all that is great about this profession.

Yvonne Thomas

- In memory of Dr Linda Wilson who inspired and mentored me
  as a new academic, to achieve more than I thought possible.
- I dedicate this book to all occupational therapists
  in Aotearoa New Zealand, and to the profession
  that works for equitable wellbeing for Māori.

Ema Tokolahi

- 'Ofa lahi atu and thanks to my family, particularly
  my children Aisea, Anthony, Lesieli, my husband
  Siaki, and my parents John and Margaret.
- Ngā mihi nui to the colleagues (near and far) who stepped
  up, stood back, and enabled me to contribute to this book.

Contents

About the editors

Ted Brown completed his undergraduate occupational therapy education in Canada in 1986 and his doctoral education in occupational therapy at the University of Queensland in 2003. He worked as an occupational therapy clinician for 16 years in Canada and Australia, primarily in the area of paediatrics. In 2005, he moved into the higher education sector, taking up an academic position in the Department of Occupational Therapy at Monash University – Peninsula Campus in Australia. Professor Brown has published four edited books, 35 book chapters, and over 400 journal manuscripts. He has supervised 65 honours, 25 masters, and 15 doctoral students to completion. He was made an inaugural fellow of the Occupational Therapy Australia Research Academy in 2017 and was inducted into the American Occupational Therapy Association Roster of Fellows in 2019. Professor Brown served as an associate editor of the *American Journal of Occupational Therapy* for 11 years (2010–2021) and the *Australian Occupational Therapy Journal* for 16 years (2005–2021). His research areas have primarily focused on occupational therapy assessment and practice with children and families, evidence-based practice in occupational therapy practice, social justice, occupational intersectionality, and evidence-based education in the healthcare professions.

Helen Bourke-Taylor completed her occupational therapy education at La Trobe University in 1990. Helen completed her Master of Science in Occupational Therapy in the USA in 2000 and her PhD at La Trobe in 2010. Helen worked clinically with children with disability, in neurorehabilitation, and with mothers of children with disability in her evidence-based programme Healthy Mothers Healthy Families. Helen is a fellow of the Occupational Therapy Australia Research Academy and is dedicated to contributing to the evidence base and advancing the profession to meet the needs of all people. Helen's research is mainly in the area of childhood disability, families, services, and instrument development. Her particular focus is centred on elevating enjoyment in healthy occupations via evidence-based approaches, strategies, and interventions. Helen is grateful to have been involved in three editions of the current book, 14 chapters, and 102 scientific papers and is the recipient of over 7.5 million dollars in grant funding. Helen has supervised many honours, master, and PhD theses and values encouraging occupational therapists to pursue research.

Louise Gustafsson is Academic Lead of Occupational Therapy at Griffith University in Queensland. She commenced her occupational therapy career in 1992 and worked in predominantly hospital-based rehabilitation services before moving to an academic career in 2002. She received her PhD in 2006, and her research is predominantly in collaboration with older adults and people living with neurological conditions and injury. She is most interested in how to better support and empower people to engage in their occupations long after the acute event, injury, or diagnosis. Professor Gustafsson has received over $14 million in research funding, published approximately 190 papers, and supported over 65 undergraduate and 18 postgraduate research students to completion. Her commitment and contribution to research and teaching have been recognised by a range of honours, including Fellow of the Occupational Therapy Australia Research Academy (2019) and Senior Fellow of the Higher Education Academy (2021).

Stephen Isbel completed his undergraduate and doctoral qualifications at Sydney University. Stephen has worked in the USA, the UK, and Australia as an occupational therapist, primarily in the areas of aged care, community care, and adult neurological rehabilitation. Stephen has research interests in aged care, post-stroke rehabilitation, driver rehabilitation, public health, and occupational therapy education. He teaches into the bachelor and masters programmes and supervises masters and doctoral candidates at the University of Canberra. Stephen lives and works in Ngunnawal country in Canberra, the federal capital of Australia.

Yvonne Thomas has been an occupational therapy educator and researcher in Australia, the United Kingdom, and New Zealand for more than 30 years. As a practitioner, Yvonne worked in a wide range of practice areas, with a particular interest in mental health recovery. She has extensive experience of curriculum design and delivery and supporting the expansion of the occupational therapy professional. Her research interests include innovative practice education, health professional education, wellbeing through occupation, and social justice for marginalised populations. Yvonne has published widely and supervises master's and doctoral students in New Zealand and the United Kingdom.

Ema Tokolahi is of English/Welsh decent, trained and practiced as an occupational therapist in the United Kingdom, and immigrated to Aotearoa New Zealand in 2005. Ema primarily practiced in mental health settings, across inpatient and community contexts, and with children, adolescents, and adults. She has taught at Otago Polytechnic since 2017, after completing her doctoral research at Auckland University of Technology. Ema is an associate professor and has led a Health Research Council–funded study to determine the research priorities for occupational therapy; a community-funded initiative to develop and implement an interprofessional student-assisted health service in partnership with iwi/community organisations; building workforce capacity to promote children's mental health; trauma-informed practice; and role emerging placements. Ema has published widely in peer-reviewed literature, served as associate editor for the *New Zealand Journal of Occupational Therapy* for the last four years, and supported several masters ākonga through to completion. Ema's research interests include culturally responsive practices and teaching, work-augmented learning as a delivery mode for occupational therapy degrees, and how we evidence occupational therapy practice.

Contributors

Lynne Adamson
Health Academic, Global Health Consultants
Sydney, New South Wales, Australia

Rebecca Allen
Professional Adviser Program Accreditation
Occupational Therapy Council of Australia Ltd.
South Perth, Western Australia, Australia

Kylie Angelou
Lecturer in Occupational Therapy
Sydney School of Health Sciences
Faculty of Medicine and Health
University of Sydney – Camperdown Campus
Sydney, New South Wales, Australia

Tammy Aplin
Conjoint Research Fellow
School of Health and Rehabilitation Sciences
Faculty of Health and Behavioural Sciences
University of Queensland
Brisbane, Queensland, Australia

Jess Archer
Lecturer
Department of Occupational Therapy
School of Primary and Allied Health Care
Faculty of Medicine, Nursing and Health Sciences
Monash University – Peninsula Campus
Frankston, Victoria, Australia

Samantha Ashby
Associate Professor of Occupational Therapy & Head of Discipline
School of Health Sciences
The University of New Castle
New Castle, New South Wales, Australia

Zainab Badat
Functional Family Therapist, Kia Puāwai
Former Practicum Leader at AUT
Auckland, New Zealand

Linda Barclay
Associate Professor and Higher Degree Research Coordinator
Department of Occupational Therapy
School of Primary & Allied Health Care
Faculty of Medicine, Nursing and Health Sciences
Monash University – Peninsula Campus
Frankston, Victoria, Australia

Jacqui Barfoot
Postdoctoral Research Fellow
Child Health Research Centre
Faculty of Medical and Behavioural Sciences
The University of Queensland
South Brisbane, Queensland, Australia.

Karen Below
Kaitakawaenga Māori Cultural Practice Supervisor
Victoria University
Wellington, New Zealand

Tori Bensemann
Occupational Therapist
Active Plus
Whanganui, New Zealand

Angela Berndt
Professor of Occupational Therapy & Academic Lead
School of Health Sciences
College of Health & Medicine
University of Tasmania
Launceston, Tasmania, Australia

Thomas Bevitt
Senior Lecturer & Professional Practice Program Convener in Occupational Therapy
Faculty of Health, University of Canberra,
Bruce, Australian Capital Territory, Australia

Anoo Bhopti
Senior Lecturer and Course Director for the Master of Occupational Therapy Practice
Department of Occupational Therapy
School of Primary & Allied Health Care
Faculty of Medicine, Nursing and Health Sciences
Monash University – Peninsula Campus
Frankston, Victoria, Australia

Michelle Bissett
Associate Professor, Course Coordinator – Occupational Therapy & Deputy Chair of
    Discipline – Allied Health, Midwifery & Community
Faculty of Health
Southern Cross University
Gold Coast, Queensland, Australia

Adriana Bootten (Sāmoan)
Occupational Therapist/Kaiwhakaora Ngangahau
Central Auckland Specialist School/Tāmaki Makaurau Te Kura Motuhake
Tāmaki Makaurau/Auckland,
Aotearoa/New Zealand

Helen Bourke-Taylor
Professor and Research Honours Course Coordinator
Department of Occupational Therapy
School of Primary & Allied Health Care
Faculty of Medicine, Nursing and Health Sciences
Monash University – Peninsula Campus
Frankston, Victoria, Australia

Julie Brayshaw
Immediate Past Chair of the Occupational Therapy Board of Australia &
Senior Lecturer & Course Coordinator – Bachelor of Occupational Therapy (Honours)
Curtin School of Allied Health
Faculty of Health Sciences
Curtin University
Bently, Western Australia, Australia

Jennie Brentnall
Lecturer
Faculty Medicine and Health
The University of Sydney
Sydney, New South Wales, Australia

Tiffany Brooke
Senior Lecturer and Fieldwork Team Associate
Otago Polytechnic
Dunedin, New Zealand

Kieran Broome
Senior Occupational Therapist and Director
Good to Better Pty Ltd
Imbil, Queensland, Australia

Georgia Brown
Ngāpuhi, Ngāti Hine, Ngāti Whatua, Ngāti Wai, Te Waiariki
Kaiwhakaora Ngangahau/Mental Health and Addictions
Tāmaki Makaurau, Aotearoa New Zealand

Ted Brown
Professor of Occupational Therapy & Undergraduate Course Director
Department of Occupational Therapy, School of Primary and Allied Health Care
Faculty of Medicine, Nursing and Health Sciences
Monash University – Peninsula Campus
Frankston, Victoria, Australia

Chloe Bryant
Lecturer
Division of Occupational Therapy
School of Health & Rehabilitation Sciences
The University of Queensland
St. Lucia, Queensland, Australia.

Angus Buchanan
Professor of Occupational Therapy
Curtin School of Allied Health
Curtin University, Perth, Western Australia, Australia

Rosalind Bye
Associate Professor Occupational Therapy
School of Health Sciences
Faculty of Health
Western Sydney University, Campbelltown Campus
Campbelltown, New South Wales, Australia

Liana Cahill
Senior Lecturer
Department of Occupational Therapy
School of Allied Health
Faculty of Health Sciences
Australian Catholic University – Melbourne Campus
Fitzroy, Victoria, Australia

Anne-Maree Caine
Program Director – Occupational Therapy
School of Health Sciences and Social Work
Griffith University, Queensland, Australia

Libby Callaway
Associate Professor
Department of Occupational Therapy
Rehabilitation, Ageing and Independent Living (RAIL) Research Centre
School of Primary and Allied Health Care
Faculty of Medicine, Nursing and Health Sciences
Monash University (Peninsula Campus)
Frankston, Victoria, Australia

Lauren J. Christie
Senior Implementation Science Research Fellow – Allied Health
Allied Health Research Unit
St Vincent's Fellow Network Sydney
Darlinghurst, New South Wales, Australia &
Clinical Fellow
School of Allied Health and Nursing Research Institute
Faculty of Health Sciences
Australian Catholic University – North Sydney Campus
North Sydney, New South Wales, Australia

Marina Ciccarelli
Professor of Occupational Therapy, Dean Learning and Teaching
Faculty of Health Sciences
Curtin University
Perth, Western Australia, Australia

CONTRIBUTORS

Emma Clark
Lecturer in Occupational Therapy
School of Health and Social Development
Faculty of Health
Deakin University – Waterfront Campus
Geelong, Victoria, Australia

Melinda Cooper
Senior Product Manager – Therapeutics
Pearson Clinical Assessment
Melbourne, Victoria, Australia

Emma Crawford
Lecturer
Discipline of Occupational Therapy
School of Health and Rehabilitation Science
Faculty of Health, Medicine, and Behaviour Sciences
Brisbane, Queensland, Australia

Michael Curtin
Associate Professor and Head of School
School of Allied Health, Exercise and Sports Sciences
Charles Sturt University
Albury, New South Wales, Australia

Anne Cusick
Professor and Chair in Occupational Therapy
School of Health Sciences
Faculty of Medicine and Health
The University of Sydney
Sydney, New South Wales, Australia

Susan Darzins
Senior Lecturer & National Course Coordinator, Bachelor of Occupational Therapy
Interprofessional Education Lead
School of Allied Health
Faculty of Health Sciences
Australian Catholic University
Fitzroy, Victoria, Australia

Vagner Dos Santos
Senior Lecturer & Head of Discipline for Occupational Therapy
School of Allied Health, Exercise and Sports Sciences
Charles Sturt University
Port Macquarie, New South Wales, Australia

Marina Elisara (Sāmoan)
Primary Mental Health Occupational Therapist
Independent Practitioner
Kirikiriroa | Hamilton, Aotearoa New Zealand

Priscilla Ennals
Senior Manager – Research and Evaluations
Neami National
Preston, Victoria, Australia

Renee Fitisemanu
Te Arawa (Tapuika, Waitaha)
Kaiwhakahaere Whakaora Ngangahau/Kawhakahaere at Te Wānanga Aronui o Tāmaki
    Makau Rau
Tāmaki Makaurau, Aotearoa New Zealand

Tracy Fortune
Associate Professor of Occupational Therapy
School of Allied Health, Human Services and Sport
La Trobe University
Bundoora, Victoria, Australia

Jessica Francis
Occupational Therapist & Director
The Training Club Pty Ltd
Sydney, NSW, Australia

Gelya Frank
Professor Emeritus
Chan Division of Occupational Science and Occupational Therapy
University of Southern California
Los Angeles, California, United States

Kate Garam
Lecturer
Department of Occupational Therapy, School of Primary and Allied Health Care
Faculty of Medicine, Nursing and Health Sciences
Monash University – Peninsula Campus
Frankston, Victoria, Australia

Ali Gebhardt
Lecturer in Occupational Therapy
School of Health Sciences
Faculty of Health
Western Sydney University, Campbelltown Campus
Campbelltown, New South Wales, Australia

Emma Gee
Lived experience consultant, occupational therapist, and author
Emma Gee Pty Ltd
Surrey Hills, Victoria, Australia

Emma George
Associate Professor and Program Director Occupational Therapy
School of Allied Health Science and Practice
Faculty of Health and Medical Sciences
University of Adelaide
Adelaide, South Australia, Australia

Erin Georgiou
Occupational Therapist
The Royal Children's Hospital
Melbourne, Victoria, Australia

Kate Gledhill
Lecturer & Third Year Undergraduate Coordinator
Department of Occupational Therapy, School of Primary and Allied Health Care
Faculty of Medicine, Nursing and Health Sciences
Monash University – Peninsula Campus
Frankston, Victoria, Australia

Emily Glennon (Cook Island)
Practice Supervisor
Health New Zealand, Te Whatu Ora.
Tamaki Makaurau | Auckland, Aotearoa New Zealand

Craig Greber
Associate Professor of Occupational Therapy
School of Health
University of the Sunshine Coast – Sippy Downs Campus
Sippy Downs, Queensland, Australia

Louise Gustafsson
Professor & Academic Lead, Discipline of Occupational Therapy
School of Health Sciences and Social Work
Griffith University – Nathan Campus
Nathan, Queensland, Australia

Tenelle J. Hodson
Lecturer
Discipline of Occupational Therapy
School of Health Sciences and Social Work
Griffith University – Nathan Campus
Nathan, Queensland, Australia

Jessica Holding
Lecturer
Discipline of Occupational Therapy
School of Health Sciences and Social Work
Griffith University
Brisbane, Queensland, Australia

Aiko Hoshino
Lecturer
Graduate School of Medicine & School of Health Sciences
Nagoya University, Japan

Stephen Isbel
Professor, Discipline of Occupational Therapy
Faculty of Health, University of Canberra Hospital
University of Canberra
Canberra, Australian Capital Territory, Australia

Carole James
Professor of Occupational Therapy
Sydney School of Health Sciences
University of Sydney
Sydney, NSW, Australia

Helen Jeffery
Principal Lecturer
School of Occupational Therapy
Otago Polytechnic
Dunedin, Otago, New Zealand

Dan Johnson
Occupational Therapy New Zealand – Whakaora Ngangahau Aotearoa (OTNZ-WNA)
    Council member
OTNZ-WNA – Tangata Tiriti (Non-Indigenous) Delegate, World Federation of
    Occupational Therapists
Wellington, New Zealand

Laura Jolliffe
Allied Health Research and Knowledge Translation Lead
Peninsula Health
Frankston, Victoria, Australia &
Adjunct Senior Research Fellow
Department of Occupational Therapy
School of Primary & Allied Health Care
Faculty of Medicine, Nursing and Health Sciences
Monash University – Peninsula Campus
Frankston, Victoria, Australia

Anna Joy
Lecturer
Department of Occupational Therapy
School of Primary & Allied Health Care
Faculty of Medicine, Nursing and Health Sciences
Monash University – Peninsula Campus
Frankston, Victoria, Australia

Rachel Kapa-Vivian (Te Aupōuri and Ngāti Kahungunu o Wairoa)
Health & Wellbeing Advisor
ASB Bank
Tamaki Makaurau | Auckland, Aotearoa New Zealand

Penelope Kinney
Head of Programmes
Te Kura Whakaora Ngangahau | The School of Occupational Therapy
Otago Polytechnic
Dunedin, Otago, New Zealand

Rhondda Knox
Chief Executive and Registrar |Tumu Whakarae me te Kairēhita
Occupational Therapy Board of New Zealand |Te Poari Whakaora Ngangahau O Aotearoa
Wellington, New Zealand

Aislinn Lalor
Senior Lecturer, Department of Occupational Therapy
Senior Research Fellow, Rehabilitation, Ageing and Independent Living (RAIL)
   Research Centre
School of Primary and Allied Health Care
Faculty of Medicine, Nursing and Health Sciences
Monash University – Peninsula Campus
Frankston, Victoria, Australia

Natasha Layton
Senior Research Fellow
Rehabilitation, Ageing and Independent Living (RAIL) Research Centre
School of Primary and Allied Health Care
Faculty of Medicine, Nursing and Health Sciences
Monash University (Peninsula Campus)
Frankston, Victoria, Australia

Simon Leadley
Lecturer & First Year Undergraduate Coordinator
Department of Occupational Therapy, School of Primary and Allied Health Care
Faculty of Medicine, Nursing and Health Sciences
Monash University – Peninsula Campus
Frankston, Victoria, Australia

Krista Lenders
Lecturer
Department of Occupational Therapy
School of Primary and Allied Health Care
Faculty of Medicine, Nursing and Health Sciences
Monash University – Peninsula Campus
Frankston, Victoria, Australia

Monica Leo
Department of Occupational Therapy, School of Primary and Allied Health Care
Faculty of Medicine, Nursing and Health Sciences
Monash University – Peninsula Campus
Frankston, Victoria, Australia

Jessica Levick
Lecturer
School of Health and Medical Sciences
University of Southern Queensland
Ipswich, Queensland, Australia

Joanne Lewis
Senior Lecturer in Occupational Therapy
Sydney School of Health Sciences
Faculty of Medicine and Health
University of Sydney – Camperdown Campus
Sydney, NSW, Australia

Jacki Liddle
Conjoint Research Fellow in Occupational Therapy
University of Queensland and Princess Alexandra Hospital
Brisbane, Queensland, Australia

Adam Lo
2nd Alternate Delegate (Occupational Therapy Australia)
World Federation of Occupational Therapists &
Senior Mental Health Clinician, Disaster Recovery Flood Team – Metro South
  Health
Brisbane, Queensland, Australia

Alexandra Logan
Senior Lecturer
School of Health Sciences
Australian Catholic University
Brisbane, Queensland, Australia

Sue Lukersmith
Associate Professor of Disability and Health Implementation Research
Health Research Institute
University of Canberra
Canberra, ACT, Australia

Claire Lynch
Senior Lecturer
School of Allied Health
Australian Catholic University
Melbourne, Victoria, Australia

Jenni Mace
Senior Lecturer
Occupational Science and Therapy
Auckland University of Technology
North Shore Campus, Auckland, Aotearoa New Zealand

Lynette Mackenzie
Professor in Occupational Therapy
Sydney School of Health Sciences
Faculty of Medicine and Health
University of Sydney – Camperdown Campus
Sydney, New South Wales, Australia

Ana Paula Serrata Malfitano
Associate Professor
Occupational Therapy Department and Post-Graduate Program in Occupational Therapy
Federal University of São Carlos
São Carlos, Brazil

Haylee Martell
Tainui, Ngāi Tāmanuhiri
Kaiwhakahaere Whakaora Ngangahau/Kawhakahaere ki Te Kura Matatini ki Ōtepoti
Kirikiriroa, Aotearoa New Zealand

Kathryn Martin
Discipline of Occupational Therapy
School of Health and Rehabilitation Science
Faculty of Health, Medicine, and Behaviour Sciences
Brisbane, Queensland, Australia

Tomomi McAuliffe
Lecturer
Discipline of Occupational Therapy
School of Health and Rehabilitation Science
Faculty of Health, Medicine, and Behaviour Sciences
The University of Queensland
Brisbane, Queensland, Australia

Carol McKinstry
Professor of Occupational Therapy, Chair of Academic Board & Deputy Dean
La Trobe Rural Health School
La Trobe University
Bendigo, Victoria, Australia

Keri McMullan
Senior Lecturer in Occupational Therapy
The School of Occupational Therapy/Te Kura Whakaora Ngangahau
Otago Polytechnic/Te Kura Matatini ki Otago

Matthew McShane
Project Coordinator-Disability Design
Griffith University
Gold Coast, Queensland, Australia

Ben Milbourn
Curtin School of Allied Health
Associate Professor of Occupational Therapy
Curtin University, Perth, Western Australia, Australia

Darren Mills
Principal Lecturer
Te Kura Whakaora Ngangahau/School of Occupational Therapy
Te Kura Matatini ki Otago/Otago Polytechnic
Dunedin, Otago, New Zealand

Matthew Molineux
Professor and Deputy Head of School (Learning and Teaching)
Discipline of Occupational Therapy
School of Health Sciences and Social Work, Griffith University
Gold Coast, Queensland, Australia

Monica Moran
Associate Professor
Western Australian Centre for Rural Health
The University of Western Australia
Geralton, Western Australia, Australia

CONTRIBUTORS

Tracy Murphy
Clinical and Academic Lead, Health Equity
Health NZ
Napier, New Zealand

Shoba Nayar
Senior Associate Editor
Journal of Occupational Science
Chennai, Tamil Nadu, India

Lisa O'Brien
Professor Emeritus
Occupational Therapy
Department of Nursing and Allied Health
School of Health Sciences
Swinburne University of Technology
Hawthorn, Victoria, Australia

Tracey Parnell
Associate Head of School & Senior Lecturer in Occupational Therapy
School of Allied Health, Exercise and Sports Sciences
Faculty of Science and Health
Charles Sturt University
Albury/Wodonga, Victoria/New South Wales, Australia

Dave Parsons
Associate Professor of Occupational Therapy
Campus Lead (Fremantle) – Occupational Therapy
School of Health Sciences
Faculty of Medicine, Nursing & Midwifery and Health Sciences
The University of Notre Dame Australia
Fremantle, Western Australia, Australia

Lachlan Pascoe
Lecturer
Discipline of Occupational Therapy
School of Health Sciences and Social Work
Griffith University
Brisbane, Queensland, Australia

Suzanne Patterson
Lecturer
Faculty of Occupational Science and Therapy
Auckland University of Technology
Auckland, Aotearoa New Zealand

Bronwyn Paynter
Founder/Occupational Therapist
Nature OT
Adelaide, South Australia, Australia

Claire Pearce
Assistant Professor of Occupational Therapy
Faculty of Health, University of Canberra Hospital
University of Canberra,
Bruce, Australian Capital Territory, Australia

Annette Peart
Senior Research Fellow
Addiction Studies, Turning Point
Eastern Health Clinical School
Faculty of Medicine, Nursing & Health Sciences
Monash University
Melbourne, Victoria, Australia

Merrolee Penman
Associate Professor
Curtin School of Allied Health
Curtin University, Perth, Western Australia, Australia

Genevieve Pepin
Professor and Higher Degree by Research Director
School of Health and Social Development
Deakin University
Victoria, Australia

Judy Ranka
Lecturer in Occupational Therapy
Sydney School of Health Sciences
Faculty of Medicine and Health
University of Sydney – Camperdown Campus
Sydney, New South Wales, Australia

Sarah Redfearn
Health Improvement Practitioner, Trainer
WellSouth
Dunedin, Otago, New Zealand

Heleen Reid
Head of Department
Department of Occupational Science and Therapy
AUT University
Auckland, New Zealand

Caleb Rixon
Chief Vision Officer
Genyus Network
Geelong, Vic, Australia

Andrea Robinson
Occupational Therapist
Response Assessment Discharge (RAD) Team
Frankston Hospital, Peninsula Health
Frankston, Victoria, Australia

Luke Robinson
Senior Lecturer, Deputy Course Director BOccTher(Hons) & Fourth Year Undergraduate
  Coordinator
Department of Occupational Therapy
School of Primary & Allied Health Care
Faculty of Medicine, Nursing and Health Sciences
Monash University – Peninsula Campus
Frankston, Victoria, Australia

Sandy Rutherford
Senior Research Officer for the Centre for Person Centred Research
Faculty of Health and Environmental Sciences
Auckland University of Technology
Auckland, New Zealand

Yasmin Sadler
Ngāpuhi, Ngai Te Rangi
Kaiwhakaora Ngangahau/Community Occupational Therapist
Tairāwhiti, Aotearoa New Zealand

Justin Scanlan
Associate Professor in Occupational Therapy
Sydney School of Health Sciences
Faculty of Medicine and Health
University of Sydney – Camperdown Campus
Sydney, New South Wales, Australia

Emma J. Schneider
Senior Lecturer
Department of Allied Health
School of Health Sciences
Swinburne University of Technology – Hawthorn Campus
Hawthorn, Victoria, Australia
Grade 4 Occupational Therapist – Research and Quality
Occupational Therapy Department
Alfred Health – The Alfred Hospital
Melbourne, Victoria, Australia

Ben Sellar
Lecturer and Program Director, Occupational Therapy
UniSA Allied Health & Human Performance
University of South Australia
Adelaide, South Australia, Australia

Loretta Sheppard
Associate Professor in Occupational Therapy
School of Allied Health
Australian Catholic University
Melbourne, Victoria, Australia

Mary Silcock
Principal Advisor
Ministry of Health
Wellington, New Zealand

Diane L. Smith
Professor Emeritus of Occupational Therapy
MGH Institute of Health Professions
Boston, Massachusetts, United States

Kaitlyn Spalding
Lecturer
Discipline of Occupational Therapy
School of Health Sciences and Social Work
Griffith University
Brisbane, Queensland, Australia

Claire Squires
Senior Lecturer
Otago Polytechnic
Dunedin, New Zealand

Mandy Stanley
Honorary Professor
Edith Cowan University
Perth, Western Australia, Australia

James Sunderland
Principal Lecturer
School of Occupational Therapy
Otago Polytechnic
Dunedin, Otago, New Zealand

Vicky Tariau (Cook Islands)
Senior Occupational Therapist
Regional Forensic Psychiatry Services: Work Rehabilitation, Waitematā District, Te
    Whatu Ora/HealthNZ

Leigh Tesch
Executive Officer
Inscape Tas
Hobart, Tasmania, Australia

Yvonne Thomas
Professor and Research Coordinator
The School of Occupational Therapy/Te Kura Whakaora Ngangahau
Otago Polytechnic/Te Kura Matatini ki Otago
Dunedin, New Zealand

Kerrie Thomsen
Associate Professor
Occupational Therapy Department
First Peoples Curriculum Pedagogy Coordinator
School of Allied Health
Faculty of Health Sciences
Australian Catholic University
Fitzroy, Victoria, Australia

Ema Tokolahi
Associate Professor
The School of Occupational Therapy/Te Kura Whakaora Ngangahau
Otago Polytechnic/Te Kura Matatini ki Otago
City Campus, Wintec, Hamilton, New Zealand

Stacey Touma
Belongside Families
Sydney, New South Wales, Australia

Merrill J. Turpin
Associate Professor
Division of Occupational Therapy
School of Health & Rehabilitation Sciences
The University of Queensland
St. Lucia, Queensland, Australia.

Carolyn Unsworth
Professor and Head of Discipline
Institute of Health and Wellbeing
Federation University Australia,
Ballarat, Victoria, Australia

Narinder Verma
Fieldwork Team Lead & Principal Lecturer
Otago Polytechnic
Dunedin, Otago, New Zealand

Kim Walder
Lecturer
Discipline of Occupational Therapy
School of Health Sciences and Social Work
Griffith University – Nathan Campus
Brisbane, Queensland, Australia

Kylie Wales
Senior Lecturer, School of Allied Health
Australian Catholic University
North Sydney, New South Wales, Australia

Kim Weigle-Reese
Lecturer
Department of Occupational Therapy
School of Primary and Allied Health Care
Faculty of Medicine, Nursing and Health Sciences
Monash University – Peninsula Campus
Frankston, Victoria, Australia

Huhana Whautere
Fieldwork Associate
Otago Polytechnic
Taranaki, New Zealand

Nicole Young
Teaching Associate
Department of Occupational Therapy
School of Primary and Allied Health Care
Faculty of Medicine, Nursing and Health Sciences
Monash University – Peninsula Campus
Frankston, Victoria, Australia

Mong-Lin Yu
Senior Lecturer & Practice Education Coordinator
Department of Occupational Therapy
Deputy Director of Education – Work Integrated Learning in School of Primary and
 Allied Health Care
Faculty of Medicine, Nursing and Health Sciences
Monash University – Peninsula Campus
Frankston, Victoria, Australia

Tables

Figures

Acronyms included in book chapters

2SLGBTTQQIA	Two Spirit, Lesbian, Gay, Bisexual, Transgender, Queer, Questioning, Intersex, and Allies
AAC	Alternative Communication
AAOT	Australian Association of Occupational Therapists
ABS	Australian Bureau of Statistics
ACA	Accident Compensation Act
ACC	Accident Compensation Corporation
ACCHO	Aboriginal Community Controlled Health Organisations
ACS	Activity Card Sort
ACSQHC	Australian Commission on Safety and Quality in Health Care
ACU	Australian Catholic University
ADL	Activities of Daily Living
AEDC	Australian Early Developmental Census
AFL	Australian Football League
AHPRA	Australian Health Practitioner Regulation Agency
AI	Artificial Intelligence
AIHW	Australian Institute of Health and Welfare
AIT	Auckland Institute of Technology (Now AUT)
ALRC	Australian Law Reform Commission
AMSTAR 2	A MeaSurement Tool to Assess Systematic Reviews
AMT	Animated Movie Test
ANTAR	Australians for Native Title and Reconciliation
ANZCERTA	Australia–New Zealand Closer Economic Relations Trade Agreement
ANZCOTE	Australia New Zealand Committee of Occupational Therapy Educators

ANZOTPEA	Australia and New Zealand Occupational Therapy Practice Education Academics
AOTA	American Occupational Therapy Association
APA	Australian Physiotherapy Association
APEASE CRITERIA	Affordability, Practicability, Effectiveness and Cost-Effectiveness, Acceptability, Side Effects and Safety, Equity
APTOS	Applied Principles and Tables of Support
AQF	Australian Qualifications Framework
ASOS	Australasian Society of Occupational Scientists
AT	Assistive Technology
AUSLAN	Australian Sign Language
AUT	Auckland University of Technology
BCW	Behaviour Change Wheel
BHSc	Bachelor of Health Sciences
BLM	Black Lives Matter
BOT–3	Bruininks–Oseretsky Test of Motor Proficiency – Third Edition
CALD	Culturally and Linguistically Diverse
CanMOP	Canadian Model of Occupational Participation
CAOT	Canadian Association of Occupational Therapy
CAPE/PAC	Children's Assessment of Participation and Enjoyment/Preferences of Activities of Children
CASP	Critical Appraisal Skills Programme
CCMHT	Calgary Cambridge Model of History Taking
CFIR	Consolidated Framework for Implementation Research
ChiPPA	Child–Initiated Pretend Play Assessment
CIT	Central Institute of Technology
CLASS	Child Leisure Assessment Scale
CLIP	Checklist of Leisure, Interests, and Participation
CM	Case Management
CMHT	Community Mental Health Team
CMTAXONOMY	Case Management Taxonomy
CMOP–E	Canadian Model of Occupational Performance and Engagement
COM–B	Capability, Opportunity, Motivation Behaviour
COPE	The Care of People with dementia in their Environments
COPM	Canadian Occupational Performance Measure
COSMIN	COnsensus-based standards for the Selection of Health Measurement INstruments
COTIPP	Canadian Occupational Therapy Inter-Relational Practice Process
CPD	Continuing Professional Development
CPHP	Community and Population Health Practice
CPPF	Canadian Practice Process Framework
CUS	I am Concerned; this makes me Uncomfortable; this is a Safety issue
DESC	Describe the specific situation or behaviour using concrete data; Express the concerns you have and how the situation

	makes you feel; Suggest alternatives and seek agreement; and Consequences
DRH	Departments of Rural Health
DSF	Dynamic Sustainability Framework
EBP	Evidence-Based Practice
EDI	Equity, Diversity, and Inclusion
EPOC	Cochrane Effective Practice and Organisation of Care
ERIC	Expert Recommendations for Implementing Change
ERQ	Environmental Restriction Questionnaire
FCP	Family-Centred Practice
GDP	Gross Domestic Product
GEM	Graduate-Entry Master's
GenX	Generation X
GP	General Practitioner
GRADE	Grading of Recommendations, Assessment, Development and Evaluations
HIPs	Health Improvement Practitioners
HOME FAST	Home Falls and Accidents Screening Tool
HOME	Home Observation for Measurement of the Environment
HPCAA	Health Practitioners Competence Assurance Act
HSNA	Home Support Needs Assessment
IAHA	Indigenous Allied Health Australia
ICF	International Classification of Functioning, Disability and Health
IDT	Interdisciplinary Team
I-HOPE	In-Home Occupational Performance Evaluation
IMPACT–S	ICF-Measure of Participation and Activities Screener
IPA	Impact on Participation and Autonomy
IPE	Interprofessional education
IQIPP-AH	Improving Quality in Practice Placements – Allied Health
IRM	Intentional Relationship Model
ISBAR	Identify; Situation; Background; Assessment and Actions; Responsibility and Referral
ISLAGIATT PRINCIPLE	'It Seemed Like A Good Idea At The Time'
ISOS	International Society for Occupational Science
IT	Information Technology
JEDI	Justice, Equity, Diversity, and Inclusion
KAWA	Kawa Model
kg	Kilograms
KOTS	Koori Occupational Therapy Scheme
KT	Knowledge Translation
KTA FRAMEWORK	Knowledge to Action Framework
LCT	Life Course Theory
LGBTQIA+	Lesbian, Gay, Bisexual, Trans, Queer, Intersex, Asexual/ Aromantic and Other Diverse Genders and Sexualities
LGBTQIAP2S+	Lesbian, Gay, Bisexual, Transsexual, Queer, Intersex, Asexual, Pansexual, Two–Spirited Plus

MDT	Multi-disciplinary team
MeSH	Medical Subject Headings
MMM	Modified Monash Model
MND	Motor Neurone Disease
MOH	Ministry of Health
MOHO	Model of Human Occupation
MOHOST	Model of Human Occupation Screening Tool
Movement ABC-3	Movement Assessment Battery for Children – Third Edition
NCOIS	National Centre of Implementation Science
NDIA	National Disability Insurance Agency
NDIS	National Disability Insurance Scheme
NGO	Non-Governmental Organisation
NHMRC	National Health and Medical Research Council
NIH	National Institute of Health
NPT	Normalisation Process Theory
NRHA	National Rural Health Alliance
NSQHS	National Safety and Quality Health Service
NSW	New South Wales
NZ	New Zealand
NZSL	New Zealand Sign Language
OECD	Organisation for Economic Co-operation and Development
OP	Occupational Performance
OPI	Occupational performance issue
OPIC	Occupational Performance Issues and Challenges
OPM	Occupational Performance Model
OPMA	Occupational Performance Model (Australia)
ORCA	Organisational Readiness for Change Assessment
OTA	Occupational Therapy Australia
OTAFC	Occupational Therapy Assessment of Functional Capacity
OTBA	Occupational Therapy Board of Australia/Te Poari Whakaora Ngangahau o Aotearoa
OTBNZ	Occupational Therapy Board of New Zealand (Te Poari Whakaora Ngangahau)
OTBNZ TE POARI	Occupational Therapy Board of New Zealand Te Poari Whakaora Ngangahau O Aotearoa
OTBNZ/TPWNA	Occupational Therapy Board of New Zealand/Te Poari Whakaora Ngangahau o Aotearoa
OTBNZ	Occupational Therapy Board of New Zealand
OTC	Occupational Therapy Council of Australia Limited
OTCA	Occupational Therapy Council of Australia Ltd.
OTIPM	Occupational Therapy Intervention Process Model
OTNZ-WNA	Occupational Therapy New Zealand – Whakaora Ngangahau Aotearoa
OTPED	Occupational Therapy Practice Education Development
OTPF-4	Occupational Therapy Practice Framework – 4th edition
PAR	Participatory Action Research
PD	Professional Development

PE	Practice Education
PEDI-CAT	Pediatric Evaluation of Disability Inventory Computer Adaptive Test
PEM-CY	Participation and Environmental Measure for Children and Youth
PEO	Person Environment Occupation
PEO fit	Person–Environment–Occupation fit
PEOP	Person–Environment–Occupation–Performance Model
PEPA	Programme for Engagement, Participation and Activities
PhD	Doctor of Philosophy
PHO	Primary Health Organisations
PICO	Patient/Population/Problem; Intervention/Issue; Comparison; Outcome
RACF	Residential Aged Care Facility
RBMT-3	Rivermead Behavioural Memory Test Third Edition
RCM	Rehabilitation Case Manager
RCT	Randomised Controlled Trial
RE–AIM	Reach, Effectiveness, Adoption, Implementation, and Maintenance
RoB	Risk of bias
ROM	Range of Motion
RSL	Returned and Services League Clubs
RUDAS	Rowland Universal Dementia Assessment Scale
RUSH	Regional University Study Hubs
SARRAH	Services for Australian Rural and Remote Allied Health
SCED	Single Case Experimental Design
SCI	Spinal Cord Injury
SDH	Social Determinants of Health
SEWB	Social and Emotional Well-Being
SFA	School Function Assessment
SIL	Supported Independent Living
SOAP	Subjective Objective Assessment Plan
SP-2	Sensory Profile 2
SPEF-R2	Student Practice Evaluation Form – Revised (Second Edition)
SPHERE	Sydney Partnership for Health, Education, Research and Enterprise
SSI	School Setting Interview
STC	Sydney Training Centre
T–CAST	Theory Comparison and Selection Tool
TDF	Theoretical Domains Framework
TeamSTEPPS	Strategies and Tools to Enhance Performance and Patient Safety
TEQSA	Australian Tertiary Education Quality and Standards Agency
TRP	Therapeutic Reasoning Process
TTCP	Transitional Therapy and Care Program
TTTA	Trans–Tasman Travel Arrangement
UN	United Nations

UQ	University of Queensland
USC	University of Southern California
USER-PARTICIPATION	Utrecht Scale for Evaluation of Rehabilitation–Participation
VAHS	Victorian Aboriginal Health Service
Vineland-3	Vineland Adaptive Behavior Scales, Third Edition
VOTPEA	Victorian Occupational Therapy Practice Education Alliance
WeHSA	Westmead Home Safety Assessment
WEIRD	Western, Education, Industrial, Rich, and Democratic
WEIS	Work Environment Impact Scale
WFOT	World Federation of Occupational Therapists
WHO	World Health Organization
WHO-EUR	World Health Organization European Regional Office
WINTEC	Waikato Institute of Technology
WW2	World War Two
Y–PEM	Youth/Young adult Participation and Environment Measure

Respectful and inclusive terminology for health care professionals when engaging with Aboriginal and Torres Strait Islander peoples

Aboriginal Community Controlled Health Services (ACCHSs)[1]
Aboriginal Community Controlled Health Sector[1]
Aboriginal and Torres Strait Islander[2]
Aboriginal and Torres Strait Islander Health Worker[2]
Aboriginal and Torres Strait Islander People(s)[2]
Aboriginal and Torres Strait Islander Health Branch (A&TSIHB)[2]
Acknowledgement of Traditional Owners[2]
Acknowledgement of Country[1]
Aunty and Uncle[1]
Anangu – usually used by Aboriginal people in and from Central Australia[2]
Clan[1,2]
Community[1,2]
Country[1–3]
Custodian[1]
Deceased Person/s Warning[1]
Dreaming/Dreamtime[4]
Elder[1,2]
Goori – usually used by Aboriginal people in northern NSW coastal regions[1,2]
First Australians[1]
First Nations[3]
First Peoples[1]
Koori – usually used by Aboriginal people in parts of NSW and Victoria[1,2]
Land[1,2,4]
Men's Business[1]
Mob[1,2,4]
Murri – usually used by Aboriginal people in northwest NSW and Queensland[1,2]

Nation[1,2,4]

Ngarrindjeri – usually used by Aboriginal people in South Australia whose ancestral country is the Lower Murray River, Lakes, and Coorong region[2]

Noongar – usually used by Aboriginal people in south-west Western Australia[1,2]

Nunga – usually used by Aboriginal people in South Australia[1,2]

Palawa – usually used by Aboriginal people in and from Tasmania[1,2]

Torres Strait Islander/Person/People[1,4]

Traditional Custodians[2,3]

Traditional Owners[1,3]

Reconciliation[4]

Sorry Business[1,2]

Welcome to Country[1,2]

Women's Business[1]

Yarning[1]

Yarning Circle[1]

Yolngu – usually used by Aboriginal people in and from Northern Territory (northeast Arnhem Land)[2]

References

1 Centre for Aboriginal Health. (2019). *Communication positively: A guide to appropriate Aboriginal terminology*. Centre for Aboriginal Health, NSW Ministry of Health. https://www1.health.nsw.gov.au/pds/ActivePDSDocuments/GL2019_008.pdf

2 Australian Indigenous HealthInfonet. (n.d.). *The Australian Indigenous Healthinfonet guidelines for Aboriginal and Torres Strait Islander terminology*. https://healthinfonet.ecu.edu.au/healthinfonet/getContent.php?linkid=675466&title=The+Australian+Indigenous+HealthInfoNet+guidelines+for+Aboriginal+and+Torres+Strait+Islander+terminology&contentid=44676_1

3 Narragunnawali: Reconciliation in Education. (2019). *A guide to using respectful and inclusive language and terminology*. Canberra: Reconciliation Australia.

4 Australians Together. (2020). *Australians together language and terminology guide*. https://creativecommons.org/licenses/by-nc-nd/3.0/

Glossary of Māori terms included in the book

Ākonga – learner or student
Aotearoa – New Zealand
Hapū – subtribe, kinship group
Hauora Māori – Māori wellbeing
Hui – gathering, meeting
Iwi – tribe
Kaimahi – worker, staff member or employee
Kaiwhakaora Ngangahau – Te Tauara Whiri i te Reo Māori | Māori Language Commission gifted this term for occupational therapist along with Whakaora Ngangahau for occupational therapy in 2020. The terms convey the reawakening or restoration to health of one's activeness, spiritedness, and zeal
Karakia – incantation
Kaumatua – elders
Kaupapa – topic, purpose, or guiding principle
Kōrero – speech, narrative, discussion, conversation
Mahi – work
Manaakitanga – hospitality
Māori – Indigenous people of Aotearoa/New Zealand, normal, natural
Marae – a Māori communal or sacred meeting place
Mātauranga – knowledge, wisdom, understanding, skill, education
Noho marae – a stay on a marae, usually for cultural learning and immersion
Pākēhā – non-Māori
Pepeha – ancestry
Rangatira – chiefly, esteemed
Tane – man / male
Tangata – people
Tangata Tiriti – people in Aotearoa by grace of Te Tiriti o Waitangi

Tangata whaiora – a person seeking health
Tangata Whenua – Indigenous people born of the land
Tauiwi – foreigner or non-Māori person
Te Ao Māori – the Māori world
Te Reo Māori – the Māori language
Tikanga – customs, correct procedure, the correct way of doing something
Tino rangatiratanga – self-determination, full authority, autonomy, or self-governance
Waiata – songs
Wairua – many waters or a place of many streams
Wairuatanga – spirituality
Whai ora – pursuing or achieving wellbeing/health
Whakapapa – genealogy, lineage
Whakarongo – to listen or to hear
Whānau – family, extended family, community
Whanaungatanga – relationality
Whare – house
Whenua – land, placenta

Bookcover photograph: Stargazing as an occupation

The cover of the third edition of the book was selected due to an occupation that people around the world have engaged in for aeons, that being stargazing. Stargazing is the act of observing the night sky, whether you're casually scanning for constellations like Orion or the Big Dipper or using a telescope to explore distant celestial bodies. Unless you're a professional astronomer, this activity is considered stargazing. It encompasses looking up at stars and other cosmic phenomena for leisure, scientific inquiry, or even astrological interpretation. Whether done with the naked eye or aided by instruments, stargazing invites us to connect with the universe above.

The image on the book cover is of the Seven Sisters, also known as the Pleiades, which form a striking open star cluster in the Taurus constellation, renowned for their luminous bluish hue and the surrounding veil of nebulosity. These stars lie within a cloud of interstellar gas and dust that reflects their light, producing a soft, ethereal blue glow. This phenomenon is known as a reflection nebula, where starlight is scattered by nearby cosmic particles, enhancing the cluster's visual brilliance. Even without a telescope, the brightest members of the Pleiades can be seen as a small, misty grouping in the night sky.

Across cultures and continents, the Pleiades have inspired rich mythologies and enduring folklore. From Greek legends to Japanese traditions, and among Aboriginal and Torres Strait Islander and Māori communities, the cluster holds deep cultural significance. These stories reflect humanity's long-standing fascination with the celestial beauty and mystery of the Seven Sisters.

As editors, we invite the occupational therapy and occupational science community in Australia and Aotearoa New Zealand to engage in the reflective occupation of stargazing – an imaginative lens through which to explore our profession's history, current practices, and future directions. We hope this third edition of *Occupational Therapy in Australia and Aotearoa New Zealand: Professional and Practice Issues* serves as an informative companion in that journey, offering insights and provocations to support critical examination and forward-thinking dialogue within our discipline.

Acknowledgements

As the six book editors, we want to extend our sincere gratitude and thanks to all the contributing chapter authors. Without their generosity, tenacity, good will, collegiality, enthusiasm, teamwork, creativity, occupational engagement, constructive feedback, exceptional conceptual thinking, and visionary forethought, the scope, breadth, depth, and critical commentary included in this book would not have been possible. Mr David Stevens is acknowledged for his formatting of the PowerPoint slides that accompany each of the chapters and his creation of the list of figures, pictures, and tables located within the book's 41 chapters. Finally, we as editors would like to extend our thanks to Mr Russell George, Senior Commissioning Editor, Health & Social, Routledge Publishers, for his support and guidance throughout the publishing process.

Editors' collective reflections on current and future editions of occupational therapy in Australia and Aoteoroa New Zealand

We acknowledge that more inclusive and consultative approaches – grounded in cultural safety, self-determination, humility, and open-mindedness – should have guided the process of initiating this edition of *Occupational Therapy in Australia and Aotearoa New Zealand*. Our decision to proceed followed a familiar Western process, involving discussions with the publisher and an agreement to move forward with building the editorial and authorship teams.

We recognise that our approach to inviting contributors did not adequately reflect culturally grounded practices that prioritise relationship-building, dialogue, and shared decision-making with Aboriginal and Torres Strait Islander, Māori, and Pacific Peoples. These practices are essential to ensuring respectful and meaningful engagement.

We acknowledge that engagement with occupational therapists who identify as Aboriginal and Torres Strait Islander, Māori, and Pacific Peoples should have occurred prior to any formal agreement with the publisher. This would have supported shared ownership and understanding of the book's purpose and content. We recognise that our actions may have contributed to omissions in this edition.

We are grateful to the Aboriginal and Torres Strait Islander, Māori, and Pacific contributing authors whose voices and expertise are represented in several chapters of this edition. Moving forward, we are committed to learning from this experience. As editors, we will actively engage in open, respectful, and reciprocal dialogue with occupational therapists who identify as Aboriginal and Torres Strait Islander, Māori, and Pacific Peoples to inform the development of future editions.

The Australian and Aotearoa New Zealand context

An introduction to occupational therapy in an Australian and Aotearoa New Zealand context

Ted Brown, Yvonne Thomas, Stephen Isbel,
Louise Gustafsson, Helen Bourke-Taylor,
and Ema Tokolahi

Authors' positionality statement

We are Western-educated occupational therapists with postgraduate qualifications working in leadership positions in Australia and Aotearoa New Zealand. We are white cisgender able-bodied English-speaking individuals. We acknowledge our white privilege, our Global North outlook, and the impacts of colonial hegemony on the Aboriginal and Torres Strait Islander peoples of Australia and Māori communities in Aotearoa New Zealand. We support decolonisation, indigenisation, racial equality, queer inclusivity, cultural sensitivity, social and occupational justice, and gender-affirmative and culturally safe and responsive health care and education. We believe in the importance of building respectful relationships with Aboriginal and Torres Strait Islander peoples of Australia and Māori communities in Aotearoa New Zealand underpinned by seeking truth, recognition and reconciliation. This impacts our world view, how we understand the perspectives of others, and our scholarly writing.

Key terms
- Occupational therapy
- Australia
- Aotearoa New Zealand

Objectives
This chapter will allow the reader to:

- Outline the history of the two first editions of *Occupational Therapy in Australia: Professional and Practice Issues*
- Describe the structure of the third edition of *Occupational Therapy in Australia and Aotearoa New Zealand: Professional and Practice Issues*
- Articulate the similarities between occupational therapy professional practice in Australian and Aotearoa New Zealand contexts

DOI: 10.4324/9781003495666-2

1.1 Background to the third edition of *Occupational Therapy in Australia and Aotearoa New Zealand: Professional and Practice Issues*

The third edition of this textbook marks a decision to expand the focus on occupational therapy in both Australia and Aotearoa New Zealand. The aim of the first two editions of *Occupational Therapy in Australia* was to provide an introductory text about the professional and practice aspects of the occupational therapy discipline in the Australian context written by Australian occupational therapy authors for an Australian occupational therapy student audience. The first two editions were adopted by many of the occupational therapy university courses in Australia as an educational resource and reference.

Given the long-shared connections and collaborations of the Australian and Aotearoa New Zealander occupational therapy professional communities, the third edition of the book will reflect the collegiality, reciprocity, respect, and affiliation between the two countries. Occupational therapy in Australia and Aotearoa New Zealand share strong professional, educational, and regulatory connections, shaped by their geographic proximity and similar healthcare structures. Therefore, including New Zealand as a partner in the drafting of the third edition, now titled *Occupational Therapy in Australia and Aotearoa New Zealand: Professional and Practice Issues,* is a natural mutually beneficial evolution. The editors of the third edition are Ted Brown, Helen Bourke-Taylor, Stephen Isbel, Louise Gustafsson, Yvonne Thomas, and Ema Tokolahi.

Since the first edition there have also been changes in the editorial group and publishers. The first edition of *Occupational Therapy in Australia: Professional and Practice Issues* (2017) was edited by Ted Brown, Helen Bourke-Taylor, Stephen Isbel, and Reinie Cordier and consisted of 27 chapters. The second edition of *Occupational Therapy in Australia: Professional and Practice Issues* (2021) was edited by Ted Brown, Helen M. Bourke-Taylor, Stephen Isbel, Reinie Cordier, and Louise Gustafsson and consisted of 30 chapters.

Occupational Therapy in Australia and Aotearoa New Zealand is divided into three sections and includes 41 chapters. There is a combination of chapters in the third edition that are general to both country contexts, some Australian-specific chapters, and some chapters only focusing on Aotearoa New Zealand topics. Each chapter is formatted to facilitate the reader's learning by including authors' positionality statements, chapter learning objectives, key words, introduction, chapter topic sections and subsections, conclusion, summary dot points, review questions, and reference list. Many chapters also include vignettes where key concepts are applied to occupational therapy settings.

In chapters that were related to both Australian and Aotearoa New Zealand contexts, authorship teams included both Australian and Aotearoa New Zealand authors who collaborated in writing the chapters. As with the first two editions of the book, the chapters in *Occupational Therapy in Australia and Aotearoa New Zealand: Professional and Practice Issues* are written by teams of experienced occupational therapists and have all gone through an internal peer-review process whereby each chapter was reviewed by two other contributing authors who had written other chapters. Chapters composed by Māori, Pasifika, and Aboriginal and Torres Strait Islander authors underwent peer review by fellow contributing authors of their respective communities to ensure cultural safety. The intent of the internal peer-review process was to add a level of rigor, credibility, integrity, and accuracy to the chapters included in the third edition of the book.

1.2 Australia and Aotearoa New Zealand: similar but also distinct

Australia and Aotearoa New Zealand have long-shared, but also distinct social, cultural, and economic histories. Both countries have rich cultural Māori, Pasifika, and Aboriginal and Torres Strait Islander histories that existed long before colonisation took place. Both nations value the unique contributions and cultural richness of their Indigenous populations – Aboriginal and Torres Strait Islander peoples in Australia, and Māori in Aotearoa New Zealand. There is a mutual emphasis on reconciliation and cultural recognition. It is important to recognise that First Nations peoples in both countries have also experienced many impacts of colonisation (Axelsson et al., 2016; Moewaka Barnes & McCreanor, 2019; Smallwood et al., 2020).

The history and development of occupational therapy in both countries have followed a similar trajectory and was initially introduced during the 1940s from overseas (e.g., the United States and United Kingdom, where the profession was quickly growing). The first Occupational Therapy Training School in Australia opened in February 1942 in Sydney, New South Wales with an initial enrolment of 20 initial students (Cameron, 1977; Docker, 1959). The first occupational therapy education course was started at the Auckland Mental Hospital in 1940 with an initial enrollment of four students (Gordon et al., 2009). The Australian Association of Occupational Therapists (AAOT) was officially formed in 1945 and the New Zealand Registered Occupational Therapists Association was established in 1949. The World Federation of Occupational Therapy (WFOT) was founded in 1952 by ten occupational therapy associations including those from Australia and New Zealand (Anderson & Bell, 1988; Mendez & Greenberg Harris, 1998).

Today, there is free flow between Australia and Aotearoa New Zealand of occupational therapy practitioners, educators, researchers, and students. Two agreements have been put in place to facilitate the alliances, free movements, and trade and cultural linkages between the two countries: the Trans-Tasman Travel Arrangement (TTTA) and the Australia-New Zealand Closer Economic Relations Trade Agreement (ANZCERTA) (Scollay et al., 2010). Established in 1973, the TTTA allows citizens of both countries to live, work, and travel freely in each other's territories without the need for a visa. It fosters strong people-to-people connections and exchanges of culture. The ANZCERTA, signed in 1983, eliminates tariffs and trade barriers, promotes mutual recognition of goods and services, and facilitates economic integration. Together, these agreements strengthen the close ties between the two nations. Australia and Aotearoa New Zealand share numerous similarities across cultural, societal, and environmental dimensions due to their geographic proximity and historical connections. These similarities are also reflected in the occupational therapy professions in both countries. A few key parallels include:

- Both countries have a shared colonial history as former British colonies, which influences their legal, political, and educational systems. Australia and Aotearoa New Zealand became independent countries in 1901 and 1947, respectively.

- Both countries are constitutional monarchies within the British Commonwealth and have parliamentary democracies based on the Westminster system with a prime minister as the head of government.
- English is the primary language in both countries, making communication and cultural exchange relatively easy. Indigenous languages like Te Reo Māori in Aotearoa New Zealand and various Aboriginal and Torres Strait Islander languages in Australia are also embraced.
- Both countries have public health care systems and public education systems where many occupational therapists are employed.
- Australia and Aotearoa New Zealand are both immigrant nations that celebrate and encourage cultural diversity.
- Both nations have similar sets of social values, human rights, and social safety nets for citizens. They both have a strong focus on equality, diversity, inclusion, social justice, environmental conservation, and promoting egalitarianism within their societies. The occupational therapy disciplines in Australia and Aotearoa New Zealand embrace these social values as well (Whiteford et al., 2022).
- Both countries are known for their love of sports, with strong national teams in various sports like rugby, cricket, and netball. The fierce sporting rivalry between them, particularly in rugby and cricket, is well known.
- Both countries have a strong outdoor culture, with people enjoying activities like hiking, swimming, surfing, bushwalking/tramping, and camping due to their diverse and compelling landscapes. This no doubt impacts the play and leisure occupations that Australians and New Zealanders engage in.

While Aotearoa New Zealand and Australia share many similarities, they also have distinct differences that set them apart. Australia, known as the world's smallest continent and largest island, is a vast landmass with diverse landscapes including deserts, rainforests, and mountains. Its sheer size leads to diverse climates, ecosystems and unique wildlife such as kangaroos, koalas, wombats, emus, echidnas, and platypuses. In contrast, Aotearoa New Zealand is an archipelago comprising two main islands (North and South) and numerous smaller ones. It is known for its mountains, glaciers, lakes, fjords, rolling green hills, and forests home to the kiwi bird, tuatara, kākāpō, and wētā. The climates of the two countries differ significantly: Australia experiences a broad range of temperatures with its continental climate, from hot, humid tropical temperatures in the north to arid deserts in the interior and cooler southern winters, while Aotearoa New Zealand has a more temperate maritime climate with milder conditions year-round, although the South Island does receive snowfall during winter.

1.3 Similarities between Australian and Aotearoa New Zealand occupational therapy practice

The legal, political, and systemic differences between Australia and Aotearoa New Zealand directly influence the way occupational therapy is funded and has led to a range of similar but different areas of practice emerging for the profession. Occupational therapy practices in both countries share several similarities due to their shared professional standards and cultural contexts (see Table 1.1).

Table 1.1 Points of Comparison: Australian and Aotearoa New Zealand Occupational Therapy Practice

Core philosophy	Both Australian and New Zealander occupational therapists aim to enhance people's participation in daily occupations to improve their health, well-being, and social outcomes (see Chapter 21).
Focus on occupation	Occupational therapists in both countries recognise the importance of occupation as a means of promoting health and well-being, and they work to facilitate meaningful engagement in daily activities (see Chapters 31 and 32).
Client-centred approach	Occupational therapists in both countries prioritise the client's needs, preferences, and goals in the therapeutic process tailoring interventions and services to individual circumstances where feasible. Clients can include individuals, families, communities, collectives, and populations (see Chapters 10, 11, and 26).
Evidence-based practice	Both countries emphasise the importance of evidence-based approaches in occupational therapy, ensuring that interventions and services provided are grounded in research and best practices. Collaborative research initiatives strengthen the profession, with universities and institutions frequently exchanging knowledge on rehabilitation, disability support, and emerging areas like telehealth and the use of artificial intelligence with special needs populations (see Chapter 23).
Social justice orientation	The profession in both countries has a strong social justice orientation that recognise the importance of occupational justice, diversity, inclusion and belonging along with acknowledging the potential impacts of colonisation, injustice, oppression, discrimination, prejudice, bias, and marginalisation (Hocking, 2017; Whiteford et al., 2022) (see Chapter 13).
Commitment to inclusion, engagement, respect, and cultural sensitivity of Indigenous Peoples	Occupational therapists in both nations engage with Māori, Pasifika, and Aboriginal and Torres Strait Islander communities with respect, cultural humility, sensitivity and awareness, and strength-based approaches. Both countries prioritise cultural competence, with New Zealand's practice deeply influenced by Māori health models (see Chapter 16) and Australia integrating Indigenous perspectives into occupational therapy education (see Chapter 15) (Emery-Whittington, 2025a, 2025b). These commitments highlight the growing emphasis on holistic, culturally responsive care, cultural safety and humility, and mutual respect.
Interdisciplinary and multidisciplinary collaboration	Occupational therapists in both nations often work collaboratively with other healthcare professionals (including doctors, nurses, social workers, speech therapists, physiotherapists, psychologists, and others) to provide comprehensive holistic care and services to clients, families, collectives, communities, and organisations.
Working with diverse populations	Occupational therapists in both countries work with a wide range of individuals, including those with physical, cognitive, social, mental health, and developmental needs.
Professional frameworks, theories and models	Frameworks and practice models like the Person-Environment-Occupation Model, Model of Human Occupation, Canadian Model of Occupational Participation, Person-Environment-Occupation-Participation model, Kawa Model, Occupational Performance Model (Australia), Occupational Therapy Intervention Process Model, and Occupational Therapy Practice Framework 4th edition, are commonly taught in occupational therapy education courses in both Australia and Aotearoa New Zealand (Turpin et al., 2024) (see Chapter 25). Professional reasoning models are also taught in both countries.

(Continued)

Table 1.1 (Continued)

Academic education of occupational therapy students	Occupational therapy education in Australia and Aotearoa New Zealand shares many similarities due to their commitment to high-quality training and adherence to shared professional standards. Both nations implement rigorous accreditation processes to ensure programmes meet ethical and professional requirements and emphasise evidence-based practices to prepare students for integrating research into professional work. The Occupational Therapy Council of Australia Limited accredits occupational therapy courses in Australia, while the accreditation body for occupational therapy courses in Aotearoa New Zealand is the Occupational Therapy Board of New Zealand (see Chapters 6, 18, 19, and 20). The Australian and New Zealand Council of Occupational Therapy Educators is an unincorporated association that supports collaboration and development in occupational therapy education across both countries.
Practice education of occupational therapy students	As part of their education, occupational therapy students in Australia and Aotearoa New Zealand complete a range of practice education experiences in a range of professional practice settings and environments during their entry-to-practice education (see Chapters 19 and 20). Practical experience is a cornerstone of occupational therapy education in both Australia and New Zealand, with students required to complete extensive fieldwork and clinical placements to develop hands-on skills. Furthermore, occupational therapy qualifications from these two countries hold global recognition, enabling graduates to pursue careers in various international settings. The Australian and New Zealand Occupational Therapy Practice Education Academics (ANZOTPEA) group focuses on advancing fieldwork education and exploring innovative models to support occupational therapy students during their professional placements.
Professional registration boards	Both countries have professional registration bodies (Occupational Therapy Board of Australia [OTBA] and Occupational Therapy Board of New Zealand/Te Poari Whakaora Ngangahau o Aotearoa [OTBNZ/TPWNA]) that set standards for registration, protection of the public and continuing professional development (Brown et al., 2021). The OTBA and OTBNZ/TPWNA have published sets of professional competency standards for occupational therapists in both jurisdictions (see Chapter 6).
Professional associations	Both countries are professional associations that represent the disciplines at the national and international levels (Occupational Therapy Australia [OTA] and Occupational Therapy New Zealand – Whakaora Ngangahau Aotearoa [OTNZ–WNA]) (Adamson et al., 2021) (see Chapter 6). Both countries are also full members of the World Federation of Occupational Therapists (WFOT) (Mendez & Greenberg Harris, 1998). Conferences and professional networks organised by OTA and OTNZ–WNA further enhance this relationship, ensuring that occupational therapists in both nations remain informed about advancements, policy changes, and best practices.

1.4 Paradigm shifts: The occupational therapy profession in Australia and Aotearoa New Zealand moving forwards since the second edition of the book

Several paradigm shifts have occurred since 2021 when the second edition of *Occupational Therapy in Australia* was published. An important paradigm shift for the occupational therapy in Australia and Aotearoa New Zealand is decolonisation of the profession, including professional practice and occupational therapy student education. Occupational therapy is founded on Euro-Western ideology and colonial systems of care, law, and education that have failed to deliver equitable health, economic, social, and education outcomes for Indigenous communities (Davis & Came, 2022). There is an urgent need to decolonise and indigenise occupational therapy practice (Rudman et al., 2021) and education curricula that can only be achieved by dismantling the colonial structure that 'maintains privilege, controls occupational opportunities, determines laws, and disfigures justice' (Emery-Whittington, 2021, p. 155). Gibson (2020) describes decolonisation as a praxis, a personal and collective action to change that which has been accepted as an unjust norm in society. A six-part, strengths-based approach to decolonise occupational therapy has been proposed (Gibson, 2020; Ryall et al., 2021):

1. Listening respectfully to the person
2. Using appropriate communication skills
3. Building authentic partnerships
4. Critically reflecting on political, social, and historical contexts, as well as the professional context
5. Applying a human rights-based approach and
6. Evaluating processes and outcomes

Engaging in decolonisation as praxis is likely to be challenging, especially for those of us who are non-indigenous and have benefited from the privileges of colonisation (Ryall et al., 2021). A commitment to decolonisation requires a decentring of coloniality, identifying the systems that afford privilege to some and disadvantage others, and consciously refusing to support and participate in colonising ways (Emery-Whittington, 2025a). While Māori and Aboriginal or Torres Strait Island occupational therapists are already doing this work, non-indigenous occupational therapists have an important role and responsibility in decolonising occupational therapy. The challenge is to use our individual and collective power to 'step up' and do the work of advocating and supporting the rights of indigenous colleagues, clients, students and communities, and to 'step back' and provide space for indigenous colleagues and communities to take the lead in moving the profession towards indigenisation (Bell, 2024). Notably, decolonisation and indigenisation are the most important paradigm shifts now and for the future of the profession.

Another issue impacting the occupational therapy discipline is globalisation. Globalisation has significantly influenced healthcare professions (including occupational therapy) by reshaping education, scope of practice, professional registration requirements, and portability and recognition of credentials (Jesus et al., 2023). As some borders become less restrictive, occupational therapists engage in cross-cultural exchanges that foster professional innovations, international collaboration and information sharing (Ergin & Akin, 2017). This interconnectedness enables practitioners to adopt best practices from diverse healthcare systems, improving client care and driving advancements in occupational therapy research and evidence-based interventions. One notable effect of globalisation is the consistency of occupational therapy education standards via global frameworks, such as those set by the WFOT's (2016) Minimum Standards for the Education of Occupational Therapists, the application of the World Health Organization's (2001) International Classification of Functioning, Disability and Health, and the adoption occupational-based practice models and theories (e.g., Model of Human Occupation, Person-Environment-Occupation Model, Canadian Model of Occupational Participation).

Globalisation also introduces economic and ethical challenges, including disparities in healthcare access where high-income countries recruit skilled professionals from other jurisdictions, exacerbating shortages in lower-income nations – a phenomenon known as 'brain drain' (Leitão et al., 2024). In addition, restrictive policies and regulatory standards can inhibit the mobility and integration of international occupational therapy practitioners (Veras et al., 2013). For example, some jurisdictions require foreign-educated therapists to write a certification examination or meet local language requirements. Globalisation's influence continues to shape the future of occupational therapy practice and education worldwide (Jesus et al., 2023).

The current paradigm shift is the emergence of artificial intelligence (AI) and all its permutations and combinations. This will no doubt impact all aspects of our occupational lives. AI is poised to transform the occupational therapy profession by enhancing efficiency, expanding service delivery, and refining professional documentation. AI-driven tools can assist therapists in assessing clients' needs, informing therapists professional reasoning processes, and providing real-time recommendations based on evidence-based practice knowledge (Stover & Jacobs, 2025). Machine learning algorithms may optimise individualised treatment plans, thus improving client outcomes through predictive analytics. Additionally, AI-powered assistive technologies, such as smart prosthetics and adaptive communication systems, can increase accessibility for clients with disabilities. Telehealth and virtual rehabilitation platforms integrated with AI can also extend occupational therapy services to remote or underserved populations, improving inclusivity (Lanne & Leikas, 2021). However, ethical considerations remain, including concerns about AI replacing human-centred care and data security in automated systems (Harishbhai Tilala et al., 2024). While AI will enhance occupational therapists' capabilities, maintaining the profession's foundational principles – such as empathy, sound professional reasoning, and client-centred practice – will be crucial (Kaelin et al., 2024). Overall, AI offers substantial advancements, but its integration must align with the core values of occupational therapy practice.

1.5 Conclusion

Occupational Therapy in Australia and Aotearoa New Zealand: Professional and Practice Issues will be the first book of its kind written collaboratively by Australian and New Zealander occupational therapy authors. It is a unique edited publication and hopefully be used as a key education resource for the education of occupational therapy students in both jurisdictions. The occupational therapy professions in Australia and Aotearoa New Zealand are both similar but also distinct. However, it is the commonality, respect, collegiality, and democratic egalitarian worldview of the discipline in both countries that ensures that the bond between occupational therapists in Australia and Aotearoa New Zealand is resilient, respectful, collegial, and enduring.

The occupational therapy professions in both jurisdictions also recognise and acknowledge the effects of colonial hegemony on the Aboriginal and Torres Strait Islander peoples of Australia and the Māori communities in Aotearoa New Zealand. The professional, registration, accreditation, and education bodies in both countries in response to the impacts of colonisation on First Nations communities strongly support and advocate for decolonisation, indigenisation, racial equality, cultural sensitivity, and social and occupational justice (Curtin, 2025). Occupational therapy education courses in Australia and Aotearoa New Zealand are taking action to decolonise their curricula and recruit students from Aboriginal and Torres Strait Islander and Māori communities (Project Advisory Group to the Occupational Therapy Council of Australia Limited et al., 2023; Rudman et al., 2021).

At a time in the world that is focused on political, social, economic, and cultural difference, division, and competition, the substantive, reciprocal, mutual, and interconnected relationship between Australia and Aotearoa New Zealand is to be valued and not taken for granted. The impact of colonisation on the Aboriginal and Torres Strait Islander and Māori communities must be recognised and actions taken to promote reconciliation, recognition, inclusivity, and truth telling (Emery-Whittington & Te Maro, 2018). Australia and Aotearoa New Zealand occupational therapists must also continue to take leadership roles on the international stage to promote social and occupational justice, along with protecting the tenants of diversity, equality, and inclusion. Overall, Australia and Aotearoa New Zealand's occupational therapy professions maintain a dynamic, cooperative relationship, fostering continuous growth and knowledge development. Hopefully, *Occupational Therapy in Australia and Aotearoa New Zealand: Professional and Practice Issues* can contribute to ensuring those issues are heard and responded to within the occupational therapy profession and beyond.

1.6 Summary

- The focus of this book is to provide an introductory text about occupational therapy discipline in the Australian and Aotearoa New Zealand context.
- Occupational Therapy in Aotearoa New Zealand and Australia began at a similar time and was influenced by the development of the profession in Europe and the United States.
- With a shared colonial history as former British colonies, Australia and Aotearoa New Zealand have similar legal, political, public educational, and public health care systems where many occupational therapists are employed.
- Indigenous communities in both countries have been discriminated against and disadvantaged as a result of colonisation, resulting in many health, education, economic, and social inequities that still exist today.
- Occupational therapy is a continually evolving profession. Current and future changes include decolonisation of occupational therapy practice, philosophy and education, globalisation, and the increasing use of AI.

1.7 Review questions

- What are the two agreements that facilitate the movement of occupational therapists between Australia and Aotearo New Zealand?
- Identify and explain five shared concepts and values that underpin occupational therapy in Australia and Aotearoa New Zealand.
- What are the key registration, professional, and educational bodies that represent the occupational therapy discipline in Australian and Aotearoa New Zealand contexts?
- What is meant by a 'paradigm shift', and how might the three paradigm shifts described in the chapter change occupational therapy practice and education in the next 15 years?

References

Adamson, L., Allen, R., Brayshaw, J., Hunter, S., Lo, A., McKinstry, C., & Volkert, A. (2021). The role of occupational therapy professional associations and regulatory bodies in Australia. In T. Brown, H. Bourke-Taylor, S. Isbel, R. Cordier, & L. Gustafsson (Eds.), *Occupational therapy in Australia: Professional and practice issues* (pp. 50–60). Routledge.

Anderson, B., & Bell, J. (1988). *Occupational therapy: Its place in Australia's history.* New South Wales Association of Occupational Therapist.

Axelsson, P., Kukutai, T., & Kippen, R. (2016). The field of Indigenous health and the role of colonisation and history. *Journal of Population Research, 33*(1), 1–7. https://doi.org/10.1007/s12546-016-9163-2

Bell, A. (2024). *Becoming Tangata Tiriti: Working with Māori, honouring the Treaty.* Auckland University Press.

Brown, T., Bourke-Taylor, H., Isbel, S., & Cordier, R. (2017). *Occupational therapy in Australia: Professional and practice issues.* Allen & Unwin.

Brown, T., Bourke-Taylor, H., Isbel, S., Cordier, R., & Gustafsson, L. (2021). *Occupational therapy in Australia: Professional and practice issues* (2nd ed.). Routledge.

Cameron, B. S. (1977). *The work of our hands: A history of the occupational therapy school of Victoria.* B. S. Cameron.

Curtin, M. (2025). The continuing evolution of the occupational therapy profession. In M. Curtin, M. Egan, Y. Prior, T. Parnell, R. Galvaan, K. Sauve-Schenk, & D. Cezar Da Cruz (Eds.), *Occupational therapy for people experiencing illness, injury or impairment: Promoting occupational participation* (pp. 93–108). Elsevier.

Davis, G., & Came, H. (2022). A pūrākau analysis of institutional barriers facing Māori occupational therapy students. *Australian Occupational Therapy Journal, 69*(4), 414–423. https://doi.org/10.1111/1440-1630.12800

Docker, S. (1959). Development of occupational therapy in Australia. *Australian Occupational Therapy Journal, 6*(1), 2–8. https://doi.org/10.1111/j.1440-1630.1959.tb00824.x

Emery-Whittington, I. G. (2021). Occupational justice – Colonial business as usual? Indigenous observations from Aotearoa New Zealand. *Canadian Journal of Occupational Therapy, 88*(2), 153–162. https://doi.org/10.1177/00084174211005891

Emery-Whittington, I. G. (2025a). Decoloniality in occupational therapy preparation: Preparation and readiness. In M. Curtin, M. Egan, Y. Prior, T. Parnell, R. Galvaan, R. Sauve-Schenk, & D. Cezar Da Cruz (Eds.), *Occupational therapy for people experiencing illness, injury or impairment: Promoting occupational participation* (pp. 2–17). Elsevier.

Emery-Whittington, I. G. (2025b). Undoing coloniality: An Indigenous occupation-based perspective. In T. Brown, S. Isbel, L. Gustafsson, D. Powers Dirette, B. Collins, & T. Barlott (Eds.), *Human occupation: Contemporary concepts and lifespan perspectives* (9th ed., pp. 191–208). Routledge.

Emery-Whittington, I. G., & Te Maro, B. (2018). Decolonising occupation: Causing social change to help our ancestors rest and our descendents three. *New Zealand Journal of Occupational Therapy, 65*(1), 12–19.

Ergin, E., & Akin, B. (2017). Globalization and its reflections for health and nursing. *International Journal of Caring Sciences, 10*(1), 607–613. https://www.internationaljournalofcaringsciences.org/docs/66_ergin_review_10_1.pdf

Gibson, C. (2020). When the river runs dry: Leadership, decolonisation and healing in occupational therapy. *New Zealand Journal of Occupational Therapy, 67*(1), 11–20.

Gordon, B., Riordan, S., Scaletti, R., & Creighton, N. (2009). *Legacy of occupation. Stories of occupational therapy in New Zealand 1940–1972.* The Bush Press of New Zealand.

Harishbhai Tilala, M., Kumar Chenchala, P., Choppadandi, A., Kaur, J., Naguri, S., Saoji, R., & Devaguptapu, B. (2024). Ethical considerations in the use of artificial intelligence and machine learning in health care: A comprehensive review. *Cureus, 16*(6), e62443. https://doi.org/10.7759/cureus.62443

Hocking, C. (2017). Occupational justice as social justice: The moral claim for inclusion. *Journal of Occupational Science, 24*(1), 29–42. https://doi.org/10.1080/14427591.2017.1294016

Jesus, T. S., Mani, K., von Zweck, C., Bhattacharjya, S., Kamalakannan, S., & Ledgerd, R. (2023). The global status of occupational therapy workforce research worldwide: A scoping review. *American Journal of Occupational Therapy, 77*(3), 7703205080. https://doi.org/10.5014/ajot.2023.050089

Kaelin, V. C., Nilsson, I., & Lindgren, H. (2024). Occupational therapy in the space of artificial intelligence: Ethical considerations and human-centered efforts. *Scandinavian Journal of Occupational Therapy, 31*(1), 2421355. https://doi.org/10.1080/11038128.2024.2421355

Lanne, M., & Leikas, J. (2021). Ethical AI in the re-ablement of older people: Opportunities and challenges. *Gerontechnology, 20*(2), 1–13. https://doi.org/10.4017/gt.2021.20.2.26-473.11

Leitão, C. A., Salvador, G. L. de O., Idowu, B. M., & Dako, F. (2024). Drivers of global health care worker migration. *Journal of the American College of Radiology, 21*(8), 1188–1193. https://doi.org/10.1016/j.jacr.2024.03.005

Mendez, A. M., & Greenberg Harris, R. (1998). *A chronicle of the World Federation of Occupational Therapists.* World Federation of Occupational Therapists.

Moewaka Barnes, H., & McCreanor, T. (2019). Colonisation, hauora and whenua in Aotearoa. *Journal of the Royal Society of New Zealand, 49*(Supp 1), 19–33. https://doi.org/10.1080/03036758.2019.1668439

Project Advisory Group to the Occupational Therapy Council of Australia Limited, Ryan, A., Gibson, C., & Hummell, J. (2023). *Aboriginal and Torres Strait Islander health curriculum implementation project – Occupational therapy program accredition.* Occupational Therapy Council of Australia Limited.

Rudman, M. T., Flavell, H., Harris, C., & Wright, M. (2021). How prepared is Australian occupational therapy to decolonise its practice? *Australian Occupational Therapy Journal, 68*(4), 287–297. https://doi.org/10.1111/1440-1630.12725

Ryall, J., Ritchie, T., Butler, C., Ryan, A., & Gibson, C. (2021). Decolonising occupational therapy through a strengths-based approach. In T. Brown, H. Bourke-Taylor, S. Isbel, R. Cordier, & L. Gustafsson (Eds.), *Occupational therapy in Australia: Professional and practice issues* (2nd ed., pp. 130–142). Routledge.

Scollay, R., Findlay, C., & Kaufmann, U. (2010). *Australia New Zealand Closer Economic Relations Trade Agreement (ANZCERTA) and regional integration.* Institute of Southeast Asian Studies (ISEAS).

Smallwood, R., Woods, C., Power, T., & Usher, K. (2020). Understanding the impact of historical trauma due to colonization on the health and well-being of Indigenous young peoples: A systematic scoping review. *Journal of Transcultural Nursing, 32*(1), 59–68. https://doi.org/10.1177/1043659620935955

Stover, A. D., & Jacobs, K. (2025). Embracing artificial intelligence (AI) in occupational therapy practice: Bridging workforce gaps and redefining care. *WORK*. OnlineFirst. https://doi.org/10.1177/10519815241312447

Turpin, M., Garcia, J., & Iwama, M. K. (2024). *Using occupational therapy models in practice: A fieldguide*. Elsevier.

Veras, M., Pottie, K., Cameron, D., Dahal, G. P., Welch, V., Ramsay, T., & Tugwell, P. (2013). Assessing and comparing global health competencies in rehabilitation students. *Rehabilitation Research and Practice, 2013*, 208187. https://doi.org/10.1155/2013/208187

Whiteford, G. E., Parnell, T., Ramsden, L., Nott, M., & Vine-Daher, S. (2022). Understanding and advancing occupational justice and social inclusion. In P. Liamputtong (Ed.), *Handbook of social inclusion* (pp. 181–210). Springer. https://doi.org/10.1007/978-3-030-89594-5_10

World Federation of Occupational Therapists. (2016). *Minimum standards for the education of occupational therapists*. WFOT. https://wfot.org/resources/new-minimum-standards-for-the-education-of-occupational-therapists-2016-e-copy

World Health Organization. (2001). *International classification of functioning, disability and health (ICF)*. WHO. https://www.who.int/standards/classifications/international-classification-of-functioning-disability-and-health

CHAPTER 2

Occupational therapy in Australia's history

Anne Cusick, Ali Gebhardt, and Rosalind Bye

Authors' positionality statements

Anne Cusick is a woman of predominantly Irish and Scottish heritage whose ancestors arrived in Australia in the early 1800s. She currently lives on unceded Gundungurra and Dharawal Country and works on unceded lands of the Gadigal People of the Eora Nation. She has been an occupational therapist for 45 years. Anne is committed to professionalisation of occupational therapy through evidence-based-practice, which includes evidence from history, multi-directional historical scholarship, truth-telling, and historical acceptance.

Ali Gebhardt is an Aboriginal Woman with over 20 years' experience working as an occupational therapist in metropolitan, rural and remote areas, a PhD student with more than 8 years' experience teaching within the occupational therapy programme at a metropolitan university. Ali is devoted to increasing the number of Aboriginal and Torres Strait Islander practitioners and the development of culturally competent occupational therapy students.

Rosalind Bye is a white Australian woman, living and working on Dharawal Country, with over 30 years' experience as an occupational therapy educator and researcher, primarily at Western Sydney University. Ros is committed to ensuring occupational therapists and occupational therapy students learn from Australia's history and understand the impact of colonialism on present day occupational therapy practice, and commit to culturally sensitive practice with clients, families, and communities.

Acknowledgements

Thank you to Professor Susan Page, pro vice-chancellor, Indigenous Education at Western Sydney University, for her guidance and review of this chapter.

Key terms
- Occupational therapy
- Philosophy

DOI: 10.4324/9781003495666-3

- History of ideas, ideologies, and social movements
- Enduring issues

Objectives
This chapter will allow the reader to:

- Recognise philosophical roots of occupational therapy concepts and practice
- Describe intellectual and social movements shaping the emergence and practice of occupational therapy in Australia
- Explain how Australia's history influences occupational therapy today
- Apply an historical perspective to your own experience of occupational therapy in Australia

2.1 Introduction

In 2037, occupational therapy will celebrate 100 years in Australia. It was 1937 when Ethel May Francis returned to Sydney after studying occupational therapy in the United States and United Kingdom, becoming the first Australian to hold an occupational therapy qualification. Her occupational therapy practice, her leadership in education and research, and the contribution of occupational therapists who followed, would evolve into something uniquely Australian, shaped by the broader history of this land and its people.

The history of the ideas that underpin Australian occupational therapy begins in the late 1700s when Western ideas literally landed on the shores of a continent already home to Aboriginal and Torres Strait Islander peoples. They had lived in Australia for more than 65,000 years, developing, sustaining, and invigorating cultural practice, traditional law, and community life over many generations. They had their own beliefs about health and their own practices to maintain wellbeing through daily occupations and connection to lands and waterways, which we acknowledge today as 'Country'. In 1788, British invasion of land brought new ideas about ways of living and meanings of health that disrupted and derided Aboriginal and Torres Strait Islander knowledge. New diseases and forced removal of people from Country, and failure to respect or recognise traditional law and cultural practice were only some of the adverse consequences of British colonialisation. Aboriginal peoples responded to these challenges in the short and long term with resistance, resilience, advocacy and leadership to better inform Australian health practice and in time, the practice of occupational therapy.

Since the ideological roots of occupational therapy were planted by British colonisers, a big part of the history of occupational therapy in Australia is therefore understanding, acknowledging and reconciling what happened in colonial times. It is understanding the legacy of colonialism and its impact today, and how the profession can work for change to decolonise occupational therapy practice now and into the future. Another aspect of the uniquely Australian history of occupational therapy is the diversity of beliefs, daily occupations and patterns of participation that come from a national population overwhelmingly composed of first, second, or third-generation migrants.

This chapter examines how ancient ideas of occupation were incorporated into Western approaches to health and recovery. It explores how these ideas were introduced in Australia and how they led to the development of occupational therapy in this country. Throughout the chapter, forces that shaped the emergence and practice of occupational therapy in Australia are identified. The chapter ends by asking you to think about your history, your place in Australia as it was and now is, and what you might do as an occupational therapist to make history yourself.

2.2 Occupation for health and wellbeing – an idea across time

Two Ancient Greek philosophers, Hippocrates and Aristotle, most influenced the 'western philosophical tradition' underpinning all health professions. Hippocrates (~460BCE–370BCE), the *father of medicine* (Tsiompanou & Marketos, 2013), is well known for the *Hippocratic Oath* which states principles of good health practice, including confidentiality and the obligation to avoid harm and to try to do good. He developed a rational approach to care, using observational evidence to identify causes of disease, individualise treatment, and implement a wholistic approach to health using nutrition, exercise, and activity (occupations). Aristotle (384 BCE–322 BCE) proposed concepts still relevant in occupational therapy today, namely *practical wisdom* (learning by *doing*), the need for *purpose* in daily life, and the notion of *habits* that, once learned, we do without much thought (Aristotle, Book II, 1103.a33, ca 350 BCE/1925).

These ancient ideas were lost in Europe for hundreds of years. Western health practice was thus rarely rational, evidence based, or wholistic. But writings of these ancient philosophers, preserved by Arabic scholars, were translated into European languages and studied in the medieval period (500–1400 CE), and the ideas again became popular in Western medicine and law (Marenbon, 2024). During the Renaissance (1400–1600s CE), exploration of these classical ideas led to a form of thinking called *humanism* which emphasised the value of human beings and their potential to use reason, logic, and free enquiry to improve society and the physical world (Luebering, 2023). Humanism underpins many social movements today and is a foundation philosophy of occupational therapy.

Humanism was core to the Enlightenment, an intellectual movement that swept European and British empires (1600s to early 1800s). Leaders in society proposed reason, logic, and scientific methods could solve human problems and change the physical world to better suit human needs. A scientific approach to health and disease was used: observation, collection of evidence, and use of reason to deduce causes of ill health were championed. Broad reform in law and health characterised this period. Reforms in two types of institutions, asylums and prisons, have particular bearing on the emergence of occupational therapy.

2.2.1 Enlightenment asylum reform – occupation to ease mental illness

Before the Enlightenment, people with mental illness were treated terribly, and many entered asylums that were like prisons, with people locked up or shackled, their humanity abused, and their health neglected. The ability of inmates to move about or engage in daily occupations was restricted. Then in the 1790s, two asylums, one in York, England, and one in Paris, France, drew upon Enlightenment humanistic principles, recognising inmates' basic human rights for food, light, movement, safe shelter, and daily occupations. It was observed that inmates with a routine of daily occupations improved, and thus the idea of 'therapeutic use of occupation' emerged. This was a precursor of modern occupational therapy. The English and French approaches were a little different even though they both used occupation as part of the asylum treatment regimen. These differences are now explained.

The Quaker-founded York Asylum adopted *moral treatment*, where inmates were required to behave and dress in line with social and moral norms, participating in regular daily routines. Carers were asked to be kind, encouraging, and instructive. Occupations were proposed to bring order to disordered minds. Occupations included self-care, attending formal meals, and social and purposeful activities (gardening, work tasks, or creative arts). Positive patient results meant moral treatment was soon considered best practice.

In Paris, Enlightenment principles and values were applied in an asylum for the 'insane', whereby the superintendent Jean-Baptiste Pussin and wife Marguerite removed physical restraints; increased food rations; provided fresh air, daylight, and physical movement; and introduced routines and daily occupations. Inmates demonstrated dramatic improvements (Bewley, 2008). Pinel, the *father of modern psychiatry* in France, wrote about these innovations and recommended their incorporation into psychiatry. The Paris asylum reforms were based on humanistic principles that were sweeping all parts of society at that time during the French Revolution. For this reason, the approach was called *humane treatment*. This approach emphasised patient rights, scientific method, accurate observation and reporting, treatment trials, and evaluation of effect. Humanistic treatment and moral treatment were both influential in the early years of occupational therapy practice in Australia.

2.2.2 Enlightenment prisons – humane conditions and purposeful occupations

Enlightenment English reformers argued that convicts should also be treated humanely. The most dedicated proponent, John Howard, identified the lack of occupation in prisons as a significant problem. His report to British Parliament exposed prison conditions to the public: 'there are very few [prisons] . . . in which any work is done or can be done. The prisoners have neither tools, nor materials of any kinds; but spend their time in sloth' (John Howard, 1777). New laws resulted, giving prisoners' rights in relation to living conditions and opportunities for occupation. But overcrowding and underfunding in prisons meant these reforms were slow to enact. Further, the British government had become accustomed to exporting their prisoners as forced labour to British colonies around the world. When the American Revolution cut off that convict destination, a new site was sought. Land now known as Australia had been claimed by Captain James Cook for the British Empire in 1770, so the decision was made to set up the first of many convict colonies there.

Prison ships, prisons, and prison colonies were governed by British Parliament, and therefore Howard's prison reform laws applied to all. A fleet of 11 ships was sent (including five male and one female prison ship) with convicts and crew coming from different cultural, racial, and faith backgrounds (United Kingdom, Europe, North America, West Indies, India, and Africa). The fleet captain, Arthur Phillip, followed the new prison laws and prioritised health of all aboard so convicts could perform occupations essential to the colony's survival when they arrived. The prison ships had remarkably few convict deaths, in part because of improved conditions, including a routine of daily occupations. The fleet set ashore in Sydney Harbour on 26 January 1788, and Captain Phillip raised the British flag. More ships followed, and British colonisation of the Australian continent was unstoppable.

2.2.3 British territorial expansion: invaded, conquered, ceded – it matters

Many Aboriginal and Torres Strait Islander peoples today view the British arrival as an invasion. The British presented their territorial expansion as 'settlement'. Despite evidence to the contrary (Bowler et al., 2003; O'Connell & Allen, 2004), the British justified land their acquisition using the doctrine of 'terra nullius' (no-one's land). Lands and waterways were seized for colonial settlement and *sovereignty* of the Crown asserted over Australia without a declaration of war or negotiation of a treaty. Sovereignty is supreme authority over all people, lands, waterways, living creatures, and plants.

The impact of territorial expansion on Aboriginal peoples went far beyond dispossession; they were in effect stripped of all rights because in British law the rights and laws of a settling power *extinguish* pre-existing laws (Blackstone, 1765). If, however, territorial expansion occurred through conquering force legally recognised as war, then under British law Aboriginal people would have at least had their customary law recognised, because laws of original inhabitants *continued* until the invading power repealed them (Australian Law Reform Commission [ALRC], 2010a). Captain James Cook was instructed by the Royal Navy to take possession of country only with consent of original inhabitants unless the land was uninhabited.

Despite evidence of inhabitation and clear demonstrations by Aboriginal peoples that they did not consent to the British on their land (Higgins & Collard, 2020), Captain Cook made the false claim of 'terra nullius', 'nobody's land', which resulted in *settlement* being used to justify possession. The colonists did not recognise Aboriginal people as original inhabitants, let alone the existing leadership structures, 'institutions', or customary laws. Colonial occupation occurred without treaty or agreements (ALRC, 2010b). Without agreements there was no regulation of rights and responsibilities on either side (Brennan et al., 2005). Instead, the British exercised *sovereignty*, a legal term giving authority to do what they liked with the land, people, and resources.

Aboriginal people in colonial times were subject to British law, but they could not use it to advance their own interests or safeguard their rights (ALRC, 2010b). Legal argument about war versus settlement, and whose laws should be followed, was highlighted even in the early years in the colony. In 1836, Stephens set out the contradiction, when defending an Aboriginal man in court he said:

> Neither could this territory be called a conquered country as Great Britain was never at war with the [Aboriginal people]; it was not ceded country either; it in fact came within neither of these, but was a country which had a population having manners and customs of their own, and we had come to reside among them. Therefore in point of strictness and analogy to our law, we were bound to obey their laws, not they to obey ours . . . the [Aboriginal people] were not protected by those [Great Britain] laws . . . they could not claim any civil rights, they could not obtain recovery of, or compensation for, those lands which have been torn from them, and which they had held probably for centuries
>
> (*Superior Court of New South Wales, 1836*)

Stephens set out the truth of what he and others observed first-hand; yet until recently, the view expressed by Stephens was not the position of the Crown or most Australians. His testimony; thousands of other contemporary records; and historical, archaeological, and scientific evidence have, however, shifted this understanding. The evidence reveals that there were territorial conquests and war in Australia for at least 150 years. The *Sydney Wars*, for example, raged between 1788 and 1817 (Gapps, 2018); then the Wiradyuri (the Anglicised spelling is Wiradjuri) uprisings occurred (1820s to 1841) as colonial governors in Sydney pressed for territorial expansion into the western frontier (Gapps, 2021, 2025).

Across the continent, similar sustained regional conflicts occurred in violent and sustained struggles now called the 'Australian Wars' (Perkins et al., 2025). There were individual targeted killings and guerilla warfare on both sides, field battles between Aboriginal warriors and armed settlers and/or police, and massacres of entire Aboriginal communities occurred (Ryan et al., 2025). Conservative estimates of deaths from direct violence are 20,000 Aboriginal people and settler/police deaths around 2,500 (Australian War Memorial, 2025). Estimates which include direct and indirect violence are deaths around 100,000 spanning a 150-year period (Perkins et al., 2025).

During all these conflicts and all these years, no land or waterways were ever ceded by Aboriginal and Torres Strait Islander people to the Crown. As the Uluru Statement from the Heart (2017) states, Aboriginal and Torres Strait Islander sovereignty 'has never been ceded or extinguished and co-exists with the sovereignty of the Crown'. Further, Aboriginal and Torres Strait Islander peoples 'can assert sovereignty in their day-to-day actions' (Behrendt, 2003). The Aboriginal and Torres Strait Islander concept of 'Connection to Country' is fundamental to this sovereignty. Ruska and Clayton-Dixon (2015) explain: It is

> the ancient reciprocal relationship we have with our lands. This relationship finds its roots in our connection to kin and country, manifesting in our song, dance and story, our language, ceremony and law. It is vested in the individual, the tribe and the nation. Our sovereignty has endured since the first sunrise – it cannot be handed to us or taken from us. Aboriginal sovereignty can only be expressed or suppressed.

Most of the health, education, justice, and social systems in which occupational therapists work are based in laws, regulations, and practices emerging from these colonial times. 'Colonialism' still influences what happens, where, and how in Australian health and social care. Colonialism is the technical, cultural, social, and economic domination of one group of people over another (Hodder-Williams, 2001). To remove this structural domination, transformative change needs to happen, shifting systems and policies away from *colonising* towards *decolonising* approaches. In health, decolonising strategies must 'unpack colonial approaches to health, so Aboriginal and Torres Strait Islander peoples can not only survive but thrive. This means transforming the policies, processes and practices that influenced health in the past, and which are still present today' (Mackean et al., 2024).

This can only be done if people know what really happened during colonial times. Australians for Native Title and Reconciliation (ANTAR) (2024) call this 'truth-telling and truth-listening'. They say:

> Truth-telling, then, is not just about exposing Australia's violent colonial history, but about recognising and understanding First Nations connections to and

care for Country and the vast contributions Aboriginal and Torres Strait Islander peoples have made to Australia's culture, development and society. In a broader sense, truth-telling processes involve addressing concepts of narrative and collective memory, trauma and healing, and responsibility and justice.

As occupational therapists working in Australia, truth telling, listening, and historical acceptance are an important part of our education and professional development. Australian practice standards for registered occupational therapists thus require development of cultural capabilities in practice. All registered occupational therapists must be able to incorporate and respond to 'historical, political, cultural, societal, environmental and economic factors influencing health, wellbeing and occupations of Aboriginal and Torres Strait Islander Peoples' (Occupational Therapy Board of Australia, 2018). This starts with knowing and acknowledging what happened in the past, understanding the enduring effects of colonialism in communities and systems, and working to decolonise practice. Historical awareness and historical acceptance are prerequisite to this practice behaviour.

2.2.4 Migration, transportation, and assimilation 1788–1900

The colonial period existed from 1788 to 1900. Alongside the terrible conflicts and impacts on Aboriginal and Torres Strait Islander people that are now recognised in Australia's colonial history, the British continued to expand and relied on convict labour to do so. Initially Australia was established as a collection of British colonies scattered across the continent. Most were started as prison colonies for convicts who had been sentenced by British courts to transportation for their crimes. Some were serious crimes, others petty, and some convicts were political prisoners. Men, women, and children were transported to prison colonies and assigned to work in different locations and in different roles as unpaid forced labour. In a strange twist to the prison reforms that mandated daily occupation for the wellbeing and health of inmates, the occupation regimen itself became part of the punishment.

Hard labour could involve work in chained gangs where living conditions were extremely poor, brutal punishments were suffered, and the work was so arduous that many died (Davidson et al., 2003). These labour-gangs built roads, bridges, their own prisons, government buildings, schools, and hospitals. Domestic service or work in businesses was allocated to many women and girls. Often on the long voyage from Britain to the colony, they would learn occupations that could be useful in these roles, for example, needlework, reading, grooming, and cleaning (Foxhall, 2011). Prison reformers like Kezia Hayter accompanied women on convict ships as matrons, teaching them skills on board, working tirelessly for their safety, wellbeing, and access to meaningful occupations in the colonies (Cowley & Snowden, 2013). Convicts with trades or professions could be assigned to these same roles in service of the colony by administrators. Sometimes their skills were so valued they were pardoned and given important leadership roles in government.

Once convicts served their term, they were free, and most emancipists remained in the colonies, sending for their families, establishing new ones or going 'on the wallaby'. This meant walking about the colony looking for work, carrying all possessions wrapped in a small 'swag' carried over the shoulder, living rough. These 'swagmen' would work on Crown land farms or on 'squats'. Squatters seized Aboriginal land, displaced Aboriginal people, or coerced them into forced or uncompensated labour as domestics and farm workers. Squatters were emancipists, members of the colony militia, or free migrants. The squatters, militia, and police formed an alliance of self-interest to limit Aboriginal rights and keep emancipist or migrant swagmen as a marginalised labour-force. It was this coalition that was responsible for many atrocities against Aboriginal and Torres Strait Islander people, including massacres, poisoning of water sources, abductions, and summary executions. Aboriginal people responded with passive and active resistance themselves.

In the mid-1800s, convict numbers waned, transportation ceased, and thousands of voluntary migrants came to the colonies. The 1850s goldrush years saw an explosion in unregulated migration from all over the world, with most staying even after the gold rush years petered out. During the 1800s roads, bridges, courts, town halls, hospitals, prisons, and schools had been built using convict labour where available or emancipist and migrant workers. These buildings housed legal and civic institutions which regulated colonial life and promoted colonial advancement. They were built and services were funded by churches, charities, entrepreneurs, or Crown funds accrued through taxes, sales, and lease of unceded Aboriginal land. Examples of colonial institutions that still exist today include:

- the Benevolent Society charity, which opened the first asylum for the destitute, aged, and poor in 1813 and today employs occupational therapists;
- a permanent government hospital in Sydney, completed in 1816 by entrepreneurs, staffed by convicts, and later professionalised with the appointment of 'Nightingale' nurses in 1868. In the 20th century, this hospital employed occupational therapists; and
- government 'lunatic asylums' for people with mental illness. These were one of the first places in Australia where dedicated occupational therapy positions were established. These are of particular importance in the history of occupational therapy in Australia. The next section explores this in more detail.

2.2.5 Colonial asylums and occupation as therapy 1838–1900

In the first 30 years of the colony the only places for anyone who had a mental illness, free or convict, was home, gaol, or wandering the streets and countryside homeless. To redress this, establishment of colonial asylums occurred. In the early 1800s 'rules and regulations [were] drawn up by Governor Macquarie for the conduct of the asylum with insistence on cleanliness, comfort, humane treatment, recreation, medical attention and records' (Cummins, 2003, p. 34) The influence of humanism and the Enlightenment can be seen here, with occupations in the form of recreation a central feature.

The first to open was the Castle Hill asylum in 1811, which installed a resident medical officer in 1814. This was progressive at the time, demonstrating the colony acknowledged mental illness was a health problem not a crime. The Castle Hill asylum was too small for demand. It was closed and an interim asylum was established at Liverpool in old court buildings, but these too were inappropriate. Finally, a purpose-built asylum was opened in 1838 at Tarban Creek (now Gladesville) within relatively easy reach of the township and with the specific purpose of psychiatric care. A medical superintendent was appointed in 1848 who had gained psychiatric experience at St Lukes hospital for the mentally ill in England where he was exposed to various physical treatments and use of occupation regimens. Therapy emphasised 'close and friendly association with the patient, intimate discussion of his difficulties and daily pursuit of purposeful activity' (Cummins, 2003, p. 36). At that time there were no occupational therapists, so nurses, tradesmen, and other staff and visitors were engaged to provide the purposeful activities which were considered occupation-as-therapy.

Early asylums across the country like Tarban Creek were modelled on the physical layout, staffing, and regimens of York asylum, and humane treatment was the practice model, as indicated by Governor Macquarie's direction. Once inside asylums, most patients were rarely released. Their lives were a daily routine of occupations comprising self-care (meals, hygiene) and asylum maintenance, including cleaning, laundry, and sewing repairs for women and manual labour, building repairs, grounds maintenance, and vegetable farming for asylum supplies (Garton, 1988). In well-funded asylums there were creative and productive occupations, including crafts, music, gardening-for-pleasure, carpentry, games, picnics, and sport (Royal Commission on Asylums for the Insane and Inebriate, 1886; Westmore & Monk, 2012). Asylum clerical, laundry, and manual work was routinely done by patients – this practice was so common that the term 'working patients' evolved (Westmore & Monk, 2012).

Well-funded asylums also added creative and productive occupations to usual self-care and asylum maintenance duties (Royal Commission on Asylums for the Insane and Inebriate, 1886; Westmore & Monk, 2012). Occupation was highly valued as a treatment medium in asylums. As Dr John O'Brien, 1888 medical superintendent of Kew Asylums in Victoria, stated: 'Occupational treatment was the only curative measure of any value in restoring patients to sanity' (cited in Westmore & Monk, 2012). Despite good intentions and effective outcomes of humane treatment, living conditions and health care deteriorated in the latter part of the 19th century, as government funding decreased due to a world-wide depression, influenza pandemic, severe drought, and competition for workers after the gold rush. Notwithstanding these problems, the place of therapeutic occupation as an effective treatment was cemented in the Australian approach to mental health treatment. Occupational therapy programmes were routinely offered in asylums and psychiatric hospitals led by volunteers, nurses, teachers, or tradesmen until trained and qualified occupational therapists were available. The first ever advertised dedicated *occupational therapist position* was in a psychiatric asylum in Victora in 1938, 100 years after the Tarban Creek asylum opening, and occupational therapy in mental health services has been prominent ever since.

2.2.6 End of the colonies and beginning of a nation 1901–1913

As colonies developed and became more populous and prosperous, the lack of cooperation between them became problematic. Each one had different rules and arrangements for education, health, business, and agriculture. This created problems between the colonies and across the country because there was no coordination point for areas of common interest like defence and migration. An application was thus submitted to the British Parliament proposing colonies federate into one national government

(Davidson et al., 2003). In 1901 the Constitution of Australia was approved by the British Parliament. The head of state remained the British Crown (still the case today), who had a representative, called the governor general, who provided reports to the Crown and retained various reserve powers. The states retained power over a number of functions, including health and education, while the federal government held power in other areas such as defence. The consequence of this historical decision is that occupational therapists today need to check whether their work conditions and responsibilities are framed by local state laws, by national laws, or by both. For example, registration is a national government responsibility, while working in a public hospital as an occupational therapist requires compliance with relevant state laws.

During the Federation period, British ideas, culture, and practice dominated; educated people spoke 'the King's English'; and Australians travelled on British passports. The new Constitution adopted British forms of government, the national anthem was God Save the King (later Queen, then King) (not changed until 1973 to Advance Australia Fair), and a public holiday was given to celebrate the monarch's birthday (remaining today). Class differences existed, and the more 'British' your appearance, manners, language, religion, and customs, the higher your assumed social class.

Nation-building initiatives were prominent, and the *population* was a focus, particularly relating to Aboriginal and Torres Strait Islander peoples and migrants. The 1901 Australian Constitution gave the new national government power to make laws with regard to 'people of any race', *except* Aboriginal people. This happened because some colonies were more discriminatory and restrictive towards Aboriginal people than others, and they refused to liberalise. Prior to Federation, for example, to get agreement on Federation, the more liberal colonies agreed to exclude Aboriginal and Torres Strait Islander people from national laws. This is why the conditions and rights of Aboriginal and Torres Strait Islander peoples varied so much across the country. It is also why they were 'not to be counted' in the national census (Section 127, Australian Constitution, 1901), and they were subjected to continuing disparities and disadvantage through state laws which emphasised protection and assimilation rather than self-determination, with devastating consequences for culturally meaningful occupation (Zeldenryk & Yalmambirra, 2006).

A similar issue arose in the area of migration. Some colonies permitted entry of migrants from any racial, cultural, or geographic background, but as these migrants moved across colony borders, more restrictive colonies objected. To get agreement on federation, national consistency in migration policy had to be achieved. So again, the more inclusive colonies gave way to race-based rules. As a result, the White Australia Policy became the law under the Immigration Restriction Act in December 1901. This policy was used to restrict entry on a range of grounds, including colour, ancestral heritage, and English language skills. This notorious policy was inconsistently applied in an effort to retain the 'Britishness' of the new federation. In building a new federation, some of the most abhorrent aspects of colonialism were thus built into the legal systems and social structures of the country. This is why awareness of historical wrongs is not enough; current action to decolonise systems and structures is necessary.

The population focus of the new federation coincided with *Social Darwinism*, a movement that aimed to strengthen societies and economies through application of 'survival of the fittest' principles. In population planning and social policy, this was evidenced in *eugenics*, a pseudo-scientific approach that promoted selective reproduction to enhance *population fitness*. In the first half of 20th-century Australia, a racialised and medicalised version of eugenics was imported from Europe to Australia and meant that people living with mental illness, disability, or even lifestyles different from the norm could be institutionalised without consent to keep them separated from the rest of the population (Wyndham, 2003). Aboriginal and Torres Strait Islander peoples were unjustifiably targeted under Social Darwinism with attempts to eradicate their way of life and culture through assimilation and segregation. This was a form of racist eugenics.

One policy arising from this movement that was particularly loathsome was the forced removal of Aboriginal children from their families. While it started early in the colonies, it was particularly aggressive after federation during the years of the White Australia policy and post-war migrant assimilation practices. Children were 'kidnapped and exploited for their labour', separated from their family and culture, and abused and neglected under government policies of protectionism, assimilation, and welfare (National Inquiry into the Separation of Aboriginal and Torres Strait Islander Children from Their Families, 1997, p. 22). Changes to Aboriginal child removal policies did not come into effect until the late 1970s – that amounts to a 200-year history of child removal sanctioned by government. The living legacy of this practice and generational impact remains evident today; there continues to be, for example, over-representation of Aboriginal and Torres Strait Islander children in out-of-home care. Understanding the full account of 'the Stolen Generations' is essential knowledge for all Australians. Aboriginal and Torres Strait Islander peoples occupational therapy clients could be part of the Stolen Generations or deeply impacted by its enduring effects. The *Bringing them home: Report of the National Inquiry into the Separation of Aboriginal and Torres Strait Islander Children from their Families* (1997) states:

> Nationally we can conclude with confidence that between one in three and one in ten Indigenous children were forcibly removed from their families and communities in the period from approximately 1910 until 1970. . . . Most families have been affected, in one or more generations, by the forcible removal of one or more children

(p. 31)

The Stolen Generations, their families, and all Aboriginal and Torres Strait Islander Peoples received a formal apology on behalf of the nation by then–Prime Minister Kevin Rudd on the 13th of February 2008; this was one step towards reconciliation.

2.2.7 World War one and its sequelae

The Federation years ended abruptly with the commencement of World War One in 1914. With the United Kingdom at war, 'British' Australia also considered itself at war. From a population of 4 million, 416,809 men, including over 1000 Aboriginal and Torres Strait Islander men, enlisted to serve in combat and non-combatant roles (Australian War Memorial, 2025). This was a staggering 38.7% of all Australian men aged between 18 and 44. Initially, Aboriginal and Torres Strait Islander men served despite the 1903 Commonwealth Defence Act 1903 preventing them from enlisting, but as time went by, restrictions were eased. Aboriginal and Torres Strait Islander men served under equal conditions of pay, education, and access to health services, and while many were promised full citizenship on their return, this did not occur.

The impact of the war on Australia was enormous: estimated deaths were 58,916, there were 166,811 wounded, 4,089 missing or prisoners of war, and 87,865 service personnel were made chronically ill (Education Services Australia and the National Archives of Australia, 2010). Almost every family in Australia was directly impacted by the war, even though it was on the other side of the world. A similar thing happened in World War Two (WW2). It is one of the reasons why in every town and suburb today there are memorials with the names of local service personnel inscribed on them and why ANZAC Day is a nationally important memorial occasion each year.

The repatriation of service personnel took many months, and as they came home, a world-wide influenza pandemic was brought with them. The country was economically depleted by war and overwhelmed by the demand on health, rehabilitation, and welfare systems. The government's ad-hoc approach to public healthcare of returned service personnel and victims of the pandemic meant churches and charities filled the void. At that time, no antibiotic treatments were available, so recovery relied on surgery, pain relief, casting and splinting, rest, nutrition, fresh air, exercise, and therapeutic occupation to restore abilities. Nurses or well-meaning people provided 'occupation-as-therapy', including art, sport, exercise, craft, reading, carpentry, or gardening. Veterans with *shellshock*, neurological damage, or psychological trauma were treated similarly to patients with physical problems, often confined to underfunded asylums with poor conditions. As in colonial times, patients often ended up doing work-related occupations needed for the asylum to function.

A new approach to recovery was brought back to Australia by service personnel, doctors, and nurses, who observed American *rehabilitation* approaches were active rather than passive convalescence programmes. These ideas were not put into practice until 20 years later when WW2 came about. The American concepts for rehabilitation were coordinated *repatriation* and *resettlement* schemes to promote *reintegration* of military personnel into their communities. Active *rehabilitation*, also known as *reconstruction*, was shown to accelerate recovery and community resettlement whilst being cheaper than institutional care. One of the rehabilitation therapies used was occupation. The American military had recruited and deployed *reconstruction aides*, who were precursors to occupational therapists, to provide physical and occupational rehabilitation in field hospitals in Europe (Gavin, 1997; Low, 1992). The success of reconstruction aides led to increased American support for occupation as therapy and influential advocates such as Dr William Rush Dunton (Dunton, 1918, 1919) successfully lobbied for recognition of *occupational therapy* as a distinct field. A facility in Philadelphia, United States, prescribed *occupational therapy* to *retrain or adjust* people for *gainful living*. Occupational therapy was 'not the making of an object but the making of a man' (Barton, 1919).

The professionalisation of occupational therapy in the United States was well underway by the end of World War One in 1919. Julia Lathrop, a proponent of active recovery, had linked *occupation* to *therapy* in the *mental hygiene movement*. Nurse Susan Tracy promoted occupation as therapy for patients, publishing the first book on occupational therapy (Metaxas, 2000; Tracy, 1910). A bio-psycho-social model of mental illness treatment by psychiatrist Dr Adolf Meyer and social worker Mary Brooks Meyer was used at Johns Hopkins Hospital – it featured the healing use of occupation (Lamb, 2014; Meyer, 1922). Eleanor Clarke Slagle was appointed the first director of occupational therapy at Johns Hopkins Hospital in 1912, and in 1917 the first *American Society for the Promotion of Occupational Therapy* was founded (later becoming the American Occupational Therapy Association).

Post-war Australia had neither the money, workforce, nor appetite to establish the profession of occupational therapy – the focus was on the relatively new health profession of physiotherapy. It was not until the poliomyelitis epidemic of the late 1920s and 1930s that the momentum changed. Polio, an infectious disease, could not at that time be prevented or treated, and it led to varying degrees of muscle paralysis, including the limbs and respiratory muscles used for breathing. Children were most at risk; sadly, some died, and while some fully recovered, others experienced life-long impairments. The active rehabilitation approach was applied, with new physical therapy techniques. Sylvia Docker, an Australian physiotherapist trained in occupational therapy in London, returned to Australia to play a vital role in Australia's polio response. She expanded the use of *therapeutic occupations, grading them* to increase function and psychological wellbeing. Children cared for in clinical environments received occupational therapy for their developmental and rehabilitation needs, because it was:

> a satisfactory method of hastening recovery in both mental and physical cases. Occupational Therapy is a definite and proven therapeutic measure having as its advocates a great many members of the medical and surgical professions and practically all mental specialists.
>
> (Howland, 1933)

Despite this recognition and high demand, no courses providing professional occupational therapy qualifications were available in Australia. Instead, training was informal, and people who had previously 'practiced' occupation treatments gave classes or visited patients; typically, these were nurses, ex-servicemen, teachers, or volunteers engaged in activities that were called occupational therapy but were not a professional service.

2.2.8 The Great Depression, 1929 to 1939 – the first professional occupational therapists

The Great Depression was a world-wide economic crisis that hit Australia in 1929. At that time there were limited welfare services and public health systems for a population already struggling with the effects of war and pandemics. Churches, charities, and committees of concerned citizens were called upon to assist those facing extreme poverty, health conditions, or disabilities, the latter often relying on benevolent doctors and charitable service settings for health care. In this context, the first dedicated *occupational therapist* job in Australia was funded by a charitable organisation – the Mental Hospital Auxiliary at Mont Park Hospital Victoria. A nurse, Lucy Syme, was employed in 1934, having had *on-the-job* training in nurse-administered occupation therapy at Broughton Hall Psychiatric Hospital in Sydney.

Professional occupational therapy began in 1937 when, as flagged in the introduction of this chapter, Ethel May Francis returned to Sydney after studying abroad for an occupational therapy diploma from Philadelphia, United States. She experienced American practice approaches and those of occupational therapists in England (Docker, 1959; Schemm, 1994). The same year, Tasmanian Joyce Keam studied occupational therapy in London, returning in 1939 to work in psychiatry in Victoria. By the end of the 1930s, the three Australian pioneers, Ethel May Francis, Joyce Keam, and Sylvia Docker, had introduced occupational therapy into physical rehabilitation, paediatric, psychiatric, and acute general medical services (Anderson & Bell, 1988). They put Australian occupational therapy on the international map via letter contact with professional colleagues overseas, sharing professional association journals and bulletins.

2.2.9 World War 2 – the professionalisation of Australian occupational therapy begins
Occupational therapy employment expanded globally in WW2. To support the American armed forces, army reconstruction aides were re-invigorated, called occupational therapists, and deployed as part of special medical services. Once more, Australia's troops, including many Aboriginal and Torres Strait Islander personnel, responded to the war effort. As a result, the Australian Army created dedicated occupational therapy positions that could only be secured with appropriate qualifications (Walker, 1961). With only three qualified occupational therapists in all of Australia – Francis, Docker, and Keam – in 1940 Francis successfully applied to the Hospital Commission to start an occupational therapy course. It was led by University of Sydney psychiatrist Professor Dawson, with Francis teaching occupational therapy subjects. From 1941, the diploma course was coordinated by the Australian Physiotherapy Association (APA) and later by the Australian Association of Occupational Therapists. The first graduate was Gwendoline Sims in 1941.

Sylvia Docker was appointed as occupational therapy director in 1942, overseeing the development of the new Sydney Training Centre (STC), and her first intake was 27 students (Docker, 1959). The curriculum covered biological, psychological, and social subject areas and there was specialist training in physical and psychological rehabilitation using a range of occupation-based modalities. The standard course was 18 months, and most graduates were commissioned lieutenants in the Australian Army, deployed overseas or in repatriation hospitals at home once qualified. As the first occupational therapists ever encountered by patients, doctors, and nurses, they had to carve out a professional role and reputation, eventually earning respect from all (Walker, 1961). After the war, by 1947 most females were discharged from the army, including occupational therapists, and while encouraged to resume home duties, many instead continued working in repatriation hospitals (Walker, 1961).

Returning Australian soldiers required significant rehabilitation and occupational therapy work was ongoing. Despite large enlistments from Aboriginal and Torres Strait Islander peoples in WW2, the promise of full citizenship was once more an empty one, and they were denied membership in the Returned and Services League Clubs (RSL) and faced continued restrictions on employment, education, and health care, including access to occupational therapy.

2.2.10 Post-war Australia – repatriation, rehabilitation, repopulation,
            and rights – 1950–1970
Post-war rehabilitation needs and the post-war *baby boom* offered new occupational therapy employment opportunities. Practice settings included Commonwealth

Rehabilitation Centres, tuberculosis sanatoriums, mental hospitals for veterans, civilian mental asylums, new paediatric and adult services in civilian hospitals, and new community health clinics (Anderson & Bell, 1988). The occupational therapy STC could not meet graduate demand, and a second training course opened in 1948 in Victoria (Cameron, 1977). Occupational therapists formed associations to promote the profession, encouraging high-quality practice through continuing professional learning, research, and supervision.

For most of the 1950s and 1960s employment for occupational therapists grew, diversifying occupational therapy employment specialties, improving salaries, conditions, and career opportunities. By 1961 there were four courses in New South Wales, Victoria, Queensland, and Western Australia and demand in other states. Course curricula included biomedical and behavioural sciences; assessment, planning, and implementation of treatment for a variety of conditions; use of research in practice; practical training in arts, crafts, and trades; and fieldwork in hospitals or other services. All courses used teacher expertise, information from the *Bulletin* (the precursor of the *Australian Occupational Therapy Journal*), and published sources primarily from the United States where textbooks had been available since 1911. By 1964 changed legislation meant all health professional training took place in government-accredited colleges or universities via approved courses, and assurance of public safety led to practitioner registration, with Western Australia the first state to register occupational therapists (1960) and other states and territories following, with nationwide registration occurring in 2012.

In the late 1940s to late 1960s, entry into post-secondary professional training courses was difficult for any person of any background unable to pay high fees and achieve the high school marks needed to get into small-cohort courses. A course like occupational therapy did not provide accommodation and subsidy like nursing did, and it charged full tuition fees, so this narrowed the socio-economic background of students. On top of this, the White Australia Policy and widespread practice of assimilation during the 1950s and 1960s meant training and employment opportunities were restricted for many people – even second- and third-generation migrants.

Aboriginal and Torres Strait Islander peoples faced even greater challenges, but these too were surmounted, with the 1950s and 1960s seeing two watershed moments. The first Aboriginal person known to graduate from an Australian university was Malera Bundjalung woman Margaret Williams, now Dr Margaret Weir, who in 1959 received her diploma in physical education from Melbourne University (Weir, 2014). In 1966 the first known Aboriginal person to graduate with a university degree was Arrernte and Kalkadoon man Dr Charles Perkins, who achieved a Bachelor of Arts from the University of Sydney. Aboriginal people may have graduated from universities with qualifications before this time but may not have disclosed their backgrounds due to assimilation and racism. Aboriginal and Torres Strait Islander peoples not only had challenges entering professional education, they also had difficulties accessing health services, which were all mainstream (Haebich, 2012). This means they were also unlikely to receive occupational therapy services.

During the 1960s a worldwide resurgence of human rights and social activism occurred. In Australia, all Aboriginal and Torres Strait Islander peoples were given the right to vote in Commonwealth elections in 1962. In 1965 the Dr Charles Perkins led students from the *University of Sydney's Student Action for Aborigines* group on a 15-day bus journey known as the *Freedom Ride* across regional New South Wales to raise awareness about the discrimination and marginalisation of Aboriginal and Torres Strait Islander peoples. In 1967, a referendum resulted in a landslide Yes vote of 90.7% to count Aboriginal and Torres Strait Islander peoples in the national census (Reconciliation Australia, 2024). It is important for today's occupational therapists to understand that these events and the fight for human rights and recognition are recent history, and the restricted access of Aboriginal and Torres Strait Islander peoples to receive services or become occupational therapists will be part of the lived experiences of Aboriginal and Torres Strait Islander peoples and their families encountering occupational therapy today.

2.2.11 Migration, multiculturalism, and market economies – 1970s to 1990s

In the 1970s to 1990s a series of governments shifted Australia to a market economy, deregulated employment and services, and more liberal and inclusive social perspectives emerged (Smyth & Cass, 1998). Approaches to migration and policies became less restrictive, and multiculturalism was introduced and actively promoted. The White Australia policy was renounced in the early 1970s, and in the 1990s migration from nearby Asia was actively welcomed with strategic engagement supported across all sectors. Australia's population demographics changed to be a multicultural nation, with the 2021 census revealing over 200 nationalities and nearly 80% of the population being a first- or second-generation Australian. Australia is now one of the most culturally diverse nations in the world. The most recent population census showed First Nations People formed 3.8% of the 25 million population (Australian Bureau of Statistics, 2021).

Indigenous activism continued, and on the 26th of January 1972, the Aboriginal Tent Embassy was established outside Parliament House (now known as Old Parliament House) in Canberra to protest for land rights. The Tent Embassy remains to the present, protesting for First Nations' sovereignty and self-determination (National Museum of Australia, 2024). The 1988 Australian bicentenary celebrations were met with large protests of more than 40,000 Aboriginal and Torres Strait Islander peoples and non-Indigenous supporters staging 'the largest march ever held in Sydney', held in 'the spirit of the Day of Mourning protest that took place in 1938' (Deadly Story, n.d.). A Royal Commission was held into Aboriginal Deaths in Custody, handing down its landmark report in 1991, of which the final recommendation was the need for all political leaders and parties to support the process of reconciliation. Land rights were contested in legal proceedings, and in 1992, the historic Mabo decision by the High Court of Australia overturned 'terra nullius' and ruled that native title existed and First Nations Peoples have rights to the land. In 1993, the Native Title Act was passed by the Australian Parliament.

During this period, a great deal was changing in the occupational therapy profession. In the late 1970s occupational therapy courses shifted from diploma to bachelor-level degrees. Some viewed the change as unnecessary *credential-creep* and a threat to *hands-on* experience that had earned occupational therapy a *can-do* reputation. Others saw the change as essential in an increasingly specialised and research-based health sector. When a national recession hit in the early 1980s and government jobs were cut, occupational therapy degree graduates had the skills and knowledge required to move into non-traditional, emerging, or generic roles, and the occupational therapy association promoted research-capacity building in the profession to show occupational therapists were effective, efficient, and essential regardless of employment context. By the 1990s, when the next economic recession hit Australia, occupational therapy had successfully adapted and was embedded across all sectors, with a growing research evidence base. A small but growing group of Aboriginal and Torres Strait Islander occupational therapists graduated during this time.

In 1999, Australians were asked via a national referendum about changing the Constitution to become a republic, replacing the British monarch and governor general with a president as our own head of state. The proposal for an Australian republic was defeated, with approximately 55% voting 'No', and Australia remains a constitutional monarchy.

2.2.12 Participation, inclusivity, and rights-based practice – 2000 to 2025

At the beginning of the new millennium, Australia was a more diverse country. The immensely successful 2000 Paralympic Games in Sydney was an exciting time for disability/health community stakeholders and consumers. Globally, in 2001 the World Health Organization (WHO) published the International Classification of Functioning, Disability, and Health (ICF) that embraced a bio-psycho-social approach and recognised social models of disability and social determinants of health (WHO, 2001). This model's focus on concepts of *function, activity,* and *participation* brought interdisciplinary attention to constructs that had been occupational therapy's *core business* for decades.

An increased focus on *human rights* during this period is evident. In 2007, the Closing the Gap campaign to reduce inequities between Aboriginal and Torres Strait Islander peoples and other Australians was launched and in 2009 the first Closing the Gap Report, titled *Closing the Gap on Indigenous Disadvantage: The Challenge for Australia* (Department of Families Housing Community Services and Indigenous Affairs, 2009), was tabled in the Australian Parliament, and each year a progress report is presented. Australian government Royal Commission enquiries into institutional care across the aged care (2018–2021) and disability (2019–2023) sectors provided shocking evidence of the need for reform. New consumer-directed service models were introduced (for example, the Australian Government My Aged Care https://www.myagedcare.gov.au/ or the National Disability Insurance Scheme https://www.ndis.gov.au/). OT Australia, the peak professional society; individual therapists; and consumers significantly contributed to these changes.

In *policy* and *practice*, this period saw occupational therapy at the heart of broad human rights reforms. Human rights approaches influenced the uptake of collaborative, power-sharing, equal models of care, including shared care, family, and person-centred practice; consumer directed care; and recovery-oriented care. Occupational therapists continued to be agents of cultural change, introducing these rights-based approaches in all contexts. The concept and strategy of decolonisation were described, explored, and promoted in occupational therapy scholarship, education, policy, and practice (George et al., 2024; Gibson, 2020; Gibson et al., 2015; Ryall et al., 2021). Professional networks and groups to support and advocate for the rights of Aboriginal and Torres Strait Islander peoples, improved health professional training, and service delivery began to form. The Koori Occupational Therapy Scheme (KOTS) was established by Lin Oke in 2005 to provide scholarship support for Aboriginal and Torres Strait Islander students to study occupational therapy in Victoria (Paluch et al., 2011). Kelli McIntosh, a proud Murawari and Kooma woman, became the first Aboriginal occupational therapist to lead KOTS in 2009, and the group was pivotal in the formation of Indigenous Allied Health Australia (IAHA) in 2009 (IAHA, 2025; Paluch et al., 2011).

In 2018 revised occupational therapy professional competencies were released which specified practice behaviours across four standards of professionalism, knowledge and learning, occupational therapy process and practice, and communication. Importantly, registered occupational therapists must strengthen knowledge, skills, and behaviours related to cultural responsiveness and capabilities when working with Aboriginal and Torres Strait Islander clients (Occupational Therapy Board of Australia, 2018). In 2023, the *Aboriginal and Torres Strait Islander Health Curriculum Implementation Project – Occupational Therapy Program Accreditation* report was released, providing guidance for educators, universities, programme accreditation stakeholders, and regulators regarding education requirements of occupational therapy programmes (Ryan et al., 2023).

Occupational therapy *research* and scholarship focussed on human rights, intersectionality, occupational justice and deprivation, trauma, and adaptation through occupation, adopting collaborative research approaches with consumers. Aboriginal and Torres Strait Islander occupational therapy scholars, both in Australia and around the world, led research on colonial history, demonstrating the need to critique Western ideas of occupation and generate strengths-based and inclusive conceptualisations of Aboriginal and Torres Strait Islander views about occupation, occupational therapy, leadership, partnership, and change (e.g., Emery-Whittington & Te Maro, 2018; Gibson, 2020; Gibson et al., 2015; Ryan et al., 2020). Ryall et al. (2021) proposed a strengths-based framework for advancing decolonising practices within occupational therapy. Collaboration led to non-Indigenous occupational therapy researchers partnering with Aboriginal and Torres Strait Islander researchers from different disciplines to explore occupational therapy's readiness to decolonise practice and strategies to do so (for example, George et al., 2024; Mackenzie et al., 2024; Rudman et al., 2021; Zeldenryk & Yalmambirra, 2006).

In *education*, deregulation in the 2000s removed centralised government control of course number, type, and location. Many universities embraced the opportunity to commence occupational therapy degrees, with around 30 Australian universities now offering courses. This growth and the opening up of universities for mass education has led to greater cultural, economic, and social diversity in the student population. Initiatives to increase the participation of Aboriginal and Torres Strait Islander students in studying occupational therapy have also accelerated. *Employment* of occupational therapists now occurs across all sectors of the economy in services that address health and social needs of people across the lifespan.

As Australia enters the second quarter of the 21st century, reconciliation efforts continue, but more is needed. While historical awareness, truth telling, and historical acceptance are increasing, it is not enough. For decolonisation to happen, action is needed to ensure occupational therapists, and the systems and structures in which they work, are culturally responsive (Indigenous Allied Health Australia, 2019). This is a personal and professional challenge requiring reflection, effort, and transformative action. This action is needed now. The loss of the 2023 'Australian Indigenous Voice' referendum signalled a setback in national reconciliation. This was a proposal set out in the 'Uluru Statement from the Heart' whereby an Aboriginal and Torres Strait Islander Voice to Parliament was proposed to advise on matters concerning Aboriginal and Torres Strait Islander peoples. Leading up to the referendum, Occupational Therapy Australia (OTA) published their firm support for the proposal in *OTA's Statement on the Voice Referendum for Constitutional Change* (2023), stating:

> Our standpoint is that the Voice represents the most powerful vehicle for the real-isation of participatory democracy to date. . . . Occupational Therapy Australia stands with our Aboriginal and Torres Strait Islander members, stakeholder and allies, and accepts the invitation offered through the Uluru Statement from the Heart. We support the yes vote for Constitutional change to establish a First Nations Voice.

While a referendum for a national treaty failed, state governments (some were previously the original colonies) can move their own legislation and treaty arrangements. Australia's first treaty with Aboriginal people in Victoria was signed and formalised as law on the 13th of November 2025. A news release by Ashton et al. (2025) published on the same day interviewed high-profile leaders about this milestone event. The following are illustrative of the sense of hope, accomplishment, and respect that came with this legislation. Victoria's First Peoples' Assembly co-chair Ngarra Murray said, 'today marks a turning point in our nation's history, a moment where old wounds can begin to heal and new relationships can be built on truth, justice and mutual respect'. The importance of self-determination in this turning point was identified by Elder Professor Tom Calma, who said, 'If you give Aboriginal and Torres Strait Islander people the opportunity to participate actively and equally in processes, we will see good outcomes.' The treaty negotiation process took over ten years. Premier Jacinta Allen said the treaty and law were 'founded on truth, guided by respect and carried forward in partnership to build a stronger, fairer, more equal Victoria for everyone'. As the first treaty in the nation, it is a milestone in Australia's history and, in the words of Aunty Jill Gallagher AO, a proud Gunditjmara woman, 'this is the story of the Aboriginal people's resistance'.

In March 2025, there were 34,143 registered occupational therapists, of which 234 were Aboriginal and/or Torres Strait Islander practitioners, making up 0.7% of all practitioners (Occupational Therapy Board of Australia, 2025). This is the same for physiotherapy registrations (0.7%) (Physiotherapy Board of Australia, 2024) but less than half that of nursing and midwifery registrations, which have 1.5% Aboriginal and/or Torres Strait Islander registered practitioners (Nursing and Midwifery Board of Australia, 2025). Since the latest census estimates 3.8% of the Australian popula-tion identify as Aboriginal and Torres Strait Islander peoples, there is work to be done to build a more proportionate representation of Aboriginal and Torres Strait Islander peoples within the profession. There is also more work to be done to create a profession and practice community that is culturally responsive, alert to colonial influences, and willing to take action to decolonise systems and structures where occupational therapists work and where people need occupational therapy. This will deepen engagement with Aboriginal and Torres Strait Islander Peoples in Australia's journey towards reconciliation.

2.3 What history will you make?

This chapter started with ancient Western philosophies about health and occupation. We saw how these ideas were introduced to Australia where an even older culture had thrived for tens of thousands of years. The adverse impact of colonialism on Aboriginal and Torres Strait Islander peoples, as well as their resistance and resilience, were explored. The way transportation, migration, and assimilation supported colonial aspirations for 'Britishness' were explained. Factors influencing the formation of a single federation and the implications for migrants and Aboriginal and Torres Strait Islander peoples were revealed. Key moments in Australian history that influenced the demand for, and employment of occupational therapists were presented, including the First and Second World Wars, influenza and polio pandemics, changes in migration, education, and deregulation in the economy. Milestones and set backs in reconciliation were identified and published professional perspectives on this presented. Throughout this history, the journey from colonial to decolonised approaches in thinking, practice, and professional issues has been promoted and continued action invited.

As we move into the second quarter of the 21st century, Australian occupational therapists will continue to be influenced by events as they unfold. Our history was made by people just like you. They made professional choices, acted in their practice, and helped set the direction and priorities that shaped our profession today. They had views about the past and what should happen in the future. As our profession becomes more diverse in people and practice, as the need for truth telling and listening, reconciliation, and decolonisation becomes more prominent, ask yourself what history you will be making in the years ahead. As you look forward to a future where occupational therapy's contribution to Australia and *all* its people is realised, there remains much to be done, and all occupational therapists can play their part.

2.4 Review questions

- Plot a timeline from 1788 to the present day, identifying important developments that influence contemporary Australian occupational therapy.
- What impact did colonisation have on occupations of Aboriginal and Torres Strait Islander peoples in the past and what decolonising strategies support autonomy and self-determination in their occupations today?
- Why do occupational therapists need to learn about Australian history to become registered health professionals in Australia?
- Imagine yourself as the author of this chapter in 10 years' time. What themes will continue to be relevant and what new topics do you think will be part of Australia's 21st-century history?

References

Anderson, B., & Bell, J. (1988). *Occupational therapy its place in Australia's history*. Australian Association of Occupational Therapists.

ANTAR [Australians for Native Title and Recognition]. (2024). *History of truth telling in Australia*. https://antar.org.au/issues/truth-telling/history-of-truth-telling-in-australia/

Aristotle. (1925). *Nichomachean ethics: Book II* (W. D. Ross, Trans.). The Internet Classics Archive. http://classics.mit.edu/Aristotle/nicomachaen.2.ii.html (Original work published 350 B.C.E)

Ashton, K., Fitzgerald, B., & Jash, T. (2025). Australia's first treaty with Aboriginal people signed in Victoria. *ABC*. https://www.abc.net.au/news/2025-11-13/australia-first-treaty-agreement-signed-law-victoria/106002730

Australian Bureau of Statistics. (2021). *Population: Census*. ABS. https://www.abs.gov.au/statistics/people/population/population-census/latest-release

Australian Law Reform Commission [ALRC]. (2010a). Recognition of Aboriginal customary laws at Common law: The settled colony debate. *ALRC Report 31*, Australian Government, Canberra. https://www.alrc.gov.au/publications/

Australian Law Reform Commission. (2010b). *Recognition of aboriginal customary laws (ALRC report 31) 4*. Aboriginal Customary Laws and Anglo-Australian Law After 1788/Australian Law as Applied to Aborigines. https://www.alrc.gov.au/publication/recognition-of-aboriginal-customary-laws-alrc-report-31/

Australian War Memorial. (2025). *Australians at war – the colonial period 1788–1901*. https://www.awm.gov.au/articles/atwar/colonial

Barton, G. E. (1919). *Teaching the sick: A manual of occupational therapy and re-education*. WB Saunders Co. (Digitized by Harvard University 2007).

Beaumont, J. (2001). *Australian defence: Sources and statistics in the Australian centenary history of defence* (Vol. VI). Oxford University Press. Retrieved Februrary 18, 2020, from https://trove.nla.gov.au/version/42710949

Behrendt, L. (2003). *Achieving social justice*. Federation Press.

Bewley, T. (2008). *Madness to mental illness; A history of the Royal College of Psychiatrists*. Royal College of Psychiatrists Archive. https://catalogues.rcpsych.ac.uk/

Blackstone, W. (1765). Commentaries on the law of England, 1, 107.

Blanco, C. (2024). What were the Australia Wars and why is history not acknowledged. *SBS Podcast*. https://www.sbs.com.au/language/english/en/podcast-episode/what-were-the-australian-wars-and-why-is-history-not-acknowledged/n86cyq00f

Bowler, J. M., Johnston, H., Olley, J. M., Prescott, J. R., Roberts, R. G., Shawcross, W., & Spooner, N. A. (2003). New ages for human occupation and climatic change at Lake Mungo, Australia. *Nature, 421*(6925), 837–840. https://doi.org/10.1038/nature01383

Brennan, S., Behrendt, L., Strelein, L., & Williams, G. (2005). *Treaty*. The Federation Press.

Cameron, B. S. (1977). *The work of our hands: A history of the occupational therapy school of Victoria*. Lincoln Institute, Author Published.

Cowley, T., & Snowden, C. (2013). *Patchwork prisoners: The Rajah quilt and the women who made it*. Research Tasmania. https://catalogue.nla.gov.au/catalog/10062403

Cummins, C. J. (2003). *A history of medical administration in NSW 1788–1973* (2nd ed.). NSW Health. https://www.health.nsw.gov.au/about/history/.../history-medical-admin.pdf

Cusick, A. (2001). OZ OT EBP 21C: Australian occupational therapy, evidence-based practice and the 21st century. *Australian Occupational Therapy Journal, 48*(3), 102–117. https://doi.org/10.1046/j.0045-0766.2001.00281.x

Davidson, G., Hirst, J., & Mcintyre, S. (2003). *The Oxford companion to Australian history*. Oxford University Press.

Deadly Story. (n.d.). *The 1988 Bicentenary protest*. Deadly Story.

Department of Families Housing Community Services and Indigenous Affairs. (2009). *Closing the gap on Indigenous disadvantage: The challenge for Australia*. Commonwealth of Australia.

Docker, S. (1959). Development of occupational therapy in Australia. *Australian Journal of Occupational Therapy*, 6(3), 2–8. https://doi.org/10.1111/j.1440-1630.1959.tb00824.x

Dunton, W. R. (1918). *Occupation therapy: A manual for nurses*. WB Saunders Co, Classic Reprint Series Forgotten Books 2013. Retrieved February 18, 2020, from http://www.forgottenbooks.com/

Dunton, W. R. (1919). *Reconstruction therapy*. WB Saunders Co., Classic Reprint Series Forgotten Books 2013. Retrieved February 18, 2020, from http://www.forgottenbooks.com/

Education Services Australia Ltd and the National Archives of Australia. (2010). *Australian recruitment statistics for the first world war*. Maa.gov.au.

Emery-Whittington, I., & Te Maro, B. (2018). Decolonising occupation: Causing social change to help our ancestors rest and our descendants thrive. *New Zealand Journal of Occupational Therapy*, 65(1), 12–19.

First Nations National Constitutional Convention. (2017). *Uluru: Statement from the Heart*. Central Land Council Library, Alice Springs, Northern Territory.

Foxhall, K. (2011). From convicts to colonists: The health of prisoners and the voyage to Australia, 1823–53. *The Journal of Imperial and Commonwealth History*, 39(1), 1–19. https://doi.org/10.1080/03086534.2011.543793

Gapps, S. (2018). *The Sydney wars conflict in the early colony 1788–1817*. UNSW Press.

Gapps, S. (2021). *Gudyarra: The first Wiradyuri war of resistance – the Bathurst war, 1822–1824*. UNSW Press.

Gapps, S. (2025). *Uprising War in the colony of New South Wales 1838–1844*. UNSW Press.

Garton, S. (1988). *Medicine and madness: A social history of insanity in New South Wales 1880–1940*. New South Wales University Press.

Gavin, L. (1997). Reconstruction aides. In L. Gavin (Ed.), *American women in World War 1– They also served* (pp. 101–128). University Press of Colorado.

George, E., Ritchie, T., Ryan, A., Fisher, M., Baum, F., & Mackean, T. (2024). 'Listen with your ears and eyes and heart and your minds and your soul': Implications for decolonising consultation and occupational therapy from case studies on 'Closing the Gap' policy implementation. *Australian Occupational Therapy Journal*, 71(3), 379–391. https//doi.org/10.1111/1440-1630.12960

Gibson, C. (2020). When the river runs dry: Leadership, decolonisation and healing in occupational therapy. *New Zealand Journal of Occupational Therapy*, 67(1), 11–20.

Gibson, C., Butler, C., Henaway, C., Dudgeon, P., & Curtin, M. (2015). Indigenous peoples and human rights: Some considerations for the occupational therapy profession in Australia. *Australian Occupational Therapy Journal*, 62(3), 214–218. https://doi.org/10.1111/1440-1630.12185

Haebich, A. (2012). Aboriginal assimilation and Nyungar Health 1948–72. *Health and History*, 14(2), 140–161. https://doi.org/10.5401/healthhist.14.2.0140

Higgins, I., & Collard, S. (2020, April 28). Captain James Cook's landing and the Indigenous first words contested by Aboriginal leaders. *ABC News*. https://www.abc.net.au/news/2020-04-29/captain-cook-landing-indigenous-people-first-words-contested/12195148

Hobbs, H. (2022). *Fact sheet sovereignty*. ANTAR. https://antar.org.au/wp-content/uploads/2022/11/Sovereignty-Factsheet.pdf

Hodder-Williams, R. (2001). Colonialism: Political aspects. In N. J. Smelser & P. B. Baltes (Eds.), *International encyclopedia of the social & behavioral sciences* (pp. 2237–2240). Pergamon. https://doi.org/10.1016/B0-08-043076-7/01250-X

Howard, J. (1777). *The state of the prisons in England and Wales with preliminary observations, and an account of some foreign prisons*. Classic Reprint Series, Forgotten Books. Retrieved February 18, 2020, from http://www.forgottenbooks.com/

Howland, G. (1933). Editorial. *Canadian Journal of Occupational Therapy*, I(September), 4–5.

Indigenous Allied Health Australia. (2019). *Cultural safety through responsive health practice: policy position statement*. IAHA. https://iaha.com.au/wp-content/uploads/2020/02/Cultural-Safety-Through-Responsive-Health-Practice-Position-Statement.pdf

Indigenous Allied Health Australia. (2025). *History of IAHA.* https://iaha.com.au/about-us/

Lamb, S. D. (2014). *The pathologist of the mind: Adolf Meyer and the origins of American Psychiatry.* John Hopkins University Press.

Low, J. F. (1992). The reconstruction aides. *American Journal of Occupational Therapy, 46*(1), 38–43. https://doi.org/10.5014/ajot.46.1.38

Luebering, J. E. (2023). The Renaissance: At a glance. *Encyclopedia Britannica.* https://www.britannica.com/topic/The-Renaissance-At-a-Glance-2235613

Mackean, T. J., O'Donnell, K., Sherwood, J., D'Angelo, A., Shakespeare, M., Wellington, C., Freeman, T., Ziersch, A. M., Fisher, M., Askew, D. A., Dwyer, J. M., Browne, A. J., & Baum, F. (2024). Decolonising primary health care practice: A definition and its importance. *Medical Journal of Australia, 223*(1), 9–12. https://doi.org/10.5694/mja2.52683

Mackenzie, L., Gwynn, J., & Gilroy, J. (2024). Experiences of occupational therapy students undertaking an Aboriginal and Torres Strait Islander health module: Embedding cultural responsiveness in professional curricula. *Australian Health Review, 48*(4), 374–380. https://doi.org/10.1071/AH23217

Marenbon, J. (2024). Medieval philosophy. In E. N. Zalta & U. Nodelman (Eds.), *The Stanford encyclopedia of philosophy* (Winter 2024 ed.). https://plato.stanford.edu/archives/win2024/entries/medieval-philosophy/

Metaxas, V. A. (2000). Eleanor Clarke Slagle and Susan E Tracy: Personal and professional identity and the development of occupational therapy in progressive era America. *Nursing History Review, 8,* 39–70.

Meyer, A. (1922). The philosophy of occupation therapy. Reprinted from the *Archives of Occupational Therapy,* Volume 1, pp. 1–10, 1922. *American Journal of Occupational Therapy, 31*(10), 639–642.

National Inquiry into the Separation of Aboriginal and Torres Strait Islander Children from Their Families (Australia). (1997). *Bringing them home: Report of the National Inquiry into the separation of Aboriginal and Torres strait islander children from their families.* Human Rights and Equal Opportunity Commission.

National Museum of Australia. (2024). *Aboriginal tent embassy.* National Museum of Australia. https://www.nma.gov.au/defining-moments/resources/aboriginal-tent-embassy

Nursing and Midwifery Board of Australia. (2025). *Registrant data – reporting period: 01 January 2025 to 31 March 2025.* Nursing and Midwifery Board, Ahpra.

Occupational Therapy Australia. (2023). *OTA's statement on the voice referendum for constitutional change.* https://otaus.com.au/about/reconciliation

Occupational Therapy Board of Australia. (2018). *Australian occupational therapy competency standards.* Occupational Therapy Board of Australia.

Occupational Therapy Board of Australia. (2025). *Registrant data – reporting period: 01 January 2025 to 31 March 2025.* Occupational Therapy Board, Ahpra.

O'Connell, J. F., & Allen, J. (2004). Dating the colonization of Sahul (Pleistocene Australia-New Guinea): A review of recent research. *Journal of Archaeological Science, 31,* 835–853.

Paluch, T., Allen, R., McIntosh, K., & Oke, L. (2011). Koori Occupational Therapy Scheme: Contributing to First Australian health through professional reflection, advocacy and action. *Australian Occupational Therapy Journal, 58*(1), 50–53. https://doi.org/10.1111/j.1440-1630.2010.00913.x

Perkins, R., Gapps, S., Murray, M., & Reynolds, H. (2025). *The Australia Wars.* Allen & Unwin.

Physiotherapy Board of Australia. (2024). *Registrant data. Reporting period: 01 October 2024 to 31 December 2024.* Physiotherapy Board, Ahpra.

Reconciliation Australia. (2024). *Reconciliation timeline: Key moments.* https://www.reconciliation.org.au/reconciliation-timeline-key-moments/

Royal Commission into Aboriginal Deaths in Custody. (1991). *Royal commission into aboriginal deaths in custody: National reports [Vol 1–5], and regional reports.* Australian Government Publishing Service.

Royal Commission on Asylums for the Insane and Inebriate, Victoria. (1886). *Report of the Royal Commission, minutes of evidence*, Q.5541, p. 224 (Victorian Parliamentary Papers, vol. 2).

Rudman, M. T., Flavell, H., Harris, C., & Wright, M. (2021). How prepared is Australian occupational therapy to decolonise its practice? *Australian Occupational Therapy Journal*, 68(4), 287–297. https://doi.org/10.1111/1440-1630.12725

Ruska, P., & Clayton-Dixon, C. (2015). Words of the struggle. *Black Nations Rising*, 10, 10.

Ryall, J., Ritchie, T., Butler, C., Ryan, A., & Gibson, C. (2021). Decolonising occupational therapy through a strength-based lens. In T. Brown, H. M. Bourke-Taylor, S. Isbel, R. Cordier, & L. Gustafsson (Eds.), *Occupational therapy in Australia: Professional and practice issues* (2nd ed., pp. 130–142). Routledge. https://doi.org/10.4324/9781003150732-13

Ryan, L., Debenham, J., Pascoe, B., Smith, R., Owen, C., Richards, J., Gilbert, S., Anders, R. J., Usher, K., Price, D., Newley, J., Brown, M., & Craig, H. (2025). *Colonial frontier massacres in Australia, 1788–1930* (Version 1.1) [Data set]. ADA Dataverse. https://doi.org/10.26193/L0WEID

Ryan, A., Gibson, C., & Hummell, J., Project Advisory Group, & Occupational Therapy Council of Australia. (2023). *Aboriginal and Torres Strait Islander health curriculum implementation project.* Occupational Therapy Council of Australia. https://www.otcouncil.com.au/wp-content/uploads/OTC-Aboriginal-and-Torres-Strait-Islander-Health-Curriculum-Implementation-Project-2023.1.pdf

Ryan, A., Gilroy, J., & Gibson, C. (2020). #Changethedate: Advocacy as an on-line and decolonising occupation. *Journal of Occupational Science*, 27(3), 405–416. https://doi.org/10.1080/14427591.2020.1759448

Schemm, R. L. (1994). Bridging conflicting ideologies: The origins of American and British occupational therapy. *American Journal of Occupational Therapy*, 48(11), 1082–1088. https://doi.org/10.5014/ajot.48.11.1082

Secher, U. (2005). The Mabo decision – preserving the distinction between 'settled' and 'conquered or ceded' territories. *University of Queensland Law Journal*, 24(1), 35–71.

Senate Standing Committee on Constitutional and Legal Affairs Two Hundred Years Later. (1983), para 3.46, cited in ALRC 2010.

Smyth, P., & Cass, B. (1998). *Contesting the Australian way: States, markets and civil society.* Cambridge University Press.

Superior Courts of New South Wales. (1836). *R v Murrell and Bummaree* (1836) 1 Legge 72; [1836] NSWSupC 35, 19 February 1836 Reported in the Sydney Gazette, 23 February 1836.

Tracy, S. E. (1910). *Studies in invalid occupations, a manual for nurses and attendants.* Whitcomb and Barrows, Reprint 2013, Forgotten Books. Retrieved March 7, 2016, from http://www.forgottenbooks.com/

Tsiompanou, E., & Marketos, S. G. (2013). Hippocrates: Timeless still. *Journal of the Royal Society of Medicine*, 106(7), 288–292. https://doi.org/10.1177/0141076813492945

Uluru Statement from the Heart. (2017). https://ulurustatement.org/the-statement/view-the-statement/

Walker, A. S. (1961). *Medical services of the Royal Australian Navy and Royal Australian Air Force with a section on women in the Army Medical Services.* Australia in the War of 1939–1945. Series 5 – Medical. Australian War Memorial.

Weir, M. (2014). *Dr Margaret Weir, abstract from generations of knowledge.* University of Western Sydney. https://www.westernsydney.edu.au/__data/assets/pdf_file/0009/781884/EXT5218_Yarramundi_Lecture_GOK_Book_Margaret.pdf

Wellings, B. M. E. (2002). *Crown and country: Nationalism and Britishness in Scotland, Australia and England* [Doctoral thesis, Australian National University]. https://doi.org/10.25911/5d778765701d2

Wellington, S. (2025). *Sovereignty, treaty, recognition: Voices from community.* NTV sbs.com.au

Westmore, A., & Monk, L. (2012). *Confinement & seclusion in Victorian mental health institutions.* Museum Victoria Collections. http://collections.museumvictoria.com.au/articles/11532

Wiradjuri Condoblin Corporation Ltd. (2022). WCC *language program: Wiradjuri* (Version 1.0) [Mobile App]. https://apps.apple.com/au/app/wiradjuri/id1424855887

World Health Organization (WHO). (2001). *International Classification of Functioning, Disability and Health*. World Health Organization.

Wyndham, D. (2003). *Eugenics in Australia: Striving for national fitness*. Galton Institute.

Zeldenryk, L., & Yalmambirra. (2006). Occupational deprivation: A consequence of Australia's policy of assimilation. *Australian Occupational Therapy Journal, 53*(1), 43–46. https://doi.org/10.1111/j.1440-1630.2005.00530.x

CHAPTER 3

Australia's health and health care system

Stephen Isbel, Claire Pearce, and Craig Greber

Authors' positionality statement

This chapter is authored by three academics of white, Anglo-Australian background. We acknowledge the cultural, historical, and social contexts in which we have lived have shaped our perspective of the world. We are aware of the social and institutional privileges linked to our racial and cultural identities and we acknowledge this introduces biases that may have influenced the writing of this chapter. We are committed to critically reflecting on our positionality and its influence on our work. In this chapter we have included viewpoints that extend beyond our own experience in the context of the chapter aims. Our intention is to contribute to an inclusive and equitable academic discourse by being transparent about our perspectives and actively seeking to understand and represent a broad range of experiences.

The chapter presents information on Aboriginal and Torres Strait Islander health and wellbeing. We have endeavoured to present the information objectively and without interpretation to minimise colonial bias. A further acknowledgement of our positionality precedes that section.

Key terms
- Health policy
- Australian government
- Health funding
- Primary care
- Secondary care
- Medicare
- Aboriginal and Torres Strait Islander health
- Social determinants of health

DOI: 10.4324/9781003495666-4

Objectives

Upon completion of this chapter, the reader will be able to:

- Provide an overview of the Australian health care system
- Describe major health challenges for Australians
- Describe how health care is funded in Australia
- Appreciate how the social determinants of health affect Australians
- Understand some of the areas where occupational therapists work

3.1 Introduction

Australia's healthcare system is highly regarded globally, with health outcomes, access to necessary services, facilities, and funding that compare favourably with other OECD (Organisation for Economic Co-operation and Development) countries (OECD, 2023). The system consists of multiple components, including primary care (community-based) and secondary care (hospitals and specialist services), supported by various regulatory, surveillance, and professional organisations (Australian Institute of Health and Welfare [AIHW], 2024a).

The system is complex, involving different levels of government funding and oversight depending on the service provided, with some services delivered through a parallel privately funded system. Occupational therapists play a crucial role in promoting the health of Australians at an individual, group, and community level. Occupational therapists provide services across all systems, utilising funding from all levels of government and private fee for service.

3.2 The Australian government and health care

Australia operates under a federated system of government, where the central government (the Commonwealth) oversees partially self-governing regions (states, territories, and local governments). The Commonwealth government manages the universal health insurance programme known as Medicare and the Pharmaceutical Benefits Scheme. Hospital services are primarily provided by the states and territories, with financial support from the Commonwealth for hospital operations, primary healthcare, and other recurring expenses.

Private healthcare services, hospitals, and aged care facilities are managed by independent organisations but also receive some Commonwealth funding. The Commonwealth provides funds to the states and territories for medical services and primary care, while the states are responsible for delivering hospital services and community health services, such as mental health support and immunisation. The division of responsibilities and functions complicates the development of integrated, coordinated national policies and services. This separation means that decisions made by one level of government can impact other parts of the system, often without full consideration of the broader implications (AIHW, 2024b)

3.3 The health of Australians

This section examines life expectancy, health disparities, and some social determinants of health as a foundation for understanding the healthcare system. Australia is diverse in terms of geography, culture, society, and health status, with communities that coexist and maintain unique, individualised identities. Recognising and celebrating this diversity is essential, and the healthcare system attempts to accommodate these differences.

3.3.1 Life expectancy

Australian males born in 2022 can expect to live to 81.2 years of age and females to 85.3 years (AIHW, 2024a). This is above the OECD average for both males (77.9 years) and females (83.2 years) (OECD, 2023). In 2024 the leading causes of death in Australia included cancer, dementia, respiratory diseases, and ischaemic heart disease (Australian Bureau of Statistics [ABS], 2024a).

3.4 Aboriginal and Torres Strait Islander people

It is acknowledged that this section was authored by a non-Aboriginal or Torres Strait Islander person. It is also acknowledged that it presents a colonial view, presenting Aboriginal and Torres Strait Islander people based on facts and figures. It is not aimed at being a representation of the lived experiences of First Nations people.

Aboriginal and Torres Strait Islander peoples are the Indigenous peoples of Australia, encompassing diverse nations, cultures, and languages and representing the traditional custodians of the land and sea in different regions (Australian Government, 2025). Torres Strait Islanders are the Indigenous peoples of over 274 islands located between the northern tip of Queensland and the southwest coast of Papua New Guinea (Australian Government, 2025). *Aboriginal* is a term that groups together the custodians of the land and sea of mainland Australia and most islands outside of the Torres Strait. There are about several hundred different groups, each with distinct culture and languages (AIHW, 2024c).

3.4.1 The importance of language and terminology

First Nations people may use various collective terms, such as *mob*, to refer to themselves. It is essential to engage respectfully with communities by asking about their preferred terms rather than assuming. In this text, as well as Aboriginal and Torres Strait Islander peoples, the term *First Nations people/s* will be used to honour the ongoing contributions of Aboriginal and Torres Strait Islander people to Australia's lands and seas over more than 45,000 years (Australian Public Service Commission, 2022). While *Indigenous* was used in previous editions of this text, it is acknowledged that this term may homogenise distinct groups and is now not the term to use.

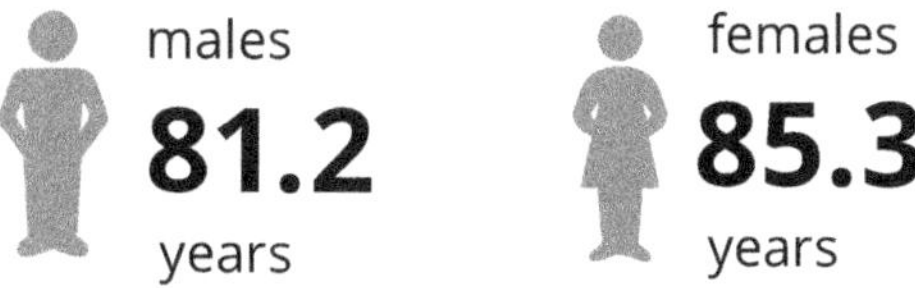

Figure 3.1 Life expectancy for a person born in Australia in 2022 (AIHW, 2024a, p. 4)

3.4.2 Population and demographics

As of June 2021, Aboriginal and Torres Strait Islander peoples made up 3.8% of Australia's total population, with approximately 984,000 individuals (AIHW, 2024c). The population is relatively young compared to non-Indigenous Australians, with a median age of 24 years. Notably, about 34% of First Nations peoples are under 15 years old, compared to 17% of the overall Australian population (AIHW, 2024c).

3.4.3 Geographical distribution of Aboriginal and Torres Strait Islander people

Figure 3.2 illustrates where First Nations people live across Australia with the following distribution:

- 41% in major cities,
- 44% in inner and outer regional areas, and
- 15% in remote or very remote areas.

The proportion of Aboriginal and Torres Strait Islander peoples within the total population increases with remoteness, ranging from 2.2% in major cities to 30% in remote and very remote areas. This distribution has implications for access to health and other essential services (AIHW, 2024c).

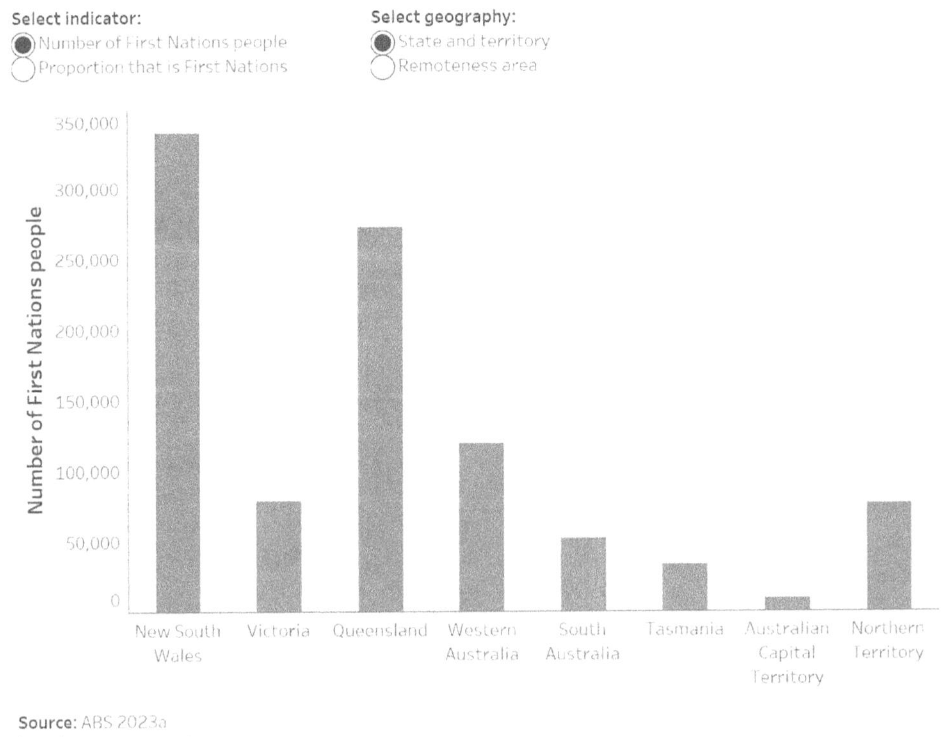

Figure 3.2 First Nations populations by state and territory

(AIHW, 2024c, Profile of First Nations people)

3.4.4 Impact of colonisation

The history of colonisation continues to negatively impact the health of First Nations people, in relation to both accessing culturally safe services and health outcomes (Meechan et al., 2024). Policies of removing children from their families, denying them cultural and spiritual experiences, including connection to country, denied Aboriginal and Torres Strait islander people self-determination (Meechan et al., 2024), leading to intergenerational trauma that exists to this day (Gibson et al., 2015).

It is important to acknowledge that Aboriginal and Torres Strait Islander people are not defined by the negative impacts of colonisation. The longest continuous culture continues to be expressed, with the awakening of language and cultural practices an important contributor to the health and wellbeing First Nations communities. As health professionals, it is imperative to understand the challenges to health, as described in in the following section, but equally important to not define individuals or communities by health statistics.

---

a. Self-determination

This definition is as defined by the Australian Human Rights Commission Aboriginal and Torres Strait Islander Social Justice Team.

Self-determination can mean different things to different groups of people. At its core, self-determination 'is concerned with the fundamental right of people to shape their own lives'. In a practical sense, self-determination means that we have the freedom to live well, to determine what it means to live well according to our own values and beliefs.

In recognising that Indigenous peoples have this right, governments are required to recognise our collective/group identities such as our nations, language groups, clans, family alliances or communities.

(Australian Human Rights Commission, 2024)

3.4.5 The health and wellbeing of Aboriginal and Torres Strait Islander people

The ongoing impacts of colonialism have resulted in significant health disparities between Aboriginal and Torres Strait Islander peoples and non-Indigenous Australians. Life expectancy provides a stark example of these inequalities. For males born between 2020 and 2022:

- First Nations males had a life expectancy of 71.9 years, 8.8 years lower than non-Indigenous males (80.6 years).
- First Nations females had a life expectancy of 75.6 years, 8.1 years lower than non-Indigenous females (83.8 years). (Australian Government, 2024a)

Although life expectancy does not capture the full scope of health and wellbeing, it highlights systemic health inequities and barriers to accessing healthcare services. Chronic diseases, those that are long-lasting and impact quality of life, are the leading cause of death, disability, and illness among Aboriginal and Torres Strait Islander people.

There has been progress in addressing these issues. For example, the rate of First Nations people accessing chronic disease management plans through GPs has been increasing. This improvement is partly due to the expansion of Aboriginal Community Controlled Health Services (ACCHS), which provide culturally appropriate and competent care. However, challenges remain. The rate of referral to medical specialists for First Nations peoples is still half that of non-Indigenous Australians, directly affecting health outcomes and perpetuating disparities (AIHW, 2020).

3.4.6 Mental health

Aboriginal and Torres Strait Islander people experience a higher rate of mental health issues than non-Indigenous Australians. Continued impacts of colonisation and subsequent polices including the forced removal of children lead to higher rates of trauma and grief, impacting both physical and mental health. First Nations people access mental health services, including community mental health services, at higher rates than non-indigenous Australians, as illustrated in Figure 3.3 (AIHW, 2020). Most mental health services are developed to address the symptoms of specific conditions. For Aboriginal and Torres Strait Islander people, access to individual services is important but equally important is community level action that supports truth telling and reconciliation, as outlined in the Uluru Statement from the Heart (The First Nations National Constitutional Convention and the Central Land Council (Australia), 2017).

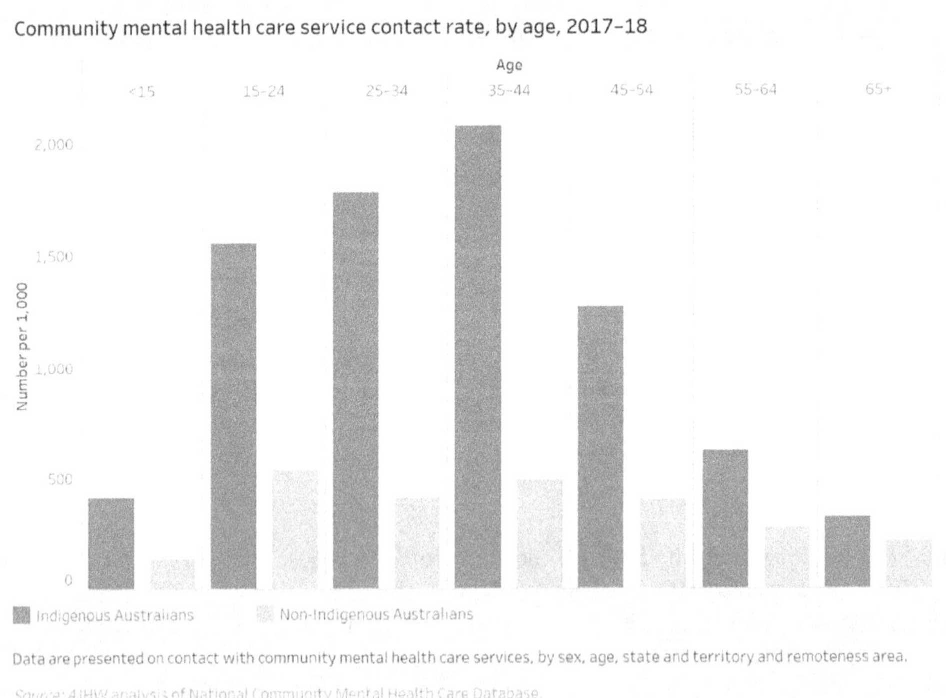

Figure 3.3 Community mental health care service contact rates, by Indigenous status and age group, 2017–18

3.4.7 Children

Infant and child mortality rates are widely recognised as key indicators of overall health. Between 2017 and 2021, the mortality rate among First Nations children aged 0–4 was 2.1 times higher than that of non-Indigenous children. These statistics highlight the persistent impacts of colonisation, which continue to contribute to systemic disadvantage.

Programs tailored specifically for First Nations women, particularly those providing continuity of care during the antenatal period, have shown success in improving health outcomes for both mothers and babies (AIHW, 2024d) To further reduce these disparities, it is essential to address broader social determinants of health, including:

- Access to stable housing,
- Quality education, and
- Culturally safe primary healthcare.

3.4.8 Policy response: Closing the gap

The Closing the Gap initiative, launched in 2008, aims to address the significant health and social disparities between Aboriginal and Torres Strait Islander peoples and non-Indigenous Australians. In 2019, the initiative was updated to place a stronger emphasis on self-determination, reflecting the importance of First Nations leadership in shaping outcomes.

Under a new agreement between the Australian Government and the Coalition of Peaks (a representative body of Aboriginal and Torres Strait Islander communities and organisations), the initiative targets key areas critical to health and wellbeing. These include:

- Life expectancy,
- Access to culturally appropriate early childhood education,
- Opportunities in vocational and higher education,
- Improved housing, and
- Reducing incarceration rates.

Additionally, the initiative incorporates cultural outcomes that are vital to First Nations identity and wellbeing. These include:

- Supporting opportunities to learn and preserve Indigenous languages, and
- Protecting relationships with land and water through legal rights.

By addressing both systemic inequalities and cultural preservation, Closing the Gap seeks to improve the health, wellbeing, and autonomy of Aboriginal and Torres Strait Islander peoples (Commonwealth of Australia, 2020).

3.5 Social determinants of health in Australia

Health is influenced by the conditions in which people live and work, often referred to as the social determinants of health. These determinants are shaped by factors such as employment, education, power, and social support. According to the World Health Organization (WHO):

> The social determinants of health (SDH) are the non-medical factors that influence health outcomes. They are the conditions in which people are born, grow, work, live, and age, and the wider set of forces and systems shaping the conditions of daily life. These forces and systems include economic policies and systems, development agendas, social norms, social policies and political systems.
> (WHO, 2024, https://www.who.int/health-topics/
> social-determinants-of-health#tab=tab_1)

In Australia, the social determinants of health reveal significant differences between various groups. Following are key statistics related to some of these determinants:

3.5.1 Socioeconomic position

Socioeconomic position is largely determined by education, income, and occupation. In 2023, some key statistics related to socioeconomic position were (ABS, 2024b) as follows:

Of people aged 15–74 years:
- 63% had not completed high school.
- 80% with a non-school qualification, and 58% without, were employed.
- 85% who finished a non-school qualification in 2022 were employed in 2023.

Of people aged 15–24 years:
- 61% were currently studying.
- 8% were not engaged in any work or study.

In relation to work and/or study (ABS, 2024c):
- 61% of people aged 15–74 years (11.9 million) were fully engaged in work, study, or both.
- 71% of men were fully engaged.
- 51% of women were fully engaged.

The average household wealth in Australia surpassed 1.04 million in 2019–2020 (ABS, 2022); however, wealth disparity exists, with the highest 20% of the wealth scale holding nearly two thirds of all wealth and those in the lowest 60% holding only 17% of wealth (lowest 20% of households owning only 1% of total wealth) (Australian Council of Social Services and University of New South Wales, 2024).

3.5.2 Early life

Conditions before birth and during early childhood affect health and wellbeing throughout life. In 2018, 78% of Australian children were on track to meet developmental indictors measured in the Australian Early Developmental Census (AEDC) (Australian Government, 2021). However, 22% of children were identified as developmentally vulnerable on 1 or more of the areas on the AEDC and 1% were vulnerable in 2 or more areas (AIHW, 2022).

3.5.3 Social exclusion

Social exclusion is defined by the United Nations (UN) as 'a state in which individuals are unable to participate fully in economic, social, political and cultural life, as well as the process leading to and sustaining such a state' (United Nations, 2016, p. 19). While Australia is generally considered an inclusive society, there are groups of people who experience social exclusion. About 4.3 million Australians experience some form of social exclusion, including older adults (44%), Aboriginal and Torres Strait Islander people (47%), and more than half of those with disabilities (Brotherhood of St Laurence & Melbourne Institute, 2020).

3.5.4 Employment and work

Employment provides not only income but also a sense of identity and purpose. Conversely, unemployment can negatively impact health and wellbeing. As of August 2024, 4.1% of Australians were unemployed, with younger people more likely to be unemployed (9.8%) (ABS, 2024b).

3.5.5 Housing and homelessness

Access to affordable, safe, and uncrowded housing is crucial for good health. Homelessness is linked to poor physical and mental health outcomes and increases the risk of social exclusion. In the 2021 Census, more than 122,000 people were recorded as homeless in Australia (AIHW, 2024e).

3.5.6 Chronic disease

Despite having a high life expectancy, many Australians are affected by chronic diseases. In 2022, 81.4% of Australians reported having at least one chronic condition, such as mental and behavioural conditions (26.1%), back problems (15.7%), and arthritis (14.5%) (ABS, 2023). These conditions are often linked to preventable factors like tobacco use, obesity, poor diet, and high blood pressure (AIHW, 2019). Government and community programmes are focused on addressing these preventable factors. Occupational therapists play a key role in promoting healthy lifestyles and can offer support through GP chronic disease management plans funded through Medicare (Australian Government, 2022).

3.6 Primary care

Health care in Australia is described across several levels based on accessibility, complexity, and specialisation. Primary care is health care people access in their community, focused on basic, everyday health needs, disease prevention, and health promotion. It often involves health screenings, general checkups, and visits for minor injuries and illnesses. Many chronic health conditions can be effectively managed in primary care settings.

Primary care is provided by general practitioners (GPs), nurses, allied health practitioners, and community health workers from across the public, private, and non-government sectors (AIHW, 2023a). It is often the first contact point for people in the community and serves as a referral point for more specialised care. A fundamental principle of primary care is the collaboration required between health care providers to meet individual health requirements. People with particular conditions can be supported in primary care through the development of care plans. GPs can refer eligible people for Medicare-subsidised allied health services within the primary care sector to manage the following conditions:

- Chronic disease
- Eating disorders
- Mental health
- Complex neurological disorders and eligible disabilities

Care plans enable coordination of primary care to avoid or reduce the need for secondary health care services and support people to navigate the primary care system. Eligible patients can receive five allied health services per calendar year, which can involve several allied health professions (Services Australia, 2024).

Attendance at GP services rose faster than population growth when comparing rates from Medicare's inception in 1984 to the end of the COVID-19 pandemic in 2022. Since then, however, attendance rates have declined sharply, and this has been attributed to a combination of increasing out of pocket expenses for the patient and decreased availability of GP appointments and socioeconomic factors (AIHW, 2023b). The average patient payment for GP visits has increased over time. In 2022, the GP attendance rate in major cities was almost twice that of those living in very remote areas. (AIHW, 2023b)

3.7 Secondary care

Secondary care provides specialised health services using more advanced diagnostic and treatment facilities. Most secondary care is provided in a hospital setting, although some specialised medical and rehabilitation services are provided within the community. Access to secondary care generally requires a referral from a primary health care worker, except when patients are admitted to hospital directly through the Emergency Department.

Because secondary care is generally more expensive, the important role of primary health care in keeping people well in their communities is often emphasised. In Australia, hospital services are provided in both public and private hospitals, accounting for 40% of total health care expenditure. In Australia during 2022–23 there were 12.1 million hospital admissions to one of 700 public hospitals or 657 private hospitals (AIHW, 2024f).

3.7.1 Public hospitals

There were 65,000 public hospital beds available in 2022–23, representing 2.5 beds per 1000 population (AIHW, 2024f). Major public hospitals are most commonly located in metropolitan areas, creating potential inequities in availability of secondary health care. In 2022–23, hospital bed availability was spread across major cities (27% of hospitals and 68% of hospital beds), regional areas (57% of hospitals and 29% of hospital beds), and remote/very remote areas (16% of hospitals and 2.9% of hospital beds) (AIHW, 2024e).

Technology has established an increased presence in health care, and hospitals are well equipped with resources to address the diverse diagnostic and treatment needs of patients. The use of technology generally increases the cost of health care provision; however technological advances can result in shorter hospital stays with associated cost savings.

Many people receive outpatient services when diagnostic or follow up care is required, or after inpatient care, without the person being admitted to hospital. In 2022–23, 48% of non-admitted services in public hospitals were provided by allied health and/ or clinical nursing staff (AIHW, 2024d). Most elective surgery is conducted in private hospitals because public hospital waiting times can be lengthy (AIHW, 2023d).

3.7.2 Private hospitals

Australians with private health insurance can choose to be treated in private hospitals with the doctor or specialist of their choice. Private hospitals contribute a third of all Australian hospital beds (AIHW, 2024f) and are regulated by state and territory governments through the granting of licences that are subject to the same accreditation requirements imposed on public hospitals. Some private hospitals also receive state funding to provide services to public patients alongside their private patient activities, and private patients can also receive services in public hospitals using their private funding. The services provided by private hospitals are important in reducing the impact of health care needs on public facilities.

3.8 Tertiary and quaternary health care

Some Australian state and territory health services distinguish further between levels of care by identifying tertiary, and even quaternary, health services that provide highly specialised medical and surgical interventions or treatment for complex or rare health conditions. Such services are provided within hospital settings and are often restricted to facilities located in capital cities or large regional centres. For that reason, patients are sometimes transferred from secondary care hospitals to more specialised tertiary hospitals or quaternary services outside of their local area to receive appropriate treatment.

3.9 Funding of health care

In 2021–22, Australia allocated 10.5% of its gross domestic product (GDP), or $241 billion, to health services (~$9300 per person) (AIHW, 2023f). During that period, $96 billion was spent on hospital service provision, including $77.2 billion for public hospitals and $18.8 billion for private hospitals. $84.1 billion was spent on primary health care. Additional expenditure of $11.7 billion was allocated to building and resourcing new hospitals (AIHW, 2024e). Public hospital funding as a share of total health expenditure is expected to grow by 21% over the next 5 years (AIHW, 2024f).

Public health service funding is a responsibility of local, state and federal governments. An example of a publicly funded health service in Australia is the National Immunisation Program that provides free vaccines to eligible Australians. The Australian government funds medical services through Medicare and provides funds to states and territories for public hospital services. It also funds some population-specific services like Aboriginal and Torres Strait Islander Health, residential aged care and veteran services. State and territory governments fund and manage public hospitals and ambulance services and deliver some community-based screening and immunisation procedures. Local governments are sometimes involved in public health initiatives and delivery of home-based health and support services.

The private system is funded by a combination of state and federal government funding, private health insurers, patients, Medicare and other sources like WorkCover. One area of pressure on health care funding due to increased demands is mental health. Approximately 1 in 5 adults and 1 in 7 young people experienced a mental health disorder in 2021–22. Almost $12.2 billion dollars was spent on mental health services during 2021–22, which equates to around 7% of total government health expenditure (AIHW, 2023f).

Pressures imposed by Australia's ageing population, rising rates of chronic disease and mental health disorders and the need to address health inequities are all forecast to impact health service funding in the foreseeable future. Given these threats to the sustainability and equity of universal health care in Australia, Angeles et al. (2023) called for substantial reforms to the funding and provision of care to secure health care access for Australians into the future. Governments and health service providers continue to work to achieve that.

Enhanced access to primary care is one proposed way of reducing pressure on secondary health care services and associated costs of health care (Department of Health and Aged Care, 2023). In 2021–22, spending on primary health care was $84.1 billion – an increase of 10.9% from the previous year – but as a proportion of total health spending it remains similar to pre-pandemic years (AIHW, 2023b).

3.10 Features of the Australian health care system

3.10.1 Medicare

Medicare is the universal health care scheme based upon the principle that all Australians should have equal access to health care. Funded through tax contributions, Medicare subsidises the costs associated with hospital care including a range of tests, imaging, and scans, and services provided by health professionals including GPs and optometrists. To be eligible for Medicare-funded services, individuals must be a citizen or permanent resident of Australia or New Zealand (Department of Health and Aged Care, 2024a).

Occupational therapists can be reimbursed through Medicare for specific services. These include:

1. Chronic disease management
2. Focused psychological services
3. Complex neurodevelopmental and eligible disability services
4. Eating disorders services

Occupational therapists wishing to access a Medicare rebate are required to register as Medicare providers. There are annual limits for how many services each individual can claim and a set rebate fee. Access requires a referral from a medical practitioner, including GPs, and completion of a GP management plan or multidisciplinary care plan (Occupational Therapy Australia, 2023).

3.10.2 Private health insurance

Australians eligible for Medicare are entitled to treatment as a public patient in public hospitals, or they can choose to self-fund or use their private health insurance to be treated as private patients. Private health insurance is also an option to part fund services not covered by Medicare including dental services, optical aids such as spectacles, and in some states and territories, ambulance services. In March 2024, 44.8% of Australians had private health insurance (APRA, 2024), but data on how many private health insurance policies provide cover for occupational therapy is not readily available.

3.11 Cost of health care

In 2021–22, Australia spent approximately $241.3 billion on health goods and services, which is an average of $9,365 per person (AIHW, 2024a). This expenditure is spread across all tiers of government and private providers, requiring collaboration across these sectors to deliver essential health services (AIHW, 2024a; Duckett, 2022) (see Figure 3.4).

The Australian and state and territory governments contributed the majority of health spending in 2021–22:

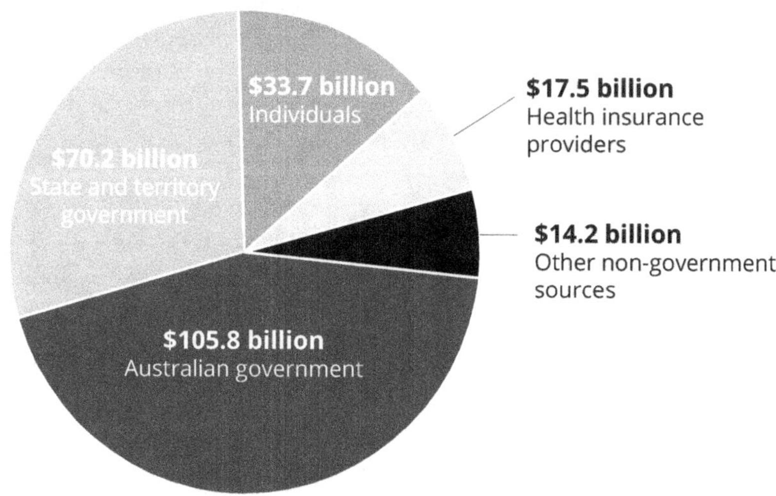

Figure 3.4 Health expenditure in Australia

(AIHW, 2024a, p. 50)

3.12 The National Disability Insurance Scheme

The National Disability Insurance Scheme or NDIS provides funding directly to people with disabilities with the aim of supporting engagement in everyday occupations. It was first trialled in 2013 and introduced across most of Australia in 2016. In 2024, 500,000 people were accessing services funded through the NDIS (National Disability Insurance Agency, 2024). The premise behind the NDIS is to give people with a disability the choice and freedom to choose care and services that are reasonable and necessary. For example, in many cases people with a disability require personal care assistance, transportation, or equipment to be able to access their home and outside environment. Recipients of the NDIS can self-manage funds that are allocated to them, or they can elect to have someone manage their funds for them choosing, who provides these services if they are a registered provider of care.

Many occupational therapists are registered providers of care which means they can charge recipients of the NDIS fees set by National Disability Insurance Agency (NDIA). Under the NDIS occupational therapists provide services such as aids and equipment, home modifications, driving assessments and a range of interventions for physical and psychosocial disabilities (Occupational Therapy Australia, 2021).

Further information on occupational therapy and the NDIS is available in Chapter 4.

3.13 Aged care

Medical services for older Australians are funded through Medicare. For those people requiring further supports or ongoing care, the options are as follows.

3.13.1 Home care packages

To support people to remain in their own homes, government funding is available for services including help with household tasks, aids and equipment, minor home modifications, and personal care. Eligible individuals may also be funded for clinical care provided by registered nurses or allied health professionals, including occupational therapy. To be eligible for a home care package, people must register with the My Aged Care platform and be referred for an assessment by an aged care assessor. This assessment will determine what level (1–4) of package the person will receive and therefore the amount of funding and services.

3.13.2 Residential aged care

For older adults who can no longer live at home, funding may be available for residential aged care, which provides accommodation and 24-hour personal care, supported by nursing and allied health. The level of financial assistance a person may receive is means tested. The government also oversees the quality of the services and sets maximum costs for services being provided (Department of Health and Aged Care, 2024b).

Occupational therapists play a key role in providing aged care services to older people – both in the community and in residential aged care facilities. Further reform is required to expand access to allied health, including occupational therapy to support older adults to both remain at home longer and to have enhanced quality of life with residential aged care settings. Further information on the role of occupational therapy in working with older adults is available in Chapter 32.

3.14 Conclusion

Australia's health care system is multifaceted, integrating public and private sectors to deliver comprehensive services across primary, secondary, and tertiary levels. While the system is globally respected for its outcomes and accessibility, significant challenges persist, particularly in addressing health inequities among Aboriginal and Torres Strait Islander peoples. Occupational therapists play a pivotal role in promoting health and wellbeing across diverse populations and settings. As Australia faces growing pressures from an ageing population and rising chronic conditions, sustainable funding and reform are essential. A continued commitment to inclusive, culturally responsive care and intergovernmental collaboration will be key to ensuring equitable health outcomes for all Australians.

3.15 Summary

- Australia's health care system is a complex mix of public and private services, with responsibilities shared across federal, state, and local governments, and supported by Medicare as the universal health insurance scheme.
- Health disparities persist, particularly for Aboriginal and Torres Strait Islander peoples, who face lower life expectancy, higher rates of chronic disease, and systemic barriers to accessing culturally safe care.
- Social determinants of health such as education, employment, housing, and social inclusion significantly influence health outcomes and contribute to inequalities across different population groups.
- Occupational therapists play a vital role in the health system, supporting individuals across the lifespan in areas such as chronic disease management, disability services (NDIS), and aged care.
- Primary care is the first point of contact for most Australians and is essential for managing chronic conditions and reducing pressure on more costly secondary and tertiary care services.
- Health funding in Australia is substantial, with over $241 billion spent in 2021–22, but rising demand from an ageing population and mental health needs calls for ongoing reform and investment.

3.16 Review and reflection questions

- How is the Australian health care system structured, and what roles do the Commonwealth and state/territory governments play in its funding and delivery?
- What are some of the key health disparities faced by Aboriginal and Torres Strait Islander peoples, and how do historical and social factors contribute to these disparities?
- Explain the concept of the social determinants of health and provide examples of how they influence health outcomes in Australia.
- What is the role of occupational therapists within the Australian health care system, and how do they contribute to addressing chronic disease and disability through programmes like Medicare and the NDIS?

References

Angeles, M. R., Crosland, P., & Hensher, M. (2023). Challenges for Medicare and universal health care in Australia since 2000. *Medical Journal of Australia, 218*(7), 322–329. https://doi.org/10.5694/mja2.51844

APRA. (2024). *Statistics. Quarterly private health insurance statistics.* Australian Prudential Regulation Authority.

Australian Bureau of Statistics. (2022). *Household income and wealth, Australia.* https://www.abs.gov.au/statistics/economy/finance/household-income-and-wealth-australia/2019-20

Australian Bureau of Statistics. (2023). *Health conditions prevalence.* https://www.abs.gov.au/statistics/health/health-conditions-and-risks/health-conditions-prevalence/latest-release

Australian Bureau of Statistics. (2024a). *Provisional mortality statistics.* https://www.abs.gov.au/statistics/health/causes-death/provisional-mortality-statistics/latest-release

Australian Bureau of Statistics. (2024b). *Labour force, Australia.* https://www.abs.gov.au/statistics/labour/employment-and-unemployment/labour-force-australia/latest-release

Australian Bureau of Statistics. (2024c). *Education and work, Australia.* https://www.abs.gov.au/statistics/people/education/education-and-work-australia/latest-release

Australian Council of Social Services and University of New South Wales. (2024). *Inequality in Australia.* https://povertyandinequality.acoss.org.au/inequality/

Australian Government. (2022). *Future focused primary health care: Australia's primary health care 10 year plan 2022–2032.* Australian Government.

Australian Government. (2025). *Aboriginal and torres strait islander peoples.* Style Manual. https://www.stylemanual.gov.au/accessible-and-inclusive-content/inclusive-language/aboriginal-and-torres-strait-islander-peoples

Australian Government, Department of Education. (2021). *Australian early development census.* https://www.aedc.gov.au/

Australian Human Rights Commission. (2024). *Aboriginal and Torres Strait Islander social justice: Self-determination.* https://humanrights.gov.au/our-work/aboriginal-and-torres-strait-islander-social-justice/self-determination

Australian Institute of Health and Welfare. (2019). *Australian burden of disease study: Impact and causes of illness and death in Australia 2015.* Australian Burden of Disease series no. 19. Cat. no. BOD 22. AIHW.

Australian Institute of Health and Welfare. (2020). *Aboriginal and Torres Strait Islander Health performance framework: Measures.* https://www.indigenoushpf.gov.au/measu

Australian Institute of Health and Welfare. (2022). *Australia's children: The transition to primary school.* https://www.aihw.gov.au/reports/children-youth/australias-children/contents/education/transition-primary-school

Australian Institute of Health and Welfare. (2023a). *Primary health care.* https://www.aihw.gov.au/reports-data/health-welfare-services/primary-health-care/overview

Australian Institute of Health and Welfare. (2023b). *Medicare funding of GP services over time.* https://www.aihw.gov.au/getmedia/05dbd806-0708-40c1-9a9c-8099c3f36faa/aihw-hwe-94.pdf?v=20240618080951&inline=true

Australian Institute of Health and Welfare. (2023c). *Admitted patients.* https://www.aihw.gov.au/reports-data/myhospitals/sectors/admitted-patients

Australian Institute of Health and Welfare. (2023d). *Elective surgery.* https://www.aihw.gov.au/reports-data/myhospitals/sectors/elective-surgery

Australian Institute of Health and Welfare. (2023e). *Health expenditure Australia 2021–22.* https://www.aihw.gov.au/reports/health-welfare-expenditure/health-expenditure-australia-2021-22

Australian Institute of Health and Welfare. (2023f). *Mental health.* https://www.aihw.gov.au/mental-health

Australian Institute of Health and Welfare. (2024a). *Australia's health 2024: In brief, Cat. no. AUS 249.* AIHW.

Australian Institute of Health and Welfare. (2024b). *Health system overview.* https://www.aihw.gov.au/reports/australias-health/health-system-overview

Australian Institute of Health and Welfare. (2024c). *Profile of First Nations people.* https://www.aihw.gov.au/reports/australias-welfare/profile-of-indigenous-australians

Australian Institute of Health and Welfare. (2024d). *Aboriginal and Torres Strait Islander Health performance framework summary report.* Australian Institute of Health and Welfare, Australian Government.

Australian Institute of Health and Welfare. (2024e). *Homelessness and homelessness services.* https://www.aihw.gov.au/reports/australias-welfare/homelessness-and-homelessness-services

Australian Institute of Health and Welfare. (2024f). *Australia's hospitals at a glance.* https://www.aihw.gov.au/reports/hospitals/australias-hospitals-at-a-glance

Australian Public Service Commission. (2022). *First Nations Vocabulary – using culturally appropriate language and terminology.* https://www.apsc.gov.au/working-aps/diversity-and-inclusion/diversity-inclusion-news/first-nations-vocabulary-using-culturally-appropriate-language-and-terminology.

Brotherhood of St Laurence & Melbourne Institute. (2020). *Who experiences social exclusion?* https://www.bsl.org.au/

Commonwealth of Australia. (2020). *National agreement on closing the gap.* Department of the Prime Minister and Cabinet.

Department of Health and Aged Care. (2023). *About primary care.* https://www.health.gov.au/topics/primary-care/about

Department of Health and Aged Care. (2024a). *Funding for aged care service providers.* https://www.health.gov.au/topics/aged-care/providing-aged-care-services/funding-for-aged-care-service-providers

Department of Health and Aged Care. (2024b). *Funding for aged care service providers.* https://www.health.gov.au/topics/aged-care/providing-aged-care-services/funding-for-aged-care-service-providers.

Duckett, S. (2022). *The Australian health care system.* Oxford University Press.

The First Nations National Constitutional Convention and the Central Land Council (Australia). (2017). *Uluru: Statement from the heart.* Alice Springs, Northern Territory.

Gibson, C., Butler, C., Henaway, C., Dudgeon, P., & Curtin, M. (2015). Indigenous peoples and human rights: Some considerations for the occupational therapy profession in Australia. *Australian Occupational Therapy Journal, 62*(3), 214–218. https://doi.org/10.1111/1440-1630.12185

Government. (2024a). *Australian Government style manual: Aboriginal and Torres Strait Islander peoples.* https://www.stylemanual.gov.au/accessible-and-inclusive-content/inclusive-language/aboriginal-and-torres-strait-islander-peoples

Meechan, E., Geia, L., Taylor, M., Murray, D., Stothers, K., Gibson, P., Devine, S., & Barker, R. (2024). Culturally responsive occupational therapy practice with First Nations Peoples – A scoping review. *Australian Journal of Rural Health, 32*(4), 617–671. https://doi.org/10.1111/ajr.13143

National Disability Insurance Agency. (2024). *What is the NDIS?* https://www.ndis.gov.au/understanding/what-ndis

National Health and Hospital Reform Commission. (2009). *A healthier future for all Australian – final report.* http://apo.org.au/node/17921

Occupational Therapy Australia. (2021). *National disability insurance agency home and living consultation – An ordinary life at home.* Occupational Therapy Australia submission.

Occupational Therapy Australia. (2023). *Medicare overview for occupational therapists.* Occupational Therapy Australia.

OECD. (2023). *Health at a glance 2023: OECD indicators.* OECD Publishing. https://doi.org/10.1787/7a7afb35-en

Services Australia. (2024). *Care plans.* https://servicesasutralia.gov.au/care-plans?context=20

United Nations Department of Economic and Social Affairs. (2016). Identifying social inclusion and exclusion. *Report on the World Social Situation.* United Nations Department of Economic and Social Affairs.

World Health Organization. (2024). *Social determinant of health.* https://www.who.int/health-topics/social-determinants-of-health#tab=tab_1

The National Disability Insurance Scheme and its relationship to occupational therapy practice in Australia

Linda Barclay, Tomomi McAuliffe, Anoo Bhopti, Libby Callaway, Stacey Touma, and Helen Bourke-Taylor

Authors' positionality statement

We are all English-speaking, university-educated professionals who identify as women. We bring personal or professional experiences of the NDIS, which inform our understanding and perspectives of both the system's strengths and the barriers faced by participants. We acknowledge the systems and structures that afford us unearned privilege and are committed to improving our understanding and practice around decolonising research, guided by people with lived experiences different than our own.

Key terms
- National Disability Insurance Scheme (NDIS)
- International Classification of Functioning, Disability and Health (ICF)
- Social policy
- Social model of disability
- Professional practice.

Objectives
This chapter will allow the reader to:

- Describe the significance, structure and function of the National Disability Insurance Scheme
- Outline the International Classification of Functioning Disability and Health and how it intersects with the NDIS
- Understand the contexts and perspectives of NDIS participants, and their families
- Explain the role, obligations, and processes for occupational therapists to collaborate successfully with participants, and deliver NDIS-funded services
- Have currency of knowledge regarding practice standards for evidence-based occupational therapy provision within the NDIS.

DOI: 10.4324/9781003495666-5

4.1 Introduction

Occupational therapists have provided services to people with disability since the profession's inception, with a growing recognition of the social model of disability and theoretical frameworks that take a focus on maximising participation (Imms et al., 2017). This practice focus aligns with the main objective of the National Disability Insurance Scheme (NDIS), which is to provide all Australians who acquire a permanent disability before the age of 65, with the reasonable and necessary supports they need to live an ordinary life (National Disability Insurance Scheme [NDIS], n.d.). Occupational therapists working within the NDIS need to understand what is considered reasonable and necessary, and should refer to the NDIS website for the most up to date information regarding this (NDIS, n.d.). The NDIS provides funding for NDIS supports that relate to the person's disability (when impairments meet the Scheme access requirements for disability, early intervention, or both), linked to their goals for social and/or economic participation. The NDIS supports goals that cover life-domains such as daily living, home, and lifelong learning and are used to determine reasonable and necessary supports to build participant capacity.

The number of NDIS participants has grown significantly since the Scheme achieved national roll out in 2020. This has resulted in an increased demand for occupational therapists who have a key role within the NDIS, providing evidence informed assessments and interventions to facilitate individualised goal-attainment.

4.2 Occupational therapy practice within the National Disability Insurance Scheme and its relationship to occupational therapy practice in Australia

4.2.1 An overview of the NDIS in Australia

The NDIS was first recommended by the Productivity Commission in 2011 following an inquiry which described the disability support system for Australians at that time as 'underfunded, unfair, fragmented, and inefficient, and gives people with a disability little choice and no certainty of access to appropriate supports' (Australian Government, 2011). At time of print there were 717,001 NDIS participants (NDIS, 2025a).

The National Disability Insurance Agency (The Agency) is the Commonwealth agency responsible for delivering the NDIS. The agency manages access to the Scheme, planning, payments, and pricing. The NDIS Quality and Safeguards Commission (The Commission) is an independent regulatory body that oversees the quality and safety of NDIS supports, by setting and enforcing standards, approving and regulating NDIS provider registration, detecting and investigating allegations of fraud, and investigating complaints about NDIS service providers (such as occupational therapists).

The Australian government appointed a panel to undertake an independent review of the NDIS in 2023, to address issues identified with the Scheme's responsiveness to participants' needs and ensure sustainability of the NDIS. Changes that have resulted from this review – and a new bill introduced in October 2024 – include impairment categories for NDIS eligibility, processes for assessment of NDIS participant status, plans and budgets, and definitions of what constitutes an NDIS support (Parliament of Australia, 2024). Given the ongoing Scheme reforms underway, the most up-to-date and reliable source of information for NDIS participants and their families, and occupational therapists working with them, is the NDIS website (NDIS, n.d.).

NDIS provider registration is also undergoing significant reform, guided by recommendations from an NDIS Provider and Worker Registration Taskforce (Department of Health, Disability and Ageing, NDIS Provider and Worker Registration Taskforce, 2025). Early reforms based on recommendations from this Taskforce include the introduction of mandatory NDIS provider registration for certain provider markets, including platform providers, support coordinators, and Supported Independent Living (SIL) providers (NDIS Quality and Safeguards Commission, n.d.). Proposals for additional reforms include a risk-proportionate, graduated NDIS registration process to be introduced for all health professionals providing NDIS-funded services (including occupational therapists). Given the NDIS provider reforms underway, the most up-to-date and reliable source of information on this is the NDIS Quality and Safeguards Commission website (NDIS Quality and Safeguards Commission, n.d.).

4.2.2 The International Classification of Functioning, Disability and Health

Whilst the World Health Organization formally endorsed the International Classification of Functioning, Disability and Health (Figure 4.1) in 2001, the ICF has more recently been embedded within, and referred to, in the NDIS rules set by the government (Australian Government, 2013; ICF Australia Interest Group [ICF-AIG], 2022). The ICF is an integration of the social model of disability (which emphasises that people are disabled by barriers in society such as steps into buildings) and the medical model (which views people as disabled due to their impairments). The ICF shifts the focus from viewing disability primarily as a problem within the individual, to a biopsychosocial model that conceives a person's functioning or disability as a dynamic interaction between the person's health condition, their environment, and their personal factors (World Health Organization, 2001).

Environmental factors in the ICF refer to the physical, social, financial and attitudinal environments in which people live and conduct their lives, while personal factors

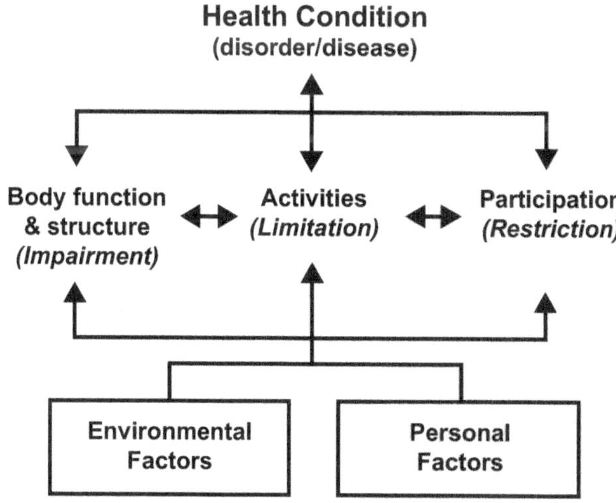

Figure 4.1 International classification of functioning, disability, and health (WHO, 2001)

refer to features that the individual may have that impact on the experience of disability, such as gender or age (World Health Organization, 2001). Disability is viewed as the result of the interaction between the health condition (e.g. spinal cord injury) and its associated body structure and function issues/consequences (e.g. paralysis, spasticity, loss of sensation, bladder or bowel incontinence), with activity (e.g. impaired mobility, inability to hold tools such as phones, or utensils for self-care) and participation in daily life (e.g. community activities, employment, socialising), within a context that includes both environmental (e.g. funding structures; built environment) and personal factors (e.g. age, gender) (World Health Organization, 2001).

While there are some differences as to how occupational therapists view and assess *participation* compared to how it is operationalised in the ICF, one of the strengths of the ICF is its conceptual approach to understanding how environmental factors can be facilitators or barriers to functioning across different areas of life (Townsend & Polatajko, 2013). This aligns with the NDIS's person-centred approach, which emphasises individualised planning and support, considering the functional capacity and goals of each participant. The ICF classifications of Activities and Participation are particularly relevant for describing a person's goals, objectives and aspirations across all relevant life areas.

Within the NDIS, supports usually relate to environmental factors (e.g. assistance, assistive technology, environmental modifications) to support functioning in particular areas of life and to build capacity, in line with the insurance principles central to the NDIS. Occupational therapy practice within the NDIS aligns closely with the ICF model because both emphasise the importance of enabling individuals to participate in meaningful activities, including the important role that the environment has in supporting or hindering this participation. Occupational therapists can use the ICF to guide their assessments and interventions, focusing on how a person's health condition impacts their ability to perform daily tasks and engage in community life (American Occupational Therapy Association [AOTA], 2020). ICF categories – such as activities, participation, and environmental factors – provide a structured way for occupational therapists to identify barriers and facilitators to function and participation.

Applying the ICF framework within occupational therapy practice can help to ensure that assessments and interventions with NDIS participants are consistent, transparent, and focused on enhancing participation and independence (ICF-AIG, 2022). More broadly, the ICF's standard language and framework also facilitates better communication between healthcare providers, NDIS planners, and participants, promoting consistency in how disability is understood and addressed across different contexts. Illustrating this, Vignette 1 provides an example of the intersect between the ICF, NDIS, and occupational therapy practice to meet the participant's person-centred goals.

4.2.2.1 Vignette 4.1: NDIS participant's experience

Peter is a 50-year-old man who sustained a C5 complete spinal cord injury (SCI) after a diving accident, while studying information technology (IT) at university. He works full-time in IT, and lives alone in an inner-city, fully modified apartment. He receives 34 hours per week of core support for personal care. Peter is on his third NDIS plan.

Peter recently needed a new power wheelchair. He selected an occupational therapist based on recommendations from the state spinal service he remains connected with. Jan, his appointed occupational therapist, developed a service agreement with Peter, proposing a total of 20 hours of occupational therapy to undertake an assessment of his goals and needs, trial power chairs and identify recommendations for the most suitable one, and write a report to the NDIA with a recommendation for a new power chair that met Peter's needs resulting from his SCI.

Jan sought consent from Peter to take a new graduate occupational therapist with her when she meets with him. This provided an excellent opportunity for the new graduate – Lewis – to develop his skills in assessing and prescribing complex high-cost assistive technology such as a power wheelchair. Jan noted in her initial meeting with Peter that he was motor and sensory complete below his lesion level. Jan utilised the ICF as a framework for her initial assessment with Peter. She noted how Peter's body function and structures (including paralysis and loss of sensation below the level of his injury, significantly impaired sitting balance, absence of hand function) impacted his activity and participation restrictions (being dependent in almost all activities of daily living and reliant on assistive technology for work, mobility, and social participation). She also identified personal factors that were strengths for him (i.e. proactive in managing his needs). They discussed Peter's goals for using the wheelchair. The influence of environmental factors was particularly important, as Peter worked from home but also liked to go to cafés and the city gardens. Jan, Lewis, and Peter trialled various wheelchairs, and once they decided on the most appropriate one that could be customised to meet Peter's needs, Lewis completed the NDIS Assistive Technology Assessment template. Jan reviewed his report and, following a few minor revisions, submitted it. The NDIA approved funding for the wheelchair, and Peter ordered it through his self-managed plan.

4.2.3 Participants and the NDIS

The NDIS supports Australian residents aged 0–65 with disability caused by permanent impairment. As of June 2025, there were 173,466 children younger than nine with an NDIS plan, and a further 23,402 children accessed early connections throughout the quarter (NDIS, 2025b). For children, the early childhood approach supports children under six with developmental concerns and children under nine with diagnosed disability, along with their families, to access timely assistance, build capacity, and promote inclusion in everyday and community settings, ensuring opportunities for growth and learning (NDIS, 2025c). Across all NDIS participant age groups, the most prevalent disability types are autism (38%), intellectual disability (13%), developmental delay (12%), and psychosocial disability (9%) (NDIS *Quarterly Reports*, 2025b). Depending on the age of the NDIS participant, or the extent of need for care and support, families and unpaid carers are important unpaid supports for NDIS participants and have a key role in enabling participation (see Vignette 4.2).

4.2.3.1 Fund management types

NDIS participants can choose from three plan-management options or a combination of the three options. These are self-managed, plan-managed, or NDIA-managed.

Box 4.1
Fund management types

<u>Self-managed funding</u> allows participants to manage their own funding, providing the flexibility and choice to decide the support they access.

<u>Plan management</u> is when a provider supports the participant to manage funding in their NDIS plan via plan managers. A plan manager can support the participants with book-keeping, including payment, and other administrative tasks such as organising required reports from multiple services.

Under <u>NDIA plan management</u> (also referred to as Agency-managed), the NDIA manages participants' records of spending. Participants can choose from a range of NDIS registered providers but not unregistered providers.

As of August 2025, 60% of NDIS participants use plan managers, 10% self-manage partly or fully, and 30% are Agency-managed (NDIS, 2025b).

4.2.3.2 Types of supports funded

Following a Support Needs Assessment, NDIS plans are developed and have a budget for funding of three possible types of supports: Core Supports for everyday activities and goals, Capacity Building Supports for skill development and independence, and Capital Supports for assistive technology and home and vehicle modifications.

Core Supports are the most flexible and can be used across any of the following four support categories; 1) consumables, 2) assistance in daily life, 3) transport, and 4) assistance with social participation. Unlike Core Supports budget, Capacity Building Supports include therapy supports such as occupational therapy and other health professional services and cannot be moved across categories. Capital Supports have three support categories: Assistive Technology, Home Modifications, and Vehicle Modifications. NDIS plan budgets, including different categories of supports, have specific funding rules and limitations. Depending on the NDIS plan, participants may receive funding for support coordination. Support coordinators or navigators can assist participants to understand their NDIS plan and connect them with NDIS providers and other community services, taking on a role like a case manager (refer to Chapter 39).

4.2.3.3 Responsibility for supports

In addition to the NDIS, many Scheme participants access other service systems. The Applied Principles and Tables of Support (APTOS) is a framework that delineates responsibilities between the NDIS and other service systems in Australia (Australian Government, 2024). It covers 11 areas, including health, education, employment, and justice. The APTOS aims to ensure coordinated support across sectors while avoiding duplication. It is guided by six general principles and includes system-specific principles and detailed tables of support for each area. This framework clarifies which system funds and provides different types of support. For example, in education, schools provide learning support, whilst the NDIS covers specialised assistive products related to disability.

4.2.3.4 Access to the NDIS

While the NDIS has aimed to support all Scheme participants to build their capacity to participate in society, unique access challenges have been experienced by particular groups. For example, in rural and remote Australia, limited availability of services hinders access to appropriate supports for NDIS participants. For people with psychosocial disability, access to and navigation of the NDIS can be complex due to the fluctuating nature of mental health conditions and complex assessment of the permanence of disability. Similarly, culturally and linguistically diverse populations may face difficulty navigating the complex system, such as the NDIS application and planning processes (Veli-Gold et al., 2023). The participation of Aboriginal and Torres Strait Islander people in the Scheme has been low, with only approximately 8% of the total participants currently identifying as Aboriginal and/or Torres Strait Islanders (NDIS, n.d.).

The NDIA engages in ongoing reviews to address the unique challenges experienced by these participant groups by co-designing strategies, including the First Nations strategy, the LGBTIQA+ strategy, and the Cultural and Linguistic Diversity strategy (NDIS, 2024). These strategies outline the Agency's commitment to facilitate equitable access to the NDIS. The First Nations Advisory Council also assists the NDIA to promote and improve cultural responsiveness of the NDIS. To best assist these groups, occupational therapists need to ensure their practice is culturally responsive and culturally safe.

4.2.4 The role of occupational therapy in the NDIS

Occupational therapists within the NDIS focus on promoting independence and participation in activities of daily living (ADLs) and enablement of social and economic participation. Their services may include NDIS-eligibility or functional capacity assessments, housing assessments, and assistive technology assessments (for more details about Allied Health Housing reports and Assistive Technology assessments, refer to Chapter 34). The assessment of functional capacity is an essential component of the NDIS, as it forms the basis of access to the Scheme and/or evidence of the need for NDIS-funded supports. Functional capacity assessments include standardised or objective assessments of physical, cognitive, and other measurable factors related to functional abilities; subjective information, including observations and information provided by the participant or their caregivers about their functional abilities and limitations (e.g., mobility/motor skills, communication, social interaction, learning, self-care, self-management); evaluation of the individual's ability to perform daily tasks such as personal care, meal preparation, and home maintenance; analysis of the individual's living environment; and any necessary home modifications or assistive technology required. A concise summary of the findings, including the participant's strengths and limitations, and recommendations for interventions and accommodations is then provided.

Intervention strategies that occupational therapists may undertake with NDIS participants include disability-related chronic disease management; prescription and implementation of assistive technology and/or environmental modifications; family-centred practice; mental health interventions; positive behaviour support; driving assessments (when specifically trained to do so); and targeted, goal-focussed skill building. Occupational therapists work within multidisciplinary teams to provide person-centred care that addresses the complex needs and goals of NDIS participants, particularly when developing and reviewing support plans. They may also liaise with NDIS local area coordinators and planners. For more detail about occupational therapy practice areas, refer to Chapters 26–39.

4.2.4.1 Vignette 4.2: Family's experience

William, a 5-year-old autistic boy, loves cars, numbers, and exploring new playgrounds. He has communication difficulties and sensory sensitivities that impact his participation in everyday activities, including preschool. His parents, Alice and Ben, sought occupational therapy to support William's development and participation. The occupational therapist adopted a family-centred practice approach by focusing on building a trusted relationship with Alice and Ben, other relevant family members (siblings), and William's educators. Recognising the family as experts on William's needs, she listened to their concerns and goals for William, such as improving his independence in self-care tasks, increasing his comfort during preschool transitions, and helping him manage sensory overload in noisy environments. After establishing a service agreement, the occupational therapist planned visits to William's home, childcare, and kindergarten in collaboration with Alice and Ben and William's educators. Therapy strategies included visual schedules, sensory regulation activities, and play-based techniques, all tailored to fit William's individual preferences and daily routines at home, at the childcare, and at his kindergarten. The therapist empowered Alice and Ben with practical skills and strategies to use between sessions, providing Alice and Ben with the tools they needed to support William and enhance the family's overall quality of life.

4.2.4.1.1 Preparing for occupational therapy practice in the NDIS

Occupational therapists that plan to work in the NDIS sector should ensure they receive appropriate education regarding the Scheme rules and guidelines, including understanding of their roles and responsibilities, adherence to the NDIS Code of Conduct in addition to their professional code of conduct, and ensuring their practice is evidence based. New graduates should seek regular supervision, have clear workload allocations and achievable session targets, and ensure they have support for complex caseloads and opportunities to shadow senior therapists at the outset. Vignette 4.3 provides an example of issues new graduates should be aware of during job seeking.

4.2.4.2 Vignette 4.3. New graduate's experience

Jenny is a recent graduate from Clever University. She has been approached by five different NDIS occupational therapy service providers offering her employment which includes incentives such as free gym memberships and meal allowances, and some offer new graduate programmes. To help her make an informed decision about where to work, Jenny reflected on the four Occupational Therapy Australia Competency Standards and asked each of the service providers the following questions:

Professionalism
- What is included in the induction process?
- Is there staff support to attend professional development opportunities?
- How is team culture fostered?

Knowledge and learning
- What model of supervision is used?
- What professional development (PD) opportunities exist?
- How will I be supported to stay up to date with occupational therapy research evidence?

Occupational therapy process and practice
- What will my caseload be for the first 12 months?
- What type of clients, complexity, and mixture will I have in my caseload?

Communication
- What meetings occur?
- What is the expectation regarding report writing?
- What are the communication processes with our clients?

Following her interviews, and consideration of these areas, Jenny chose to work at a large multi-state NDIS provider which offered excellent support and supervision during the first year of work. However, she recognised the need for a mentor separate from her employer to support her professional and personal growth and development.

4.2.5 Evidence-based occupational therapy practice within the NDIS

Occupational therapy is an evidence-based profession that requires registered practitioners to provide effective, person-centred services to NDIS participants. Practitioners have an obligation to be ahead of research evidence, uphold evidence-based practice when providing NDIS-funded services, and share such information with NDIS participants and their families to facilitate true shared decision making. Importantly, researchers play an important role in creating evidence, synthesising evidence, and translating evidence into practice that benefits NDIS participants (see Chapters 22 and 23). Furthermore, it is important for practitioners to have the skills to identify and reject low-value interventions and de-implement ineffective interventions.

Amendments to the NDIS act in 2024 clarified that only evidence-based, effective, and beneficial interventions will be funded by the Scheme. Interventions need to be cost effective compared to similar interventions and address the participant's goals. The NDIA Research and Evaluation branch, established in 2020, prioritises areas set out in the Research and Evaluation strategy 2022–2027 (NDIS, n.d.). Targeted areas included evidence-based early intervention for high volume cohorts (e.g., children with intellectual disability or autism) and the effectiveness of home and living supports and assistive technology. The Research and Evaluation branch synthesises and mobilises evidence that will result in innovative and effective services to enhance the lives of NDIS participants. Research evidence is drawn from numerous sources including research conducted by occupational therapy researchers and knowledge producers. Examples of NDIS relevant issues that occupational therapy researchers have explored include participants' experiences of the Scheme (O'Neill et al., 2024), suitability of specific interventions for NDIS-participants in early intervention (Barfoot et al., 2017), and what mentorship recent graduates need to maintain the effectiveness of the occupational therapy workforce (Jackson et al., 2023).

The World Federation of Occupational Therapists has prioritised eight areas globally to enhance the evidence base of the profession and better serve clients (Mackenzie et al., 2017). Among the most prioritised research areas internationally are: 1) effectiveness of occupational therapy interventions, 2) evidence-based practice and knowledge translation, and 3) participation in everyday life. All three priorities provide evidence that will directly impact decisions about best practice, equipment, and technology and the efficacy of interventions in the NDIS. Some examples include best approaches for specific populations such as training manual wheelchair use for adults (Charlton et al., 2024), use of virtual reality to improve functional performance of adults with acquired brain injury (Grewal et al., 2024), and effective interventions for parents of children with disability (Leo et al., 2025).

4.3 Conclusion

The National Disability Insurance Scheme provides important access to occupational therapy services for participants. The NDIS is currently undergoing significant reforms, and readers are advised to maintain currency through the NDIS website and Occupational Therapy Australia.

4.4 Summary

- The National Disability Insurance Scheme provides Australians who are born with or acquire a permanent disability before the age of 65 with the reasonable and necessary supports they need to live an ordinary life.
- There are three types of supports funded in the Scheme: Core Supports, Capacity Building Supports, and Capital Supports.
- Occupational therapy practice within the NDIS aligns closely with the International Classification of Functioning, Disability and Health.
- Occupational therapists within the NDIS focus on promoting independence in activities of daily living and enablement of social and/or economic participation.
- Occupational therapists need to implement evidence-based practice when providing NDIS-funded services.

4.5 Review and reflection questions

- How does the International Classification of Functioning, Disability and Health influence occupational therapy practice within the NDIS?
- What are the roles and responsibilities of occupational therapists within the NDIS?
- What are functional capacity assessments within the NDIS and why are they important?
- Why is evidence-based practice important for occupational therapists within NDIS practice?

References

American Occupational Therapy Association (AOTA) (2020). Occupational Therapy Practice Framework: Domain and process (4th ed.). *American Journal of Occupational Therapy*, 74(Supp 2), 7412410010p1–7412410010p87. https://doi.org/10.5014/ajot.2020.74S2001

Australian Government. (2013). *National Disability Insurance Scheme Act 2013*.

Australian Government, Department of Social Services. (2024). *The applied principle and tables of support to determine responsibilities of the NDIS and other service systems.* https://www.dss.gov.au/councils/resource/applied-principles-and-tables-support-determine-responsibilities-ndis-and-other-service-systems

Australian Government, Department of Social Services. (2025). *NDIS provider and worker registration taskforce.* https://www.dss.gov.au/disability-and-carers-standards-and-quality-assurance/ndis-provider-and-worker-registration-taskforce

Australian Government. Productivity Commission. (2011). *Disability care and support: Inquiry report.* https://www.pc.gov.au/inquiries/completed/disability-support/report

Barfoot, J., Meredith, P., Ziviani, J., & Whittingham, K. (2017). Relationship-based approaches in early childhood intervention: Are these applicable to paediatric occupational therapy under the NDIS? *Australian Occupational Therapy Journal, 64,* 273–276. https://doi.org/10.1111/1440-1630.12343

Charlton, K., Murray, C., Layton, N., Ong, E., Farrar, L., Serocki, T., & Attrill, S. (2024). Manual wheelchair training approaches and intended training outcomes for adults who are new to wheelchair use: A scoping review. *Australian Occupational Therapy Journal, 72*(1), e12992. https://doi.org/10.1111/1440-1630.12992

Department of Health, Disability and Ageing. (2025). *NDIS provider and worker registration taskforce.* https://www.health.gov.au/committees-and-groups/ndis-provider-and-worker-registration-taskforce

Grewal, J., Eng, J. J., Sakakibara, B. M., & Schmidt, J. (2024). The use of virtual reality for activities of daily living rehabilitation after brain injury: A scoping review. *Australian Occupational Therapy Journal, 71*(5), 868–893. https://doi.org/10.1111/1440-1630.12957

ICF-Health Australia Interest Group (ICF-AIG). (2022). *The ICF and its potential uses in the National Disability Insurance Scheme.* https://disability.unimelb.edu.au/__data/assets/pdf_file/0005/4817651/ICF-and-potential-uses-for-the-NDIS-FINAL87.pdf

Imms, C., Granlund, M., Wilson, P. H., Steenbergen, B., Rosenbaum, P. L., & Gordon, A. M. (2017). Participation, both a means and an end: A conceptual analysis of processes and outcomes in childhood disability. *Developmental Medicine and Child Neurology, 59*(1), 16–25. https://doi.org/10.1111/dmcn.13237

Jackson, O., Villeneuve, M., & Millington, M. (2023). The experience and role of mentorship for paediatric occupational therapists. *Australian Occupational Therapy Journal, 70*(1), 86–96. https://doi.org/10.1111/1440-1630.12839

Leo, M., Bourke-Taylor, H., Odgers, S., & Tirlea, L. (2025). Online interventions for the mental health and well-being of parents of children with additional needs: Systematic review and meta-analysis. *Australian Occupational Therapy Journal,* 1–28. https://doi.org/10.1111/1440-1630.13004

Mackenzie, L., Coppola, S., Alvarez, L., Cibule, L., Maltsev, S., Loh, S. Y., Mlambo, T., Ikiugu, M. N., Pihlar, Z., Sriphetcharawut, S., Baptiste, S., & Ledgerd, R. (2017). International occupational therapy research priorities. *OTJR: Occupation, Participation and Health, 37*(2), 72–81. https://doi.org/10.1177/1539449216687528

NDIS. (2024, April 29). *Cultural and linguistic diversity strategy.* https://www.ndis.gov.au/strategies/cultural-and-linguistic-diversity-strategy

NDIS. (2025a). *Explore data.* https://dataresearch.ndis.gov.au/explore-data

NDIS. (2025b). *Quarterly reports.* https://www.ndis.gov.au/publications/quarterly-reports

NDIS. (2025c). *The early childhood approach for children younger than 9.* https://www.ndis.gov.au/understanding/families-and-carers/early-childhood-approach-children-younger-9

NDIS. (n.d.). https://www.ndis.gov.au

NDIS Quality and Safeguards Commission. (n.d.). https://www.ndiscommission.gov.au/

O'Neill, M., Bourke-Taylor, H., Bhopti, A., & Cotter, C. (2024). The experiences of families of children with cerebral palsy and complex disability after three years accessing the National Disability Insurance Scheme. *Australian Occupational Therapy Journal, 71*(6), 910–924. https://doi.org/10.1111/1440-1630.12973

Parliament of Australia. (2024). *National disability insurance scheme amendment (getting the NDIS Back on Track No. 1)*. Bill No. 47/24, House of Representatives. https://www.aph.gov.au/Parliamentary_Business/Bills_Legislation/Bills_Search_Results/Result?bId=r7181

Townsend, E., & Polatajko, H. (Eds.). (2013). *Enabling occupation II: Advancing an occupational therapy vision for health, well-being.* CAOT.

Veli-Gold, S., Gilroy, J., Wright, W., Bulkeley, K., Jensen, H., Dew, A., & Lincoln, M. (2023). The experiences of people with disability and their families/carers navigating the NDIS planning process in regional, rural and remote regions of Australia: Scoping review. *Australian Journal of Rural Health, 31*(4), 631–647. http://doi.org/10.1111/ajr.13011

World Health Organization. (2001). *The International Classification of Functioning, Disability and Health (ICF)*. https://icd.who.int/browse/2025-01/icf/en

CHAPTER 5

Aotearoa New Zealand health care system and its occupational therapy Whakapapa

Mary Silcock, Heleen Reid, Claire Squires, Tori Bensemann, and Tracy Murphy

Authors' positionality statement

(Elizabeth) Mary Silcock identifies as a fifth-generation white tangata Tiriti Pākehā woman, originally descended from English colonial settlers. Mary is a kaiwhakaora ngangahau/occupational therapist, sociologist/social scientist, and mother. She currently works at the Ministry of Health, Aotearoa New Zealand. Contribution to this chapter has been as a private citizen and is not Ministry of Health policy.

Ko Maungaroa te maunga,
Ko Marokopa te awa,
Ko Ngati Maniapoto te iwi.
Ko Tainui te waka.
Ko Ngati Te Kanawa raua Ngati Rarua ngā hapu.
Ko Tori Bensemann toku ingoa.
Ko Adaline raua ko Briana ōku tamahine.

Tori identifies as a community engaged Māori kaiwhakaora ngangahau/occupational therapist, with a passion for working with kaumātua. She resides in Whanganui, New Zealand.

Heleen Reid is a Dutch, tangata Tiriti first generation woman living in Aotearoa New Zealand. Her personal and professional experiences in whakaora ngangahau occupational therapy have shaped her worldviews and biases, particularly towards health and education. She is reflexive of these biases in her work and strives for equity and dignity for diverse perspectives.

He uri ahau no Ngāpuhi. Ko Ngati Hinera me Te Uri Taniwha ōku hapū. Ko Tracy Murphy tōku ingoa. Tracy is a kaiwhakaora ngangahau Māori (Māori occupational therapist) and emerging kaupapa Māori researcher, with a special clinical interest in stroke care.

DOI: 10.4324/9781003495666-6

Claire Squires identifies as a first-generation Pākehā tangata Tiriti woman, descended from English and Australian parents. She is a kaiwhakaora ngangahau | occupational therapist who has worked in the public and private health settings in New Zealand and Australia since graduating in 2001. She is currently a senior lecturer at the School of Occupational Therapy in Ōtepoti | Dunedin.

Key terms
- Health policy
- Health systems
- Population and demography
- Occupational therapy practice
- History
- Te Tiriti o Waitangi

Glossary of terms (Te reo Māori)
- Kaumātua – Elders
- Kaiwhakaora ngangahau – occupational therapist
- Te ao Māori – Māori worldview
- Whakaora ngangahau – occupational therapy
- Whakapapa – genealogy, genealogical table, lineage, descent, used here to describe the history of occupational therapy
- Whānau – family group, extended family

Objectives
This chapter will allow the reader to:

- Understand the evolution of the occupational therapy profession in the Aotearoa New Zealand context
- Understand population health needs in Aotearoa New Zealand
- Identify the colonial roots of the profession's philosophies and the importance of including a te ao Māori worldview into practice
- Identify the main structures and priorities of the health system in Aotearoa New Zealand and the most common areas of occupational therapy practice

5.1 Introduction

The chapter provides an overview of health in Aotearoa New Zealand and tracks the evolution (whakapapa) of occupational therapy from its introduction through to current-day practice. The impact of colonisation and specifically the development of health services on the health and wellbeing status of the Aotearoa New Zealand population is a major factor in delivering occupational therapy and provides a framework for understanding how occupational therapy has evolved, our current scope and practice areas, and the potential direction for the profession in the future.

Links are made between the profession's philosophies, the indigenous te ao Māori worldview, and health inequities facing Māori. A brief overview of key influences on health outcomes and disparities in health and life expectancy for the main ethnic groups is presented. A summary of the current health system and the main practice settings for occupational therapists is provided. The chapter concludes with a snapshot of where occupational therapy is in 2025.

5.1.1 Te Tiriti o Waitangi and health

Aotearoa New Zealand became part of the British Empire's colonial settlement project in 1840 when a treaty, te Tiriti o Waitangi, was signed by representatives of the British Crown and a number of Māori leaders (Orange, 2015). Te Tiriti o Waitangi is accepted as a constitutional document that guides the relationship between the Crown (embodied by the New Zealand government) and Māori (Ministry of Justice, 2025). Te Tiriti o Waitangi affirmed the sovereignty of Māori as the Indigenous people of the land (tangata whenua) while granting the Crown the right to govern their subjects (tangata Tiriti) (Waitangi Tribunal, 2014). Te Tiriti o Waitangi provided Māori equal access to the rights and privileges of British citizenship, including healthcare (Cram et al., 2019; Kidd et al., 2025).

The colonial government quickly built hospitals in the main towns of Auckland, New Plymouth, Wanganui, and Wellington. Healthcare was provided primarily by British trained medical doctors and nurses (Armstrong, 2009). Occupational therapy was introduced to the health system in the 1950s by British occupational therapists and has been part of the health system since then.

As a result of the colonial influence, systemic and structural racism within the health system has existed since its inception, resulting in significant health inequities for Māori (Ministry of Health, 2024d). Māori identity and wellbeing have been eroded through occupational deprivation, loss of cultural knowledge, and loss of access to cultural practices (Emery-Whittington, 2021; Hopkirk & Wilson, 2014). Māori approaches to health prioritise wellbeing through strengthening self-determination, identity, and connection with the environment (Wilson et al., 2021). Occupational therapy aligns well to te ao Māori due to its holistic, client-centred practice and a shared emphasis on the importance of context, environment, and meaningful engagement in daily activities (Hopkirk & Wilson, 2014).

5.2 Occupational therapy within Aotearoa New Zealand

5.2.1 Occupational therapy whakapapa in Aotearoa

In Aotearoa New Zealand occupation was first used as a therapeutic tool in mental health services (Skilton, 1981). Occupational therapy was almost entirely confined to mental hospitals until after World War II. Occupational therapists then worked in a wide range of settings including non-government community based organisations as well as occupational health, social services, education, and justice services (Wilson, 2003). An Occupational Therapy Training School was established in 1946, and the Occupational Therapy Act (1949) established a regulatory authority and process for legal recognition and registration as a profession (Silcock et al., 2016). The New Zealand Association of Occupational Therapists (now named Occupational Therapy New Zealand – Whakaora Ngangahau Aotearoa (OTNZ-WNA)) was also established in 1949 and was a founding member of the World Federation of Occupational Therapists in 1952 (Silcock et al., 2016). The profession has slowly grown in size since this time, and in 2024 there were 3,555 practising occupational therapists (Occupational Therapy Board of New Zealand, 2024).

From the early 1990s occupational therapists have advocated for cultural competency and the incorporation of Māori frameworks into practice (Henare, 1992, 1993; Jungerson, 1992). The Occupational Therapy Board of New Zealand (OTBNZ) responded by embedding cultural safety into professional standards from the mid 2000s (Silcock et al., 2016) and continues to prioritise this expectation as a key competency for practice in the profession (Occupational Therapy Board of New Zealand, 2024). The OTBNZ competencies, with a strong focus on equity and cultural safety, have reinforced the profession's long-standing commitment to valuing and prioritising the influence of Indigenous worldviews and te Tiriti o Waitangi. For several decades, these principles have shaped and guided professional practice.

5.3 Health services in Aotearoa

Occupational therapists work across a variety of settings, including the public health system, primary health organisations (PHOs), private practices, whanau-ora, school, and community-based services. In the public health system occupational therapists are employed in hospitals, rehabilitation centres, and community health services. The public health system in Aotearoa New Zealand is predominantly financed with around 80% from general taxation (Tenbensel et al., 2023). Community-based non-governmental primary care entities (PHOs) were established in the early 2000s throughout the country (Tenbensel et al., 2023). These PHOs enabled occupational therapists to work outside the public hospital system more easily. Occupational therapists work in primary care alongside general practice physicians, pharmacies, home-based personal and social care, rehabilitation practitioners, counselling, and health promotion (Mackenzie et al., 2013; Tse et al., 2003) focussing on preventative care and early intervention.

The introduction of the Pae Ora (Healthy Futures) Act (2022) has had a notable impact on occupational therapy practice (Tenbensel et al., 2023). Pae Ora aims to create a more equitable, accessible, and cohesive health system (Ministry of Health, 2024c). As part of this reform whaikaha, a new Ministry of Disabled People was created. Whaikaha sits outside the health system as part of the Ministry of Social Development (Whaikaha Ministry of Disabled People, 2024). These reforms have been subsequently amended due to a change in political government and as at early 2025 the reforms are still bedding in and settling into a stable system. For occupational therapy, Pae Ora means greater involvement in multi-disciplinary teams and highlights the importance of addressing health inequities, particularly for Māori and other underserved populations.

5.3.1 Accident Compensation Corporation

At the same time as the public health system was being established New Zealand introduced a limited 'no-fault' accident and injury legislation to provide an insurance cover for injured workers very early in the health systems development. In 1900 a Workers Compensation Act introduced mandatory insurance for employers to financially support injured or compensate for fatal accidents at work. Over time this legislation has been amended and modified coverage was expanded to include all injuries that workers sustained whether at work or not, as well as motor vehicle injuries and to self-employed workers. The Accident Compensation Act (ACC) (1972) superseded the original legislation and the right to sue was removed for any type of injury. Along with compensation for wages, health related services are paid for through the ACC scheme including treatment, rehabilitation, and transport costs. (Accident Compensation Corporation, 2024).

Occupational therapy has provided services through the ACC insurance schemes throughout its existence in Aotearoa New Zealand. Rehabilitation programmes funded by ACC progressed from the hospital to community settings and into paid employment. (New Zealand Registered Occupational Therapy Association & Accident Compensation Commission, 1974). Criteria for eligibility continues to expand for access to the scheme with work-related gradual process injuries or infections and treatment injuries now covered, as well as mental trauma and self-harm after an accident. Occupational therapists started moving into private practice to deliver assessment, rehabilitation, and vocational rehabilitation as enabling legislative changes were introduced (Accident Compensation Corporation, 2024), with 14% of the workforce in 2024 now employed through this scheme (Occupational Therapy Board of New Zealand, 2024).

5.3.2 Private practice

Private occupational therapy practice in Aotearoa New Zealand has evolved alongside the broader development of the profession. Private occupational therapists have diversified their practice beyond publicly funded hospital settings and ACC contracts into other niche areas for fee-paying consumers (Occupational Therapy Board of New Zealand, 2018).

5.4 Life expectancy and health in Aotearoa New Zealand

The population of Aotearoa New Zealand was counted at 4,993,923 in 2023 (Statistics New Zealand, 2024). The population continues to diversify, and while European ethnicities made up the majority of the population (67.8 %), Māori (17.8%), Asian (17.3%), Pacific peoples (8.9%), and Middle Eastern/Latin American/African (1.9%) ethnic groups grew significantly faster since 2018 than the European ethnic group (with some people identifying with more than one ethnicity).

Like many other developed countries, people are living longer, and fertility rates are falling, meaning that there is a higher proportion of people aged over 65 years. By 2028 an estimated 1 in 5 people will be 65+ years, and by 2050 it is estimated this will have risen to 1 in 4, with a much greater proportion of over–85-year-olds (Statistics New Zealand, 2022). The median age of the population is now 38.1 years; however, Māori and Pacific ethnic populations have a lower age profile, with the median age for people who identify as Māori descent 27.2 years and of Pacific ethnic descent 24 years (Statistics New Zealand, 2024).

Overall life expectancy in Aotearoa New Zealand is increasing, with an average life expectancy of 82 years; New Zealanders are ranked 16th compared to other countries (Health New Zealand – Te Whatu Ora, 2024a). However, there remains a persistent life expectancy gap between people who identify as Māori and Pacific Island ethnicities compared to non-Māori (see Table 5.1).

There are increasing and disparate rates of chronic preventable diseases and disabilities between groups within the population. People who identify as Māori or Pacific

Island ethnicities have higher rates of avoidable mortality from conditions which are preventable than people who identify as European or Asian (Health New Zealand – Te Whatu Ora, 2024a). The rural population (19%) also has a lower life expectancy. Rural areas have a higher proportion of Māori (23%) compared to urban areas (16%) and a higher proportion of people aged 65 years and over (22% versus 16%), and 69% of people living in rural areas are European ethnicities, but in the South Island, this is greater (81%) (see Table 5.2) (Health New Zealand – Te Whatu Ora, 2024b). In 2013 there were an estimated 1.1 million people who had a disability or impairment, and approximately 60% of people aged over 65 have a disability (Statistics New Zealand, 2014).

Table 5.1 Life expectancy by sex and ethnicity in Aotearoa New Zealand (adapted from Health New Zealand, 2024b)

Ethnicity	Average life expectancy (2020–2022)	Life expectancy gap (calculated from non-Māori non-Pacific average)
Asian females	89.1 years	+4 years
Asian males	86.3 males	+5.4 years
European females	84.7 years	3 years
European males	81.2 years	0.5 years
Pacific females	79.2 years	5.9 years
Pacific males	75.5 years	6.2 years
Māori females	78.8 years	6.3 years
Māori males	74.8 years	7.1 years
Non Māori non-Pacific females	85.1 years	
Non-Māori non-Pacific males	81.7 years	

Table 5.2 Top 10 avoidable contributors to life expectancy gap for Māori, Pacific people compared to non-Māori/non-Pacific populations (adapted from Health New Zealand, 2024c)

Top 10 avoidable contributors for life expectancy gap for Māori		To 10 avoidable contributors to life expectancy gap for Pacific peoples	
Coronary heart disease	0.8	Diabetes	0.7
Cancers – trachea, bronchus, lung	0.8	Coronary heart disease	0.7
Diabetes	0.4	Cancers – trachea, bronchus, lung	0.3
COPD	0.4	Cerebrovascular accident	0.3
Injuries – land transport	0.3	Valvular heart disease	0.2
Injuries suicide	0.3	Perinatal complications	0.2
Stroke	0.2	Cancers – stomach	0.1
Injuries – other accidental	0.2	Cancers – uterine	0.1
Valvular heart disease	0.1	Cancers – female breast	0.1
Cancers – liver	0.1	Cancers – liver	0.1

5.5 Addressing health outcomes – priorities

5.5.1 Health outcomes for Māori and Pacific peoples

Timely access to healthcare is a significant issue for the health system, and since the mid-1990s, Māori and Pacific health providers have increased their role in the delivery of community-based health and social services. Many of these are contracted to PHOs and/or are independent community providers. During the COVID-19 pandemic these organisations were significantly strengthened and leaned on by the public health system for community leadership and management of COVID-19 in the community (Cassim & Keelan, 2023).

To address the systemic causes of health inequities for Māori in 2009 a kaupapa Māori-driven holistic model called Whānau Ora was instituted, driven by the late Dame Tariana Turia. Whānau Ora continues to provide wraparound services for all aspects of Māori wellbeing (Te Puni Kōkiri, 2025). As well as this model, kaupapa Māori initiatives for many health, education, and social services have been developed over the last three decades. The Ministry of Health and Health New Zealand both have Māori health strategies and action plans focussed on Māori health outcomes (Health New Zealand – Te Whatu Ora, 2024c; Ministry of Health, 2023a)

Pacific communities and Pacific health providers also have mobilised over the last decade to address health disparities for their people (for example, see Ratuva et al., 2021; Tu'akoi et al., 2022). The Ministry for Pacific Peoples has published several reports focussed on Pacific wellbeing (Ministry of Pacific Peoples, 2025), and the Ministry of Health and Health New Zealand have dedicated Pacific Health strategies and operational plans (Health New Zealand – Te Whatu Ora, 2024d; Ministry of Health, 2023b).

Occupational therapists work for Māori and Pacific health providers, and occupational therapy is adapted to fit under the cultural health models appropriate for these services. As of December 2024 there were 249 (7%) of the occupational therapy workforce who identified as Māori and 95 (3%) who identified as a Pacific ethnicity (Occupational Therapy Board of New Zealand, 2024). As well as these responses to health inequities, there are other social determinants of health that occupational therapists often must accommodate in their practice. Two of these main structural drivers are housing and poverty.

5.5.2 New Zealanders homes and housing

Poor-quality housing, including poor physical living conditions, overcrowding (a deficit of one or more bedrooms), and lack of heating, constitutes a significant health risks and health outcomes in Aotearoa New Zealand. In 2018, 11.2% of people lived in crowded households. Crowding is more common among Māori (21%), Pacific people (40%), and Asian people (19%) than European/Other people (4.5%) and is likely contributing to lower health outcomes for some of these populations (Health New Zealand – Te Whatu Ora, 2024a). In rural areas there are often poorer standards of housing due to higher social deprivation (Health New Zealand – Te Whatu Ora, 2024b). Occupational therapists often deal with housing and built environments in their work, and this is a key policy area for public health initiatives such as rheumatic fever prevention.

5.5.3 Socio-economic conditions

Socio-economic deprivation and material hardship are rising in Aotearoa New Zealand. There are large disparities between regions of the country. Some regions have an estimated 40% of the population living in areas with the highest levels of deprivation. Counties Manukau, a city within the greater Auckland region, had the most people living in the highest levels of socio-economic deprivation. The large rural region of the Waikato in mid-central North Island has the next highest (Health New Zealand – Te Whatu Ora, 2024a). Child poverty in Aotearoa New Zealand also increased in 2023, with the national census estimating 12.5% of all children live in material hardship. This figure nearly doubles for disabled children, with 22.3% of disabled children living in material hardship compared to 11.15% of non-disabled children (Ministry of Health, 2024b). There are also significant ethnic disparities in socioeconomic deprivation. Compared to people who identify as a European ethnicity, more than twice as many people who identify as Māori and almost three times as many people who identify as a Pacific ethnicity live in socio-economically deprived areas (Health New Zealand – Te Whatu Ora, 2024a). Occupational therapists frequently need to address conditions of poverty as part of their interventions. Poverty and material hardship is an emerging area of scholarship in the profession (Leadley, 2024).

5.6 Where is occupational therapy in 2025?

Occupational therapy is one of 26 regulated health professions in Aotearoa New Zealand and is referred to as an allied health profession (Ministry of Health, 2024a). There are currently two undergraduate education programmes, and a master's entry-level graduate qualification has recently been approved by the OTBNZ. Successful completion of an approved education programme is required for registration. Under the Trans-Tasman Mutual Recognition Act 1997, Aotearoa New Zealand–registered occupational therapists are eligible to be registered in Australia, and vice versa. In 2024, most practising occupational therapists were trained in Aotearoa New Zealand (76%). There is an upward trend of overseas-trained therapists moving to Aotearoa New Zealand. In 2024 there were 257 overseas-qualified therapists registered, up from 176 in 2023 and 77 in 2022.

As of December 2024, the two most common employment roles were rehabilitation (36%) and mental health practitioner (11%). Occupational therapists work across the life course, with 41% of therapists working with children or adolescents, 35% with adults, and 24% with older people (Occupational Therapy Board of New Zealand, 2024). Occupational therapy remains a highly feminised profession, with only 296 therapists (8.2%) who identified as men practising in 2024 (Occupational Therapy Board of New Zealand, 2024).

5.7 Conclusion

Occupational therapy in Aotearoa New Zealand continues to evolve and expand in roles and settings where it is practised. There are many options and opportunities to practice in private, public, culturally specialised, and not-for-profit community organisations as an occupational therapist. The influence of indigenous worldviews and te

Tiriti o Waitangi on the way the profession is practised has been valued and prioritised by the profession for several decades. It is well placed to contribute to addressing the significant health disparities between Māori and Pacific peoples living in New Zealand. Occupational therapists often work with people in the population who have less equitable health outcomes and as such need to incorporate social determinants of health such as access to healthcare, housing, and poverty into their practice.

5.8 Summary

- Occupational therapy was introduced as part of a colonial health system.
- The health system is made up of three key pillars: Health New Zealand, Primary Health Organisations, and Accident Compensation Corporation.
- Occupational therapists work across the life course and most often in rehabilitation practice settings.
- Occupational therapy approaches align well to te ao Māori health models, and practise is expected to incorporate Māori health worldviews in all settings.

5.9 Review and reflection questions

- What was the constitutional document signed in 1840?
- What is the insurance scheme called which funds healthcare after an accident?
- Which ethnic groups have the youngest population?
- What are the main social determinants of health occupational therapists come across in Aotearoa New Zealand?
- How would barriers to accessing occupational therapy impact health and wellbeing?
- What occupational therapy intervention could be provided to address material hardship?

References

Accident Compensation Corporation. (2024). *Our history.* https://www.acc.co.nz/about-us/who-we-are/our-history

Armstrong, J. (2009). *Under one roof: A history of Waikato Hospital.* Waikato District Health Board.

Cassim, S., & Keelan, T. J. (2023). A review of localised Māori community responses to Covid-19 lockdowns in Aotearoa New Zealand. *AlterNative: An International Journal of Indigenous Peoples, 19*(1), 42–50. https://doi.org/10.1177/11771801221124428

Cram, F., Te Huia, B., Te Huia, T., Williams, M. M., & Williams, N. (2019). *Oranga and Māori health inequities, 1769–1992.* Katoa Limited.

Emery-Whittington, I. G. (2021). Occupational justice – Colonial business as usual? Indigenous observations from Aotearoa New Zealand. *Canadian Journal of Occupational Therapy, 88*(2), 153–162. https://doi.org/10.1177/00084174211005891

Health New Zealand – Te Whatu Ora. (2024a). *Health status report.* https://www.tewhatuora.govt.nz/publications/health-status-report

Health New Zealand – Te Whatu Ora. (2024b). *Life expectancy in Aotearoa New Zealand: An analysis of socioeconomic, geographic, sex and ethnic variation from 2001 to 2022.* https://www.tewhatuora.govt.nz/publications/life-expectancy-in-aotearoa-an-analysis-of-socioeconomic-geographic-sex-and-ethnic-variation-from-2001-to-2022

Health New Zealand – Te Whatu Ora. (2024c). *Māori Health – Hauora Māori*. https://www. tewhatuora.govt.nz/health-services-and-programmes/maori-health

Health New Zealand – Te Whatu Ora. (2024d). *Ola Manuia interim Pacific Health Plan 2022– 2023*. https://www.tewhatuora.govt.nz/health-services-and-programmes/pacific-health/ola-manuia-pacific-health-plan

Henare, D. (1992). Occupational therapy in Aotearoa: Part 1. The challenge. *New Zealand Journal of Occupational Therapy, 43*(2), 10–13.

Henare, D. (1993). Occupational therapy in Aotearoa: Part 2. The steps to biculturalism. *New Zealand Journal of Occupational Therapy, 44*(1), 4–9.

Hopkirk, J., & Wilson, L. H. (2014). A call to wellness–Whitiwhitia i te ora: Exploring Māori and occupational therapy perspectives on health. *Occupational Therapy International, 21*(4), 156–165. https://doi.org/10.1002/oti.1373

Jungerson, K. (1992). Culture, theory, and the practice of occupational therapy in New Zealand/Aotearoa. *American Journal of Occupational Therapy, 46*(8), 745–750. https://doi. org/10.5014/ajot.46.8.745

Kidd, J., Tipa, Z., Arnet, H., & Rēnata, H. (2025). Hauora Māori: Aspirations of Māori health practitioners for a culturally relevant health system. *Ethnographic Edge, 8*(1), 57–76. https:// doi.org/10.24135/ee.v8i1.294

Leadley, S. (2024). *Tamaiti/child poverty: The ways in which poverty shapes tamariki/children's patterns of participation in occupations, their potential and wellbeing*. Auckland University of Technology. https://openrepositorydev.aut.ac.nz/items/69b7bedc-0e26-4b64-a49b-3e77d9deef53/full

Mackenzie, L., Clemson, L., & Roberts, C. (2013). Occupational therapists partnering with general practitioners to prevent falls: Seizing opportunities in primary health care. *Australian Occupational Therapy Journal, 60*(1), 66–70. https://doi.org/10.1111/1440-1630.12030

Ministry of Health. (2023a). *Pae Tū: Hauora Māori Strategy*. https://www.health.govt.nz/ strategies-initiatives/health-strategies/pae-tu-hauora-maori-strategy

Ministry of Health. (2023b). *Te Mana Ola: The Pacific Health Strategy*. https://www.health. govt.nz/strategies-initiatives/health-strategies/te-mana-ola-the-pacific-health-strategy

Ministry of Health. (2024a). *Hauora Haumi allied health report 2024*. https://www.health. govt.nz/publications/hauora-haumi-allied-health-report-2024

Ministry of Health. (2024b). *Health and independence report – Te Pūrongo mō te Hauora me te Tū Motuhake 2023*. https://www.health.govt.nz/publications/health-and-independence-report-2023

Ministry of Health. (2024c). *Pae Ora (healthy futures) act*. https://www.health.govt.nz/about-us/ new-zealands-health-system/overview-and-statutory-framework/pae-ora-healthy-futures-act

Ministry of Health. (2024d). *Tatau Kahukura: Māori health chart book 2024*. https://www. health.govt.nz/publications/tatau-kahukura-maori-health-chart-book-2024

Ministry of Justice. (2025). *Te Tiriti o Waitangi – Treaty of Waitangi*. Retrieved January 20, 2025, from https://www.justice.govt.nz/about/learn-about-the-justice-system/how-the-justice-system-works/the-basis-for-all-law/treaty-of-waitangi/

Ministry of Pacific Peoples. (2025). *Reports*. https://www.mpp.govt.nz/publications-resources/ reports/

New Zealand Registered Occupational Therapy Association & Accident Compensation Commission. (1974). *Occupational therapy and accident compensation*.

Occupational Therapy Board of New Zealand. (2018). *The occupational therapist workforce. Making sense of the numbers*. https://www.otboard.org.nz/document/4797/OTB-18299-Making-sense-of-the-numbers-report-WEB.pdf

Occupational Therapy Board of New Zealand. (2024). *Pūrongo ā-Tau – annual report*. https:// www.otboard.org.nz/document/8264/2024%20OTBNZ%20Annual%20Report%20 FINAL.pdf

Orange, C. (2015). *The Treaty of Waitangi*. Bridget Williams Books.

Ratuva, S., Crichton-Hill, Y., Ross, T., Basu, A., Vakaoti, P., & Martin-Neuninger, R. (2021). Integrated social protection and COVID-19: Rethinking Pacific community responses in Aotearoa. *Journal of the Royal Society of New Zealand*, 51(Supp 1), S37–S54. https://doi.org/10.1080/03036758.2020.1861033

Silcock, M., Campbell, M., & Hocking, C. (2016). How Western structures shape our practice: An analysis of the Competencies for Registration for occupational therapists in Aotearoa New Zealand 1990–2014. *New Zealand Journal of Occupational Therapy*, 63(2), 4–12.

Skilton, H. (1981). *Work for your life: The story of the beginning and early years of occupational therapy in New Zealand*. Hudlo Printers.

Statistics New Zealand. (2014). *Disability survey: 2013*. https://www.stats.govt.nz/information-releases/disability-survey-2013

Statistics New Zealand. (2022). *One million people aged 65+ by 2028*. https://www.stats.govt.nz/news/one-million-people-aged-65-by-2028/

Statistics New Zealand. (2024). *Place and ethnic group summaries*. https://www.stats.govt.nz/tools/place-and-ethnic-group-summaries/

Tenbensel, T., Cumming, J., & Willing, E. (2023). The 2022 restructure of Aotearoa New Zealand's health system: Will it succeed in advancing equity where others have failed? *Health Policy*, 134, 104828. https://doi.org/10.1016/j.healthpol.2023.104828

Te Puni Kōkiri. (2025). *Whānau Ora Kaupapa*. Retrieved January 20, 2025, from https://www.tpk.govt.nz/en/nga-putea-me-nga-ratonga/whanau-ora/whanau-ora-kaupapa2

Tse, S., Wilson, L., Ford, J., & Clair, V. W.-S. (2003). Challenges and opportunities: Occupational therapy and primary health organisations in New Zealand. *New Zealand Journal of Occupational Therapy*, 50(2), 24–27.

Tu'akoi, S., Ofanoa, M., Ofanoa, S., Lutui, H., Heather, M., Jansen, R. M., van der Werf, B., & Goodyear-Smith, F. (2022). Co-designing an intervention to prevent rheumatic fever in Pacific People in South Auckland: A study protocol. *International Journal for Equity in Health*, 21(1), 101. https://doi.org/10.1186/s12939-022-01701-9

Waitangi Tribunal. (2014). *The report on stage 1 of the Te Paparahi o Te Raki Inquiry. He Whakaputanga me te Tiriti: The declaration and the treaty*. Waitangi Tribunal. https://forms.justice.govt.nz/search/Documents/WT/wt_DOC_85648980/Te%20Raki%20W.pdf

Whaikaha Ministry of Disabled People. (2024). *Our whakapapa*. https://www.whaikaha.govt.nz/about-us/who-we-are/our-whakapapa

Wilson, D., Moloney, E., Parr, J. M., Aspinall, C., & Slark, J. (2021). Creating an Indigenous Māori-centred model of relational health: A literature review of Māori models of health. *Journal of Clinical Nursing*, 30(23–24), 3539–3555. https://doi.org/10.1111/jocn.15859

Wilson, L. H. (2003). *Role differentiation in a professionalising occupation: The case of occupational therapy, New Zealand* [Doctorate, Otago]. http://hdl.handle.net/10523/1483

The role of occupational therapy professional associations and regulatory bodies in Australia and New Zealand

Rebecca Allen, Julie Brayshaw, Priscilla Ennals, Dan Johnson, Rhondda Knox, Adam Lo, and Genevieve Pepin

Authors' positionality statement

We bring a diverse and complementary range of experiences and perspectives to our collaborative work across Australia and New Zealand. Collectively, our careers span clinical practice, leadership, management, research, education, policy, and regulatory activities, providing us with a comprehensive understanding of the complex and evolving nature of occupational therapy. Through this chapter, we aim to share insights that inform students and graduates of professional and regulatory structures which support and shape current and future occupational therapy practice. We advocate for a profession that remains dynamic, reflective, and responsive to the diverse needs of individuals, communities, and systems.

Key terms
- Professional association
- Regulation
- Accreditation
- Standards of practice

Objectives

Upon completion of this chapter, the reader will be able to:

- Describe the role of professional associations Occupational Therapy New Zealand Whakaora Ngangahau Aotearoa, and Occupational Therapy Australia, and their relationship with World Federation of Occupational Therapists
- Discuss the registration of occupational therapy practitioners in Australia and New Zealand and the bodies that participate in the process of registration
- Describe the accreditation of occupational therapy education programmes
- Discuss the importance of professional and regulatory bodies to occupational therapists and the interrelationship between these organisations and practitioners

DOI: 10.4324/9781003495666-7

6.1 Introduction

This chapter describes the role of six interrelated independent Australasian organisations which support the practice of occupational therapy. The organisations are:

- Occupational Therapy New Zealand Whakaora Ngangahau Aotearoa (OTNZ-WNA) and Occupational Therapy Australia (OTA), the national professional associations;
- the World Federation of Occupational Therapists (WFOT), the international professional association;
- the Occupational Therapy Board of New Zealand (OTBNZ Te Poari) and Occupational Therapy Board of Australia (OTBA), the profession's registration boards; and
- the Occupational Therapy Council of Australia Ltd (OTC), the body responsible for the accreditation of occupational therapy education programmes in Australia and elements of the assessment of internationally qualified practitioners wishing to practise in Australia.

Effective working relationships enhance the role of each entity and the contributions they bring to the profession and practice of occupational therapy in Australia and New Zealand. The role and relationship of these organisations are outlined.

6.2 Introducing the organisations

6.2.1 The national professional associations

6.2.1.1 Occupational therapy New Zealand Whakaora Ngangahau Aotearoa and Occupational Therapy Australia

Professional associations play a role in leading the profession, guiding standards of practice and facilitating knowledge dissemination (Stokes, 2016).

The Occupational Therapists Club formed in Sydney, Australia, in 1944 became the Australian Association of Occupational Therapists in 1945, with individual state/territory associations. In 2010 all state and territory associations merged into one nationwide organisation, now called Occupational Therapy Australia. OTNZ-WNA was formed in 1949. Both organisations have executive leaders and a board of directors that oversee leadership and management. OTNZ-WNA has a co-governance model referred to as the Tiriti Relationship Governance Model, ensuring the voices of Māori members are represented.

As member-based organisations, the professional associations provide a range of services and support for therapists across their careers. These include learning and development activities, professional support, advocacy on issues impacting the profession, networking, and connection to other occupational therapists. Membership includes students, new graduates, experienced practitioners, and affiliate members. The associations have strong links with other professional organisations. For OTA, these include Allied Health Professions Australia, Indigenous Allied Health Australia, Speech Pathology Australia, and the Australian Physiotherapy Association.

6.2.2 The international professional association

6.2.2.1 *World Federation of Occupational Therapists*

The WFOT is the official international organisation representing the occupational therapy profession. It was formed in 1951 with ten member countries. Today the WFOT has 111 member organisations representing over 633,000 occupational therapists and contributes to international initiatives through the long-standing relationship with the World Health Organization. The mission of the WFOT is to advance 'global health and wellbeing through the development, use and practice of occupational therapy' (WFOT, 2024). The WFOT is a distinctive international organisation, unparalleled among other allied health professions, that fosters a cohesive and collaborative culture among member country representatives through a shared vision and commitment to advancing the profession globally. The WFOT strategic priorities and goals rest on the following four pillars:

- Leading as the global professional association for occupational therapy
- Advocating for health and wellbeing through occupational engagement
- Furthering access to occupational therapy
- Advancing and promoting occupational therapy

The WFOT supports the development, use and practice of occupational therapy worldwide, demonstrating the profession's relevance and contribution to society. An important activity led by the WFOT to promote the profession is the international occupational therapy congress held every four years and hosted by member countries across all continents. The WFOT sets the minimum education standards for entry-level occupational therapy programmes worldwide. In both Australia and New Zealand, members of OTA and OTNZ-WNA automatically belong to the WFOT, as the two associations pay an annual organisation membership fee.

The WFOT is managed by a Board of Directors, comprising the president, president elect, director education, director finance, director practice, director research, member at large, and a non-elected executive director (ex-officio). Governance includes a general assembly, with an official delegate from each member organisation or country supported by an alternate delegate and at times, a second alternate delegate. OTNZ-WNA has a unique arrangement and is the only WFOT member organisation with two equal delegates, an Indigenous (tangata whenua) and non-Indigenous (tangata tiriti) delegate, sharing one vote.

6.2.3 The registration and accreditation authorities

Professional registration of occupational therapists is essential to uphold standards of practice and ensure the protection of the public in accessing health services. There is a legal requirement that anyone who uses the title or practices as an 'occupational therapist' in Australia or New Zealand must be registered by the registration board. The functions of the OTBA and OTBNZ include:

- registering occupational therapy practitioners and students
- assessing the qualifications of internationally qualified occupational therapists to determine a pathway for registration

- deciding the requirements for registration
- developing standards, codes, and guidelines for the profession
- approving programme accreditation standards and accredited programmes of study
- considering and making decisions on notifications (complaints) made against registered practitioners.

6.2.3.1 Occupational Therapy Board of Australia

Occupational therapy is one of 16 health professions regulated by nationally consistent legislation under the National Registration and Accreditation Scheme (NRAS). Australian practitioners are required to comply with the Health Practitioner Regulation National Law Act 2009 (the National Law). The OTBA includes six board members who are occupational therapists and three community members, all of whom are appointed by the Ministerial Council. To fulfil its responsibilities, the OTBA works closely with the Australian Health Practitioner Regulation Agency (AHPRA) which oversees the regulation of all registered health professions in Australia.

Under the National Law, all students enrolled in an approved occupational therapy programme of study must be registered with the OTBA. There are no fees for student registration and students do not need to apply for registration. Each education provider provides details of new and continuing occupational therapy students to AHPRA which manages student registration on behalf of the OTBA. After completing their studies, graduates must apply to the OTBA for registration as an occupational therapist before they commence practice. The OTBA has currently assigned the Occupational Therapy Council of Australia Ltd the roles of accrediting programmes of study and assessing internationally qualified practitioners who apply to register to practice in Australia when their qualifications are deemed relevant but not substantially equivalent to an approved Australian qualification.

6.2.3.2 Occupational Therapy Council of Australia Ltd

The OTC is an independent, not for profit organisation, established as a public company limited by guarantee. Its operation is overseen by a board of directors, comprising experienced occupational therapists as well as independent and community representatives. The OTC:

- undertakes accreditation of occupational therapy programmes offered by Australian education providers. This role includes developing and reviewing accreditation standards for occupational therapy education. These standards outline what is expected of the education providers that deliver entry-level occupational therapy education. Accreditation standards ensure occupational therapy entry-level programmes meet the expectations of the profession and the public so that graduates will be competent and safe to practice.
- contributes to the assessment of internationally qualified occupational therapists seeking to migrate to Australia and providing a practical assessment of competence (through a period of supervised practice) for practitioners whose qualification is deemed relevant but not substantially equivalent to an approved Australian qualification.

6.2.3.3 Occupational Therapy Board of New Zealand Te Poari Whakaora Ngangahau O Aotearoa

Occupational therapy whakaora ngangahau is one of 18 health professions regulated by nationally consistent legislation under the Health Practitioners Competence Assurance Act (2003) (HPCAA). Practitioners are required to comply with the HPCAA. Defined in legislation as a 'responsible authority', the functions of the Board are listed in Section 118 of the HPCAA. To meet these OTBNZ develops secondary legislation as identified in the HPCAA.

The Board has six practitioner members who are occupational therapists and three lay members, all of whom are Ministerial appointees. A co-governance model (Tangata Whenua and Te Tiriti) is in place. To fulfil its responsibilities, the Board works closely with the Ministry of Health Manatū Hauora in liaising with the Minister, shaping and supporting national policy, regulatory review and undergoing a five-yearly responsible authority performance review.

Under the HPCAA, on completing their studies, graduates must make an application to the Board for registration as an occupational therapist before they commence practice. Guidance and support for new graduates applying for registration and a practicing certificate are available through staff and online.

The roles of the OTBNZ include approving programmes of study as meeting the standards required for students to graduate with the knowledge, skills, and professional attributes to practice and conducting assessments of occupational therapists who hold an international qualification not approved by the OTBNZ. Occupational therapists wishing to work in New Zealand are required to have their qualifications assessed and undertake a period of supervised practice before gaining general registration status. This process assists practitioners to understand New Zealand health care settings and ensures New Zealand competency standards are met.

6.2.4 How regulatory, accreditation, and professional organisations support practice

The roles of the occupational therapy organisations described in this chapter facilitate:

- knowledge: sharing and professional learning,
- professional practice: standards and research, and
- change: lobbying and advocacy.

6.2.4.1 Facilitators of knowledge sharing and professional learning

Each organisation contributes to the development of practitioner knowledge.

6.2.4.1.1 CONTINUING PROFESSIONAL DEVELOPMENT

The OTBNZ and OTBA registration standards require practitioners to engage in continuous learning through their careers to ensure they maintain their competence and provide safe and effective services. Practitioners are required to plan, record, and reflect on their practice and professional development activities.

The OTBNZ's mandated learning post registration is a formal portfolio framework aligned to regulated competencies along with supervision. The OTBA requires practitioners to plan, record and reflect on their professional development activities. Practitioners are also expected to participate in interactive learning with others.

The accreditation standards in both countries require education providers to ensure graduates are prepared for life-long learning through continuous professional development (CPD) and capacity for reflection on their practice. Provision of CPD is core to the mission of professional associations and is a benefit of membership. OTA and OTNZ-WNA deliver CPD programmes including national scientific conferences, practice-oriented events, and an extensive range of workshops and webinars. CPD programmes are targeted at qualified occupational therapists, building contemporary knowledge and skills for advancing practice. Several offerings are particularly useful and relevant for new graduates and early career therapists.

The associations also share knowledge and information through their respective scientific journals, communiques and member only resources on their website. Member services include networking and learning opportunities via special interest and regional/local area groups, issue-based forums, and online access to practice-area-based communities of practice.

The WFOT promotes professional knowledge through collaborative international activities to develop competency standards, position papers and international congresses. Online educational opportunities reflect the international nature of the profession and create possibilities for wider sharing of knowledge and cross-cultural learning. The WFOT Bulletin was the official publication of the WFOT and was published biannually but ceased publication in 2024. Past issues are still freely available to individual WFOT members via the WFOT website.

6.2.4.2 *Facilitators of professional practice – standards and research*

All organisations have significant, albeit different, roles to play in the development of professional standards. They agree that standards must align with the diversity of occupational therapy practice and be updated as practice changes, addressing emerging health care needs, technological advances, and public expectations.

6.2.4.2.1 REGISTRATION STANDARDS

A key function of the OTBA and the OTBNZ is to establish registration standards which a practitioner must meet to become and remain registered as an occupational therapist. Enforceable by law, registration standards ensure therapists are qualified, competent, and safe to deliver occupational therapy services. In Australia, the National Law requires the Board to establish standards for:

- professional indemnity insurance which must be maintained by occupational therapists,
- how it will consider any criminal history when deciding if it is relevant to professional practice,
- continuing professional development,
- English language skills for people applying for registration, and
- recency of practice which determines eligibility for practice.

In New Zealand, the HPCAA (2003) requires the Board to establish standards in relation to requirements for registration of practitioners and authorisations of scope of practice. Requirements for registration of practitioners are contained in Section 15 and fitness for registration in Section 16 of the HPCAA. The initial application for registration and annual renewal processes in both countries require practitioners to make declarations about whether they meet the mandatory registration standards.

In addition to registration standards, the Boards have developed codes and guidelines for the profession. In Australia these include a Code of Conduct, Competency Standards, a social media policy, and guidelines for advertising regulated health services. In New Zealand, these include a Code of Ethics and Conduct, guidelines for health disclosure, standards for driver assessment, Supervision Standards, and guidance for new graduates.

Both Boards have guidelines for mandatory notifications outlining the process of informing the Board about a health practitioner who may be putting public safety at risk. The OTBA and OTBNZ audit a proportion of occupational therapists each year, requesting and assessing evidence that they have met the registration standards. Audits provide an assurance of public protection by ensuring that occupational therapists are meeting the registration standards.

6.2.4.2.2 COMPETENCY STANDARDS

The professional competencies describe the standards expected for competent practice by occupational therapists for registration and for regulation of the profession by the Boards.

The Australian Occupational Therapy Competency Standards (OTBA, 2018) focus on four conceptual areas of occupational therapy practice:

- professionalism,
- knowledge and learning,
- occupational therapy process and practice, and
- communication.

The New Zealand Competencies for Registration and Continuing Practice for Occupational Therapists (Occupational Therapy Board of New Zealand, 2022) describe the five areas an occupational therapist must be competent in to be registered with OTBNZ:

- applying whakaora ngangahau occupational therapy knowledge, skills, and values;
- responsiveness to te Tirit o Waitangi;
- developing and sustaining partnerships;
- practicing in a safe, legal, ethical, sustainable and culturally competent way; and
- practicing responsively and upholding the occupational therapy profession.

In both Australia and New Zealand, each competency standard is further described by a number of practice behaviours. The practice behaviours communicate to practitioners and the public the expected behaviours an occupational therapist should demonstrate under each competency standard. The competency standards apply to all occupational therapists whether they work clinically, in research, education, management, or other roles not involving direct contact with clients. They have been designed for regulatory use and are the benchmark for the standard of practice deemed suitable by the profession.

Competency standards are developed within a cultural and social timeframe. The need for respectful, collaborative, safe, and culturally responsive practice is supported in the competency standards in both countries, where occupational therapists are expected to recognise that historical, political cultural, societal, environmental, and economic factors influence clients' health, wellbeing and occupational participation.

The OTBA standards specifically acknowledge the need for occupational therapists to enhance their cultural responsiveness and capabilities for practice with Aboriginal and Torres Strait Islander peoples.

The standards in New Zealand specifically acknowledge Te Tiriti o Waitangi and the need for occupational therapists' responsiveness to Te Tiriti in their practice. Occupational therapists are required to aim to enhance tino rangatiratanga (self-determination), ensure equity, and enable occupational justice. They are required to practice professionally, with a commitment to addressing both individual and systemic barriers to people's participation in occupation. These barriers can be cultural, educational, environmental, or social; related to health, disability, or spirituality.

Te Tiriti o Waitangi is the founding document of New Zealand. It shapes the diverse historical and sociopolitical realities of Māori and all other settlers and their descendants. Understanding how Te Tiriti affects all lives is essential for helping people participate in their desired occupations. Such understanding helps occupational therapists see how systemic and individual issues can breach people's rights and limit their opportunities to participate in their chosen occupations.

6.2.4.2.3 ACCREDITATION STANDARDS FOR EDUCATION PROVIDERS

To be eligible to apply for registration as an occupational therapist, students need to graduate from an education programme approved by the registration board.

In Australia, the National Law mandates that for each registered profession there will be standards which determine the requirements for an educational programme to ensure its graduates are provided with the knowledge, skills, and professional attributes to practice that profession. The National Law requires that education programmes are accredited by an accreditation committee established by the registration board or an external accreditation entity. In Australia, occupational therapy accreditation is carried out by the OTC, and the OTBA subsequently approves (or not) the accreditation decision.

In New Zealand, the HPCAA mandates that OTBNZ prescribes the qualifications required for scopes of practice within the profession, and for that purpose accredits and monitors educational institutions and degrees, courses, studies, or programmes. OTBNZ is responsible for accrediting and monitoring schools of occupational therapy to ensure education programmes continue to meet competencies to enable registration in the professions scope of practice. The OTBNZ develops national accreditation and re-accreditation standards that incorporate and build on the WFOT minimum standards and the OTC standards. As part of its international commitment, OTA assesses Australian accredited education programmes against the WFOT standards. OTA also contributes to programme accreditation through regular liaison with education programmes, students, graduates and other professional organisations.

In New Zealand, the WFOT delegates have the responsibility to ensure education programmes are accredited against the WFOT standards as and when required by WFOT.

The most recent re-accreditation in 2023 had OTNZ-WNA WFOT delegates on the reaccreditation committee as part of the OTBNZ led accreditation process.

Setting, reviewing, and monitoring standards are important professional activities, requiring liaison between the regulatory bodies, professional associations, education providers, practitioners, students, and community members. Educators and accreditors will seek participation of students and graduates in both ongoing programme review, as well as the formal accreditation process.

6.2.4.2.4 STANDARDS TO ENHANCE PRACTICE

A role of professional associations is to develop standards to enhance practice. OTA contributes to this function through the development of Capability Frameworks (i.e. a framework of what best practice looks like in a particular area at the foundational, inter-mediate or senior practitioner level), Guides to Good Practice, and a Code of Ethics. Both OTA and OTNZ-WNA provide CPD to support the requirement of CPD for ongoing registration.

The associations also present the official stance of the organisations through position papers developed in response to an issue, concern or need of members. Position papers outline the profession's view on important issues and indicate what the profession regards as good practice which can guide practice and advise stu-dents, practitioners, the public, and other stakeholders. For example, the WFOT position statement on Occupational Therapy and Disaster Management (WFOT, 2024) outlines the significant role of occupational therapists in disaster management for enabling individuals and communities to identify and participate in valued occu-pations, promote wellbeing, and reduce the impact of a changed life context brought about by disaster.

Another example: OTA is responsible for assessing occupational therapists as Better Access to Mental Health endorsed occupational therapists within the Australian Medicare Benefits Scheme. This Scheme provides people with mental health con-cerns access to a defined number of low cost or free allied health services (Australian Government Department of Health and Aged Care, 2024). Criteria to provide services under this scheme are set by the Australian Department of Health and include a two-year minimum of supervised mental health experience, OTA membership, OTBA reg-istration, and ongoing supervision. Applicants submit a portfolio which is assessed by a panel of experienced occupational therapists.

6.2.4.2.5 SUPPORTING RESEARCH

Research is integral to a profession's development and is imperative to improve the quality of services provided by the profession. The OTBNZ, OTBA, and OTC use evidence and best practice to support their standards. OTA and OTNZ-WNA actively support research development and dissemination in the profession. Their internation-ally recognised journals, the *Australian Occupational Therapy Journal* and the *New Zealand Journal of Occupational Therapy*, publish high-quality, peer-reviewed infor-mation. Each journal has an editorial board of skilled and internationally renowned researchers, educators, and clinical experts.

In addition to research published in journals, occupational therapy professional associations at national and international level hold scientific meetings where new research and practice innovations can be shared. These conferences attract researchers, practitioners, employers, service recipients, and other occupational therapy stakeholders.

These occur every two years for OTA and OTNZ-WNA and every four years for the WFOT Congress. The regional groups of the WFOT, such as the Asia Pacific Occupational Therapy Regional Group, which includes Australia and New Zealand, also hold a congress every four years, between the WFOT Congresses. In 2024, the 8th Asia Pacific Occupational Therapy Congress was held in Japan, and the next is due to be held in Korea in 2028. Students are encouraged to attend and often participate as volunteers. Students and new graduates have presented findings from their honours theses and other projects at these events.

An Occupational Therapy Australia Research Foundation was launched in 2013 to support and build research capacity in the profession in Australia through providing research grants and awards. OTA also established the Occupational Therapy Australia Research Academy in 2017 to recognise outstanding scholarship and foster capacity building in occupational therapy research. Fellows are inducted into the Academy biannually. In New Zealand, an independent Research and Education Trust have been established with the support of OTNZ-WNA. This trust accepts applications for grants towards the costs of research and training, with annual awards available. The WFOT recently developed a programme area devoted to research. The programme team focuses its activities on the priority areas for research that are determined from the international occupational therapy community.

6.2.4.3 Facilitators of change

While the focus of the professional bodies and the registration authorities differs, the standards they set facilitate change. For example, the OTBA (2018) competency standards specifically require all occupational therapists to enhance their cultural responsiveness and capabilities for practice with Aboriginal and Torres Strait Islander Peoples. The OTC accreditation standards for education providers support this expectation as one of the ways occupational therapy can contribute to the National Scheme's Aboriginal and Torres Strait Islander Health and Cultural Safety Strategy 2020–2025 (AHPRA, 2020).

Similarly, the OTBNZ influences and embeds change through regulation and makes policy submissions that have relevance to the HPCAA (professional and public safety). For example, the OTBNZ (2022) competency standards specifically require all occupational therapists to ensure cultural responsiveness to Te Tiriti O Waitangi. The Board's Strategic Plan Te Pae Tawhiti 2024–2029 directs an equity focus for the organisation and regulation and supports Pae Ora (Healthy Futures) Act 2022 and the Government Policy Statement on Health (Minister of Health, 2024).

6.2.4.4 Increasing the profile of the profession – lobbying and advocacy

Lobbying and advocacy are core functions of professional associations and can influence policy and practice. Occupational therapy practice is influenced by government policy. Professional associations provide a collective voice to positively impact policy that relates to the profession. OTA and OTNZ-WNA actively engage in policy and advocacy by building relationships with politicians and government department representatives and through submissions and government hearings.

The WFOT is actively involved with lobbying and advocating at the international level. Key relationships include those with the United Nations, World Health Organisation, Rehabilitation International, World Bank, and other non-government organisations. Some of the areas of advocacy at the international level include human rights, mental health, and disaster preparedness and response.

Advocacy and promotion of the profession also occurs through sharing stories of occupational therapy and its impact for people across diverse media platforms. OTA and OTNZ-WNA celebrate and promote the profession during OT Week, which is the third week of October each year. World Occupational Therapy Day is the opportunity to heighten the visibility of the profession's development work and to promote the activities of WFOT locally, nationally, and internationally. It is held on October 27th each year. Celebrations are held around the world and on social media.

6.3 Conclusion

It is important for students and practitioners to understand the role and responsibilities of key external organisations which shape their education and practice. Each of the organisations described in this chapter has a role in facilitating knowledge sharing and professional learning, professional practice standards, research, and change. While these organisations intersect, their roles are unique in the way they support the profession, raise the profile, and enhance occupational therapy practice.

6.4 Summary

In this chapter, the organisations that shape and represent the occupational therapy profession have been profiled.

- OTBNZ is the national registration body for all occupational therapists who wish to practice in New Zealand and is tasked with developing mechanisms to ensure competent and safe practice to protect the public.
- OTBNZ also accredits the occupational therapy education programmes in New Zealand and reviews all international applicants seeking a review of their occupational therapy education for parity purposes with the New Zealand education of occupational therapists.
- OTBA is the national registration body for all occupational therapists who wish to practice in Australia and is designed to ensure competent and safe practice to protect the public.
- OTC accredits the occupational therapy education programmes in Australia and assesses internationally qualified practitioners who apply to register to practice in Australia when their qualifications are relevant but not substantially equivalent to an approved Australian qualification.
- OTA and OTNZ-WMA are the peak bodies that represent the occupational therapy profession in Australia and New Zealand respectively, while the WFOT advocates for the profession at the international level.

6.5 Review questions

- Summarise the key distinctions between professional associations (OTNZ-WNA and OTA) and regulation/registration authorities (OTBNZ and OTBA).
- Why do these organisations need to have distinct roles?
- What is the key purpose of accreditation standards for occupational therapy programmes of study?
- What are the benefits to you of belonging to your professional association?
- Why is registration important for a profession?
- What are the benefits of being part of the WFOT for a national professional group and an individual practitioner?

Websites for the organisations

- Occupational Therapy Australia: www.otaus.com.au
- Occupational Therapy Board of Australia: www.occupationaltherapyboard.gov.au
- Occupational Therapy Council of Australia Ltd: www.otcouncil.com.au
- World Federation of Occupational Therapists: www.wfot.org
- Occupational Therapy Board of New Zealand: https://otboard.org.nz/
- Occupational Therapy New Zealand – Whakaora Ngangahau Aotearoa: https://www.otboard.org.nz/index.html

References

Australian Government Department of Health and Aged Care. (2024). *Better access initiative.* https://www.health.gov.au/our-work/better-access-initiative

Australian Health Practitioner Regulation Agency. (2020). *National Scheme's Aboriginal and Torres Strait Islander health and cultural safety strategy, 2020–2025.* https://www.ahpra.gov.au/About-AHPRA/Aboriginal-and-Torres-Strait-Islander-Health-Strategy.aspx

Health Practitioner Regulation National Law Act. (2009). https://www.legislation.qld.gov.au/view/whole/html/inforce/current/act-2009-045

Health Practitioners Competence Assurance Act. (2003). https://www.legislation.govt.nz/act/public/2003/0048/latest/DLM203312.html

Minister of Health. (2024). *Government policy statement on health 2024–2027.* Ministry of Health. https://www.health.govt.nz/publications/government-policy-statement-on-health-2024-2027

Occupational Therapy Board of Australia. (2018). *Australian occupational therapy competency standards.* https://www.occupationaltherapyboard.gov.au/Codes-Guidelines/Competencies.aspx

Occupational Therapy Board of New Zealand. (2022). *Competencies for registration and continuing practice for occupational therapists.* https://otboard.org.nz/document/6151/7569%20OTBNZ%20%E2%80%93%20Competencies%20for%20practice%20FINAL.pdf

Pae Ora (Health Futures) Act. (2022). https://www.legislation.govt.nz/act/public/2022/0030/latest/LMS575405.html

Stokes, G. (2016). Relevance and professional associations in 2026: Towards a new role for thought leadership. In J. Guthrie, E. Evans & R. Burritt (Eds.), *Relevance and professional associations in 2026* (pp. 44–47). RMIT University & Chartered Accountants, Australia & New Zealand. https://www.psc.gov.au/sites/default/files/Relevance%20and%20Prof%20Associations%20in%202026.pdf

WFOT. (2024). *Position statement on occupational therapy and disaster management.* https://wfot.org/resources/disaster-management-for-occupational-therapists

Scope of practice of occupational therapists in Australia and Aotearoa New Zealand

Kieran Broome, Kim Walder, Jessica Levick, and Yvonne Thomas

Authors' positionality statement

We are Western-educated occupational therapists with postgraduate qualifications working in leadership positions in Australia and New Zealand. We are white cisgender, able-bodied, and English-speaking and acknowledge our white privilege, our Global North outlook, and the impacts of colonisation on Indigenous people of both countries. We support decolonisation, equity and inclusivity through cultural safe and responsive health care and education, partnerships, advocacy, and personal development.

Key terms
- Extended scope
- Advanced scope
- Interprofessional practice
- Competency
- Professional roles and responsibilities
- Supervision

Objectives
This chapter will allow the reader to:

- Describe the scope of occupational therapy across health and social care systems
- Differentiate between extended scope of practice and advanced scope of practice
- Reflect on occupational therapy roles within interprofessional teams
- Identify the limits to occupational therapy scope of practice

7.1 Introduction

While all occupational therapists share a professional focus on occupation and a structured educational programme, the day-to-day practice of occupational therapists can

DOI: 10.4324/9781003495666-8

be quite diverse. The term scope of practice refers to who we work with, what occupational therapists do, where we work, and the tasks and duties that we are qualified to undertake. In this chapter we will explore the current scope of practice of occupational therapists in Australia and Aotearoa New Zealand and the key questions of who, what, when, where, why, and how.

7.2 Who

Occupational therapists work with individuals and collectives, across the lifespan. Occupational therapists work with newborns on safe positioning to preserve and maximise functional movement and to support occupations both now (for example feeding) and in the future. Some occupational therapists working solely with children and their families (Odgers et al., 2024) often focus on the development of self-care occupations like dressing or eating and the occupation of play, which fosters the development of new capacities, including physical, cognitive, and social skills (Novak & Honan, 2019). Occupational therapists address challenges some children face in the school environment due to the interplay between environmental factors and/or physical, psychological, developmental, sensory processing, or neurodiversity factors (Jeremy et al., 2024).

An occupational therapist working in a mental health setting may work with people who have acute or chronic psychiatric conditions that are impacting their ability to participate in meaningful occupation. Working with adults, occupational therapists frequently focus on maximising independence and safe and satisfying participation in occupations including self-care, paid or volunteer work, or leisure. Occupational therapists work with people at times of transition such as becoming a parent, leaving school, and retirement as they try out new occupations and restructure their daily lives (Eagers et al., 2016).

For older adults, the focus can include preventing decline and maintaining meaningful occupational participation. Occupational therapists can enhance home safety (providing home modifications), organise appropriate services, address loneliness or change of roles, and explore assistive technology (a mobility scooter to support) (Hughes et al., 2023). Occupational therapists also have an established role in palliative care, enabling dignity, quality of life, and participation in valued occupations as long as possible during the terminal phase of a person's illness. Intervention strategies include prescribing assistive technology and symptom management (Chow & Pickens, 2020).

Occupational therapy clients may have a broad range of physical and mental health conditions, disabilities, and inequities. Some occupational therapists have a diverse caseload, and others focus their expertise on a narrower range of conditions or area of need. All occupational therapists working in Australia and New Zealand have a professional requirement to develop cultural safety and responsiveness to the specific needs of Māori, Aboriginal, and Torres Strait Islander peoples. Some occupational therapists develop advanced skills to best serve populations with particular needs or ways of viewing health and wellness (Gray & McPherson, 2005; Reweti, 2023). Such populations include Māori, Aboriginal or Torres Strait Islander Peoples, Pacific People, people from culturally and linguistically diverse backgrounds, refugees and asylum seekers, and people who identify as LGBTQIAP2S+. Occupational therapists need to consider the health inequities and occupational injustices that specific populations can experience and tailor their approach to match (Ramugondo, 2025). Occupational therapists have a role in advocacy to address systemic and environmental factors contributing to such inequities (Restall & Egan, 2022).

Some occupational therapists also work with collectives. This might be a therapeutic group within a rehabilitation, paediatric, aged care, or mental health setting where group members have common goals or needs. Occupational therapists also work in community development, public health, or organisational contexts where interventions are targeted at a community rather than individual level.

7.2.1 Vignette 7.1: A day in the life of an occupational therapist

Sam is a rural generalist occupational therapist. Their first visit of the day was to Peter, an adult living with an intellectual disability. He lives with his parents and wants to be an active contributor to the household. After talking to Peter's parents about their expectations and hopes, incorporating a list of skills Peter was interested in developing, Sam selected cooking a stir fry as an assessment task. They engaged Peter in the cooking, assessing risks needing to be managed, identifying strategies to encourage Peter to slow down and think about what he was doing, and demonstrating to the support worker how to grade their assistance towards developing Peter's independence.

Next, Sam visited Nancy, who was experiencing fluctuating functional neurological disorder symptoms. Nancy had been avoiding going out in the community, as her legs would unpredictably give way, causing her to collapse to the ground. Sam helped Nancy to explore online a range of lightweight power wheelchairs that might allow her to access the community. After conducting a precautionary cognitive screening tool and taking Nancy's measurements to shortlist suitable wheelchairs, Sam arranged to take Nancy to a supplier to trial a wheelchair. Nancy had almost run out of food, and Sam was concerned as Nancy was already limiting what she was eating. After considering referral to a meal delivery service, they remembered that Nancy's children were local and would be willing to help if they knew of Nancy's predicament. Nancy felt embarrassed asking her children for assistance with groceries, so Sam used psychological strategies to explore and address those feelings, giving Nancy the confidence to phone her son.

Sam then returned to the office to document that day's sessions and continue working on a care needs assessment report for a previous client until their final clinic visit with 8-year-old Lucy, who had deafness and developmental delay. Sam played a board game and ball game with Lucy to build communication and turn-taking skills.

7.3 What

Occupational therapists undertake generic health professional activities, core occupational therapy skills (including occupational and activity analysis and use of occupation as a therapeutic medium) and extended skill sets in particular areas (see Table 7.1). Within the competency requirements of various health professions, there are shared practices. For example, all health professionals must be able to develop a therapeutic relationship through effective communication and rapport building, engage in collaborative goal setting, use professional reasoning to make decisions, document client progress, prepare reports, liaise with key stakeholders (parents, employers, or other providers), and refer to other health professionals when clients have needs beyond their scope of practice or when collaborative care could benefit the client. Health professionals must continually monitor and improve their service delivery through activities such as participating in reflective practice, supervision, evaluating programmes, critically appraising research and its relevance to practice, or establishing new services.

Additionally, occupational therapists bring specific unique skills that are core to occupational therapy practice. These include:

- Identifying where a person's current patterns of occupational engagement enhance or diminish their overall health and wellbeing.
- Analysing a person's occupational performance and engagement through information gathering approaches including observation, interviews, and standardised and non-standardised assessment.
- Through occupational, activity and task analysis, identifying strengths and challenges related to the person (e.g., their motivation, capabilities or skills), the occupation (how they do the activity), and their environment (including the physical environment and the people, culture, and systems surrounding them).
- Engaging people in graded or adapted occupations to build capacities and skills.
- Exploring adapted ways of doing things (e.g., to conserve physical energy).
- Making changes to the environment around a person such as training caregivers; designing modifications to the home, school, or work environment; or recommending and providing training in the use of assistive technologies such as wheelchairs or kitchen aids.

A therapist may learn advanced assessment techniques, gain certification for specific assessments or interventions, or be credentialed for prescription of assistive technologies or housing modifications.

Many occupational therapists take on roles performed by a range of health professionals; however, each profession will bring their own unique lens to the role. For

Table 7.1 Scope of practice in interprofessional, advanced, and extended practice

Scope concept	Interprofessional practice	Advanced scope of practice	Extended scope of practice
What occupational therapists do	Skill sharing with other health professionals with support/training	Undertake specific training in a particular area	Undertake activities usually associated with another health profession
How occupational therapists practice	Considers skill set and reasoning required for skill sharing/delegation	Gains experience in the advanced area over time	Requires further specialised training
Examples	Skill sharing or delegation across professions in a rural or remote team, i.e. Calderdale framework (Smith & Duffy, 2010)	Driving assessment for people post-stroke or with a disability	Making requests for x-rays in emergency department following a fall

example, falls education could be delivered by an occupational therapist, nurse, or physiotherapist in a community health team. The occupational therapist would specifically focus on the interaction between a person's fall risk, the environment, and occupational performance and engagement. Other shared roles are also found in mental health case management or aged care assessment. A lymphoedema practitioner may be a nurse, physiotherapist, or occupational therapist who has completed additional training to develop specific skills and draws on shared professional training in anatomy and physiology. International differences in practice exist, with many occupational therapist lymphoedema practitioners in Australia but few in New Zealand.

Occupational therapists adopt a holistic approach to understanding a person's context and needs. Sometimes the client's specific needs fall within the scope of occupational therapy. At other times, it is more appropriate to refer on to another health professional. An occupational therapist may be asked to run diversional activities in an aged care facility which have no therapeutic benefit or meaning for the residents. However, this decision can sometimes be less clear cut. For example, a person who needs to carry groceries upstairs could work with an occupational therapist or be referred to a physiotherapist. It is important that occupational therapists take careful consideration of what is and isn't within their scope of practice.

7.4 When

Occupational therapists work with people at many points along their health and well-being journey. Some occupational therapists work with people in a health promotion or preventative capacity before issues arise. Examples include working in ergonomics, a university student well-being service, or adventure therapy. Occupational therapists can be primary health practitioners, where clients may access occupational therapists as the first point of contact. For instance, a person with a hand injury may choose to go to see a hand therapist (who may be an occupational therapist or physiotherapist) with or without a referral from another health practitioner. Occupational therapists may also be frontline health care providers: for example, in acute mental health services, in emergency departments or intensive care units, in disaster recovery after a flood or cyclone, with a police or ambulance officer providing healthcare alongside an emergency response, or in general practice as health improvement practitioners (see Chapter 36).

Occupational therapists also play a role in discharge planning or coordination of services to assist a person transitioning home from hospital or after discharge from a health service. This might include organising assistive technology and providing mental health support or referrals to support services.

Some therapeutic relationships can extend across various times over the years as the client's needs change. Others may work intensively with clients over a shorter period, for example, during neurological rehabilitation or acute mental health treatment. Other therapists may practice in a limited component of the occupational therapy process, such as only assessment and/or intervention planning rather than intervention delivery.

7.4.1 Vignette 7.2: A client journey

Ali is 18 years old and lives at home with her parents in Auckland, New Zealand. She achieved good grades in high school and recently completed her first trimester of university study. She has a few close friends, but lately, she hasn't made plans to see them, instead spending a lot of time in her bedroom. Typically a highly motivated student, Ali found the first trimester challenging and failed one course. Recently she felt distracted, tired, and low in mood. Ali's maternal grandmother experienced schizophrenia and her mother post-natal depression.

Ali's lecturer Russel noticed she had missed multiple classes and reached out repeatedly to find out why. Finally, Ali replied saying she had been oversleeping her alarm and felt overwhelmed trying to organise herself for morning class. Russel referred Ali to Student Wellbeing Services, where an occupational therapist, Keaghan, provided support. After a few sessions with little improvement, Ali disclosed to Keaghan she had been hearing unusual sounds over recent weeks like scratching and an alarm bell but couldn't locate the sound. More recently an unfamiliar female voice was dictating her actions such as 'you are walking' or 'you are looking in the mirror'. Ali was highly distressed by this and punched the mirror, leading to a broken right fourth metacarpal and lacerated extensor digitorum.

Ali required a tendon repair at the Emergency Department and was referred to an outpatient occupational therapist for hand therapy and to the mental health assessment team. She was seen by Jess, a mental health occupational therapist, who spoke to Ali and her mother Narelle about what led up to the accident including her current mental state, challenges with her recent occupational performance, the home environment, and typical function. Post surgery, Ali was admitted to the mental health inpatient unit for assessment of an early psychosis. Ali was treated by a team of psychiatrists, nurses, occupational therapists, and psychologists. Due to the significant change in Ali's occupational performance, the occupational therapist on the inpatient unit completed a functional assessment.

7.5 Where

Humans engage in occupations in a wide range of settings, and therefore occupational therapists can be found almost everywhere. Three of the more common healthcare settings are hospitals, clinics, and community health. Many therapists work in a domiciliary model (i.e., visiting people in their home), given that people live much of their lives at home. However, you'll also find occupational therapists visiting or being based in schools, workplaces (for injury prevention, ergonomics, and return to work rehabilitation), prisons, court rooms (or more broadly doing a medicolegal assessment and report to support lawyers and the judiciary system), or other community settings.

Some innovative practices will bring occupational therapists and their clients to places such as sporting fields, adventure play spaces, or the wilderness to enable participation in a broad range of health-giving occupations. Telehealth also provides opportunities for therapists to connect with clients and their everyday environments remotely and is an expected skillset for contemporary practitioners. Opportunities are limitless, with therapists supporting individuals and collectives, and through social media, podcasts, videos, and books.

7.6 Why

Occupational therapists bring a unique lens that makes a valuable contribution to health and social services and the wider community. The central principle underpinning all occupational therapy practice is the link between health and well-being and the ability to participate in occupations which give life meaning and purpose. Why each therapist practices so differently depends on a wide range of factors.

Some therapists may develop interest in particular areas and develop focussed skills and expertise, especially through further training or self-directed learning and reflection. Supervision also plays a key role in ensuring competent practice and extending a therapist's skillset.

Funding systems will play a major role. A key focus of occupational therapy in hospitals will be discharge home, and therefore occupational therapists will often focus on essential self-cares such as showering and dressing and ensuring that appropriate services and equipment are in place when the person returns home. Some funding systems may also restrict the types of interventions and assessments that they will fund occupational therapists to do or require that the occupational therapist focusses on particular outcomes (such as return to work in workplace rehabilitation).

There may also be differences in expectations and roles of occupational therapists across nations, states, and even individual workplaces. What may be common practice for occupational therapists in one service may be the role of another health profession in a different service.

7.7 How

How occupational therapists deliver occupational therapy is governed by several factors. Professional and registration bodies set scope of practice standards and codes of ethics. Key documents guiding practice in Aotearoa New Zealand are the Occupational Therapy Board of New Zealand's Scope of Practice, Code of Ethics for Occupational Therapists, and Competencies of Registration and Continuing Practice (Occupational Therapy Board of New Zealand, 2022). In Australia, standards and guidelines include the Australian Occupational Therapy Competency Standards (Occupational Therapy Board of Australia, 2019), Code of Conduct (AHPRA, 2022), and Scope of Practice Framework (Occupational Therapy Australia, 2017). Occupational Therapy Australia also has a Code of Ethics, position statements, and capability frameworks for various practice areas.

Occupational therapists' practice will also be governed by workplace policies, procedures, and practices. Such guidelines might determine the clients we can work with, how often we can see them, and the frameworks and tools used. Some occupational therapists work from one specific theoretical model or frame of reference due to organisational requirements, practice context, and/or personal preference. Evidence also informs practice (Hoffmann et al., 2023). Therapists need to consider the best available relevant research evidence and weigh this up in terms of the client's specific context, the practice context, and the clinical expertise of the therapist with support from more senior therapists if required.

It is important that occupational therapists adopt a person-centred approach, which includes being whānau/family centred. This requires therapists to consider the client's unique context and preferences and to work collaboratively with clients and their family, fostering choice and informed decision-making in terms of their needs and occupational therapy services. At times, there may be tension between a client's preferences and a therapist's scope of practice, necessitating careful ethical reasoning. For example, a client may seek therapist interventions to enable engagement in a non-health promoting occupation. When working with communities, the entire community is the 'client', necessitating a collaborative and collective-centred approach, which adds complexity.

The daily lives of occupational therapists can be highly diverse depending on the practice context. Many therapists work with individual clients in direct service delivery. Others may work through a third party or in a consultative capacity, for example, working with teachers, providing medico-legal reports, delivering training for support workers, or consulting around public building accessibility. Some occupational therapists work alone as sole practitioners, structuring their days around individual appointments, report writing, and other solitary activities, whereas other therapists work in multidisciplinary practice running individual or group sessions with other professionals such as social workers or speech pathologists. As the allied health assistant or therapy assistant workforce increases, there are opportunities for occupational therapists to delegate tasks. For example, an occupational therapist might complete an initial assessment, develop a therapy programme for the allied health assistant to implement, and monitor and review that programme with the assistant, enabling the therapist to reach more people or focus on higher-level activities.

7.8 Conclusion

It is clear there are a wide range of factors informing an occupational therapist's scope of practice. Some determinants are external, such as professional standards and organisational requirements. Other factors are internal, including the therapist's competencies and level of experience. It is critical that all occupational therapists be aware of and comply with their scope of practice within their specific practice context. This ensures practice is safe, ethical, and legal. Importantly, determining scope of practice may not always be clear cut. There can be a gradual slope between what is within and outside of scope, and what may be acceptable in one context may not be in another. Seek support through supervisors, professional bodies, or registration boards for guidance as required. However, despite the diversity of practice contexts in which we might work, the one centralising factor uniting all occupational therapy roles is our underpinning occupational perspective as the foundation of our practice.

7.9 Summary

- Occupational therapists work with a range of people across the lifespan to improve occupational performance and engagement in valued occupations.
- Regardless of the practice setting, occupational therapists have a unique skill set they utilise to support a client's ability to participate such as analysing occupational performance, grading and adapting occupations, and modifying a person's environment or equipment.
- The context in which an occupational therapist works will impact their scope of practice and who they work with.
- The amount of time an occupational therapist will spend with a client is dependent on client occupational needs, the context (acute vs community), and therapist scope of practice within their role.
- As well as working with individuals, occupational therapists can also work with collectives.
- Within Australia and New Zealand, occupational therapists have scope of practice frameworks that provide clear guidelines for safe clinical practice.

7.10 Review and reflection questions

- Describe the various roles and responsibilities of occupational therapists when working with clients at different life stages, from neonates to older adults.
- What is the difference between advanced scope and extended scope, using examples of each?
- When do you refer to another professional within and outside your profession?
- What is the difference in the scope of practice of an occupational therapist and occupational therapy assistant?
- Reflect on the vignette about Sam's day as an occupational therapist. What challenges do you think they faced in balancing the diverse needs of their clients?

References

Australian Health Practitioner Regulation Agency (AHPRA) and National Boards. (2022). *Code of conduct.* https://www.occupationaltherapyboard.gov.au/Codes-Guidelines/Code-of-conduct.aspx

Chow, J. K., & Pickens, N. D. (2020). Measuring the efficacy of occupational therapy in end-of-life care: A scoping review. *American Journal of Occupational Therapy*, 74(1), 7401205020p1–7401205020p14. https://doi.org/10.5014/ajot.2020.033340

Eagers, J., Franklin, R. C., Broome, K., & Yau, M. K. (2016). A review of occupational therapy's contribution to and involvement in the work-to-retirement transition process: An Australian perspective. *Australian Occupational Therapy Journal*, 63(4), 277–292. https://doi.org/10.1111/1440-1630.12300

Gray, M., & McPherson, K. (2005). Cultural safety and professional practice in occupational therapy: A New Zealand perspective. *Australian Occupational Therapy Journal*, 52(1), 34–42. https://doi.org/10.1111/j.1440-1630.2004.00433.x

Hoffmann, T., Bennett, S., & Del Mar, C. (2023). *Evidence-based practice across the health professions.* Elsevier Health Sciences.

Hughes, S., Murray, C. M., McMullen-Roach, S., & Berndt, A. (2023). A profile of practice: The occupational therapy process in community aged care in Australia. *Australian Occupational Therapy Journal*, 70(3), 366–379. https://doi.org/10.1111/1440-1630.12860

Jeremy, J., Spandagou, I., & Hinitt, J. (2024). A profile of occupational therapists working in school-based practice in Australian primary schools. *Occupational Therapy International*, 2024(1), 2077870. https://doi.org/10.1155/2024/2077870

Novak, I., & Honan, I. (2019). Effectiveness of paediatric occupational therapy for children with disabilities: A systematic review. *Australian Occupational Therapy Journal*, 66(3), 258–273. https://doi.org/10.1111/1440-1630.12573

Occupational Therapy Australia. (2017). *Occupational Therapy Australia scope of practice framework* [position paper]. https://otaus.com.au/publicassets/725829df-2503-e911-a2c2-b75c2fd918c5/Occupational%20Therapy%20Scope%20of%20Practice%20Framework%20(June%202017).pdf

Occupational Therapy Board of Australia. (2019) *Australian occupational therapy competency standards.* https://www.occupationaltherapyboard.gov.au/Codes-Guidelines/Competencies.aspx

Occupational Therapy Board of New Zealand. (2022). *General scope of practice: Kaiwhakaora ngangahau occupational therapist.* https://otboard.org.nz/document/5885/Jan%202022%20Scope%20of%20Practice.pdf

Odgers, S., Thomas, Y., & Tokolahi, E. (2024). Mothering occupations: A review identifying mothering occupations. *Australian Occupational Therapy Journal*, 71(2), 352–363. https://doi.org/10.1111/1440-1630.12921

Ramugondo, E. L. (2025). Occupational consciousness: Theorising to dismantle systemic racism and dehumanisation. *Journal of Occupational Science*, 32(1), 5–21. https://doi.org/10.1080/14427591.2024.2429681

Restall, E., & Egan, G. (2022). Collaborative relationship-focused occupational therapy. In G. Egan & E. Restall (Eds.), *Promoting occupational participation: Collaborative relationship-focused occupational therapy: 10th Canadian Occupational Therapy Guidelines* (pp. 99–117). Canadian Association of Occupational Therapists.

Reweti, A. (2023). Understanding how whānau-centred initiatives can improve Māori health in Aotearoa New Zealand. *Health Promotion International, 38*(4). https://doi.org/10.1093/heapro/daad070

Smith, R., & Duffy, J. (2010). Developing a competent and flexible workforce using the Calderdale Framework. *International Journal of Therapy and Rehabilitation, 17*(5), 254–262. https://doi.org/10.12968/ijtr.2010.17.5.47844

Ethical and legal responsibilities of occupational therapy practice in Australia and Aotearoa New Zealand

Dave Parsons, Ben Milbourn, Merrolee Penman, and Angus Buchanan

Authors' positionality statement

We are doctorally qualified, registered occupational therapists from Anglo Saxon backgrounds who have trained in Australia and the United Kingdon (UK) and work in the Australian university education sector. Collectively, we have experience working and teaching in Australia, Aotearoa New Zealand, and the United Kingdom across multiple sectors including academia, acute and primary health, disability, community, private practice, and leadership and management roles. We bring our own unique lived experiences and are committed to modelling the highest standards of ethical and professional practice. We believe that a profession is only strengthened when it considers morally right and acceptable behaviour and encompasses values like honesty, integrity, fairness, responsibility, respect, and confidentiality.

Key terms
- Ethics
- Ethical practice
- Legislation
- Professional practice

Objectives
This chapter will allow the reader to:

- Provide details of the general ethical responsibilities of health care professionals including occupational therapists
- Explain the legal responsibilities of being a health care practitioner
- Provide an overview of the regulatory authorities relevant to Australian and Aotearoa New Zealand occupational therapy practice
- Identify key legislation that impacts Australian and Aotearoa New Zealand occupational therapy practice

DOI: 10.4324/9781003495666-9

8.1 Introduction and practice context

This chapter introduces ethical principles, the codes of conduct and relevant legislation that govern the practice of occupational therapy in Australia and Aotearoa New Zealand. Ethics, the codes of conduct and relevant legislation provide all health professionals with a guiding framework for their practice. Broadly speaking, ethics provide a general set of principles that guide and influence an occupational therapist's judgement in their practice, while a code of conduct is more focused, providing targeted guidance for how occupational therapists should act in specific situations related to occupational therapy practice. Legislation refers to laws that have been enacted, are legally binding and must be followed. Breaches in ethical principles, a code of conduct, and the law (legislation) can have a considerable impact on an occupational therapist's career, and thus must be understood and adhered to by all registered occupational therapists. Understanding ethical principles, codes of conduct, and relevant laws is also critical to the practice of occupational therapy students who are required to demonstrate the highest levels of behaviours in their classes, assessments, fieldwork practice, and personal life.

It can be difficult to define exactly what an ethical issue is. Every occupational therapy student must be able to articulate an ethical framework that guides their thinking and reasoning when considering the range of potential issues that may be encountered. Students place themselves at significant risk of investigation of their professional conduct if they are unable to identify situations that might be unethical and even illegal in all aspects of their lives. Clients and their families may also be placed in considerable jeopardy if students who work with them engage in unethical activities, particularly where clients may be in vulnerable situations.

To work legally as occupational therapists in Australia or Aotearoa New Zealand, practitioners must be registered with their respective regulatory authority Board. The role and functions of each Board are determined by each country's laws related to the regulation of health professions. In Aotearoa New Zealand, this is the Health Practitioners Competence Assurance Act (2003) and in Australia, the Health Practitioner Regulation National Law Act (2009).

On completion of tertiary studies, graduates register with the relevant National Boards are not able to commence practice until approval is received and this registration needs to be renewed annually. For Australian occupational therapists, this is the Occupational Therapy Board of Australia (OTBA), and for Aotearoa New Zealand occupational therapists, this is the Occupational Therapy Board of New Zealand/ Te Poari Whakaora Ngangahau o Aotearoa (OTBNZ). The core role of the National Boards and the Australian Health Practitioners Regulatory Agency is to protect the public. It is imperative that practitioners understand that the key role of the OTBA and OTBNZ is to protect the public, not to uphold the individual needs of registered occupational therapists

In Australia, students enrolled in an approved programme of study in occupational therapy will be registered by their enrolling institution with the OTBA. Registered occupational therapists must conduct their duties and responsibilities in a manner that is professional, ethical, and legal. There are severe penalties that may be imposed by the National Boards, employers, and/or the legal system if an occupational therapist (or occupational therapy student) is found to be knowingly or unknowingly engaging in unethical or illegal behaviours. While not a breach of professional ethics per se, occupational therapy students may face severe penalties for breaches in university policies, for example, academic misconduct, general misconduct, or the student charter.

Registration Boards publish documents that guide the ethical and legal practice of Australian and Aotearoa New Zealand occupational therapists: these are the Australian Health Practitioners Regulatory Agency & National Boards Code of Conduct (2022) and the Code of Ethics for Occupational Therapists (2022) (Australian Health Practitioners Regulatory Agency and National Boards, 2022; Occupational Therapy Registration Board of New Zealand/Te Poari Whakaora Ngangahau o Aotearoa, 2022). The principles outlined in the codes are designed to guide occupational therapists' professional reasoning, ethical and legal decision-making. The principles also support the establishment of effective ongoing working relationships with clients and their families. All occupational therapy students and practitioners should be using the codes as a foundation for ethically appropriate professional practice as well as their clinical reasoning and decision-making.

8.2 Overview of ethics

Ethics is a broad area of philosophy too expansive to fully address in this chapter; however, there are specific facets that are essential for a practising occupational therapist to understand and engage with. The principles of normative ethics (how people should behave morally), and more specifically *bioethics,* are the most relevant for the practice of occupational therapy. Bioethics can be defined as the study of moral problems that impact human well-being (Freegard, 2012). Before examining the nature of ethics, it is important to understand why it is relevant to occupational therapy practice.

Occupational therapists have a fiduciary obligation to clients. A fiduciary obligation is where a professional has: i) special duties due to trust and confidence placed in them by their client, ii) the ability to dominate and influence the client due to their status in the relationship, and iii) a duty to serve their clients' welfare without abusing their special status in the relationship (Kutchins, 1991; Lohman & Brown, 1997). This special ethical obligation to clients is in addition to the everyday morality that members of society must exhibit.

The fiduciary obligation is often greater for health professionals than for other types of workers. For example, if an occupational therapist was completing a home visit and their client disclosed that they were experiencing mental health issues, the occupational therapist has the professional obligation to encourage their client to seek the appropriate help and support. If the client shares the same information with a tradesperson working at their home, the tradesperson has no such fiduciary obligation.

The most common and widely recognised practical implementation of the bioethical principles is the Four Principles Approach as described by Beauchamp and Childress (2019). This approach provides a set of four core principles that all health professionals, including occupational therapists, should follow throughout their practice. The four principles – autonomy, non-maleficence, beneficence, and justice – are outlined:

8.2.1 Autonomy

Health professionals should espouse the principle of autonomy: To respect an autonomous agent is, at a minimum, to acknowledge that person's right to hold views, to make choices, and to take actions based on personal values and beliefs (Beauchamp & Childress, 2019). Clients have the right to their personal values, views, and beliefs and these come before the values, views, and beliefs of the therapist regarding decisions made about the client's care or because of the interaction with the occupational therapist. As part of this process, it is critical that the occupational therapist be aware of their own values, views, and beliefs and understand how these may influence their own decision-making and behaviour. The occupational therapist must recognise their own influence in the context of providing a service to their clients.

8.2.2 Non-maleficence

The principle of non-maleficence is an obligation of the health practitioner to not inflict harm intentionally and is closely aligned with the maxim in medical ethics, 'Above all do no harm' (Beauchamp & Childress, 2019). While simple in definition, in practice, this principle can be quite complex, with numerous ambiguities in the definitions of harm and injury (Beauchamp & Childress, 2019). Occupational therapists might also cause harm or injury to their clients without intent; however, due to a duty of care, they might still unintentionally breach this ethical principle (Beauchamp & Childress, 2019). Occupational therapists must be mindful of the consequences of their actions and their behaviour and any potential harm or injury to their client, regardless of their original intent.

8.2.3 Beneficence

The principle of beneficence is an active process by which occupational therapists must take positive steps for the benefit of their clients. This principle outlines that occupational therapists are not only obligated to respect their client's autonomy and cause no harm or injury but must contribute to their welfare (Beauchamp & Childress, 2019). Beneficence also encompasses the kindness and empathy that occupational therapists should have for their clients. Occupational therapists must do all in their power to actively engage with often vulnerable populations, to enhance client health and well-being throughout the therapeutic process.

8.2.4 Justice

The principle of justice can be broadly described as the 'fair, equitable, and appropriate treatment considering what is due or owed to persons' (Beauchamp & Childress, 2019). This principle is complex and can be understood on a number of levels. Freegard (2012) identifies four ways to determine the equitable and fair distribution and allocation of scarce resources in the health sector: i) justice as fairness – those with equal needs should be served equally without discrimination or prejudice, ii) comparative justice – those with the greatest needs should receive more of the available resources without discrimination or prejudice, iii) distributive justice – resources should be allocated based on a set of societal norms that are pre-determined, and iv) compensatory justice – those who experience discrimination or prejudice should receive more resources to address this imbalance.

The most notable characteristic of the Four Principles Approach is that each principle should not conflict with another. If conflict does arise, practitioners need to consider the reasoning that may elevate one principle over another. No principle is inherently superior to another, and all are interrelated (Freegard, 2012). The framework then acts as a guide to decision-making with consideration of each particular principle, acknowledging that every ethical situation is unique, and there is no one formula or hierarchy that can be applied that will work in all instances.

These principles form part of a code of ethics or conduct that occupational therapists and other health professionals are required to implement within their practice.

8.3 Code of ethics/conduct for occupational therapists

A code of ethics or code of conduct is a transparent disclosure that provides guidance as to how a profession or organisation is expected to behave and function and is intended to be a reference for users in their decision-making. However, all practitioners must also understand their legal obligations, acting in accordance with these. For any conflict between Australian or Aotearoa New Zealand laws and the codes, then the relevant laws always take precedence (Australian Health Practitioners Regulatory Agency and National Boards, 2022; Occupational Therapy Registration Board of New Zealand/Te Poari Whakaora Ngangahau o Aotearoa, 2022).

For Aotearoa New Zealand occupational therapy practice, there are three Mātāpono or principles. Each leads with the word relationships, as outlined in Table 8.1, with further detail about what each of these refers to provided in the Code of Ethics document.

Table 8.1 Principles Outlined in the Countries Respective Code of Conduct/Ethics

Australia	*Aotearoa New Zealand*
Code of Conduct (2022, p. 4)	Code of Ethics for Occupational Therapists (2022, p. 5)
■ Put patients first – safe, effective, and collaborative practice	■ Relationships with people receiving occupational therapy services
■ Aboriginal and Torres Strait Islander health and cultural safety	■ Relationships with communities and people who may require occupational therapy services
■ Respectful and culturally safe practice for all	■ Relationships with colleagues and the profession
■ Working with patients	
■ Working with other practitioners	
■ Working within the health care system	
■ Minimising risk to patients	
■ Professional behaviour	
■ Maintaining practitioner health and well-being	
■ Teaching, supervising, and assessing	
■ Ethical research	

The Code of Conduct published by the Australian Health Practitioners Regulatory Agency and National Boards (2022) is more detailed, outlining 11 principles, each with further explanation provided in their publication.

Despite the differences in how the two codes are presented, both are underpinned by the four ethical principles of autonomy, non-maleficence, beneficence, and justice (Beauchamp & Childress, 2019). Aligned with these four principles are expected behaviours and professional qualities, such as principles promoting the values of respect (collaboration and communication); those promoting the values of trust (honesty, fairness, accountability and transparency) (College of Occupational Therapists of Ontario, 2019); ensuring service users right to privacy and confidentiality; and acting with integrity, truthfulness, and dependability (Doherty, 2023).

All occupational therapists (and occupational therapy students) must be aware of their relevant code of ethics/code of conduct and have a working understanding of how the code applies to their own specific practice context. Implementation of a code of ethics/conduct in practice is dynamic and will raise ethical issues that need to be explored and resolved (Bourne et al., 2013). Examples of ethical issues experienced by occupational therapy students and occupational therapists have included resource and systemic issues (e.g. perpetuating social inequities, interpersonal conflicts (e.g. intimidating interactions), practice management (e.g. being asked to undertake tasks outside of scope of practice), clinical decision making (e.g. disagreement with supervisors or management), or client safety (e.g. use of outdated practices) (Bourne et al., 2013; Bushby et al., 2015; Howard et al., 2023; McArdle et al., 2023).

To assist practitioners in exploring and resolving ethical issues, several ethical decision-making frameworks have been proposed in the literature (see, for example: (Kornblau & Burkhardt, 2024; Swisher & Royeen, 2019; VanderKaay et al., 2020) or by professional organisations (see, for example: (College of Occupational Therapists of Ontario, 2019). Irrespective of their origin, ethical-decision making frameworks are designed to be a 'how-to' guide to assist professionals with negotiating ethical quandaries (Swisher & Royeen, 2019). Generally, the frameworks consist of a series of steps such as:

1. recognising the ethical quandary
2. gathering relevant data, considering all contributing factors
3. consulting with others to gain as broader picture as possible
4. analyse using ethical principles
5. consider all solutions, weighing up the relative merits and challenges,
6. determining the 'best' solution
7. evaluating and reflecting on the outcomes
    (College of Occupational Therapists of Ontario, 2019; Doherty, 2023)

8.4 Legal responsibilities of being a health care practitioner

Occupational therapists in Australia and Aotearoa New Zealand must meet nationally consistent registration standards to practise occupational therapy (Australian Health Practitioners Regulatory Agency, 2024; Occupational Therapy Registration Board of

New Zealand/Te Poari Whakaora Ngangahau o Aotearoa, 2024). The OTBA and OTBNZ have mandatory standards, which include:

- continuing professional development (CPD)
- criminal history disclosure
- English language skill competency
- professional indemnity insurance; and
- recency of practice

The OTBA and OTBNZ (Australian Health Practitioners Regulatory Agency, 2024; Occupational Therapy Registration Board of New Zealand/Te Poari Whakaora Ngangahau o Aotearoa, 2024) provide clear guidance for registered occupational therapists and occupational therapy students transitioning into practitioners. This includes:

- Occupational therapists must demonstrate how they are maintaining and improving their competence in occupational therapy practice through CPD and/or supervision.
- Occupational therapists must disclose their complete criminal history when applying for occupational therapy registration.
- Occupational therapists must be able to provide evidence of English language skills that meet the English language skills registration standard.
- Registered occupational therapists must consider that they have appropriate indemnity insurance.
- Occupational therapists must demonstrate recency and relevance of their practice.
- Occupational therapists must be aware of their responsibility under the National Law to notify the Boards in relation to certain impairments.

Occupational therapists also have a legal obligation to make a mandatory notification if they have formed a reasonable belief that a health practitioner has behaved in an unethical or illegal manner. This constitutes notifiable conduct in relation to the practice of their profession. Types of notifications fall under three broad areas:

- **Competency** – This relates to the ability to practise to the standard reasonably to be expected of an occupational therapist and where there are significant departures from accepted professional standards, for example, not having the skills to practice a clinical area competently.
- **Conduct** – This relates to concerns about the appropriateness of the professional behaviours and conduct. For example, this could include practising while intoxicated by alcohol or drugs, inappropriate client relationships, and/or sexual misconduct.
- **Health** – This relates to a health condition(s) that impairs an occupational therapist's ability to carry out practice safely. For example, this could include physical and/or mental health conditions.

The purpose of the mandatory notification requirements is to prevent the public from being placed at risk of harm. The Australian Health Practitioners Regulatory Agency and OTBNZ should be notified if a health professional believes that an occupational therapy student or practitioner has behaved in a way that presents a serious risk to the public. In Australia and Aotearoa New Zealand, an occupational therapist may be suspended and possibly struck off the professional register for failing to recognise and manage risks within their caseload, breaching professional boundaries, and failing to act within the scope of practice as an occupational therapist.

Unlike Aotearoa New Zealand, students enrolled in an approved Australian occupational therapy programme of study must be registered with the OTBA. Registration is automatically completed by the student's respective tertiary institution. The Australian Health Practitioners Regulatory Agency can be notified for student breaches of the same ethical and conduct standards expected of qualified practitioners. This includes if the education provider reasonably believes, 'a student has an impairment that, in the course of the student undertaking clinical training, may place the public at substantial risk of harm' (Australian Health Practitioners Regulatory Agency, 2020, p. 11). In both Australia and Aotearoa New Zealand, the respective Board receives new graduate lists from the relevant educational providers. These lists confirm which students have been awarded an accredited occupational therapy qualification. In Aotearoa New Zealand this is also accompanied by a statement highlighting if there are any reportable issues such as criminal history, English competency and health conditions that may impact practice. Students should be aware that in Aotearoa New Zealand, formal disciplinary orders that have occurred at university are required to be reported to OTBNZ at the time of graduation.

Further to registration with OTBA and OTBNZ, occupational therapy students and practitioners have a responsibility to ensure they are aware and have a working knowledge of the laws and legislation that impact their practice care provided to clients. In both Australia and Aotearoa New Zealand there are legislation and laws that address a wide range of issues that impact an occupational therapist's work. These laws are in place to both support consumers and to guide practitioners in their workplaces. For example, there is legislation in both countries that addresses disability and sexual discrimination, health and safety, mental health, and employment rights. In most contexts, places of employment will have policies and procedures that implement these laws. Failure to uphold these laws may result in both legal proceedings against a practitioner and being reported to the respective Board, placing their registration at risk.

8.4.1 Vignette 8.1: Australian occupational therapy Student in a community organisation
        with clients accessing National Disability Insurance Scheme funding

Isla-Mae is a final-year graduate entry occupational therapy student on a placement with a community organisation providing occupational therapy interventions for children. Isla-Mae has been shadowing her occupational therapy supervisor Wendy. Tomorrow, they have an appointment to see Derek, a teenager diagnosed with autism, and his mum, Linda, to undertake an occupational therapy functional assessment to support a disability support funding request. Wendy must rush out of the office and arranges to meet Isla-Mae at the family home the next day. Wendy asks Isla-Mae to collect Derek's paperwork (confidential details including health professional reports) to bring to the meeting. Isla-Mae collects the paperwork and decides rather than coming back to the office in the morning, she will take the paperwork home with her. Isla-Mae puts the paperwork in her backpack and catches public transport home. Midway through her journey home, she gets a text message from her friend who asks to meet at the pub. Isla-Mae has several drinks and forgets her backpack. The next morning before the meeting she realises her mistake and is distressed.

Questions to consider based on the case study

1. Which of the four ethical principles has Isla-Mae not considered in her actions?
2. How has Isla Mae acted in a maleficent way?
3. How might Isla Mae approach the situation differently next time?
4. What are the potential consequences of Isla-Mae's actions as a student?
5. What are the potential consequences of Isla-Mae's actions if she was a registered occupational therapist?

8.4.2 Vignette 8.2: Aotearoa New Zealand occupational therapy student visiting an aged care facility

Joyce is first-year undergraduate occupational therapy who attends a placement in an aged care facility. Her occupational therapy supervisor, Ming, appears very busy and is only on site every second day. Ming asks Joyce to spend her time in the common lounge area when she is not on site, with a focus on getting to know the staff and residents. Joyce provides support to Ken, who is using a wheeled walker to move into the living room area. Ken is unsteady on his feet and falls over mid-journey to the sofa. Ken appears unhurt but Joyce calls out for help to get him back on his feet. A care assistant (Pete) comes into the room, sees Ken on the floor and comes over to lift him up from the ground. Pete looks at Joyce, winks, and says, 'You didn't see that', with Ken laughing. Later in the day, Ken complains he is in pain with his hip.

Questions to consider based on the case study:

1. From a perspective of beneficence, in what ways has Ken benefited from Pete or Joyce's actions?
2. What are the consequences (justice) of Joyce not telling other staff that Ken had a fall?
3. What choices (autonomy) did Ken have in the decision-making process?
4. How might Joyce approach the situation differently next time?

8.5 Conclusion

Ethics help health professionals make decisions about what are the right and wrong things to do in both simple and complex situations. Occupational therapists will be faced with making ethical decisions every day of their working lives. All health professionals need a strong theoretical understanding of ethics and how they can be used to support their clinical practice. All occupational therapists should be able to articulate an ethical framework based on ethical principles and then demonstrate practice that meets the expectations of employers and professional and regulatory bodies. In Australia and Aotearoa New Zealand, there are important documents that guide and govern occupational therapy practice – The Australian Health Practitioners Regulatory Agency & National Boards Code of Conduct (2022) and the Code of Ethics for

Occupational Therapists. It is the responsibility of all occupational therapists to have a working knowledge of how these documents apply to their own specific practice context. Occupational therapists need to be fully aware of their legal responsibilities associated with professional registration and other specific legislation that impacts on their practice. There are significant implications if an occupational therapist engages in unethical behaviours, dubious decision making, or illegal practices.

8.6 Summary

- Understanding and upholding ethical principles and relevant laws is critical to the practice of occupational therapy.
- The most common and widely recognised practical implementation of the bioethical principles is the Four Principles Approach.
- Occupational therapists working in Australia and Aotearoa New Zealand have a legal requirement to meet national registration standards to practice occupational therapy. The Occupational Therapy Board of Australia and the Occupational Therapy Board of New Zealand/Te Poari Whakaora Ngangahau o Aotearoa enforce these standards in their respective jurisdictions.
- The Occupational Therapy Board of Australia and Occupational Therapy Board of New Zealand/Te Poari Whakaora Ngangahau o Aotearoa's key role is to protect the public, not to uphold the individual needs of registered occupational therapists.

8.7 Review and reflection questions

- What are the ethical principles that can help guide occupational practice?
- How can a Code of Ethics/Conduct improve ethical practice in occupational therapy?
- What is some legislation that is most relevant to occupational therapy practice?

References

Australian Health Practitioners Regulatory Agency. (2020). *Guidelines for mandatory notifications*. http://www.occupationaltherapyboard.gov.au/Codes-Guidelines/Guidelines-for-mandatory-notifications.aspx

Australian Health Practitioners Regulatory Agency. (2024). *Registration*. Retrieved October 11, 2024, from http://www.occupationaltherapyboard.gov.au/Registration.aspx

Australian Health Practitioners Regulatory Agency and National Boards. (2022). *Code of conduct*. Ahpra. https://www.ahpra.gov.au/Resources/Code-of-conduct/Shared-Code-of-conduct.aspx

Beauchamp, T. L., & Childress, J. F. (2019). *Principles of biomedical ethics* (8th ed.). Oxford University Press.

Bourne, E., Sheepway, L., Pollard, N., Kilgour, A., Blackford, J., Alam, M., & McAllister, L. (2013). Ethical awareness in allied health students on clinical placements: Case examples and strategies for student support. *Journal of Clinical Practice in Speech-Language Pathology*, 15(2), 94–98. https://doi.org/10.1007/s10805-023-09479-3

Bushby, K., Chan, J., Druif, S., Ho, K., & Kinsella, E. A. (2015). Ethical tensions in occupational therapy practice: A scoping review. *British Journal of Occupational Therapy*, 78(4), 212–221. https://doi.org/10.1177/0308022614564770

College of Occupational Therapists of Ontario. (2019). *Critical thinking and professional judgement through an OT lens*. https://www.coto.org/docs/default-source/prep-modules/

prep-module-critical-thinking-and-professional-judgement-through-an-ot-lens-2019.pdf?sfvrsn=81510fff_2

Doherty, R. F. (2023). Ethical practice. In G. Gillen & C. Brown (Eds.), *Willard and Spackman's occupational therapy* (pp. 454–467). Lippincott Williams & Wilkins.

Freegard, H. (2012). Ethics in a nutshell. In H. Freegard & L. Isted (Eds.), *Ethical practice for health professionals* (pp. 11–24). Cengage Learning.

Howard, B. S., Govern, M., Gambrel, A. M., Haney, M., Ottinger, H., Rippe, T. W., & Earls, A. (2023). Encounters with ethical problems during the first 5 years of practice in occupational therapy: A survey. *The Open Journal of Occupational Therapy*, *11*(3), 1–14. https://doi.org/10.15453/2168-6408.2078

Kornblau, B., & Burkhardt, A. (2024). *Ethics in rehabilitation: A clinical perspective.* Routledge.

Kutchins, H. (1991). The fiduciary relationship: The legal basis for social workers' responsibilities to clients. *Social Work*, *36*(2), 106–113. https://doi.org/10.1093/sw/36.2.106

Lohman, H., & Brown, K. (1997). Ethical issues related to managed care: An in-depth discussion of an occupational therapy case study. *Occupational Therapy in Health Care*, *10*(4), 1–12. https://doi.org/10.1080/07380579709168827

McArdle, H., Barlott, T., McBryde, C., Shevellar, L., & Branjerdporn, N. (2023). Navigating ethical tensions when working to address social inequities. *American Journal of Occupational Therapy*, *77*(1), 7701205160. https://doi.org/10.5014/ajot.2023.050071.

Occupational Therapy Registration Board of New Zealand/Te Poari Whakaora Ngangahau o Aotearoa. (2022). *Code of ethics for occupational therapists.* Occupational Therapy Registration Board of New Zealand/Te Poari Whakaora Ngangahau o Aotearoa. https://www.otboard.org.nz/site/ces/codeofethics?nav=sidebar

Occupational Therapy Registration Board of New Zealand/Te Poari Whakaora Ngangahau o Aotearoa. (2024). *Registration.* Retrieved October 11, 2024, from https://www.otboard.org.nz/site/rp/registration?nav=sidebar

Swisher, L. L., & Royeen, C. B. (2019). *Rehabilitation ethics for interprofessional practice: Beyond principles, individualism, and professional silos.* Jones & Bartlett Learning.

VanderKaay, S., Letts, L., Jung, B., & Moll, S. E. (2020). Doing what's right: A grounded theory of ethical decision-making in occupational therapy. *Scandinavian Journal of Occupational Therapy*, *27*(2), 98–111. https://doi.org/10.1080/11038128.2018.1464060

Professional issues

Skills for effective communication in occupational therapy practice

Luke Robinson, Andrea Robinson, Nicole Young, and Krista Lenders

Authors' positionality statement

All authors acknowledge the traditional owners of the land on which they wrote this chapter: Bunurong Country. The authors are from predominantly middle-class families and acknowledge their white privilege. The authors all live in Australia, identify as cisgender, and are part of the Millennial generation. All authors are occupational therapists who bring diverse knowledge and experiences as practitioners, researchers, and educators, and they value effective communication and what this brings to practice. The authors position themselves as aspiring allies to communities of diverse perspectives, including western/non-western, Indigenous, disability, inter/multigenerational, neurodiverse, and LGBTQIAP2S+.

Author notes

- Throughout this chapter we use the word 'client' to capture terms such as patient and service user along with consideration of consumers' families, carers, and support persons. We recognise the complexity that each of these words hold and the preferences of different occupational therapists.
- Again, we use 'verbal' and 'non-verbal' to discuss communication. We recognise the complexity that each of these words hold and the preferences of different occupational therapists, including spoken and non-spoken.

Key terms
- Communication
- Therapeutic use of self
- Therapeutic relationship
- Rapport building
- Teamwork
- Team communication
- Inclusive communication
- Cultural sensitivity

DOI: 10.4324/9781003495666-11

Objectives

This chapter will allow the reader to:

- Articulate the importance of communication in occupational therapy practice
- Describe the communication cycle and define the different types of communication (verbal, non-verbal, and written) involved
- Summarise and apply various strategies and frameworks that can assist therapists in developing and refining verbal, non-verbal, and written communication skills
- Outline strategies to build and enhance the therapeutic use of self in occupational therapy service
- Explain methods to promote effective communication when working with individuals and collectives from diverse backgrounds
- Identify and apply skills, frameworks, and strategies to promote effective communication in health care and professional teams

9.1 Introduction

Communication, the cornerstone of human interactions and the foundation of our social existence, enables us to express our thoughts, feelings, and ideas, fostering understanding, connection, collaboration, and knowledge exchange. Effective communication is crucial for building relationships, resolving conflicts, and achieving personal and professional goals. As occupational therapists, we must communicate using verbal, non-verbal, and written messages, which is essential for the effectiveness of our service provision with clients, their carers or family, colleagues, and other professionals.

Communication is one of the four standards of competent practice expected of Australian occupational therapists (Occupational Therapy Board of Australia [OTBA], 2018). It is embedded within the Aotearoa New Zealand occupational therapy Competencies, specifically *Applying Whakaora Ngangahau Occupational Therapy Knowledge, Skills and Values* for Registration and Continuing Practice for Occupational Therapists in New Zealand (Occupational Therapy Board of New Zealand, 2022). Therefore, it is fundamental for a practising or student occupational therapist to be aware of the purpose of communication, its key elements, and the skills required for appropriate communication when providing, evaluating, or promoting safe and quality occupational therapy services. Further, it is essential to understand and apply the skills required to work within health care or professional teams and use culturally responsive, safe and relevant communication tools and strategies to ensure the best outcomes for individuals or groups receiving occupational therapy services (National Safety and Quality Health Service [NSQHS], 2021).

This chapter explores the key elements and skills required for effective communication in client interactions and in healthcare and professional teams. It also defines and explores the therapeutic use of self when communicating in occupational therapy practice, considerations, and strategies to promote effective and inclusive communication with individuals from diverse backgrounds.

9.2 Defining communication

Human communication is the product of several physiological, psychological, social, and environmental influences (Van Servellen, 2020). It is a complex process involving the purposeful exchange or transmission of information interpreted by one or more individuals or parties (Henderson, 2019). At its core, communication involves the interaction of five fundamental elements: the sender, the message, the transmission medium, the receiver, and feedback (Tamparo & Lindh, 2017).

As demonstrated in the communication cycle presented in Figure 9.1, communication is a two-way process that can involve various methods of *transmission* (for example, spoken, written, or non-verbal) by a *sender* of a *message* to a *receiver* (for example, client, client's family, colleagues). While this view of communication appears straightforward, several factors must be considered. For example, the ability of multiple messages to be transmitted simultaneously through verbal and non-verbal means, or the ability to involve multiple senders and receivers, must be thought through when describing communication (White et al., 2023; Wright et al., 2013).

To ensure open, respectful, and effective communication when providing occupational therapy services, presenting at team meetings and communicating in other professional contexts, it is essential to recognise the two-way nature of communication between the sender and the receiver to ensure mutual understanding (refer to Figure 9.1). Generally, misunderstandings or issues in communication between the sender and receiver in health care settings can result in errors, inappropriate treatment, adverse outcomes, damage to the therapeutic relationship and even permanent disability, or, in extreme cases, death (Iedema et al., 2015; Taylor, 2020). For example, without a mutual understanding during an occupational performance assessment of a functional transfer to communicate concerns about instability, fatigue, or weakness, a client may fall on a therapist, leading to potential injury for both parties. In this example, clarifying any client concerns about feeling unsteady, nauseous, dizzy, or weak

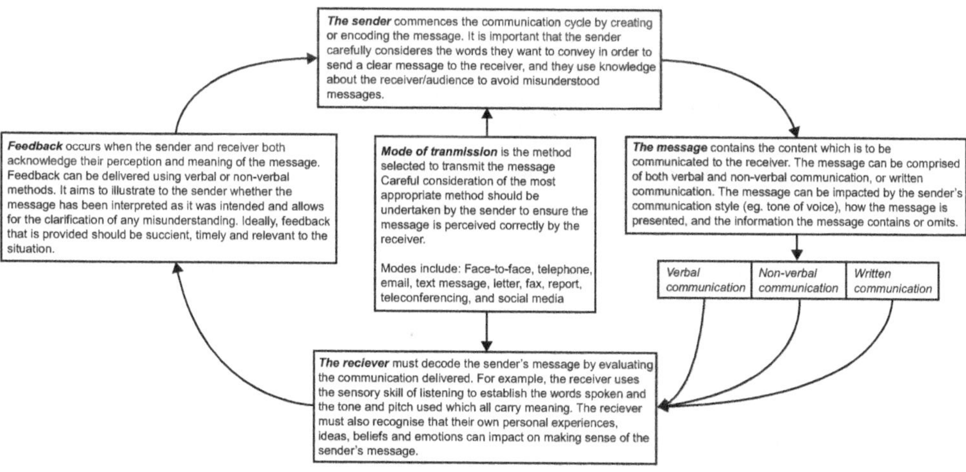

Figure 9.1 The communication cycle

(Adapted from Tamparo & Lindh, 2017)

in the legs or adapting communication to meet the client's needs can help to reach a mutual understanding and avoid injury for both parties.

Further, it is essential to recognise the inherent power imbalance between health care professionals and the individual(s) receiving health care services and their families and/ or carers and the impact this can have on communication (Stevens et al., 2021). Factors that lead to feelings of powerlessness in a health care setting include the removal of independence, social status and responsibility, a lack of information sharing and basic comforts, and inability to express identity (Askew et al., 2021). Occupational therapists must, therefore, employ effective communication skills and strategies to establish, maintain, and conclude therapeutic relationships with clients and relevant parties. This approach can help minimise perceived or actual power imbalances and foster collaborative partnerships (Stevens et al., 2021).

9.3 Types of communication

In occupational therapy practice, three primary types of communication are employed: *verbal*, *non-verbal*, and *written*. *Verbal* communication is crucial in practice and essential for building a therapeutic relationship (O'Brien & Conners, 2024). This communication mode involves using spoken, augmentative and alternative communication (AAC), or sign language to transmit information (Henderson, 2019; McMahon et al., 2024). The construction of phrases, as well as the pitch, tone, volume, and speed of speech, all play a significant role in ensuring the message is effectively conveyed to the recipient and that there is a mutual understanding of the message (O'Toole, 2024).

Non-verbal communication involves messages conveyed through intentional or unintentional gestures and body language that occur alongside or without spoken words (O'Toole, 2024). Broadly, non-verbal communication can be classified into four different categories:

- *Kinesics*: head and body movements (for example, smiling, nodding, leaning postures, facial expressions)
- *Vocalics*: non-linguistic vocal cues (for example, sound pitch, use of appropriate silence)
- *Haptics*: body contact (for example, handshake, appropriate supportive touch)
- *Proxemics*: spatial cues (for example, distance between an occupational therapist and the client) (Bhat & Kumar Kingsley, 2020)

In addition, professional presentation (for example, clothing, name badge, personal hygiene), gestures, and the time and place (for example, a private, quiet environment) of communication can influence how the receiver interprets and understands the message transmitted by the sender (Henderson, 2019). For instance, if a therapist attempts to convey empathy and compassion through verbal communication, but their arms are crossed, and they are consistently glancing at the clock on the wall, the receiver might not perceive the therapist as empathetic or compassionate. Alternatively, if a therapist is showing excessive direct eye contact, it may appear confrontational and, in some circumstances, be considered culturally inappropriate (Purnell, 2018).

Written communication refers to using written sources to communicate information, observations or events (Jordan & Halle, 2023). Written communication can vary from client service records, team meeting agendas or minutes, instructions, reports, and formal or informal notes. In some instances, organisational or legal requirements must be adhered to when using written communication in practice (Ahpra, 2022; OTBNZ, 2022). An example of written communication in occupational therapy service provision is documentation that serves as a record or account of verbal communication with clients and accompanying events (Henderson, 2019). This form of written communication aims to communicate information about a client and/or other involved parties, the rationale for occupational therapy service provision, and a chronological record of outcomes or other significant events (Australian Commission on Safety and Quality in Health Care, 2021; Health Information Standards Organisation – New Zealand, 2018).

9.4 Skills for effective communication

9.4.1 Skill for effective verbal communication

Effective language is crucial to ensure that a message is Clear, Correct, Complete, Concrete, Concise, Considered, and Courteous – an approach referred to as the Seven Cs (Krishna, 2018). In addition to the Seven C's, a message's sender must ensure they use language that safely promotes engagement in the communication cycle (refer to Figure 9.1). For example, rather than a therapist saying to a client: 'I need to see you go to the toilet' as part of an assessment, an alternative could be: 'As part of my occupational therapy assessment, I would like to assess how much you can do for yourself and any risks to your safety when sitting down on and standing up from the toilet. Is it okay if I complete this assessment with you now?' Additional skills to promote responsive and appropriate verbal communication are discussed in Table 9.1.

Occupational therapists can use several client-centred and evidence-based tools to enhance communication during the therapeutic process. One such tool is the Canadian Occupational Performance Measure (COPM), which helps the therapist and client identify key occupational performance issues that are personally important to the client. It also allows clients to self-assess their occupational performance over time (Law et al., 2019). The COPM focuses on self-care, productivity, and leisure occupations, providing therapists with a semi-structured interview schedule and rating scales to collect relevant information while ensuring that the client actively participates in the communication exchange.

An alternative tool for understanding a client's perspective on their occupational performance is the occupational profile (American Occupational Therapy Association [AOTA], 2020). This profile summarises the client's occupational history, experiences, daily living patterns, interests, values, habits, and needs. Through both formal interview techniques and informal conversations, therapists gather information that helps them understand what is meaningful and important to the client. This understanding aids in identifying the client's current occupational performance issues and collaboratively designing occupation-based goals and interventions (AOTA, 2020).

Another tool that could assist in effective verbal communication with clients in health care settings is the Calgary Cambridge Model of History Taking (CCMHT) (Silverman et al., 2013). Although initially designed to take a medical history, this guide can be modified for occupational therapists when constructing an occupational profile or an individual's narrative. Furthermore, it can assist students and therapists in comprehending the fundamental elements of conducting successful communicative cycles by exploring five stages (refer to Table 9.2).

Table 9.1 Skills to promote responsive and appropriate verbal and non-verbal communication

Skill		Description	Purpose
Observation skills		Observing the person(s) in a given environment and noticing their presentation, verbal and non-verbal communication, social skills, tone of voice, behaviour, and motor skills (O'Brien & Conners, 2024).	Useful when gathering information, determining cognitive or physical capacities, or hypothesis testing.
Active listening skills		Non-verbal skills, including body language, facial expression, posture, eye contact, and gestures, should convey interest and understanding (McKenna et al., 2020).	Useful to encourage, build therapeutic relationships and trust, ensure accurately recalled information, convey empathy, and ask relevant questions. Encourages connection and presence in being there with the person.
Questioning skills	Open-ended questions	Verbal questions which give the person(s) answering control over the information provided and allow the therapist to listen, observe and learn (O'Toole, 2024). Typically involve 'who', 'what', 'where', 'when', 'why', or 'how'.	Useful when the information required is not discreet and may need a thorough discussion of memory, elaboration, opinion, detail, and/or description of experiences and feelings. Generally, they are less threatening because they allow the person(s) answering to control the information they provide; however, they may be time consuming or result in unnecessary information.
	Closed-ended questions	Verbal questions used to elicit discrete information that is short, definite, and to the point (O'Toole, 2024). Typically, they result in 'yes', 'no', or concise answers to check or clarify something.	Useful when the required information is discrete or only one answer is desired. These questions demand little of the person(s) and can save time and provide the exact answer without resulting in overthinking or using too many words. However, they can result in incomplete answers that lack detail or wrong conclusions.

(Continued)

Table 9.1 (Continued)

Skill		Description	Purpose
Clarifying and facilitating skills	Reflection	Trying to clarify the thoughts and feelings the person(s) has sent in their message by asking questions to let the person confirm or reject the interviewer's suggestions based on the discussion so far (Curtin et al., 2017).	Useful to explore and share emotions, convey listening and empathy, explore values and beliefs, build a therapeutic relationship, individualise experiences to allow the person(s) to make sense of information, and encourage in-depth exploration of feelings.
	Paraphrasing	Providing a summary or comment of the person(s) own words to show understanding of the message (Curtin et al., 2017).	Useful to confirm understanding and accuracy of information provided, convey empathy, demonstrate active listening, build the therapeutic relationship, and advance the conversation.
	Summarising	Providing a recap or verification of understanding of what the person(s) has said so that both parties are clear at the end of a conversation and to signpost the completion of the interaction (O'Toole, 2024).	Useful to allow the person(s) to correct interpretation or provide further information, build trust and therapeutic relationship, establish future directions and lay the foundation for collaboration. Also, useful during communication when there is a change of theme, or large amounts of information have been shared.
	Clarifying	Verify the person(s) message if it is unclear or needs further elaboration for understanding (Curtin et al., 2017).	Useful to ensure that the interviewer correctly understands the person(s) words, meanings, goals, actions, values or beliefs. Continues to build the therapeutic relationship by deepening trust as feelings are shared and explored.
	Focusing	Helping the person(s) to identify one or more priority issues for exploration and attention (Curtin et al., 2017).	Useful to give the individual control of the agenda, ensure client-centred practice by identifying the client's priorities, allow further information to be gathered and given, and allow for the articulation of values and beliefs.

Table 9.2 Use of the Calgary Cambridge Model of History Taking (CCMHT) with an occupational focus (Adapted from Baptiste, 2017; Silverman et al., 2013)

Stage	Actions
1. Initiate the session	Create a welcoming space that fosters open dialogue, builds genuine connections, and understands the individual's goals and expectations for occupational therapy intervention.
2. Gathering information	Explore the person's occupational profile by considering the environments in which they engage in occupations, personal resources, barriers, and facilitators to occupational performance regarding their health and well-being or use an assessment tool such as the COPM to identify occupational performance issues.
3. Providing structure	Make the therapeutic process and role of an occupational therapist in the given practice setting clear to the person. Ensure that the communication cycle flows logically and comfortably.
4. Building the relationship	Be present with the person and ensure appropriate non-verbal communication is used in response to non-verbal behaviours or cues. Involve the person in the conversation by ensuring open and honest communication. When making plans, ensure they are person-centred and incorporate identified occupational performance issues, barriers, and facilitators relevant to the person. This essential process requires a shared understanding that will result in shared decision-making.
5. Closing the session	Ensure that the communication cycle ends in a timely and respectful manner. Consider asking the client to paraphrase the key points of discussion. Summarise the key points and clearly articulate any plans for further interviews, assessments, and/or interventions as appropriate to the person.

9.4.2 Skills for effective non-verbal communication

In occupational therapy practice, non-verbal communication skills are equally important. Occupational therapists can use various tools to guide effective non-verbal communication. For instance, Egan (1975) created the SOLER model specifically for health care professionals. This model aims to enhance active listening, which involves receiving, interpreting, and responding to spoken and non-verbal messages (Egan, 1975; Weger et al., 2014). The SOLER model provides prompts and considerations to improve communication and has five key components (refer to Table 9.3). In response to several limitations of the SOLER model (for example, cultural appropriateness and practice area considerations), several revisions have been proposed, including SOLVER, which prompts the sender to vary their voice appropriately, and SURTEY, which allows for cultural variations (refer to Table 9.3).

However, it should be noted that many of these models are designed for Western culture and may not fully address the diverse cultural variations and expectations in communication (O'Toole, 2024). Table 9.3 outlines additional skills and considerations to enhance effective non-verbal communication.

When communicating during practice using verbal or non-verbal methods, one must be aware of contextual considerations that may impact how the message is transmitted to the receiver. These include client factors, such as a cognitive, motor, or psychological impairment; environmental factors, such as noise, lighting, or distractions; and ethical considerations, such as the level of privacy available (O'Toole, 2024).

Table 9.3 SOLER and SURTEY models for improving non-verbal communication

Soler *(Egan, 2007)*	*Surtey* *(Stickley, 2011)*
Squarely: sit squarely (opposite) to the other person.*	Sit at an angle to the client.
Open posture: adopt a posture where neither arms nor legs are crossed.	Uncross legs and arms.
Lean towards the other: position the body towards the other person to communicate interest in what they are talking about.**	Relax.
Eye contact: use eye contact to project engagement and interest in a conversation, ensuring it is not confrontational or culturally inappropriate.	Give appropriate touch.
Relax: avoid fidgeting or demonstrating nervousness.	Provide eye contact. Trust your intuition: pay attention to your internal cues.

Notes:

* This position may feel threatening to some people or not feasible due to the environment; therefore, an angle between chairs may be preferred (Egan, 2007).

** This should be done when appropriate and culturally acceptable.

9.4.3 Skills for effective written communication

All written health care communication must be accurate, understandable, well-constructed, succinct, and professional (Australian Commission on Safety and Quality in Health Care, 2021; Health Information Standards Organisation – New Zealand, 2018). High-quality documentation requires dedication, time, and practice (Hammoud et al., 2012; Hay et al., 2020). O'Toole (2024) outlines five steps to create written communication that is accurate, suitable, and of high quality.

1. *Consider the purpose:* The purpose should direct the content and inform the focus, details, and length.
2. *Consider the audience:* The content should be written with the specific audience in mind. For example, other health professionals, compensable bodies such as WorkCover/Accident Compensation Corporation (ACC) (compensation systems for individuals injured at work), or clients. The writer must also ensure that the language used is tailored to the audience, for example, medically focused language or language suitable for people with average literacy levels (Fajardo et al., 2019). Further, the writer should recognise the difference between deficit-based (e.g., the client struggles with poor attention, lacks motivation, and is unable to complete tasks independently) and strength-based language (e.g., the client benefits from structured environments, demonstrates persistence with support, and is developing independence in task completion) and ensure the correct language is used for the specified audience.
3. *Consider ethical requirements:* The content should ensure confidentiality and privacy are maintained as required to protect the rights of those discussed in the communication. This includes the use of artificial intelligence (AI) (Australian Government, 2024; Health Research Council of New Zealand, 2025).

4. *Consider content and organisation:* The content should adhere to the organisation's requirements and the code of conduct for registered health practitioners (for example, the codes outlined by the OTBA, 2018 and the Occupational Therapy Board of New Zealand, 2022). This includes the use of artificial intelligence.
5. *Consider professional writing style:* The writing style should align with the audience, adhere to relevant legal requirements, and be proofread for grammatical and spelling errors. In addition, the writer should consider the appropriateness of abbreviations (for example, when writing a report for a WorkCover or ACC, use the full term 'active range of motion' instead of the abbreviation 'AROM' (Sames, 2015)) and the use of sentence case, avoiding all capital letters to enhance accessibility.

Various other tools and frameworks are available to guide students and therapists in documenting written communication in a structured and organised way (Sames, 2015). One example is the SOAP note format (Gateley, 2024):

Subjective – experiences, personal views, or feelings of a client;
Objective – data from the client encounter such as assessment findings;
Assessment – a synthesis of the subjective and objective evidence; and
Plan – actions to be taken following interaction.

While this format is commonly used in acute and sub-acute settings, the basics for composing notes can be adapted and applied in other ways of recording client care (Gateley, 2024). While the SOAP note format provides one option for the documentation of written information, a therapist must consider the requirements of each practice setting to adhere to legal and organisational requirements.

9.5 Considerations for effective health care communication in Australia and Aotearoa New Zealand

To develop a shared understanding of the fundamental considerations and skills required to implement person-centred, safe communication in health care in Australia and Aotearoa New Zealand, White et al. (2023) developed a framework for enhancing effective health care communication (refer to Figure 9.2). The framework presented depicts six concentric rings, with the outer three capable of independent rotation to create various combinations of factors relevant to specific settings. At the centre are the Core Values, emphasising that health care communication should be equitable, inclusive, evidence-based, collaborative, and reflective. Surrounding this core are two static rings – Tailored Communication and Collaborators – indicating that all elements within these circles are always relevant in health care interactions. The outer three rings – modality, context, and purpose – are designed to rotate, showcasing how different combinations of these aspects must be considered alongside the core principles. While this framework was designed to start conversations to form the foundation of a dialogue about the priorities and key considerations for developing teaching curricula, professional development, and research programmes related to health care communication, it also provides a set of values and considerations specifically for the unique contexts of Australia and Aotearoa New Zealand.

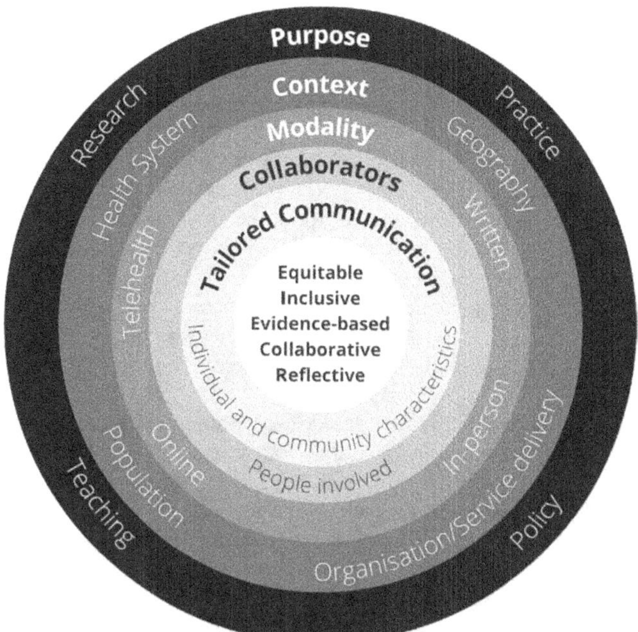

Figure 9.2 Framework for enhancing effective communication in Australia and Aotearoa New Zealand (White et al., 2023)

Use of the framework can be illustrated by considering an occupational therapist supporting a stroke survivor's discharge planning who lives in a remote area. The therapist's communication can be guided by the framework's layers: clarifying the *purpose* (to ensure a safe discharge transition home to a rural area and continuity of care [practice]), considering the *context* (health system processes for transitioning between acute and rural community care with the use of telehealth follow up due to geographical access), and selecting the most effective *modality* (a combination of spoken (telehealth consultation) and online written communication). By collaborating with the client, caregiver(s), and other members of the healthcare team supporting the survivor, the therapist ensures that all information is accurate, coordinated, and meaningful. Through communication that is equitable, inclusive, evidence-based, collaborative, and reflective, the therapist delivers care that is both person centred and responsive to the broader service environment.

9.6 Therapeutic use of self

The therapeutic use of self is a valuable skill that enhances effective communication with clients. This concept dates to the late 1700s during the moral treatment era. It refers to how therapists interact with clients by utilising their own personalities, insights, perceptions, and judgments to motivate clients and facilitate the therapeutic process (AOTA, 2020; Taylor, 2020). In essence, the therapeutic use of self involves paying attention to the client's needs and responding in a way that promotes the client's goals. This is achieved by building a solid therapeutic relationship during the therapeutic process that is underpinned by mutuality and authenticity to ensure that both parties are present, committed, and able to co-participate in a relationship that

Table 9.4 Strategies to build and enhance the therapeutic use of self in occupational therapy service delivery

Skill	*Strategies to build and enhance*
Self-awareness	■ Keep a reflective journal to document your feelings and reactions to life events. Gibbs' (1988) reflective cycle offers one model to help identify strengths and areas for improvement. The Intentional Relationship Model (IRM) can be used to reflect on the therapeutic relationship process (Taylor, 2020). ■ Ask for feedback from consumers and colleagues to understand your strengths and areas for improvement better. ■ Ask for specific feedback about your verbal and non-verbal communication skills.
Developing trust	■ Ensure commitments made are within time frames specified when feasible. ■ Be authentic, honest, and transparent. ■ Do not overpromise outcomes that you cannot deliver. ■ Always maintain confidentiality. ■ Use language that is clear, precise and appropriate. ■ Ensure client-centred practice.
Developing empathy	■ Read stories about others who have been through significant life events. ■ Listen deeply to the life narratives of others. ■ Participate in activities of other cultures. ■ Reflect on the stories of clients, peers, and other people. ■ Participate in a lived-experience activity (i.e., spend time in a wheelchair and experience the barriers and challenges faced). ■ Try to imagine the injury, condition, or circumstances faced from the perspective of the client and/or their family.
Verbal communication	■ Practice and role-play a variety of interviews to gain experience and feedback. ■ Identify the strengths and areas that can form personal goals for development. ■ Ask for feedback from colleagues on your strengths and areas for further development.
Non-verbal communication	■ Observe an occasion of service provision and identify the types of non-verbal skills used (use the CCMHT checklist to guide observation). ■ Practice expressing your emotions without talking. ■ Practice and role-play a variety of interviews to gain experience and feedback. ■ Play charades to tune into your style of non-verbal communication. ■ Ask for feedback on your non-verbal skills during a conversation with peers or colleagues.
Active listening	■ Observe other therapists and recognise the active listening techniques used. ■ Practice and role-play a variety of interviews and try to summarise the key points expressed. ■ Do not always think about the most apparent or practical solution to a problem instead of listening to the client's communication. ■ Aim to stay present within the conversation. ■ Develop techniques to improve listening by setting self-directed goals.
Use of therapeutic modes	■ Be aware of your preferred therapeutic mode(s) and the importance of adapting modes to best suit the needs of a client(s) at each moment. The six modes include empathising, collaborating, encouraging, problem-solving, instructing, and advocating (Taylor, 2020).

facilitates the implementation of professional reasoning (Taylor, 2020; Pendleton & Schultz-Krohn, 2023).

To successfully implement the therapeutic use of self, a therapist must possess self-awareness to allow a mindful examination of their role in the intervention/service delivery process (O'Brien & Conners, 2024). This involves knowledge of one's own behaviour, emotional responses, and the effects that can be projected onto others. Second, they need to learn how to develop trust, provide support, engage in active listening, and empathise by placing themselves in a position to attempt understand the client's experience. This can be achieved by showing genuineness, respect, self-disclosure, and warmth when communicating with clients, all of which assist in developing and sustaining the therapeutic relationship (McKenna, 2017). Table 9.4 provides examples of how to build and enhance the key skills involved in the therapeutic use of self. It is suggested that supervision from a experienced therapist be used to deal with issues that arise when developing the skills of the therapeutic use of self and to provide support, consultation, skill upgrading, and opportunities for further development and feedback on personal awareness in the therapeutic process (Burnard, 2005; McKenna, 2017). In addition, reflective practice is an integral part of this process as it enhances the development of the therapeutic use of self by encouraging individuals to critically evaluate their experiences, emotions, and interactions, leading to greater self-awareness and more effective, empathetic engagement with clients.

9.7 Skills for cross-cultural communication

Many societies worldwide are characterised by cultural, ethnic, and linguistic diversity. Present-day Australia and Aotearoa New Zealand are some of the world's most multicultural and linguistically and ethnoculturally diverse nations. The most recent census data in Australia (ABS, 2021) and Aotearoa New Zealand (Stats NZ, 2024) reported that just under 30% of their populations were born overseas.

In Australia, the 2021 Census reported that there were 300 separately identified languages spoken in Australian homes, including the languages of the Aboriginal and Torres Strait Islander people (with 9.5% of Aboriginal and Torres Strait Islander people reporting speaking one of the 150 Australian Indigenous languages at home) and Australian Sign Language (AUSLAN), an important language for the deaf community. In Aotearoa New Zealand, over 150 spoken languages were reported (including New Zealand Sign Language (NZSL), and after English, the most widely spoken language was te reo Māori (Stats NZ, 2024).

As communication is fundamentally a social process that involves cooperation, negotiation, and exchange of meaning, avoiding or neglecting problems between linguistically and culturally different parties in a multicultural society is impossible if only one party is willing or able to modify their linguistic behaviour (Martin & Nakayama, 2014; Pauwels, 1995). Achieving culturally competent communication involves recognising and valuing the diverse strengths, cultural knowledge systems, lived experiences, and perspectives each individual brings, which influence their communication styles, preferences, and understandings of social structures such as power, privilege, and equity (O'Toole, 2024). Table 9.5 highlights various factors that can improve the likelihood of successful communication in therapeutic relationships or when interacting with individuals and groups from diverse cultural backgrounds.

Table 9.5 Considerations for cross-cultural communication (Adapted from Hazelwood & Shakespeare-Finch, 2011)

Considerations	
Reflect	Apply critical self-awareness by evaluating personal and cultural values, beliefs, and traditions. Be aware of your own cultural biases and tendencies to stereotype.
Learn	Investing time to understand cultural differences and similarities better (for example, cultural sensitivity training, films/books, podcasts, attending cultural experiences). Ask clients about their communication preferences to ensure that interactions are tailored to individual needs, fostering a more comfortable and effective therapeutic relationship.
Respect	Treat all people equally, regardless of difference. Respect should also be given to the environments in which the person lives and works, gender roles, and generational relationships relative to different cultural groups.
Privilege	Explore and understand your own privilege. Maintain confidentiality as a privileged learner of another person's story.
Do no harm	If you do not have the skills and competency to help another person, refer them to someone who can provide appropriate care.
Listening	Demonstrate active listening and be aware of non-verbal communication.
Promote social justice	Do not condone discrimination and ethnocentrism by remaining silent.
Social inclusion	Be aware of and respect the differences between individualist (which places greater value on perceptions of 'self' and 'I'), and collectivist (which places greater value on perceptions of 'we', 'us', or 'the group') cultures.
High- and low-context cultures	Be aware of the differences between high-context (communication is full of implicit meaning; exemplify the value placed on non-verbal communication) and low-context (does not assume shared background knowledge and understanding; almost everything is explained in words) cultures.
Use of interpreters	Use interpreters (preferably face-to-face; otherwise, consider phone interpreters) when indicated. Ensure that you are prepared, ask only a few questions at a time, and direct the communication to the person and not the interpreter to build rapport.

9.8 Skills for inclusive communication

Inclusive language in health care is a powerful way to create equitable, respectful, and accessible environments. It acknowledges and validates diverse identities, experiences, and backgrounds while avoiding terms that may marginalise or exclude individuals (Marjadi et al., 2023). This approach goes beyond simply choosing words, representing a commitment to honouring client dignity and providing person-centred care.

By respecting individual identities, abilities, cultures, and lived experiences, health care providers can foster stronger therapeutic relationships, enhance patient engagement, and deliver more effective care (Braybrook et al., 2023). Inclusive language also challenges traditional power dynamics, breaks down barriers to access, and promotes an environment where everyone feels valued and understood. This thoughtful communication is essential for cultural competency and reflects a growing societal understanding of diversity, equity, and inclusion in health care (Gill et al., 2018). Table 9.6 summarises some considerations for inclusive communication in occupational therapy

Table 9.6 Considerations for inclusive communication

Consideration	
Use neutral language, such as neutral pronouns or terms for significant others.	Use neutral pronouns such as they/them. If your client refers to a significant other as 'they/them' or as a 'partner' or 'friend', use the same words. When appropriate, ask about gender identity and pronouns during your interactions so that patients feel comfortable sharing their information. For example, you might say, 'I want to ensure I am using your name and pronouns correctly. My name XXXXXX, and my pronouns are YYY/yyy. What about you?' When discussing gender history, do so privately and frame your questions clearly and justifiably.
Consider the messages your non-verbal signals might send	When discussing sexual orientation, gender identity, and life preferences, be mindful of the impact of potential non-verbal signals of discomfort. For example, your facial expression or volume/tone of voice may suggest surprise/disapproval or physical expressions such as posture/eye contact shifts may suggest discomfort.
Avoid using negative language that contains euphemisms, is derogatory, or implies only those without a disability or impairment are 'normal' or 'able-bodied'	Avoid framing disability as a limitation (e.g., 'suffers from,' 'disabled,' 'wheelchair-bound,' 'special,' 'normal') unless the community has preference (e.g., deaf community). Instead, consider saying 'child or young person with a disability', 'child or young person who uses a wheelchair for mobility', or 'child or young person without a disability'.
Avoid using language that is not neurodiversity affirming.	Neurodiversity-affirming language encompasses terminology that respects and accurately represents neurodivergent individuals from an objective, strengths-based perspective, rather than emphasising deficits. This approach is crucial when describing or referring to neurodivergent individuals. For example, instead of using terms like 'red flags' or 'symptoms,' one might refer to 'traits.' Rather than saying someone is 'suffering from' a condition, it is more appropriate to state that they 'are' neurodivergent. Terms such as 'obsession' can be replaced with 'special interest' or 'deep interest,' while 'fix' or 'cure' should be substituted with 'support.' Additionally, instead of labelling someone as 'low functioning' or 'high functioning,' it is better to specify that they 'have X and Y support requirements.'
Avoid using language based on assumptions that are inappropriate, discriminatory or offensive.	Don't make assumptions about someone's ancestry based on their physical features.

practice which can be used in conjunction with the People with Disability Australia (2021) and the New Zealand Ministry of Social Development (2021) guides to language about disability and accessibility.

9.9 Skills for team communication and interprofessional practice

Communication is fundamental to effective teamwork in health care and other occupational therapists' professional settings. Effective teams in health care or other professional settings are characterised by trust, respect, collaboration, and open communication (Buljac-Samardzic et al., 2020). The degree of open communication is reflected by a team's ability to communicate accurately and respectfully, with the freedom to express opinions and ask questions.

Poor communication within health care organisations is cited as a significant factor in patient safety incidents (Australian Commission on Safety and Quality in Health Care, 2021). To avoid poor team communication, all health professionals must develop constructive professional behaviours to communicate with clients and other health professionals involved in the service provision process (Henderson, 2019). Several frameworks, such as the *Team Strategies and Tools to Enhance Performance and Patient Safety (TeamSTEPPs)*, have been developed to encourage successful team communication and collaboration (Clancy & Tornberg, 2007). This framework focuses on the importance of team structure by recognising the need for individual roles within the team, a structured process where team members clearly and accurately exchange information, a designated leader(s) who can organise the team and review processes, situation monitoring to maintain awareness to support team functioning, and mutual support amongst team members (King et al., 2008). In addition to the skills explored in this chapter's previous sections, therapists can utilise several tools and strategies to achieve and maintain effective team communication and enhance interprofessional practice.

9.9.1 Briefing, monitoring, and debriefing

Briefings are short sessions before the start of team involvement with a client and provide an opportunity to share the plan, discuss team roles and responsibilities, establish expectations, anticipate outcomes, and consider contingencies (Ryan et al., 2019). A briefing should be viewed as a primer to ensure the team is united and understands individual roles. After a team has begun its collaboration with the client, they may choose to monitor their plan by having a team huddle, which usually is an ad hoc meeting to re-establish situational awareness and review, adjust, and reinforce any plans in place. The monitoring process can occur once or several times during a team's involvement with a client. Following the cessation of the client-team therapeutic relationship, team members can debrief about improving team performance and effectiveness by discussing lessons learnt and reinforcing positive behaviours that lead to team success (Clancy & Tornberg, 2007; Kolbe et al., 2021).

9.9.2 ISBAR

One tool to assist in transferring client information and communicating outstanding issues and tasks to a team within a health care setting is the ISBAR handover tool (Burgess et al., 2020). The tool was initially developed to aid communication by offering

Table 9.7 Explanation and example of the ISBAR acronym

	Step	Considerations and example
I	Identification	Client, staff members *Sarah Jones, a 45-year-old female, admitted to the rehabilitation ward following a right sided stroke.*
S	Situation	Symptoms/problem, patient stability/level of concern *She is currently ten days post stroke, experiencing left-sided weakness and difficulty with daily activities.*
B	Background	History of presentation, date of admission and diagnosis, relevant past medical history *She lives alone in a single-story home, works as an accountant, and was previously independent in all activities. Medical history includes hypertension and type 2 diabetes.*
A	Assessment and Actions	What are the findings of your assessments/impressions of the situation? What have you done so far? ■ *Upper limb function: moderate weakness on the left side, scoring 3/5 strength* ■ *Requires moderate assistance with personal care tasks* ■ *Independent with bed mobility* ■ *Independence in toilet transfers using over-toilet-frame* ■ *Cognitive function intact* ■ *Motivated to return home and work*
R	Responsibility and Referral	What you want to be done, interventions underway or that need monitoring, who is responsible for a review and when it needs to occur, and a plan depending on results/outcomes. ■ *Continue daily OT sessions focusing on upper limb rehabilitation* ■ *Progress ADL training with emphasis on one-handed techniques* ■ *Home assessment scheduled for next week* ■ *Family education sessions are recommended* ■ *Referral to community OT services for work rehabilitation*

a pattern of transferred information, so errors or omissions become clear and avoidable. Use of the ISBAR tool: Identify, Situation, Background, Assessment and Actions, Responsibility and Referral (refer to Table 9.7) has shown to improve team communication substantially and result in fewer adverse events (Thompson et al., 2011). This tool is frequently used in multidisciplinary medical handover meetings in acute, sub-acute, and community settings to ensure a transparent picture of health professional involvement and professional reasoning.

9.9.3 DESC Script and the two-challenge rule

The DESC Script is a template for assertive communication that provides a constructive process for resolving team conflicts (Bower & Bower, 2009). The script: Describe the specific situation or behaviour using concrete data, Express the concerns you have and how the situation makes you feel, Suggest alternatives and seek agreement, and Consequences should be stated in terms of impact on established team goals. Promote a timely discussion that avoids blaming statements and focuses on *what* is right rather than *who* is right (Bower & Bower, 2009).

When information conflicts arise among team members, an alternative communication strategy is the two-challenge rule, implemented using the CUS Script (Pian-Smith et al., 2009). This rule prompts the user to express their concern at least twice, using the CUS script format: 'I am Concerned; this makes me Uncomfortable; this is a Safety issue.' If the initial assertion is disregarded, the concerned individual should repeat the process. If the issue persists or remains unacceptable, they should escalate the matter by speaking with a supervisor or the next person in the chain of command. By employing this strategy, the concerned person ensures that their expressed concern is heard, understood, and acknowledged, even when advocating for a client.

9.10 Conclusion

Effective communication is crucial for delivering occupational therapy services across all professional environments. Occupational therapists must utilise verbal, non-verbal, and written communication when interacting with individuals, their families, groups, and team members. By understanding and applying various skills, strategies, and frameworks, therapists can work towards achieving effective communication with people from diverse backgrounds, different roles in the therapeutic process, and varying levels of occupational performance capabilities.

9.11 Summary

- All occupational therapists are required to possess skills for achieving effective communication.
- Various skills, strategies, and frameworks can assist therapists in developing and refining verbal, non-verbal, and written communication skills that can be used with individuals receiving occupational therapy services and health professional team members.
- Knowledge of and strategies to develop active listening and the therapeutic use of self can assist in the therapeutic process by developing a therapeutic relationship.
- Occupational therapists providing services in Australia and Aotearoa New Zealand work with individuals from diverse cultural backgrounds and need to utilise ways to enhance successful communication and understanding between parties.
- Effective team communication is vital to enhance safety and performance in health care and professional settings.

9.12 Review questions

- What are the five basic elements of the communication cycle?
- What two skills or strategies can assist occupational therapists in achieving effective verbal communication?
- What are four strategies to build and enhance the therapeutic use of self in occupational therapy service delivery?
- What three strategies could occupational therapists consider to ensure effective communication with individuals from culturally and linguistically diverse backgrounds?
- When would an occupational therapist consider using the DESC Script, and what does it promote?

References

American Occupational Therapy Association. (2020). Occupational Therapy Practice Framework: Domain and process (4th ed.). *American Journal of Occupational Therapy*, 74(Supp 2), 7412410010p1–7412410010p87. https://doi.org/10.5014/ajot.2020.74S2001

Askew, D. A., Foley, W., Kirk, C., & Williamson, D. (2021). 'I'm outta here!': A qualitative investigation into why Aboriginal and non-Aboriginal people self-discharge from hospital. *BMC Health Services Research*, 21(1), Article 907. https://doi.org/10.1186/s12913-021-06880-9

Australian Bureau of Statistics. (2021). *Cultural diversity: Census*. ABS. https://www.abs.gov.au/statistics/people/people-and-communities/cultural-diversity-census/latest-release

Australian Commission on Safety and Quality in Health Care. (2021). *National safety and quality health service standards* (2nd ed.). https://www.safetyandquality.gov.au/sites/default/files/2021-05/national_safety_and_quality_health_service_nsqhs_standards_second_edition_-_updated_may_2021.pdf

Australian Government. (2024). *Safe and responsible artificial intelligence in health care – Legislation and regulation review public consultation [Public consultation]*. https://consultations.health.gov.au/medicare-benefits-and-digital-health-division/safe-and-responsible-artificial-intelligence-in-he/supporting_documents/Consultation%20on%20Safe%20and%20Responsible%20AI%20in%20Health%20Care.pdf

Australian Health Practitioner Regulation Agency. (2022). *Code of conduct*. https://www.ahpra.gov.au/docs/default-source/default-document-library/code-of-conduct.pdf

Baptiste, S. (2017). Communication in occupational therapy practice. In M. Curtin, M. Egan, & J. Adams (Eds.), *Occupational therapy for people experiencing illness, injury or impairment: Promoting occupation and participation* (7th ed., pp. 79–89). Elsevier.

Bhat, B. V., & Kingsley, M. K. (2020). Effective non-verbal communication. In S. Parija & B. Adkoli (Eds.), *Effective medical communication* (pp. 39–47). Springer. https://doi.org/10.1007/978-981-15-3409-6_4

Bower, S. B., & Bower, G. H. (2009). *Asserting yourself: Updated edition: A practical guide for positive change*. Hachette.

Braybrook, D., Bristowe, K., Timmins, L., Roach, A., Day, E., Clift, P., Rose, R., Marshall, S., Johnson, K., Sleeman, K. E., & Harding, R. (2023). Communication about sexual orientation and gender between clinicians, LGBT+ people facing serious illness and their significant others: A qualitative interview study of experiences, preferences and recommendations. *BMJ Quality & Safety*, 32(2), 109–120. https://doi.org/10.1136/bmjqs-2022-014792

Buljac-Samardzic, M., Doekhie, K. D., & van Wijngaarden, J. D. H. (2020). Interventions to improve team effectiveness within health care: A systematic review of the past decade. *Human Resources for Health*, 18(1), 2–42. https://doi.org/10.1186/s12960-019-0411-3

Burgess, A., van Diggele, C., Roberts, C., & Mellis, C. (2020). Teaching clinical handover with ISBAR. *BMC Medical Education*, 20(Supp 2), Article 459. https://doi.org/10.1186/s12909-020-02285-0

Burnard, P. (2005). *Counselling skills for health professionals* (4th ed.). Nelson Thornes.

Clancy, C. M., & Tornberg, D. N. (2007). TeamSTEPPS: Assuring optimal teamwork in clinical settings. *American Journal of Medical Quality*, 22(3), 214–217. https://doi.org/10.1177/1062860607300616

Curtin, M., Egan, M., & Adams, J. (2017). *Occupational therapy for people experiencing illness, injury or impairment: Promoting occupation and participation* (7th ed.). Elsevier.

Egan, G. (1975). *The skilled helper: A systematic approach to effective helping*. Brooks/Cole.

Egan, G. (2007). *Skilled helping around the world: Egan's the skilled helper* (8th ed.). Thomson Brooks/Cole.

Fajardo, M. A., Weir, K. R., Bonner, C., Gnjidic, D., & Jansen, J. (2019). Availability and readability of patient education materials for deprescribing: An environmental scan. *British Journal of Clinical Pharmacology*, 85(7), 1396–1406. https://doi.org/10.1111/bcp.13912

Gateley, C. (2024). *Documentation manual for occupational therapy*. Taylor & Francis.

Gibbs, G. (1988). *Learning by doing: A guide to teaching and learning methods*. Oxford Polytechnic.

Gill, G. K., McNally, M. J., & Berman, V. (2018). Effective diversity, equity, and inclusion practices. *Healthcare Management Forum, 31*(5), 196–199. https://doi.org/10.1177/0840470418773785

Hammoud, M. M., Dalymple, J. L., Christner, J. G., Stewart, R. A., Fisher, J., Margo, K., Ali, I. I., Briscoe, G. W., & Pangaro, L. N. (2012). Medical student documentation in electronic health records: A collaborative statement from the Alliance for Clinical Education. *Teaching and Learning in Medicine, 24*(3), 257–266. https://doi.org/10.1080/10401334.2012.692284

Hay, P., Wilton, K., Barker, J., Mortley, J., & Cumerlato, M. (2020). The importance of clinical documentation improvement for Australian hospitals. *Health Information Management Journal, 49*(1), 69–73. https://doi.org/10.1177/1833358319854185

Hazelwood, Z., & Shakespeare-Finch, J. (2011). *I'm listening: Communication for health professionals*. Inn Press.

Health Information Standards Organisation (New Zealand). (2018). *HISO 10065:2018 allied health data standard*. Te Whatu Ora.

Health Research Council of New Zealand. (2025). *2025 artificial intelligence in healthcare application guidelines*. https://gateway.hrc.govt.nz/

Henderson, A. (2019). *Communication for health care practice*. Oxford University Press.

Henderson, S. (2003). Power imbalance between nurses and patients: A potential inhibitor of partnership in care. *Journal of Clinical Nursing, 12*(4), 501–508. https://doi.org/10.1046/j.1365-2702.2003.00757.x

Iedema, R., Piper, D., & Manidis, M. (2015). *Communicating quality and safety in health care*. Cambridge University Press.

Jordan, K., & Halle, A. (2023). Administrative and operational considerations. In S. Dahl-Popolizio, K. Smith, M. Day, S. Muir, & W. Manard (Eds.), *Primary care occupational therapy* (pp. 15–29). Springer. https://doi.org/10.1007/978-3-031-20882-9_3

King, H. B., Battles, J., Baker, D. P., Alonso, A., Salas, E., Webster, J., Toomey, L., & Salisbury, M. (2008). TeamSTEPPS™: Team strategies and tools to enhance performance and patient safety. In *Advances in patient safety: New directions and alternative approaches (Vol. 3: Performance and tools)*. Agency for Healthcare Research and Quality (US).

Kolbe, M., Schmutz, S., Seelandt, J. C., Eppich, W. J., & Schmutz, J. B. (2021). Team debriefings in healthcare: Aligning intention and impact. *BMJ, 374*, n2042. https://doi.org/10.1136/bmj.n2042

Krishna, D. K. (2018). Decoding 7Cs in effective communication. *International Journal of Communication, 28*(1–2), 37–46.

Law, M., Baptiste, S., Carswell, A., McColl, M. A., Polatajko, H., & Pollock, N. (2019). *COPM: Canadian occupational performance measure* (5th ed. rev.). COPM Inc.

Marjadi, B., Flavel, J., Baker, K., Glenister, K., Morns, M., Triantafyllou, M., Strauss, P., Wolff, B., Procter, A. M., Mengesha, Z., Walsberger, S., Qiao, X., & Gardiner, P. A. (2023). Twelve tips for inclusive practice in healthcare settings. *International Journal of Environmental Research and Public Health, 20*(5), 4657. https://doi.org/10.3390/ijerph20054657

Martin, J. N., & Nakayama, T. K. (2014). *Experiencing intercultural communication: An introduction* (5th ed.). McGraw-Hill.

McKenna, J. (2017). Psychosocial support. In M. Curtin, M. Egan, & J. Adams (Eds.), *Occupational therapy for people experiencing illness, injury or impairment*. Elsevier.

McKenna, L., Brown, T., Oliaro, L., Williams, B., & Williams, A. (2020). Listening in health care. In D. L. Worthington & G. D. Bodie (Eds.), *The handbook of listening* (pp. 373–383). Wiley Blackwell. https://doi.org/10.1002/9781119554189.ch25

McMahon, L. F., Shane, H. C., & Schlosser, R. W. (2024). Using occupational therapy principles and practice to support independent message generation by individuals using AAC instead of facilitated communication. *Augmentative and Alternative Communication, 40*(1), 12–18. https://doi.org/10.1080/07434618.2023.2258398

Ministry of Social Development. (2021). *Accessibility guide: Leading the way in accessible information* (3rd ed.). Ministry of Social Development.

O'Brien, J. C., & Conners, B. (2023). *Introduction to occupational therapy* (6th ed.). Elsevier.

Occupational Therapy Board of Australia. (2014). *Code of conduct.* https://www.occupationaltherapyboard.gov.au/Codes-Guidelines/Code-of-conduct.aspx

Occupational Therapy Board of Australia. (2018). *Australian occupational therapy competency standards 2018.* https://www.occupationaltherapyboard.gov.au/codes-guidelines/competencies.aspx

Occupational Therapy Board of New Zealand. (2022). *Competencies for registration and continuing practice for occupational therapists.* https://www.otboard.org.nz/competencies

O'Toole, G. (2024). *Communication e-book: Core interpersonal skills for healthcare professionals.* Elsevier Health Sciences.

Pauwels, A. (1995). *Cross-cultural communication in the health sciences: Communicating with migrant patients.* Macmillan Education Australia.

Pendleton, H. M., & Schultz-Krohn, W. (2023). The Occupational Therapy Practice Framework and the practice of occupational therapy for people with physical disabilities. In H. M. Pendleton & W. Schultz-Krohn (Eds.), *Pedretti's occupational therapy* (pp. 31–66). Elsevier.

People with Disability Australia. (2021). *PWDA language guide: A guide to language about disability* (Version 2). https://pwd.org.au/resources/disability-info/language-guide/

Pian-Smith, M. C. M., Simon, R. D., Minehart, R., Podraza, M., Rudolph, J., Walzer, T., & Raemer, D. (2009). Teaching residents the two-challenge rule: A simulation-based approach to improve education and patient safety. *Simulation in Healthcare, 4*(2), 84–91. https://doi.org/10.1097/SIH.0b013e31818cffd3

Purnell, L. (2018). Cross-cultural communication: Verbal and non-verbal communication, interpretation and translation. In M. Douglas, D. Pacquiao, & L. Purnell (Eds.), *Global applications of culturally competent health care: Guidelines for practice* (pp. 131–142). Springer. https://doi.org/10.1007/978-3-319-69332-3_14

Ryan, S., Ward, M., Vaughan, D., Murray, B., Zena, M., O'Connor, T., Nugent, L., & Patton, D. (2019). Do safety briefings improve patient safety in the acute hospital setting? A systematic review. *Journal of Advanced Nursing, 75*(10), 2085–2098. https://doi.org/10.1111/jan.13984

Sames, K. (2015). *Documenting occupational therapy practice* (3rd ed.). Pearson.

Silverman, J., Kurtz, S. M., & Draper, J. (2013). *Skills for communicating with patients* (3rd ed.). Radcliffe Publishing.

Stats NZ. (2024). *Census results reflect Aotearoa New Zealand's diversity.* https://www.stats.govt.nz/news/census-results-reflect-aotearoa-new-zealands-diversity

Stevens, E. L., Hulme, A., & Salmon, P. M. (2021). The impact of power on health care team performance and patient safety: A review of the literature. *Ergonomics, 64*(8), 1072–1090. https://doi.org/10.1080/00140139.2021.1906454

Stickley, T. (2011). From SOLER to SURETY for effective non-verbal communication. *Nurse Education in Practice, 11*(6), 395–398. https://doi.org/10.1016/j.nepr.2011.03.021

Tamparo, C. D., & Lindh, W. Q. (2017). *Therapeutic communication for health care professionals* (4th ed.). Cengage Learning.

Taylor, R. R. (2020). *The intentional relationship: Occupational therapy and use of self* (2nd ed.). F. A. Davis.

Thompson, J. E., Collett, L. W., Langbart, M. J., Purcell, N. J., Boyd, S. M., Yuminaga, Y., Ossolinski, G., Susanto, C., & McCormack, A. (2011). Using the ISBAR handover tool in junior medical officer handover: A study in an Australian tertiary hospital. *Postgraduate Medical Journal, 87*(1027), 340–344. https://doi.org/10.1136/pgmj.2010.105569

Van Servellen, G. (2020). *Communication skills for the health care professional: Context, concepts, practice, and evidence* (3rd ed.). Jones & Bartlett Learning.

Weger, H., Castle Bell, G., Minei, E. M., & Robinson, M. C. (2014). The relative effectiveness of active listening in initial interactions. *International Journal of Listening, 28*(1), 13–31. https://doi.org/10.1080/10904018.2013.813234

White, S. J., Condon, B., Ditton-Phare, P., Dodd, N., Gilroy, J., Hersh, D., Kerr, D., Lambert, K., McPherson, Z. E., Mullan, J., Saad, S., Stubbe, M., Warren-James, M., Weir, K. R., & Gilligan, C. (2023). Enhancing effective healthcare communication in Australia and Aotearoa New Zealand: Considerations for research, teaching, policy, and practice. *PEC Innovation*, *3*, 100221. https://doi.org/10.1016/j.pecinn.2023.100221

Wright, K. B., Sparks, L., & O'Hair, D. (2013). *Health communication in the 21st century* (2nd ed.). Wiley-Blackwell.

CHAPTER 10

Occupational therapists working with individuals and families

Person-centred and relational occupation-based practice

Simon Leadley, Monica Leo, Jacqui Barfoot, and Priscilla Ennals

Authors' positionality statement

The authors acknowledge the traditional owners of the land on which they wrote this chapter: Bunurong Country, Turrbal and Jagera Country, Wurundjeri. We are from predominantly middle-class families/whānau and Western university educated and acknowledge our white privilege. We currently live in Australia and come from Aotearoa New Zealand and Australia, with European and Asian ancestries. We identify as cisgender and aspire to ally with the 2SLGBTTQQIA community. Authors acknowledge we are primarily from GenX. We are occupational therapists who bring diverse knowledge and experiences and value collaborative relational practice, occupational justice, human rights, and the contribution this brings to practice.

Key terms
- Person-centred
- Family-centred
- Collaboration
- Relationship-focused
- Cultural safety
- Rights-based
- Self-determination
- Equity
- Contextual relevance

Objectives
This chapter will allow the reader to:

- Develop an understanding of what person-centred, family-centred, and collaborative relationship-focused practice is and why it matters in occupational therapy practice.

DOI: 10.4324/9781003495666-12

- Outline some approaches to support person-centred, family-centred, and collaborative relationship-focused practice.
- Demonstrate application of person-centred, family-centred, and collaborative relationship-focused practice to support people to participate in occupations.
- Identify barriers to implementing person-centred, family-centred, and collaborative relationship-focused practice and how to navigate these issues.

10.1 Introduction

Person and family-centred, collaborative relationship-focused practice is an emerging yet vital concept in occupational therapy and broader health care. This approach requires occupational therapists to be mindful and self-aware, considering their values, beliefs, attitudes, biases, and privilege, and how these influence therapeutic relationships with individuals, whānau/mob/families, groups, and communities (de las Heras de Pablo & Muñoz, 2024; Egan & Restall, 2022).

This practice is crucial as it aligns with occupational therapy tenets such as partnership, hope, respect, compassion, and fostering positive therapeutic relationships aimed at achieving equitable occupational outcomes. It effectively supports occupational therapy goals, empowering individuals to participate fully in occupations and communities, benefiting their health and wellbeing (de las Heras de Pablo & Muñoz, 2024; Egan & Restall, 2022).

This chapter explores key elements of person/family-centred and collaborative relationship-focused practice, its alignment with occupational therapy, particularly in Aotearoa New Zealand and Australia, the shift from client-centred to person and family-centred practice, supporting models and approaches, illustrative vignettes, and potential facilitators and barriers to implementation.

10.2 What is person/family-centred and collaborative relationship-focused practice?

Person and family-centred practice places the person, whānau/mob/family, group, or community at the centre of the therapeutic relationship. Collaborative relationship-focused practice considers the therapist's positionality and its influence on therapeutic partnerships. It also acknowledges the economic, political, cultural, and social systems impacting engagement in meaningful occupations and emphasises building equitable, authentic relationships (Egan & Restall, 2022). This aligns with humanist philosophy and ethical values, promoting autonomy, dignity, collaboration, and agency.

Recognised as best practice in occupational therapy (Bourke-Taylor et al., 2024; Egan & Restall, 2022), person and family-centred practice values the strengths, choices, and decisions of the person or whānau/mob/family. It involves collaboration as equal partners in therapy, moving beyond an individual approach to include family and community contexts. Terms like 'patient' or 'client' are replaced with 'individual', 'person', 'whānau/mob/family', 'groups', or 'community' (Egan & Restall, 2022).

A key aspect of this approach is focusing on the quality and dynamics of the therapist-person/family relationship. Therapists must ensure clear communication (e.g., active listening processes, professional record keeping), professional behaviour, ethical and culturally safe practice, and adherence to best practices. They should support

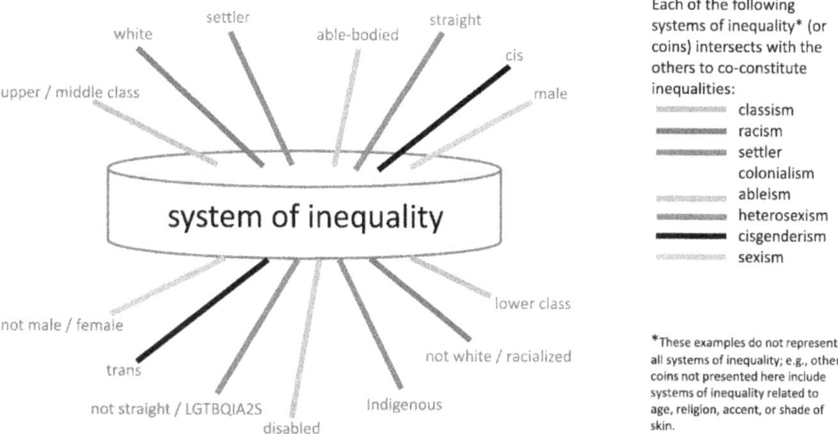

Figure 10.1 The coin model of privilege and critical allyship

(Nixon, 2019)

people's autonomy and agency, address power dynamics, and be mindful of their positionality, biases, and privilege to achieve the best outcomes (de las Heras de Pablo & Muñoz, 2024; Egan & Restall, 2022).

Occupational therapists must recognise historic and ongoing inequities faced by people with disabilities, Indigenous peoples, migrants, refugees, the 2SLGBTTQQIA community, and those living in poverty. They should be allies in support of change to achieve equity in society (Egan & Restall, 2022). Therapists should examine their biases and privileges to enhance equitable outcomes, challenging assumptions and understanding structural factors that influence participation in occupations, and therapeutic relationships. For example, if someone is late or disagrees with a recommendation, therapists should consider factors like socioeconomic status, cultural misunderstandings, stressors, feeling unheard, or past negative experiences in the health system. Refer to Figure 10.1 (Nixon, 2019), which underscores the need for occupational therapists to reflect on their biases, privileges, and attitudes to foster equitable outcomes through a person/family-centred and collaborative relationship-focused approach.

10.2.1 Why a person/family-centred, collaborative relationship-focused approach is important for occupational therapy practice

Person/family-centred, collaborative relationship-focused approaches are foundational in occupational therapy, prioritising the unique needs, preferences, and values of individuals, whānau/mob/families, collectives, and their support networks. These approaches recognise the person or collective as experts in their own lives, emphasising lived experiences, shared decision-making, equitable partnerships, co-design principles, strengths-based approaches, and fostering shared power, mutual respect, and competence.

While occupational therapy values vary and are influenced by cultural and contextual factors (Thomas et al., 2019), professional values such as holism, person-centred care, respect for autonomy, cultural safety, and the transformative power of meaningful occupations align with person/family-centred, collaborative relationship-focused practices (Egan & Restall, 2022; Hooper & Wood, 2024). Relational practice is integral to building trust and rapport to address occupational performance and participation goals within broader social, cultural, political, institutional, and physical contexts (Egan & Restall, 2022).

This approach is recommended as best practice, supporting optimal occupational participation and performance by focusing on needs and enabling agency in the therapeutic process. Practices like trauma-informed care, family-centred practice (FCP), and the recovery approach align with collaborative principles, respecting autonomy, fostering partnerships, collaboration, empowerment, hope, and ensuring safety (Barbic & Glowacki, 2024; Bourke-Taylor et al., 2024; Connor, 2024; Egan & Restall, 2022).

10.2.2 What are the key principles of person/family-centred and collaborative relationship-focused practice?

Key principles consistent with a person/family-centred and collaborative relationship-focused practice include taking account of context, cultural humility and safety, awareness of practitioner's own positionality, active listening and safe communication, respect for autonomy and self-determination, and equitable collaboration and partnerships. The key aspects of a relationship-focused practice approach, as outlined in the Canadian Model of Occupational Performance (CanMOP), are portrayed in Figure 10.2, and the primary principles involved in person/family-centred and collaborative relationship-focused practice described in more depth in Table 10.1. Collaborative relationships are nuanced, support safety and self-determination, and are contextualised, meaning that therapists are attuned to the needs of individuals and communities, from their perspective, and that a shared understanding of need and context builds over time (Egan & Restall, 2022).

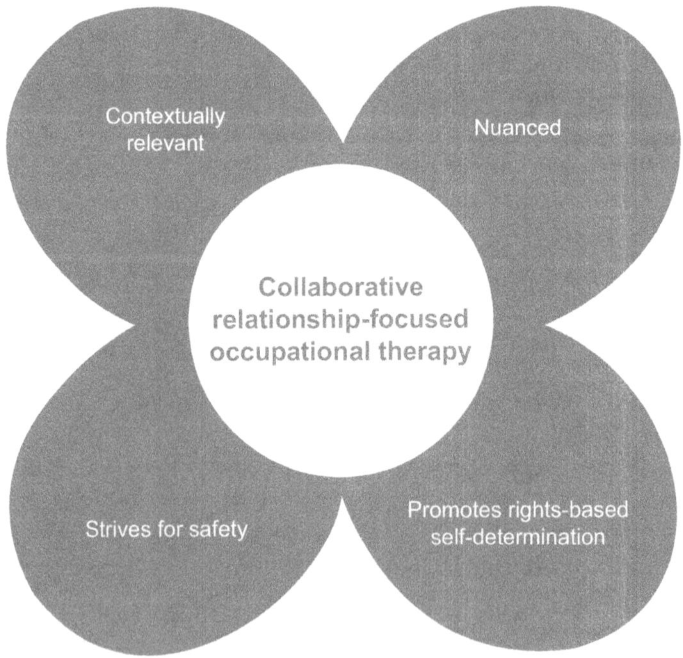

Figure 10.2 Key characteristics of relationship-focused practice

(Restall & Egan, 2022, p. 101)

Table 10.1 Primary principles involved in person/family-centred and collaborative relationship-focused practice

Principle	Description
Awareness of one's own positionality, power, and context	Therapists are critically aware of their own identities, power, privilege, and biases and that of the system in which any service is offered. Efforts are made to foster people's ability to exercise their power and to reduce power inequalities. Therapists are alert to the fact that choices and possibilities may be constrained by social contexts and inequalities (Egan & Restall, 2022).
Cultural humility and curiosity, and cultural safety	Therapists recognise their own world views and how dominant perspectives shape institutions. They remain open to diverse world views (Egan & Restall, 2022). Cultural safety involves critically examining power dynamics and acknowledging colonial impacts on health and social outcomes, especially for Indigenous peoples. It goes beyond cultural awareness to actively address inequities (Curtis et al., 2019).
Seeking to understand the practice context and wider social context	Therapists consider social determinants and systemic factors impacting individuals, families, and communities (Restall et al., 2022). They address inequities in their practice. For example, when supporting employment goals, therapists examine how historical, social, economic, and political structures affect work opportunities, self-worth, and engagement.
Active listening and safe, professional communication	Therapists genuinely listen to and understand nuanced perspectives, ensuring people feel heard and respected. They use effective communication to provide accessible information and support understanding. Recognising language's role in safety and inclusivity, therapists use respectful and humble language, both verbally and nonverbally (Egan & Restall, 2022). For example, using familiar language communicates respect and supports informed choices and consent (Restall et al., 2022).
Striving for safety	To prevent harm, therapists must avoid errors, omissions, and inappropriate interventions. Emotional safety is ensured through deep listening, curiosity, positionality awareness, and trauma-informed principles (Egan & Restall, 2022). Therapists should prioritise people's needs and be vigilant about boundary violations. Effective supervision helps prevent unconscious boundary violations. Parallel process describes how supervisor-practitioner dynamics mirror practitioner-person relationships (Prasko et al., 2024). Supportive supervision fosters nurturing, collaborative relationships, enhancing outcomes through relational quality (Prasko et al., 2024).
Respect for autonomy and self-determination	Rights-based self-determination involves applying rights, equity, and justice lenses (Restall et al., 2022), in line with the Universal Declaration of Human Rights (United Nations, 1948). Respecting people's life choices can challenge therapists when perspectives clash with their values, or policies. For example, differing views on risk may arise if a person prefers to be discharged home despite safety concerns.
Equitable collaboration and partnerships	Therapists prioritise connection to understand individuals, families, and collectives, focusing on their aspirations and concerns. Actions are based on shared knowledge and respect for self-determination (Restall et al., 2022). This approach values mutual competence, combining personal skills and experiences with professional expertise to achieve meaningful goals.

10.2.3 History of the development of 'client-centred practice' to 'person/family-centred collaborative relationship-focused practice' in occupational therapy

Since occupational therapy's inception, building a relationship with the person, family or group, and understanding what values and occupations are meaningful to them have been core principles of the therapeutic approach (Egan & Restall, 2022). Table 10.2 details the historical development of these core principles towards person/

Table 10.2 Timeline of development of 'client-centred practice' to 'collaborative relationship-focused practice' in occupational therapy

Period	Events
1983	The first client-centred practice guidelines were published in 1983 by the Department of National Health and Welfare and the Canadian Association of Occupational Therapists, focusing on client strengths and active participation. The Occupational Performance Model (Reed & Sanderson, 1983) placed the 'individual' at the centre.
1990s	Further clarification on guidelines for occupation-specific client-centred practice included: ■ Collaborative client assessments ■ Focus on client-identified priorities ■ Emphasis on autonomy, partnership, and accessibility ■ Importance of active participation in goal-setting.
2000–2010	The Canadian Model of Occupational Performance (CMOP) was published in 1997, updated in 2000, and further revised in 2007 and 2013 as the Canadian Model of Occupational Performance and Engagement (CMOP-E). Key features include: ■ Respect for client values, knowledge, abilities, and experiences ■ The right to make choices reflecting their needs ■ Collaborative goal setting and outcome measures (Townsend & Polatajko, 2013) ■ The Kawa model was developed and framed the therapist-person relationship as culturally nuanced, subjective, and based on non-western (Japanese and collectivist) worldviews (Iwama & Matsubara, 2024).
2010–2020	Client-centred practice was endorsed by the World Federation of Occupational Therapists in 2010. Emerging themes included: ■ Recognition of power structures in therapist-client relationships ■ Awareness of social, political, and institutional influences on relationships ■ Criticism of 'client-centred' terminology and the omission of the therapist's role and relational context in current models. Updates to models like the Model of Human Occupation (MOHO) incorporate principles of person-centred practice, such as collaborative goal setting (Taylor & Kielhofner, 2017).
2022	The newly developed Canadian Model of Occupational Participation emphasised collaborative, relationship-focused practice and shifted the focus from occupational performance to participation. It highlighted historical and structural inequities affecting outcomes and reinforced the need for therapists to develop contextually relevant, nuanced, safe, and rights-based relationships with individuals, families, groups, and collectives (Egan & Restall, 2022).

Note: Refer to Chapter 25 for more information on CanMOP.

family-centred and collaborative relationship-focussed practice and extends these ideas to consider the broader contextual factors that impact opportunities for individuals or collectives to engage in occupations.

10.2.4 Occupational therapy frameworks and approaches that support person/family-centred and collaborative relationship-focused practice

Occupational therapy practice utilises various models and approaches to support person/family-centred and collaborative relationship-focused practice. Table 10.3 summarises evidence-informed occupational therapy models incorporating these approaches.

Table 10.3 Occupational therapy models/approaches that support person/family-centred and collaborative relationship-focused practice

Approach	Description of how it relates to person/family-centred collaborative relational practice	How this aligns with occupational therapy practice
CanMOP/ Collaborative relationship-focused practice (Egan & Restall, 2022)	▪ Expands person/family-centred practice to build relationships promoting safety, rights, and self-determination ▪ Recognises relationships as contextually and temporally nuanced ▪ Promotes justice, equity, and human rights ▪ Starts with the therapist acknowledging their role in the relational context of therapy	▪ Raises awareness of the therapist's social positionality, beliefs, and systemic context, and their influence on therapy ▪ Considers the individual's or collective's therapy needs, emphasising broader factors affecting engagement in meaningful occupations
Kawa Model (Iwama & Matsubara, 2024)	▪ Developed by Japanese occupational therapists to provide a non-western, collectivist, subjective, and holistic model, with a culturally responsive approach to achieving occupation and well-being goals	▪ Promotes a culturally safe, narrative-based therapeutic relationship with a person/family/collective, to enhance participation in occupations and wellbeing based on their cultural worldview
Model of Human Occupation (MOHO) (Taylor & Kielhofner, 2017)	▪ Emphasises the interaction between volition (personal values, beliefs, interests and motivations), habituation (roles, habits and routines), performance capacity (abilities), occupational identity/ competence/adaptation, and the environment. Each of these impacts how an individual engages in meaningful occupations	▪ Uses strategies like validation, negotiation, coaching, and support to enable change ▪ Empowers individuals/groups to participate in goal setting and intervention planning
Occupational performance coaching (Graham et al., 2020)	▪ Prioritises personal agency ▪ Builds high-trust partnerships through mindful listening, non-judgmental acceptance, and authentic empathy ▪ Sets meaningful goals, promoting autonomy, relatedness, and competence	▪ Prioritises building high-trust partnerships ▪ Emphasises deep listening to understand and engage with the person's (child, parent/s, guardian) needs, enhancing their abilities and capacity

(Continued)

Table 10.3 (Continued)

Approach	Description of how it relates to person/family-centred collaborative relational practice	How this aligns with occupational therapy practice
Intentional Relationship Model (IRM)	■ Sustains helpful relationships with individuals/families/groups using collaborative and reflexive communication ■ Frames the therapeutic relationship through 'Interpersonal events' (e.g., strong emotions) and 'Interpersonal characteristics' (e.g., communication style) ■ Promotes therapeutic modes: advocating, collaborating, empathising, encouraging, instructing, and problem-solving (de las Heras de Pablo & Muñoz, 2024)	■ Helps therapists understand the impact of their interactions on the therapeutic relationship ■ Offers strategies to enhance and sustain a positive therapeutic relationship
Therapeutic use of self	■ Deliberately applies the therapist's skills and experiences to maximise occupational outcomes for individuals, families, and groups ■ Focuses on person/family/group-centred care, shared decision-making, and collaborative processes, while addressing power imbalances and sharing power (de las Heras de Pablo & Muñoz, 2024; Gillen, 2024)	■ Utilises problem-solving, rapport building, motivation, empathy, mutuality, reciprocity, active listening, co-creation, storytelling, respect, hope, trust, and safety ■ Requires practitioners to practice self-awareness

Note: Refer to Chapter 25 for more information on models of practice.

This approach is crucial across the life course, from infancy to older adulthood. For example, in early life, family-centred and relational approaches shift focus from child-practitioner relationships to strengthening parent-child dynamics, increasing family involvement, and enhancing children's skills and participation in occupations, especially with disabilities (Barfoot et al., 2024; Bourke-Taylor et al., 2024). Vignette One showcases this approach with a child and their parent. Throughout all life stages and professional fields, promoting positive relationships and a collaborative occupational therapy style is valued and supported by evidence (de las Heras de Pablo & Muñoz, 2024; Egan & Restall, 2022). Vignette Two highlights this approach in an adult mental health setting, achieving positive outcomes for the individual and their whānau/family.

10.2.4.1 Vignette 10.1: Child-parent intervention using a family-centred
collaborative relationship-focused approach

Shelly, a 20-month-old girl with cerebral palsy, had been receiving occupational therapy since she was six months old. Jane, Shelly's mother, struggled with the home programme due to Shelly's distress. Recognising the developmental approach wasn't effective, the therapist referred them to another therapist using a collaborative relational approach.

The new therapist explored Jane's parenting values, aiming for Shelly's independence and support. Jane shared that Shelly's distress – hair pulling and headbanging – made therapy difficult. They set goals: boosting Shelly's confidence in movement, expanding her diet, and using the standing frame without distress.

The therapist filmed Jane playing with Shelly and reviewed the footage together, noting Shelly's subtle cues. Over five sessions, they enhanced Jane's ability to understand and respond to Shelly's signals, improving their interactions and reducing distress. This made daily activities smoother. Shelly progressed significantly using single words, crawling, and engaging in pretend play. Her distress behaviours decreased, and Jane found it easier to read and respond to Shelly's needs.

This vignette highlights the value of relationship-based practices in family-centred care, enhancing developmental progress and strengthening the parent's ability to support their child in daily activities.

10.2.4.2 Vignette 10.2: Adult mental health using a collaborative relationship-focus practice approach

As a kaiwhakaora ngangahau/occupational therapist in Aotearoa New Zealand, I worked with many tangata whaiora (individuals receiving mental health care) in a secure mental health forensic unit. Despite institutional barriers, we maintained a person/family-centred, collaborative, strengths-based, and culturally safe approach.

One young man, Aleki, from Samoa, was admitted after experiencing bipolar disorder and unsafe behaviour leading to his arrest. As part of the occupational therapy and interdisciplinary team (IDT), I met Aleki in a time and space of his choice, giving him control over the process. Using the culturally responsive Kawa model, Aleki shared his story, strengths, and ambitions, such as returning to rugby, education, and family life.

With Aleki's permission, we connected him to a Pasifika health service, supporting his recovery journey. This approach facilitated Aleki's return to his family, tertiary education, and eventually paid employment.

10.2.5 Barriers to implementing person/family-centred and collaborative relationship-focused practice and how to navigate these issues

Several factors influence person/family-centred, collaborative relationship-focused practice. At the micro level, individual or collective values, beliefs, cultural influences, age, gender, language preferences, socio-economic status, cultural or religious beliefs, and experiences of trauma or discrimination need to be considered. Also important are the therapist's training in person/family-centred, collaborative, culturally competent approaches, and their own context and wellbeing (Egan & Restall, 2022).

At the macro level, government policies, funding, laws, and healthcare regulations can impact therapists' ability to work collaboratively. Western health systems often follow a biomedical model that can create power imbalances. Inconsistent definitions of collaborative practice also pose practical challenges (Lage et al., 2024). Codes of Ethics from the Occupational Therapy Board of New Zealand (2022) and Occupational Therapy Australia (2014) offer guidelines on person/family-centred, collaborative relationship-focused practice.

Given these challenges, occupational therapists should engage in reflective practices like individual and group supervision, and self-reflection. Reflective supervision involves a trusting relationship with a skilled peer, colleague, or supervisor, allowing open discussion without fear of judgment (Dancza et al., 2022). Critical reflexivity involves questioning how practice is influenced by professional discourses and social, political, and economic forces and requires attention to these broader factors (Egan & Restall, 2022).

Reflective practices enhance therapists' ability to work collaboratively and build relationships. This includes reflecting on privilege, beliefs, communication styles, and systemic factors. Self-awareness fosters authentic partnerships (Egan & Restall, 2022). Reflective supervision helps therapists explore motivations and alignment to values. Developing person/family-centred, collaborative relationship-focused practice skills requires ongoing learning. Reflection areas include:

- Effective practices and challenges
- Impact of actions or inactions on interactions
- Managing positional power
- Engaging with cultural humility or safety
- Use of language and attention to context (Dancza et al., 2022)

10.3 Conclusion

This chapter explored the evolution and importance of collaborative relationship-focused practice in occupational therapy. It emphasises therapists' self-awareness, positionality, and reflection on power dynamics, values, and systemic influences. The approach involves partnering with individuals, whānau/mob/families, groups, and communities to address barriers to participation in occupations, and to promote self-determination and equity. Embracing this practice helps therapists challenge inequities, foster cultural safety, and ensure their work is responsive, relevant, and meaningful.

10.4 Summary

- Person/family-centred collaborative relationship-focused practice in occupational therapy is evolving and is now considered best practice.
- It centres on the person, family, or community, honouring their preferences, autonomy, and self-determination, and prioritises compassionate, hopeful relationships.
- Working relationally requires therapists to build self-awareness, be mindful of power, privilege, and biases, and maintain curiosity about those they support. This approach is contextually relevant, nuanced, safe, promotes rights-based self-determination, and addresses historical and structural inequities.
- Supportive spaces for reflection, like supervision, aid in developing self-awareness.

10.5 Review and reflection questions

- How might your perspectives, experiences, and positionality influence your clinical/professional practice?
- How would you explain collaborative relationship-focused practice and its key principles?
- What values, knowledge, and skills help you foster collaborative, respectful, and competent therapeutic relationships?
- What factors or barriers might affect implementing a person/family-centred, collaborative relationship-focused approach, and how would you navigate these challenges?

References

Barbic, S., & Glowacki, K. (2024). Recovery model. In G. Gillen & C. Brown (Eds.), *Willard & Spackman's occupational therapy* (14th ed., pp. 632–646). Wolters Kluwer.

Barfoot, J., Meredith, P., Whittingham, K., & Kerley, L. (2024). Including a relationship-focus in paediatric occupational therapy interventions: Introducing the PAIR Model. *Journal of Occupational Therapy, Schools, & Early Intervention, 17*(2), 331–347. https://doi.org/10.1080/19411243.2023.2203416

Bourke-Taylor, H., Sim, S. S., & Rassafiani, M. (2024). An occupational therapy perspective on families, occupation, health, and disability. In G. Gillen & C. Brown (Eds.), *Willard & Spackman's occupational therapy* (14th ed., pp. 180–198). Wolters Kluwer.

Connor, E. (2024). Providing occupational therapy services for persons with childhood trauma. In G. Gillen & C. Brown (Eds.), *Willard & Spackman's occupational therapy* (14th ed., pp. 1197–1212). Wolters Kluwer.

Curtis, E., Jones, R., Tipene-Leach, D., Walker, C., Loring, B., Paine, S.-J., & Reid, P. (2019). Why cultural safety rather than cultural competency is required to achieve health equity: A literature review and recommended definition. *International Journal for Equity in Health, 18*(1), 174–181. https://doi.org/10.1186/s12939-019-1082-3

Dancza, K., Volkert, A., & Tempest, S. (2022). *Supervision for occupational therapy: Practical guidance for supervisors and supervisees.* Taylor & Francis.

de las Heras de Pablo, C. G., & Muñoz, J. P. (2024). Therapeutic relationships and person-centered collaboration: Applying the Intentional Relationship Model. In G. Gillen & C. Brown (Eds.), *Willard & Spackman's occupational therapy* (14th ed., pp. 468–481). Wolters Kluwer.

Egan, M., & Restall, G. (2022). Collaborative relationship-focused occupational therapy. In M. Egan & G. Restall (Eds.), *Promoting occupational participation: Collaborative relationship-focused occupational therapy. 10th Canadian occupational therapy guidelines* (pp. 97–117). Canadian Association of Occupational Therapists.

Gillen, G. (2024). Occupational therapy interventions for individuals. In G. Gillen & C. Brown (Eds.), *Willard & Spackman's occupational therapy* (14th ed., pp. 343–365). Wolters Kluwer.

Graham, F., Kennedy-Behr, A., & Ziviani, J. (2020). *Occupational performance coaching: A manual for practitioners and researchers.* Taylor & Francis.

Hooper, B., & Wood, W. (2024). A philosophy of occupational therapy. In G. Gillen & C. Brown (Eds.), *Willard & Spackman's occupational therapy* (14th ed., pp. 38–53). Wolters Kluwer.

Iwama, M. K., & Matsubara, A. (2024). The Kawa (river) model. In G. Gillen & C. Brown (Eds.), *Willard & Spackman's occupational therapy* (14th ed., pp. 599–616). Wolters Kluwer.

Kinsella, N., Pentland, D., & McCormack, B. (2022). How context influences person-centred practice: A critical-creative case study examining the use of research evidence in occupational therapy with people living with dementia. *Scandinavian Journal of Occupational Therapy, 30*(3), 398–414. https://doi.org/10.1080/11038128.2022.2119162

Lage, C. R., Wright, S., Monteiro, R. G. S., Aragao, L., & Boshoff, K. (2024). Collaborative practice with parents in occupational therapy for children: A scoping review. *Australian Occupational Therapy Journal, 71*(5), 833–850. https://doi.org/10.1111/1440-1630.12974

Nixon, S. A. (2019). The coin model of privilege and critical allyship: Implications for health. *BMC Public Health, 19*(1), 1637–1650. https://doi.org/10.1186/s12889-019-7884-9

Occupational Therapy Australia. (2014). *Code of ethics.* https://otaus.com.au/publicassets/73509493-3865-ed11-9475-005056be13b5/OTA%20Code%20of%20Ethics.pdf

Occupational Therapy Board of New Zealand. (2022). *Code of ethics for occupational therapists.* https://otboard.org.nz/document/6150/7569%20OTBNZ%20%E2%80%93%20Code%20of%20Ethics.pdf

Prasko, J., Liska, R., Krone, I., Vanek, J., Abeltina, M., Sollar, T., Gecaite-Stonciene, J., Jurisova, E., Juskiene, A., Bite, I., & Ociskova, M. (2024). Parallel process as a tool for supervision and therapy: A cognitive behavioral and schema therapy perspective. *Neuroendocrinology Letters, 45*(2), 107–126.

Reed, K., & Sanderson, S. (1983). *Concepts of occupational therapy* (2nd ed.). Lippincott, Williams and Wilkins.

Restall, G., Egan, M., Valavaara, K., Phenix, A., & Sack, C. (2022). Canadian occupational therapy inter-relational practice process framework. In M. Egan & G. Restall (Eds.), *Promoting occupational participation: Collaborative relationship-focused occupational therapy. 10th Canadian occupational therapy guidelines* (pp. 119–150). Canadian Association of Occupational Therapists.

Taylor, R. R., & Kielhofner, G. (2017). Introduction to the Model of Human Occupation. In R. R. Taylor (Ed.), *Kielhofner's Model of Human Occupation* (5th ed., pp. 3–10). Wolters Kluwer.

Thomas, Y., Seedhouse, D., Peutherer, V., & Loughlin, M. (2019). An empirical investigation into the role of values in occupational therapy decision-making. *The British Journal of Occupational Therapy, 82*(6), 357–366. https://doi.org/10.1177/0308022619829722

Townsend, E. A., & Polatajko, H. J. (2013). *Enabling occupation II: Advancing an occupational therapy vision for health, well-being, & justice through occupation* (2nd ed.). CAOT Publications ACE.

United Nations. (1948). *Universal declaration of human rights (UDHR)*. https://www.un.org/en/about-us/universal-declaration-of-human-rights

Occupational therapists working with groups, families/Whānau, communities/mob, and populations

Kate Gledhill, Darren Mills, Simon Leadley, and Yvonne Thomas

Authors' positionality statement

We are Western-educated occupational therapists with postgraduate qualifications working in leadership positions in Australia and New Zealand. We are white, cisgender, able-bodied, and English-speaking and acknowledge our white privilege, our Global North outlook, and the impacts of colonisation on Indigenous people of both countries. We support decolonisation, racial equality, queer inclusivity, cultural sensitivity, social and occupational justice, and gender-affirmative and culturally safe and responsive health care and education.

Key terms
- Groups
- Group facilitation
- Families
- Community
- Population-based practice

Objectives
This chapter will allow the reader to:

- Define group, family, community, and population-based practice
- Recognise the different dimensions of family and culture
- Describe examples of occupational therapy practice with groups of people communities and populations
- Understand group theory and dynamics
- Identify concepts of community practice and engagement to address health equity

DOI: 10.4324/9781003495666-13

11.1 Introduction

Occupational therapists support health and wellbeing not only at the individual level, but also within groups, families, communities, and entire populations. This broader scope of practice reflects the profession's commitment to promoting occupational justice and addressing the social determinants of health-factors such as housing, education, income, and access to services that influence people's ability to participate in everyday life (Whiteford et al., 2021). By considering these wider influences, occupational therapists help reduce health inequities and contribute to building more inclusive and equitable societies.

In Australia and Aotearoa New Zealand, occupational therapists work in diverse settings and roles. They collaborate with families to support shared goals, engage with communities to co-design meaningful initiatives, and advocate for policy changes that benefit population health. These practices are grounded in the profession's core values of 'doing' and 'being' – recognising both the importance of meaningful activity and the lived experience of individuals and groups within their social, political, and physical environments (Pereira & Whiteford, 2022).

This chapter introduces the foundational concepts of occupational therapy practice with groups, families, communities, and populations. It explores key definitions and the unique contributions occupational therapists make in promoting participation, inclusion, and social change across different levels of society.

11.2 Working with groups

Occupational therapy has a long-standing tradition of using group work to support participation in occupations, recovery, and rehabilitation. Group interventions can help sustain and remediate performance skills; build capacity; and promote recovery, health, and wellbeing (Cole, 2025; Ikiugu, 2024). Participation in occupationally focused groups fosters a sense of doing, being, and belonging to support occupational change across the life course (Ikiugu, 2024). Group work is an efficient way to address occupational needs for diverse populations. Evidence supports the use of occupational therapy groups with children and adults (Armstrong et al., 2021), in hospital rehabilitation settings (Spalding et al., 2023), with acquired brain injury (Kotzur et al., 2024), mental health (Zedel & Chen, 2021), and with older adults through programmes like Lifestyle Redesign (Cole, 2025). In occupational therapy, therapeutic groups consist of two or more people with a shared purpose. The aim of these groups is to support participation in occupations, skill development, and occupational identity while fostering inclusion and community cohesion. They function as dynamic systems shaped by member interactions and environmental contexts, with therapeutic outcomes as the goal (Cole, 2025; Ikiugu, 2024).

Group theory informs structure and process and highlights therapeutic benefits including interpersonal learning, cohesiveness, self-awareness, altruism, resilience, and transformative change (Cole, 2025). Yalom and Leszcz (2005, as cited in Cole, 2025) describe a self-reflective loop where members integrate experiences and reflections. Group development typically follows stages: forming, storming, norming, performing, and adjourning (Tuckman, 1965, as cited in Cole, 2025; Ikiugu, 2024). While theorists like Bion and Schutz suggest different stages for groups, critiques by Yalom, Poole, and Gersick suggest these stages are dynamic and not always linear (Cole, 2025).

Additionally, groups develop unique cultures, including shared values, norms, and relationships between members and leaders. Different leadership styles include democratic or facilitative (based on democratic processes), autocratic or directive (provide more guidance), laissez-faire (greater autonomy granted to the group), or an advisory approach (group leader acts as advisor) (Cole, 2025; Ikiugu, 2024).

Effective and safe occupational therapy groups are collaboratively designed, culturally responsive, and inclusive of lived experience (Curtis et al., 2019; Egan & Restall, 2022). However, most group theory reflects Western worldviews and often excludes Indigenous perspectives (Cole, 2025; Ikiugu, 2024). In Australia, culturally safe practice includes respecting Aboriginal and Torres Strait Islander histories, knowledge, and communication styles and addressing systemic inequities (Department of Health Disability and Ageing, 2014). Similarly, in Aotearoa New Zealand, culturally safe groups should where possible have Māori leadership; be grounded in Māori values and models such as whakawhanaungatanga (relationality) or manaakitanga (hospitality); and utilise Māori health and wellbeing models such as the Hui process, Meiheina, or Te Whare Tapa Whā (Wilson et al., 2021). In both contexts, therapeutic groups should aim to reduce health inequities such as those experienced by Indigenous/First Nation peoples.

11.3 Families

Family is a central part of human life, but its meaning and structure varies widely. It can be defined through cultural, economic, moral, or statistical lenses. Families may be nuclear, extended, communal, or chosen, and their roles evolve over time. Some family members take on caregiving roles and provide resources, while others, such as children, older adults, or individuals experiencing illness or disability, contribute in diverse ways and benefit from supportive relationships that enable their participation and wellbeing (Schneider & Kreyenfeld, 2021). Contemporary constructions of family challenge traditional norms, such as the nuclear unit composed of parents, children, and close relatives. Communal living arrangements, rainbow families, gangs, and non-normative relationships reflect diverse ways people form supportive networks considered family (Sanner et al., 2021).

In occupational therapy, families, especially in caregiving roles, are a unique population; therefore, understanding how a person defines family is important. Family influences daily routines, roles, identity, and access to assistance. For example, a person' s recovery may rely on family members for transport, meal preparation, or emotional support. Occupational therapists consider internal family dynamics, such as cultural and faith-based values, health status, and economic conditions, and external factors impacting family, such as access to services and social inclusion. By recognising the varied forms and functions of family, occupational therapists can better understand the client's environment, strengths, and challenges. This supports holistic, person-centred care and promotes meaningful engagement in occupations that matter to the individual and the family (Demers, 2022).

11.3.1 Relational practice in occupational therapy

11.3.1.1 *Kinship, country, and collaboration in Indigenous Australian contexts*

Kinship is central to Aboriginal and Torres Strait Islander wellbeing, shaping identity, belonging, and social roles across generations. It extends beyond biological ties to include cultural obligations, connection to the environment, and collective responsibility. Concepts such as Yarning (sharing stories and building relationships), Dadirri (deep listening and quiet still awareness), and Country (a living entity with which people have reciprocal relationships) reflect the depth of relationality and spirituality within Indigenous worldviews (Smallwood et al., 2024). Kinship systems guide caregiving, decision-making, and healing and require recognition and integration in occupational therapy practice. Culturally responsive models, such as those informed by the Indigenous Allied Health Australia Framework, prioritise relationality, self-determination, and holistic health. Occupational therapists are expected to honour Indigenous knowledge systems and collaborate with communities to support meaningful engagement, aligning practice with principles of equity and reconciliation (Curtis et al., 2019).

11.3.1.2 Whakawhanaungatanga and Whānau-centred practice in Aotearoa
Whānau is central to Māori wellbeing, shaping identity, belonging, and intergenerational roles within te ao Māori (a Māori worldview). It encompasses hapū and iwi (extended family systems) whakapapa (connections to people past and present, land and objects), cultural obligations, and collective responsibility. Whānau-centred approaches reflect values such as manaakitanga (hospitality), whanaungatanga (relationality), and wairuatanga (spirituality), which guide caregiving, decision-making, and healing practices. Māori models of care, such as Te Whare Tapa Whā and the Tū Kahikatea framework, emphasise holistic wellbeing and relational health, integrating physical, mental, spiritual, and environmental dimensions. Occupational therapists are expected to honour and embed Te Tiriti o Waitangi principles, Māori knowledge systems, and tikanga (customs/values/rules) into practice to provide culturally safe and responsive interventions with tangata whaiora (people seeking wellness) and their whānau (family) (Wilson et al., 2021).

11.4 Communities

Occupational therapists engage with communities in diverse and meaningful ways. The concept of 'community' itself can vary depending on context. In public health, a commonly used definition describes a community as a group of individuals who share common values, interests, or social connections–regardless of whether they live in the same geographic area (MacQueen et al., 2001). For example, communities may be based on location, such as school or sporting communities, or they may be formed around shared interests across different regions, such as Occupational Therapy Australia's and the New Zealand Association of Occupational Therapists special interest groups, which connect practitioners with similar professional passions from various locations.

Just as the definition of community is flexible, so too are the ways occupational therapists work within them. Community practice in occupational therapy can be broadly understood through three approaches:

- **Community-based programmes:** These are services delivered in community settings but focused on individual needs. An example is a falls prevention programme offered at a community health centre. While the intervention targets individuals, it also promotes health education and encourages social engagement to a group of people with a similar need (Costa et al., 2024).
- **Community-level initiatives:** These aim to address broader population-level concerns. They focus on the social, economic, cultural, political, and environmental

factors that influence health and participation. These initiatives are typically designed and led by health professionals and seek to create systemic change (Egan & Restall, 2022).

- **Community-led initiatives (community development)**: This approach involves occupational therapists working collaboratively with community members. The emphasis is on supporting communities to identify and address their own priorities. Therapists act as partners rather than leaders, fostering empowerment and shared decision-making (Lauckner, 2018).

Across all levels of community practice, occupational therapists must consider the wider contexts of everyday life – such as housing, education, employment, and social inclusion. These factors are often shaped by systemic barriers and social determinants of health and addressing them is essential to promoting health equity (Egan & Restall, 2022).

Occupational therapists in community settings act as change agents, designing and advocating for initiatives that empower communities to create meaningful change. Occupational therapists address occupational deprivation – when individuals or groups are denied meaningful participation – and its impact on health and wellbeing (McKinnon et al., 2024) and contribute to shaping inclusive social policies.

However, being a change agent also requires reflexive practice. This means occupational therapists must critically reflect on their own positions of power and expertise (Irvine-Brown et al., 2021). It is important to approach community work with humility, recognising when to step back and support communities in leading their own change. Empowerment, not control, is the goal.

11.5 Populations

Occupational therapists work with populations to promote health through meaningful occupations. Populations can be defined as geographic, i.e. all people living in a region, or as a group of people with similar needs and common circumstances, for example refugees living in a specific country. A framework for population-based practice (Keller, 2004, cited in Atala et al., 2025) includes three levels of involvement:

1. Systems-level population-based practice: aims to change organisations, policies, laws, and power structures that impact health. An example of occupational therapy practice at this level is working in government, such as the Department of Education, or the Ministry of Health, where occupational therapists contribute to national or state laws and policies. Similarly, within large organisations, occupational therapists may work within health and safety teams to change organisational culture to promote health and wellbeing of all employees.
2. Community-level population-based practice: focuses on changing community attitudes, community awareness, and community behaviours (Hyett et al., 2020). There is overlap here between community-based practice and population-based practice, including health promotion and community action. An example of community level population-based practice is working with a community to promote mental resilience following a national disaster (WFOT, 2024).
3. Individual-level population-based practice: aims to change the attitudes, beliefs, and practices of individuals (and families) where the individual (and family) receives

services because they are members of a defined population, and those services contribute to the health of the population. An example of individual level population-based practice is supporting aging in place interventions for older adults (Stotz et al., 2025) or promoting social skills for people in the criminal justice system.

The occupational therapy skills and competences required for population-based practice are not different from those required for practice in other roles. Population-based occupational therapists emphasise the importance of communication skills, collaboration, consultation, and networking skills (Atala et al., 2025). Many occupational therapy programmes provide students with theoretical knowledge and practice experience in community-based practice and population focused services through alternative placements. Increasing post-registration education in population health (Domholdt et al., 2020), community development, and disaster management (Estes et al., 2024) prepares the profession for these roles.

11.6 Conclusion

Occupational therapists in Australia and Aotearoa New Zealand work across groups, families, communities, and populations to promote health, wellbeing, and occupational justice. Group work in occupational therapy supports participation, recovery, and wellbeing across diverse populations, fostering effective skill development, belonging, and social interaction. Understanding group development theory that incorporates a self-reflective loop is essential in managing group dynamics and fostering a sense of cohesion and belonging for group members. As an occupational therapist, understanding the diversity within family structures and roles is essential, as families influence routines, identity, and access to support. The diversity in family structure is particularly important to recognise in Indigenous cultures. In Australia, kinship, Country, and cultural obligations shape wellbeing, requiring culturally responsive models. In Aotearoa, whānau-centred care grounded in Māori values and models supports holistic health. Therapists must honour Indigenous knowledge and collaborate respectfully.

Community and population-based practices span individual-focused programmes, population-level initiatives, and community-led development, all of which aim to reduce systemic barriers and foster inclusion. Population-based practice further addresses health through policy, advocacy, and education. Effective practice at the group, family, community, and population levels all require strong communication, collaboration, and cultural competence. Occupational therapists are well-positioned to lead change, empower communities, and promote equitable participation for all.

11.7 Summary

- Group theory guides structure and process, highlighting therapeutic benefits such as self-awareness, resilience, and interpersonal growth.
- Group dynamics describe the interactions and relationships between members of a group, which can significantly influence how the group functions and achieves its goals.
- Family structures are unique, diverse and influence recovery, health and well-being.
- Community engagement is influenced by systemic barriers and social determinants of health. Occupational therapists work with communities to become change agents in addressing systemic barriers.

- Population-level occupational therapists work within communities, workplaces, and governments to create positive change for groups of people with a focus on communication, connection, collaboration, and networking.

11.8 Review and reflection questions

- How do you define family, and how might this be different from other people?
- What are the similarities and differences between a group and a community?
- Describe three ways that occupational therapists can honour Indigenous/First Nations ways of knowing and doing in community practice.
- What does it mean to be a change agent in community settings?
- How can occupational therapists improve their skills and competency when working with groups, communities, and populations?

References

Armstrong, J., Elliott, C., Davidson, E., Mizen, J., Wray, J., & Girdler, S. (2021). The power of playgroups: Key components of supported and therapeutic playgroups from the perspective of parents. *Australian Occupational Therapy Journal, 68*(2), 144–155. https://doi.org/10.1111/1440-1630.12708

Atala, M., Bennington, M., & Domholdt, E. (2025). Population-based practice in occupational therapy. *Occupational Therapy in Health Care, 39*(1), 162–176. https://doi.org/10.1080/07380577.2023.2243515

Cole, M. B. (2025). *Group dynamics in occupational therapy: The theoretical basis and practice application for group intervention* (6th ed.). Routledge.

Costa, N., Ambrens, M., Delbaere, K., Wilson, L., Li, A., & Sherrington, C. (2024). A systems approach to aid policy action on falls prevention among community-dwelling older people in Australia. *Public Health Research & Practice, 34*(1), e3412405. https://doi.org/10.17061/phrp3412405

Curtis, E., Jones, R., Tipene-Leach, D., Walker, C., Loring, B., Paine, S.-J., & Reid, P. (2019). Why cultural safety rather than cultural competency is required to achieve health equity: A literature review and recommended definition. *International Journal for Equity in Health, 18*(1), 174–181. https://doi.org/10.1186/s12939-019-1082-3

Demers, L. (2022). Expanding occupational therapy perspectives with family caregivers. *Canadian Journal of Occupational Therapy, 89*(3), 223–237. https://doi.org/10.1177/000841742211039

Department of Health Disability and Ageing. (2014). *Aboriginal and Torres Strait Islander Health curriculum framework*. Australian Government. https://www.health.gov.au/resources/publications/aboriginal-and-torres-strait-islander-health-curriculum-framework?language=en

Domholdt, E., Cooper, S., & Kleinhoff, R. (2020). Population health content in entry-level occupational therapy programs. *American Journal of Occupational Therapy, 74*(3), 7403205160p1–7403205160p9. https://doi.org/10.5014/ajot.2020.036392

Egan, M., & Restall, G. (2022). Collaborative relationship-focused occupational therapy. In M. Egan & G. Restall (Eds.), *Promoting occupational participation: Collaborative relationship-focused occupational therapy. 10th Canadian occupational therapy guidelines* (pp. 97–117). Canadian Association of Occupational Therapists.

Estes, R. I., Delgado, G. M., Bing, N. J., Byrne, M. E., Eady, J. S., Hollywood, K. E., & Kopp, A. B. (2024). Occupational therapists in disaster management: A survey study. *The Internet Journal of Allied Health Sciences and Practice, 22*(3), Article 4. https://nsuworks.nova.edu/ijahsp/vol22/iss3/4/

Hyett, N., Kenny, A., McKinstry, C., & Gibson, C. (2020). How do OTs practice with communities to improve community-level health, well-being and inclusion? A systematic review. *American Journal of Occupational Therapy, 74*(Supp 1), 7411505146p1. https://doi. org/10.5014/ajot.2020.74S1-PO5401

Ikiugu, M. N. (2024). Group process and group intervention. In G. Gillen & C. Brown (Eds.), *Willard & Spackman's occupational therapy* (14th ed., pp. 481–495). Wolters Kluwer.

Irvine-Brown, L., Ware, V.-A., & Malfitano, A. P. S. (2021). Exploring the praxis of occupational therapy–community development practitioners. *Canadian Journal of Occupational Therapy, 89*(1), 26–35. https://doi.org/10.1177/00084174211066662

Kotzur, C., Patterson, F., Harrington, R., Went, S., & Froude, E. (2024). Therapeutic groups run for community-dwelling people with acquired brain injury: A scoping review. *Disability and Rehabilitation, 46*(21), 4860–4876. https://doi.org/10.1080/09638288.2023.2283099

Lauckner, H., Leclair, L., & Yamamoto, C. (2020). Occupational therapists' roles in community development: Canadian perspectives. *Canadian Journal of Occupational Therapy, 87*(1), 35–45. https://doi.org/10.1177/0008417419888516

MacQueen, K. M., McLellan, E., Metzger, D. S., Kegeles, S., Strauss, R. P., Scotti, R., Blanchard, L., & Trotter, R. T., II. (2001). What is community? An evidence-based definition for participatory public health. *American Journal of Public Health, 91*(12), 1929–1938. https:// doi.org/10.2105/AJPH.91.12.1929

McKinnon, S., Petrone, N., & Tarbet, A. (2024). The role of an occupational therapy practitioner in professional advocacy: A scoping review. *Translational Science in Occupation, 1*(2). https://doi.org/10.32873/unmc.dc.tso.1.2.02

Pereira, R. B., & Whiteford, G. E. (2022). Enabling inclusive occupational therapy through the Capabilities, Opportunities, Resources, and Environments (CORE) approach. In A. Taket, B. R. Ziersch, & S. F. Baum (Eds.), *Handbook of social inclusion: Research and practices in health and social sciences* (pp. 1699–1716). Springer. https://doi.org/10.1007/978-3-030-89594-5_97

Sanner, C., Ganong, L., & Coleman, M. (2021). Families are socially constructed: Pragmatic implications for researchers. *Journal of Family Issues, 42*(2), 422–444. https://doi. org/10.1177/0192513X20905334

Schneider, N. F., & Kreyenfeld, M. (2021). Introduction: The sociology of the family–towards a European perspective. In N. F. Schneider & M. Kreyenfield (Eds.), *Research handbook on the sociology of the family* (pp. 2–20). Edward Elgar Publishing.

Smallwood, R., Usher Am, K., Marriott, R., Sampson, N., & Jackson, D. (2024). Understanding the importance of connection: An indigenous exploration of the social and emotional well-being and resilience of a rural cohort of Aboriginal young people. *Journal of Youth Studies, 27*(10), 1407–1425. https://doi.org/10.1080/13676261.2023.2213638

Spalding, K., Gustafsson, L., & Di Tommaso, A. (2023). Evaluation of an inpatient occupation-based group program using a process evaluation framework. *Australian Occupational Therapy Journal, 70*(1), 32–42. https://doi.org/10.1111/1440-1630.12829

Stotz, N. L., Steiner, V., Polavarapu, M., & Czaja, E. (2025). Occupational therapy's role in population health with older adults. *Inquiry: A Journal of Medical Care Organization, Provision and Financing, 62*, 00469580251366149. https://doi.org/10.1177/00469580251366149

Whiteford, G., Parnell, T., Ramsden, L., Nott, M., & Vine-Daher, S. (2021). Understanding and advancing occupational justice and social inclusion. In A. Taket, B. R. Ziersch, & S. F. Baum (Eds.), *Handbook of social inclusion: Research and practices in health and social sciences* (pp. 1–30). Springer. https://doi.org/10.1007/978-3-030-48277-0_10-1

Wilson, D., Moloney, E., Parr, J. M., Aspinall, C., & Slark, J. (2021). Creating an Indigenous Māori-centred model of relational health: A literature review of Māori models of health. *Journal of Clinical Nursing, 30*(23–24), 3539–3555. https://doi.org/10.1111/jocn.15859

World Federation of Occupational Therapists (WFOT). (2024). *Occupational therapy and disaster management – position statement.* https://wfot.org/resources/occupational-therapy-and-disaster-management

Zedel, J., & Chen, S.-P. (2021). Client's experiences of occupational therapy group interventions in mental health settings: A meta-ethnography. *Occupational Therapy in Mental Health, 37*(3), 278–302. https://doi.org/10.1080/0164212X.2021.1900763

CHAPTER 12

Partnering with experts by experience in occupational therapy

Louise Gustafsson, Jacki Liddle, Michelle Bissett, Priscilla Ennals, Caleb Rixon, Kim Walder, and Matthew McShane

Authors' positionality statement

The authors of this chapter are predominantly middle-class and educated, and all reside in Australia. The authorship team includes people who identify as members or are allies of the 2SLGBTTQQIA and the disability community and people who are connected to peoples and communities from other cultures. They have all been involved in leading or participating in partnering activities across practice, research, education and governance, either in their professional role or as an expert by experience. The authors acknowledge their white privilege and that they are on a continuing path of learning and understanding. They recognise that a First Nations' perspective is missing and that this is a limitation of the chapter.

Key terms
- Experts by experience
- Power-sharing
- Partnering
- Co-design
- Participatory

Chapter objectives
This chapter will allow the reader to:

- Define partnering with experts by experience
- Outline key outcomes, including anticipated benefits of partnering
- Overview the principles, barriers, and enablers of partnering
- Describe partnering in clinical contexts at individual, service delivery, organisational, and system levels
- Describe partnering in research, and educational contexts

DOI: 10.4324/9781003495666-14

12.1 Introduction

Partnering with experts by experience has origins in the emancipatory and social justice philosophy of the early 1900s (McShane & Gustafsson, 2024). Empowerment, inclusivity, and agency are prominent when partnering with individuals or collectives as active and equal contributors to identify needs and generate solutions. This participatory approach is often referred to as consumer and community involvement within Australia (National Health and Medical Research Council & Consumers Health Forum of Australia, 2016); engagement with consumers, whānau, and communities in New Zealand (Te Tāhu Hauora, Health Quality and Safety Commission, 2023); or patient and public involvement in other countries such as the United Kingdom (Health Research Authority & INVOLVE, 2024). In this chapter we use the term partnering in lieu of involvement, as we believe that it demonstrates a deeper and more authentic form of power-sharing. We also use the term expert by experience rather than consumer or community to represent the active and valuable roles of individuals with lived experience in all forms of partnering. Other terms such as lived experience expert, patient, client, and service-user may be used by other groups; however, there is no single term that is suitable or acceptable for everyone, and it is important to have conversations when setting up processes to identify preferred terms (Aplin et al., 2024). In this chapter, we introduce the reader to why partnering is important for occupational therapy, key principles, barriers, and enablers and explore partnering across clinical, research, and educational contexts.

12.2 'Nothing about us without us'

The colloquial phrase 'nothing about us without us' has been used by a range of different groups of people, including disabled people, to ensure that these often-unheard voices and opinions are included and privileged in the actions and decision making by those who may hold more power – including health professionals. We need genuine and ongoing engagement of people with living experience, alongside those who support them, and we must avoid tokenistic or tickbox approaches to partnering (Liddle et al., 2022). Much has been written to support health professionals to partner with people in relation to health service design and implementation (e.g. Greenhalgh et al., 2019; Miller et al., 2017; Rolleston et al., 2022). Partnering is considered essential for the delivery of person-centred care which focuses on building trust, mutual respect, and shared knowledge between consumers and health care providers. Services that are planned, designed, or produced through partnering are more likely to meet the needs of the people with lived experience.

Effective partnering is important to:

- Enhance quality of care to lead to better health outcomes
- Enhance consumer experience
- Promote efficient use of resources
- Lead to service innovation and improvement
- Foster inclusivity

(Australian Commission on Safety and Quality in
Health Care, 2021; Farmer et al., 2018)

12.3 'Whose voice is missing'?

One meaningful way for occupational therapists to foster deeper partnerships with individuals or groups commonly excluded is by reflecting on the phase 'Whose voice is missing?' This reflective prompt encourages therapists to actively seek out and amplify the voices of marginalised individuals or communities, ensuring their involvement throughout the occupational therapy process. When partnering with people from historically overlooked groups – often excluded due to misconceptions about their vulnerability – it is vital to approach collaboration with sensitivity. Some individuals may carry past experiences of distrust or even harm within healthcare settings, which can shape their willingness to engage, build relationships, and see value in their contributions. Taking time to build connections, carefully constructing spaces of participation, regularly acknowledging and addressing power differentials, and building capacity through training and support can play a role in building trust and respect in relationships (Spies et al., 2022).

12.4 Enablers and barriers to partnering

Organisational culture can either support or hinder partnering activities. Leadership – from managers to executives and funders – must not only acknowledge the value of partnering but also actively support it. Without this commitment, partnering risks becoming a tokenistic box-ticking exercise rather than a meaningful initiative. Additionally, excessive bureaucracy and rigid organisational processes can hinder effective engagement (Sandvin Olsson et al., 2025). Several factors can negatively affect partnering activities. Short timeframes, lack of experience among stakeholders, and failure to involve experts by experience in identifying the core need or problem can significantly weaken efforts (Soklaridis et al., 2024). Partnering activities are supported when there is power-sharing and shared decision-making; resourcing is available to support capacity building and recognition of the contributions of experts by experience through reimbursement (Spies et al., 2022). Reasonable payment, including coverage of participation expenses and ongoing capacity building (training, support etc.), is a minimum requirement of involvement. Inclusion of groups or multiple individuals is recognised as good practice to address the potential for power imbalances and lack of support.

12.5 Guiding principles

The 'nothing about us without us' mantra requires therapists to think about how they should partner with experts by experience. It is essential that experts by experience be involved in defining the need or problem and not just in the exploration of a solution for an agenda that has been set by the organisation or occupational therapist. Equally important is that shared principles for partnering be discussed and agreed upon. Caleb (lived experience activist and stroke survivor) and Priscilla (occupational therapist), who have partnered with each other and with others, in many projects in education, practice, research, and governance, provide shared views on what it takes to partner well in Table 12.1. These principles can be used to guide partnership development. Caleb and Priscilla's experiences mirror those described in the literature (for example: Cornish et al., 2023; Roper et al., 2018; Spies et al., 2022).

Table 12.1 Guiding principles

Key principles	*Practical considerations*
Relationships first	■ Work to avoid transactional or extractive relationships ■ Mutuality is key. This means you are an active part of this relationship, so you need to bring yourself ■ Find shared values and a shared vision – these are the foundation of relationship ■ Relationships take time. Make time to check-in on the relationship regularly
Positionality and power sharing	■ Understand and acknowledge who has more/less power and status in this context ■ Those with more power are responsible for reducing the imbalance – avoid posturing, speak less, elevate those with less power ■ Develop a common understanding of the issue – 'not just me looking at your problem. What is our shared problem/issue/goal?' ■ Power shifting won't happen without strong relationships ■ Think about language and power – use we/us/ours rather than yours/mine ■ Consider who benefits from this project. How can benefits be shared?
Establish working practices	■ Clarify roles and check-in on these regularly ■ Agree on the steps to the mission ■ Aim for shared decision making – agree on which decisions are key and how they will be made ■ Consider how conflict and disagreement will be navigated, and do not assume conflict will not happen ■ Create a safe enough environment for optimal participation of everyone. Check-in on this regularly – are any barriers to involvement emerging? ■ Have fun ■ Keep checking in with everyone involved. Is this working? How could we do this differently and better? What is getting in the way?
Take care with startings and endings	■ Relationships require care as they start or end in relation to project based work ■ Consider what happens to relationships when a project ends. Consider who needs what to end well ■ Celebrate the partnership and achievements ■ Make time to reflect on what was learnt and ensure this learning influences future partnering

12.6 Exploring partnering in occupational therapy

12.6.1 Partnering in contemporary practice contexts

In Aotearoa New Zealand, the Health Quality and Safety Commission (2023) has a 'Code of Expectations' that describes how health services should engage with experts by experience at the individual and organisational level. In Australia, the Australian Commission on Safety and Quality in Health Care (2021) has a standard relating to partnering with experts by experience. Like the New Zealand code, this includes partnering as an individual specific to their own health care but also in the design and evaluation of health services at a higher level. The standard gives practical advice regarding how health professionals can work with individuals to enact shared decision-making across three levels. It is important to remember that although these levels have been developed predominantly for partnering activities within a health context, they are transferable across practice contexts such as education or social contexts and when working with collectives.

12.6.1.1 Level one: partnering at the level of the individual

Client-centred or person-centred practice is a core tenet of occupational therapy and is recognised as the first level of consumer partnership (Australian Commission on Safety and Quality in Health Care [ACSQHC], 2021). Partnering at the level of the individual occurs throughout the occupational therapy practice process as therapists collaboratively seek to understand the occupational concerns, co-develop goals, and engage in shared decision-making to develop and enact an intervention plan. This level of partnering (Figure 12.1) is explored further in Chapter 10.

12.6.1.2 Level two: partnering at the level of service delivery

When therapists partner at this level, experts by experience act as a representative of the group to which they belong (Figure 12.2). The experts by experience bring the interests of the collective into the discussions including lived experience of a condition or life event and the services, identified and prioritised needs, and possible solutions. The involvement of experts by experience at this level is often related to the design,

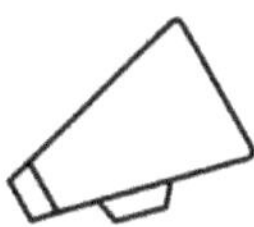

Figure 12.1 Client-centred practice

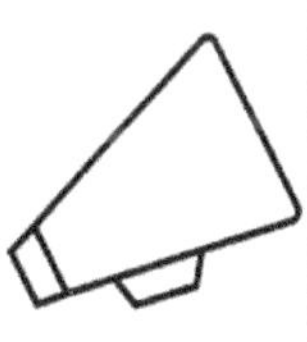

Figure 12.2 Partnering at levels two or three

organisation, and delivery of the whole or part of a programme within that service. From the perspective of occupational therapy clinical practice, this can range from partnering to co-design resources such as handouts through to co-production of a new occupational therapy service. Recent examples of partnering at this level include co-design of a personal safety tool for community based mental health settings (Francis et al., 2024), co-design of an occupation-based group for inpatient rehabilitation (Wall et al., 2024), and co-design of complex interventions for children with cerebral palsy (Massey et al., 2024).

12.6.1.3 Level three: Partnering at the level of the organisation or system

Partnering with experts by experience at an organisational or systems level is becoming more accepted and expected. Some contexts where this might occur, include health service/network boards and executive leadership groups, government departments and advisory groups, Quality and Safety Committees, ethics committees, Occupational Therapy Australia, and the Occupational Therapy Board of Australia. The involvement of experts by experience at this level ensures a different perspective – lived experience of a condition, of service access and use, of concerns and risks, of what matters and what might help – is included in the considerations, decision making, oversight, and strategy development of these groups (Hodges et al., 2023). Their lived experience perspectives are equally valued alongside their expertise in governance, strategy, and leadership. To avoid tokenism, organisations and boards must carefully consider why they are engaging with experts by experience, what they need to do differently to distribute power between all members (this might include, for example, unlearning or adjusting meeting processes), and to monitor whether the engagement is as effective as expected. Some organisations prefer to have lived experience–led groups (rather than individuals) who sit alongside their boards or committees to include a wider range of lived experience perspectives (Anderson & Bigby, 2023). If consumer advisory groups are separated, clear two-way communication and processes for influence are required.

12.6.2 Research contexts

The value of partnering in research is now well recognised, and funders and publishers often require researchers to demonstrate how partnering has or will occur. The inclusion of experts by experience as leaders of the research, as research team members, or in research advisory groups ensures that research effort is directed towards needs or problems important to the group of focus and that the generated solutions and methodology are the most appropriate. Some examples include when experts by experience:

- lead a project about an issue that is important to their community
- identify priority areas for future research
- contribute to the development of study materials so they make sense and are acceptable
- lead or support analysis of qualitative research
- share findings from research

The benefits to partnering in research include embedding real-world experiences, constraints, and priorities into the research and design of solutions to support transparent processes and meaningful and acceptable outcomes while building alliances amongst people who need to work together in an ongoing way (Greenhalgh et al., 2019). Authentic partnering in research requires personal investment; a commitment to positioning oneself as a learner (and un-learner) – someone who is curious, reflective, and reflexive and who seeks to uncover personal assumptions and blind spots. It also requires capacity building and active support of experts by experience to position themselves as leaders in the process (Roper et al., 2018).

12.6.2.1 Illustrative research example

The Florence Project is a programme of research about technology and people living with dementia (Liddle et al., 2022). Living experience experts (people living with dementia and care partners) took on various partnering roles, including those of advisor, investigator, and co-designer of technology. In reflecting about their involvement across three studies, the investigator team (including people living with dementia, care partner, occupational therapist, and interaction designer) constructed advice for those seeking to partner in research.

Four actions were recommended:

1. Agree on the value of what you are doing
2. The time to start partnering is now
3. Ask, do not assume
4. Push back on 'we always have'

Investigators noted the important role that occupational therapy skills may play in creating accessible and inclusive research processes and supporting the engagement of people with living experience in research. They also noted the importance of a personalised rather than one-size-fits-all approach to inclusive partnering.

A personal reflection on partnering in research – Caleb

As a survivor, I've often felt like researchers see me solely for my trauma narrative. But I'm so much more than that. And it's time we shook up these power imbalances in research.

The problem starts with the labels we use. If you're a professor 'professing' and I'm a 'consumer,' what do you think I'll believe my role is? Am I just here to consume?

Talk to the person you're working with – not their role. Partnering is relational, not transactional. It's about seeing the whole person, with all their experiences, skills, and insights, and recognising that they bring more to the table than just their story of survival.

They can contribute to study design, data analysis, or even writing up results. Don't just slot someone into a pre-defined 'consumer' box.

You can disrupt those power imbalances by treating people with lived experience as equal partners, not subjects or data points. When you truly partner with someone, magic happens. That's when research becomes something that can make a difference in people's lives.

I'm not just here to consume your research. I'm here to help create it.

12.6.3 Partnering in education

Partnering in higher education for curriculum design, delivery, and evaluation in health professions is becoming increasingly widespread (Scanlan et al., 2020). Indeed, it is frequently required by professional bodies and embedded in accreditation standards (Occupational Therapy Council of Australia, 2018). Partnering should occur across an entire programme ranging from engagement in advisory and/or consumer reference groups (Arblaster et al., 2018), employment by universities in lived experience academic positions (Byrne et al., 2014), and co-design and delivery of course content or assessments (Logan et al., 2018). Involvement of experts by experience in the assessment of students provides a valuable insight into development of key skills in occupational therapy practice including client and family-centred practice. Evidence-informed guidelines for partnering in education have been developed to help address potential barriers and to promote best practice (for example, Roberts et al., 2023). An example of this form of partnering is represented in the Valuing Lived Experience project at Curtin University in Western Australia (Dorozenko et al., 2016). As a result of the project, lived experience academics are responsible for coordinating courses, developing and delivering course content, developing student assessments, co-producing student assessments with industry partners, supervising research students, and leading research projects.

Research evidence reveals positive outcomes for students, including:

- Enhanced communication skills, appreciation for empathy in therapeutic relationships and person-centred practice (Cleminson & Moesby, 2013)
- A deeper applied understanding of theory (Cooper & Spencer-Dawe, 2006)
- An ability to challenge personal attitudes and pre-conceptions (Unwin et al., 2017)
- Critical reflection on power and privilege in healthcare (Collén, 2019)
- Preparing students for consumer-driven health service delivery (Byrne et al., 2014)

A personal reflection on authentic partnering for more meaningful outcomes – Matt

Partnering with experts by experience in research or education is an incredibly valuable and rewarding endeavour. But is that process equally valuable and rewarding for all parties involved?

When the experts by experience are people with disability, they often face a real lack of agency, treated like props rather than equal collaborator. They may be spoken about by their 'disability' or their persona as a 'person with a disability' rather than being recognised simply as a person.

At times, these partnerships can feel like an 'exercise' aimed at upskilling the able-bodied world-often in a way that is more about making others feel good than development of genuine understanding.

In some cases, involving people with disabilities in projects serves as a box-ticking measure to demonstrate inclusivity, rather than centring their human experience and expertise. Too often, projects focus on their 'disability' rather than recognising them as whole individuals with valuable insights beyond that aspect of their persona.

Historically, people with disabilities have been spoken about rather than spoken to. This long-standing exclusion can lead to an unconscious sense of gratitude simply for being acknowledged or included. But should we accept this as the status quo, or should we strive for something better?

12.7 Conclusion

This chapter has explored the concept of partnership and the various ways that occupational therapists should partner with experts by experience. Effective partnering is essential for better health outcomes through the development of resources, approaches, and policies that are collaboratively informed by the relevant stakeholders. Partnering may occur within contemporary occupational therapy practice concepts, research, and education. It may have a focus on the co-design of occupational therapy service delivery, or there may be a focus on organisational or system level issues including policy or strategy development. Guiding principles for partnering include relationships first, positionality and power–sharing, establishing working practices, and taking care of startings and endings. All elements of practice highlight the need to consider power sharing and authentic relationship development to position the partnership for success.

12.8 Summary

- Partnering with experts by experience is a key component of contemporary occupational therapy practice, research, and education.
- Relationships and power-sharing are at the core of all authentic partnering activities.
- In occupational therapy practice, therapists partner to understand a need and improve and develop services in response.
- Experts by experience are valued members of advisory boards or governance teams, ensuring that the voice of the collective are represented in discussions about organisational policy and guidelines, and so on.
- Barriers to effective partnering include poor organisational support, inadequate resourcing, short timeframes, and inexperience.
- Enablers to effective partnering include shared decision making, recognition and reimbursement, and capability and experience of the individuals involved.

12.9 Review and reflection questions

- Why is it important for occupational therapists to hear and consider the perspectives of experts by experience in their practice?
- What is the risk of working with only one individual expert by experience?
- What are some key principles that are relevant to partnering with experts by experience?
- What are some of the issues that can negatively impact partnering with experts by experience?
- If you are planning on partnering with experts by experience on a project, how can you set up conditions for effective partnership from the beginning? Consider who holds the power in decision making: how could this be shared more effectively?

References

Anderson, S., & Bigby, C. (2023). 'Nothing about us without us'. Including lived experiences of people with intellectual disabilities in policy and service design. In C. Bigby & A. Hough (Eds.), *Disability practice: Safeguarding quality service delivery* (pp. 225–246). Palgrave Macmillan. https://doi.org/10.1007/978-981-99-6143-6_12

Aplin, T., Russi, M., Bryant, E., Frost, D., Sam, M. A., Lund, C., Ong, E., Listopad, L., & Liddle, J. (2024). A commitment to partnering with people with lived experience: Beginning conversations by exploring preferred language. *Australian Occupational Therapy Journal*, 71(1), 1–3. https://doi.org/10.1111/1440-1630.12934

Arblaster, K., Mackenzie, L., Matthews, L., Willis, K., Gill, K., Hanlon, P., & Laidler, R. (2018). Learning from consumers: An eDelphi study of Australian mental health consumers' priorities for recovery-oriented curricula. *Australian Occupational Therapy Journal*, 65(6), 586–597. https://doi.org/10.1111/1440-1630.12518

Australian Commission on Safety and Quality in Health Care. (2021). *National safety and quality health service standards* (2nd ed.). https://www.safetyandquality.gov.au/standards/nsqhs-standards/partnering-consumers-standard

Byrne, L., Platania-Phung, C., Happell, B., Harris, S., & Bradshaw, J. (2014). Changing nursing student attitudes to consumer participation in mental health services: A survey study of traditional and lived experience-led education. *Issues in Mental Health Nursing*, 35(9), 704–712. https://doi.org/10.3109/01612840.2014.888604

Cleminson, S., & Moesby, A. (2013). Service user involvement in occupational therapy education: An evolving involvement. *Journal of Mental Health Training, Education and Practice*, 8(1), 5–14. https://doi.org/10.1108/17556221311307989

Collén, K. (2019). Education for a sustainable future? Students' experiences of workshops on ethical dilemmas. *Social Work Education*, 38(1), 119–128. https://doi.org/10.1080/02615479.2018.1543391

Cooper, H., & Spencer-Dawe, E. (2006). Involving service users in interprofessional education: Narrowing the gap between theory and practice. *Journal of Interprofessional Care*, 20(6), 603–617. https://doi.org/10.1080/13561820601029767

Cornish, F., Breton, N., Moreno-Tabarez, U., Delgado, J., Rua, M., de-Graft Aikins, A., & Hodgetts, D. (2023). Participatory action research. *Nature Reviews Methods Primers*, 3(1), 34. https://doi.org/10.1038/s43586-023-00113-3

Dorozenko, K. P., Ridley, S., Martin, R., & Mahboub, L. (2016). A journey of embedding mental health lived experience in social work education. *Social Work Education*, 35(8), 905–917. https://doi.org/10.1080/02615479.2016.1214255

Farmer, J., Bigby, C., Davis, H., Carlisle, K., Kenny, A., & Huysmans, R. (2018). The state of health services partnering with consumers: Evidence from an online survey of Australian health services. *BMC Health Services Research*, 18, 628. https://doi.org/10.1186/s12913-018-3433-y

Francis, A., Le, A., Adams-Leask, K., & Procter, N. (2024). Utilising co-design to develop a lived experience informed personal safety tool within a mental health community rehabilitation setting. *Australian Occupational Therapy Journal*, 71(6), 1076–1088. https://doi.org/10.1111/1440-1630.12988

Greenhalgh, T., Hinton, L., Finlay, T., Macfarlane, A., Fahy, N., Clyde, B., & Chant, A. (2019). Frameworks for supporting patient and public involvement in research: Systematic review and co-design pilot. *Health Expectations*, 22(4), 785–801.

Health Quality and Safety Commission. (2023). *Code of expectations for health entitites' engagement with consumers and whānau*. https://www.hqsc.govt.nz/resources/resource-library/code-of-expectations-for-health-entities-engagement-with-consumers-and-whanau/

Health Research Authority and INVOLVE. (2024). *Impact of public involvement on ethical aspects of research*. Health Research Authority. https://www.hra.nhs.uk/planning-and-improving-research/best-practice/public-involvement/impact-public-involvement-ethical-aspects-research/

Hodges, E., Leditschke, A., & Solonsch, L. (2023). *The lived experience governance framework: Centring people, identity and human rights for the benefit of all*. Prepared by LELAN (SA Lived Experience Leadership & Advocacy Network) for the National Mental Health Consumer and Carer Forum and the National PHN Mental Health Lived Experience Engagement Network. Mental Health Australia. https://www.lelan.org.au/wp-content/uploads/2023/08/Lived-Experience-Governance-Framework.pdf

Liddle, J., Worthy, P., Frost, D., Taylor, E., & Taylor, D. (2022). Partnering with people living with dementia and care partners in technology research and design: Reflections and recommendations. *Australian Occupational Therapy Journal*, 69(6), 723–741. https://doi.org/10.1111/1440-1630.12843

Logan, A., Yule, E., Taylor, M., & Imms, C. (2018). Mental health consumer participation in undergraduate occupational therapy student assessment: No negative impact. *Australian Occupational Therapy Journal*, 65(6), 494–502. https://doi.org/10.1111/1440-1630.12484

Massey, J., Tsianakas, V., Gordon, A. L., Sadler, N., & Robert, G. (2024). Co-designing complex therapy interventions with parents as partners in the care of children with cerebral palsy: An experience-based codesign study in England. *Research in Developmental Disabilities, 151,* Article 104793. https://doi.org/10.1016/j.ridd.2024.104793

McShane, M., & Gustafsson, L. (2024). Co-design: Do we need to (co-)change our (co-)thinking? *Australian Occupational Therapy Journal*, 71(4), 445–446. https://doi.org/10.1111/1440-1630.12986

Miller, C. L., Mott, K., Cousins, M., Miller, S., Johnson, A., Lawson, T., & Wesselingh, S. (2017). Integrating consumer engagement in health and medical research–an Australian framework. *Health Research Policy and Systems, 15,* Article 9. https://doi.org/10.1186/s12961-017-0171-2

National Health and Medical Research Council & Consumers Health Forum of Australia. (2016). *Statement on consumer and community involvement in health and medical research.* National Health and Medical Research Council. https://www.nhmrc.gov.au/about-us/publications/statement-consumer-and-community-involvement-health-and-medical-research

Occupational Therapy Council of Australia. (2018) *Accreditation standards for Australia entry-level occupational therapy education programs.* https://www.otcouncil.com.au/wp-content/uploads/OTC-Accred-Stds-Dec2018-effective-Jan2020.pdf

Roberts, M., Bissett, M., Gawne, H., Slattery, M., Stewart, V., & Walder, K. (2023). *Co-designing health profession education with lived experience expertise: Recommendations for university practice.* Griffith University. https://doi.org/10.25904/1912/4772

Rolleston, A. K., Korohina, E., & McDonald, M. (2022). Navigating the space between co-design and mahitahi: Building bridges between knowledge systems on behalf of communities. *Australian Journal of Rural Health*, 30(6), 830–835. https://doi.org/10.1111/ajr.12916

Roper, C., Grey, F., & Cadogan, E. (2018). *Co-production: Putting principles into practice in mental health contexts.* University of Melbourne. https://healthsciences.unimelb.edu.au/__data/assets/pdf_file/0007/3392215/Coproduction_putting-principles-into-practice.pdf

Sandvin Olsson, A. B., Haaland, M., Stenberg, U., Slettebø, T., & Strøm, A. (2025). Contextual factors affecting patient representatives in primary healthcare service development. *Tidsskrift for Omsorgsforskning, 11*(1), 1–17. https://doi.org/10.18261/tfo.11.1.1

Scanlan, J. N., Logan, A., Arblaster, K., Haracz, K., Fossey, E., Milbourn, B. T., Pépin, G., Machingura, T., & Webster, J. S. (2020). Mental health consumer involvement in occupational therapy education in Australia and Aotearoa New Zealand. *Australian Occupational Therapy Journal*, 67(1), 83–93. https://doi.org/10.1111/1440-1630.12634

Soklaridis, S., Harris, H., Shier, R., Rovet, J., Black, G., Bellissimo, G., Gruszecki, S., Lin, E., & Di Giandomenico, A. (2024). A balancing act: Navigating the nuances of co-production in mental health research. *Research Involvement and Engagement, 10*(1), Article 30. https://doi.org/10.1186/s40900-024-00561-7

Spies, R., Ennals, P., Egan, R., Hemus, P., Droppert, K., Tidhar, M., Simmons, M., Bendall, S., Wood, T., & Lessing, K. (2022). Co-research with people with mental health challenges: Transforming knowledge and power. In P. Liamputtong (Ed.), *Handbook of social inclusion: Research and practices in health and social sciences* (pp. 281–307). Springer International Publishing. https://doi.org/10.1007/978-3-030-89594-5_138

Unwin, P. F., Rooney, J. M., Osborne, N., & Cole, C. (2017). Are perceptions of disability changed by involving service users and carers in qualifying health and social work training? *Disability & Society, 32*(9), 1387–1399. https://doi.org/10.1080/09687599.2017.1322498

Wall, G., Pearce, C., Gustafsson, L., & Isbel, S. (2024). Designing an occupation-based group intervention for adult inpatient rehabilitation: Partnering with clinicians and patients using a nominal group technique design. *Australian Occupational Therapy Journal, 71*(5), 674–685. https://doi.org/10.1111/1440-1630.12950

CHAPTER 13

Social justice and intersectionality

Overview and implications for occupational therapy practice

Ted Brown, Jenni Mace, Vagner Dos Santos, Diane L. Smith, and Aiko Hoshino

Authors' positionality statement

We are all doctorally qualified occupational therapists who work in the university education sector. We come from several different countries, including Canada, Aotearoa New Zealand, United States, Japan, and Brazil. We acknowledge the impact of colonisation on First Nations peoples around the world, including Australia and Aotearoa New Zealand. We support social justice principles of access to resources, equity, participation, diversity, and human rights regardless of race, age, national origin, ability status, economic status, sexuality, gender identity, and other identities.

Key terms
- Belonging
- Diversity
- Equality
- Inclusivity
- Intersectionality
- Occupational discrimination
- Occupational enablement
- Occupational imbalance
- Occupational intersectionality
- Occupational justice
- Occupational rights
- Social justice

Objectives
This chapter will allow the reader to:

- Define the concepts of social justice, intersectionality, and related occupational terms

DOI: 10.4324/9781003495666-15

- Apply the concept of intersectionality to clients, families, and groups that occupational therapists and students may engage with
- Describe the similarities and differences between social justice and occupational justice
- Articulate strategies that occupational therapy students and clinicians can do to address social justice and intersectionality issues from an occupational perspective

13.1 Introduction

Social justice and intersectionality are increasingly relevant and significant concepts for occupational therapy students, clinicians, educators, and researchers to be aware of. We often are working with individuals, families, organisations, communities, and populations that have experienced historical or current discrimination, oppression, unfairness, and inequities in their daily occupational lives. How we respond to these issues and their impact on people's occupational engagement, health and wellbeing in a respectful, informed, sensitive, non-biased way is fundamental and requisite.

This chapter introduces the evolving ideas, theories and terminology of a social and occupational justice lens to practice and the importance of the freedom to do and be. Intersectionality is explored alongside social justice as a reminder of the complex nature of human identity and how multiple labels and social categorisations can interact to give individuals and communities different experiences of privilege or discrimination. As occupational therapists, knowing how to deal with social and institutional barriers can be challenging. We may not even recognise these barriers if we do not experience them ourselves.

Therefore, this chapter aims to equip practitioners with the language and strategies for both recognising injustice and promoting fair and equitable inclusion and participation in the occupations people and communities want and need to do.

Two illustrative vignettes are provided for readers, presenting different types of social justice issues through an occupational lens. These vignettes are grounded in the unique sociocultural, historical, and policy contexts of Australia and Aotearoa New Zealand. Finally, how occupational therapy students and practitioners can respond to social justice and intersectionality issues from an occupational perspective is outlined.

13.2 Social justice

Social justice infers that 'an ideal condition in which all members of a society have the same basic rights, protection, opportunities, obligations, and social benefits' (Barker, 2013, pp. 398–399). It recognises that inequalities from the past exist and need to be focused on to address inherent discrimination, oppression, unfairness and institutional disparities. Social justice as a process should be inclusive, participatory, cooperative, mutual, consultative, respectful, welcoming of difference, and affirming of collective agency. As professionals working with individuals, families, communities, collectives, and organisations from a range of backgrounds in the healthcare, social, educational, and justice systems, occupational therapists must focus on social justice to promote occupational enablement and equality with these groups.

13.3 Social justice movements

Occupational therapists have a professional and ethical responsibility to work towards building a society where occupations can be equitably realised. To do so, they must possess a thorough understanding of various social justice movements and their historical backgrounds. Inequality must be recognised not as a personal pathology or individual experience but as phenomena with specific causal factors that require awareness and action. Social justice movements are characterised by their participatory, collaborative, inclusive, and agency-affirming nature. Throughout history, numerous social movements have been implemented to seek social justice within countries, organisations, and communities (Brittanie, 2023).

One example of a recent social justice movement was #Black Lives Matter (BLM) that began in the United States in 2013 in response to violence towards, profiling of, and discrimination against Black individuals, particularly addressing police misconduct (Harris, 2015). The movement rapidly spread worldwide through social media and gained traction in many jurisdictions. In these countries, the movement expanded to address discrimination against immigrants, foreign workers, refugees, and ethnic minorities, with BLM protests highlighting these issues. Discrimination against racial and ethnic minorities, as well as immigrants, includes not only institutional discrimination – where societal systems and laws disadvantage specific races or groups – but also everyday subtle discriminatory acts and unconscious biases.

The #Me Too Movement is a social movement aimed at empowering victims of sexual violence and harassment to come forward and share their experiences (Quan-Haase & Mendes, 2021). Although the movement began in 2006, it gained significant momentum in 2017 when a Hollywood actress used the hashtag #MeToo on social media. This sparked a global movement that extended beyond Western countries to Asia, South America, Africa and other regions worldwide. The movement addresses the deep-seated issues of sexism, discrimination, sexual violence and coercive behaviour, as well as the oppression resulting from power, legal, and economic imbalances that affect those in weaker social positions. It highlights the importance of ensuring that survivors of sexual violence and harassment receive fair treatment and that perpetrators are held accountable, advocating for what is known as Survivor's Justice (Stubbs-Richardson et al., 2023).

The LGBTQIAP2S+ rights movement advocating for the rights of sexual minorities, specifically lesbian, gay, bisexual, transgender, queer, intersex, pansexual, two-spirit individuals, is unfolding in various forms across the globe (Dicklitch-Nelson & Rahman, 2022) Efforts are being made to secure rights such as marriage equality, healthcare access, employment opportunities, adoption rights, and recognition in various social, legal, religious and cultural contexts, however, the scope of these civil rights varies by country. When individuals with diverse gender identities intersect with other social identities such as race, class, age, appearance, or ability, which is intersectionality, the discrimination and oppression they may experience are highly individualised. Intersectionality will be discussed in more detail in Section 13.5.

First Nations and Indigenous rights is primarily centred in countries that have a history of colonisation including Canada, United States, Australia, Aotearoa New Zealand, African nations, and countries in South America. First Nations peoples seek to protect their cultural heritage and address historical injustices, and achieve social, economic, and political equality. This includes the efforts of Indigenous peoples such as Australia's Aboriginal and Torres Strait Islander, Aotearoa New Zealand's Māori, Canada's First Nations, Inuit, and Métis and Native American communities (Gussen, 2017). The importance of Indigenous peoples' rights to self-government, their own legal systems, their land, language, and cultural heritage is emphasised. Additionally, this includes efforts to protect the environment, which is closely connected to Indigenous peoples' traditional practices and spiritual beliefs.

13.4 Social justice and occupational justice

The difference between social justice and occupational justice can often be confusing. Social justice is a concept that recognises humans as social beings who engage in social relations (Stadnyk et al., 2010). It favours equitable access to opportunities and resources to reduce group differences related to characteristics such as age, ability, culture, gender, social class, and sexual orientation. Occupational justice is concerned with enabling, mediating, and advocating for environments and dynamics in which all people's opportunities to engage in occupation are just, health-promoting, and meaningful (Whiteford & Hocking, 2012). Social justice and occupational justice are joint aspirations towards an inclusive and mutually supportive world (Jakobsen, 2004).

Occupational injustice, conversely, has been defined as 'an outcome of social policies and other forms of governance that structure how power is exerted to restrict participation in the everyday occupations of populations and individuals' (Nilsson & Townsend, 2010, p. 58). Types of occupational injustice include the following.

- **Occupational deprivation** points to externally imposed barriers to valued, meaningful occupations necessary for well-being.
- **Occupational imbalance** is due to occupational patterns of being over- or underoccupied, due to excessive work demands, enforced idleness, or burdensome responsibilities to care for the environment, dependents, or oneself.
- **Occupational alienation** has been defined as 'deep feelings of incompatibility with the occupations associated with a place, situation, or others to the extent that basic needs and wants appear impossible to attain or maintain' (Wilcock & Hocking, 2015, p. 258). It may manifest as aggressive occupations associated with social unrest or self-destructive behaviours.
- **Occupational marginalisation** is usually associated with discrimination, such that people are systematically relegated to occupational opportunities and resources that are less valued within a society (Stadnyk et al., 2010).
- **Occupational apartheid** refers to the systematic segregation of groups of people and deliberately denying them access to occupations, such as quality education or well-paid work, or occupational contexts, based on prejudice about their capacities or entitlement to the benefits of culturally valued occupations (Wilcock & Hocking, 2015).

Other definitions that are important to understand when applying concepts of social and occupational justice:

- **Equity, diversity, and inclusion (EDI)** is a conceptual framework that promotes the fair treatment and full participation of all people, especially populations that have historically been underrepresented or subject to discrimination because of their background, identity, disability, and so on.

- **Equity** involves providing resources according to the need to help diverse populations achieve their highest state of health and other functioning.
- **Diversity** refers to the representation or composition of various social identity groups in a work group, organisation, or community.
- **Inclusion** strives for an environment that offers affirmation, celebration, and appreciation of different approaches, styles, perspectives, and experiences.
- **Belonging** means that everyone is treated and feels like a full member of the larger community and can thrive.

13.5 Intersectionality

Intersectionality is a term first introduced by scholar and civil rights advocate Kimberlé Crenshaw in 1989 in the United States. Originally it was used to describe the impact of multiple oppressions experienced by black women in the United States (Bauer et al., 2021). To understand intersectionality, you must look at the different parts of people's identities and how these intersecting identities can cause people to experience life differently from others, including yourself. Intersectionality recognises that intersecting and overlapping identities can be both oppressive and empowering. In addition, it creates both strengths and vulnerabilities in individuals, families, and communities. Some of our sociocultural identities help us to be resilient and productive members of our communities, but others lead to discrimination, marginalisation, and oppression (De Silva, 2020). Examples of sociocultural identities include class, primary language, race, citizenship, religion, gender identity, skin colour, and age.

The starting point for intersectionality is difference and recognising how hierarchies of race, class, gender, disability, and sexuality generate structural inequalities for particular groups. There are many intersecting identities, but more importantly intersecting systems of privilege and oppression. Many marginalised populations are groups and communities with intersecting identities and regularly experience systemic discrimination, oppression, and inequality. Intersectionality is not about defining groups as 'victims' but instead recognising the inequalities and taking practical action to remedy the societal, political, and economic power and privilege imbalances. Taking a human occupation lens, intersectionality has several relevant concepts (Ambrosio & Silva, 2022; Balanta-Cobo et al., 2022). These include:

- **Occupational Intersectionality:** the different types and layers of sociocultural identities that a person, family, community, or collective may have and how they intersect with each other in tandem to create occupational strengths and vulnerabilities;
- **Occupational Privilege:** engaging in daily occupations that are central to one's identity, that are taken for granted and assumed by one or more societal groups, and that other members of society may not have ready access to based on their multiple layered intersecting sociocultural identities;
- **Occupational Oppression:** individuals, families, communities, or collectives being denied the right to engage in fundamental daily occupations that provide

sustenance, meaning, purpose, health, and well-being based on their multiple, layered intersecting sociocultural identities; and

■ **Occupational Discrimination:** individuals, families, communities, or collectives being denied access to daily occupations based on their multiple, layered intersecting sociocultural identities (e.g., gender identity, sexual orientation, class, citizenship, physical or cognitive ability, ethnicity, race, etc.).

Vignette 13.1
From youth control towards compassion in regional Australia

Introduction

This case study examines the implementation of curfews in Australia, specifically focusing on the 2024 curfew in Alice Springs. It highlights how these measures, while justified under the guise of public safety, reflect colonial practices that reinforce intersecting disadvantages by largely affecting, youth, Aboriginal and Torres Strait Islander, and remote communities. By exploring the rationale, social context, and meanings of these curfews, this case study seeks to understand intersectionality to assess situations but also to guide our professional engagement by considering an intersecting capabilities approach.

Curfew as an impulse of control: impact on First Nations, youth, and remote communities

The control of space and the regulation of people's movement are mechanisms used to shape social dynamics, often revealing deep connections to impulses of control over specific social groups. Curfew has historically been implemented for various purposes, often to control public spaces and specific populations under the pretext of public safety. Curfews inherently curtail democratic rights, such as freedom of movement, and in democratic societies like Australia, curfews are typically justifiable only under exceptional circumstances where significant and overriding benefits can be demonstrated.

In Australia official and 'unofficial' curfews disproportionately affect Aboriginal and Torres Strait Islander people, as experienced by the young Redfern activists in the 1960s, whereby simply being on the streets of Redfern late at night was enough to contravene the 'unofficial curfew' (Lothian, 2007). It is important to note that curfews have remained relatively common in the Australian debate and are often linked to the management of Aboriginal and Torres Strait Islander youth, particularly those living in regional communities (Nakata & Bray, 2023). For instance, in 1990, Port Augusta in South Australia held a local referendum that supported a 10 pm curfew for children under 16 (Simpson & Simpson, 1993), and in 1991, Cloncurry in North West Queensland implemented a midnight-to-dawn curfew for teenagers (Jones & Marks, 1996).

While evidence suggests that broad stay-at-home measures can reduce overall crime rates, as seen during the COVID-19 pandemic (Nivette et al., 2021), the effectiveness of such restrictive measures appears inconsistent when applied to specific social groups and/or geographical areas. In fact, researchers in Australia have questioned the efficacy of youth curfews in reducing crime, finding no conclusive evidence that curfews actually lower crime rates, nor do they address the root determinants of the issue itself (Zahnow & Goldsworthy,

2017). Instead, these measures often exacerbate social injustices, reinforcing intersecting disadvantages of those most affected, in this case First Nations, youth, and remote communities.

2024 Mparntwe/Alice Springs curfew

In 2024, Mparntwe/Alice Springs implemented a youth curfew as part of an emergency declaration from 27 March to 16 April 2024. This curfew was enforced in denominated high-risk areas and applied to individuals under the age of 18 from 6 pm to 6 am, unless they had a valid reason, such as employment, accessing youth-related services, being accompanied by a responsible adult, or having a medical emergency (Northern Territory Government, 2024). Although intended to enhance public safety, this curfew reflects how the control of space and movement can disproportionately impact specific social groups, in this case First Nations youth living in remote areas.

The implementation of the Alice Springs curfew demonstrates the ongoing presence of colonial impulses of control in contemporary governance. While these measures are presented as temporary solutions to safety concerns, they reflect a continuation of historical practices that aim to regulate the lives of certain people. In other words, the discussion of public safety is placed under a higher value than youth safety. By imposing such restrictions, the curfew inadvertently impacts the perception of First Nations youth in remote areas, suggesting a need to control and manage their presence in public spaces, instead of indicating their need for protection. This reinforces structural inequalities and highlights the importance of addressing the systemic issues that lead to the implementation of such measures.

The 2024 Alice Springs curfew serves as a case study for thoughtful reflection on how such measures may fail to resolve the social issues they aim to address and may inadvertently perpetuate a legacy of intersecting disadvantages.

Final note: A shift from public safety towards youth safety

The 2024 Alice Springs curfew underscores the persistent challenges Aboriginal and Torres Strait Islander youth face in regional Australia, particularly as these measures exacerbate pre-existing exclusion rooted in colonial legacies. A broader and more humane approach is needed – one that moves beyond controlling disadvantage and instead centres on intersecting capabilities as a core ethical and professional commitment. Intersecting capabilities refers to the opportunities and freedoms that individuals have to achieve to experience well-being across various social domains, where different aspects of identity (such as race, class, and ability) interact to either expand or constrain these opportunities.

Occupational therapist jurisdiction should not support responses based on restrictive measures, instead we must apply concepts such intersecting capabilities to work towards enhancing the experiences of young people, particularly most affected by lack of protection. This requires rethinking theoretical frameworks by integrating intersectionality into our reasoning, not merely to identify disadvantages but to move towards expanding intersecting capabilities, i.e., imaging and building an 'other' social experience for First Nations youth in regional areas. Engaging with Aboriginal and Torres Strait Islander youth in the co-creation of community-led solutions is essential. Here, rights related to self-determination, social opportunities are crucial.

The shift from disadvantage to capability represents a fundamental change to understand the issue from 'public safety' to 'youth safety.' It recognises that safety is not merely the absence of risk but the presence of opportunity and self-determination. The Alice Springs curfew, presented here as a case study, serves as a call to action, encouraging occupational therapists to move away from frameworks rooted in repressive thinking and practice and/or deficit approach, but to move toward those that prioritise intersecting capabilities. This shift is not only theoretical but demands a professional and ethical commitment particularly for those most vulnerable to systemic marginalisation. By using intersectionality as a guiding framework, we can move towards a clearer understanding and, more importantly, towards solutions that foster lives and dignity.

Vignette 13.2
Finding home

Introduction

It has been noted that occupational therapists and occupational scientists have, in the past, celebrated occupations as having a positive influence on health and well-being. A social justice perspective on occupation has called attention to how social inequities and those in power influence ideas of social difference such as race, class, gender, age, sexual orientation, and disability and how this in turn impacts who can and cannot participate in various occupations (Angell, 2012). This case study highlights how assumptions about social difference, asserted in Aotearoa New Zealand housing policy over time, have not only shaped the meaning New Zealanders give to home but also the choices and opportunities people have to participate in the occupations they need, want, and are entitled to engage in.

Hegemony and the good citizen

Hegemony is a term used to describe how one dominant group's ideologies, values, and ethics become the established norm, giving power and control over other groups of people (Wilding, 2011). These processes are often subtle and disguised as a moral good. Institutions and their policies can be hegemonic, impacting the way people live their everyday lives by influencing their future goals, dreams, fears, and meaningful occupations.

Aotearoa New Zealand governments have a long history of alienating Māori from their traditional homelands through confiscation and dispossession which forced them to find a new place to work and live in urban centres (Boulton et al., 2022). Literature describing the historical impact of housing policy on Māori is where we see a more subtle assimilation to Eurocentric ideologies and morals around homemaking and how to be a good citizen (Brookes, 1997; Wanhalla, 2006).

Early housing and health policies were driven by attempts to improve Māori health after outbreaks of tuberculosis and influenza had reduced the number of Māori significantly. In the early 1900s, health officials had the power to order occupants to improve their homes on the threat of demolition. In the 1930s, surveys of Māori homes were carried out to measure the need for improvements. Homes were measured against distinctly European standards.

The importance of extended family was not recognised when homes were observed to be overcrowded. Traditional Māori architectural designs or where traditional activities and objects might be located in a home were ignored (Hall, 2008). Housing officers reported not only on the state of housing but also noted well-kept homes and families that 'lived like Europeans'.

The education system also promoted the concept of an ideal Aotearoa New Zealand citizen and the activities they should engage in (School Publications Branch, 1949). An example of this is a book called *Houses to Live in*, developed in 1949 for schools. In the story, Mr and Mrs Walton are looking to buy a new home. Mr Walton wants a home that has places for the things that enable him to do and be. For instance, a place for odd jobs, a place for a fishing rod or golf clubs, a place to work in the evenings, and a place to rest away from the noise of the children. Mrs Walton had on her list areas that would enable play for the children outside, a room for fun with the family that would not mess up the formal lounge, a place to entertain friends for dinner, and a safe place for her china (Brookes, 1997). Whilst these policies and ideologies of home were portrayed as well intentioned, the active promotion of Western occupations was used as a tool to colonise, resulting in the erosion of Māori ways of doing and being (Emery-Whittington, 2021). Memmott et al. (2003) posit the idea of spiritual homelessness for Indigenous cultures where separation from traditional lands results in a loss of connection to kin, cultural identity, and a sense of self.

Hegemony and the gendered home

When children heard the story of Mr and Mrs Walton in the 1950s, they not only learnt to read but also learnt what the gendered roles of New Zealanders should be. We learn that Mr Walton is the money earner, whilst Mrs Walton cares for the home and their children. In the 21st century, this is still a reality, with only 1% of Aotearoa New Zealand men taking up paid parental leave. The same study shows that a father's involvement for children at nine months and two years increases especially if the father is Māori or Pasifika (Hennecke et al., 2022). What has changed is that we know that it is more likely that both parents are working, with a Aotearoa New Zealand childcare survey showing 53% of preschoolers attending at least one type of formal early childhood education (Statistics New Zealand, 2010). Feminist researchers also highlight that traditional views of the family home reinforce heterosexual ideals and not gender-diverse households.

Final note: A human rights response

In 2024 we have 1 in 100 New Zealanders classified as homeless, and half of these people are under 25. This has also been driven by successive government ideologies that favour neoliberalism and a house as an investment rather than a home. Neoliberalism ideology suggests that minimising government involvement in economic and social matters, alongside the deregulation of labour and financial markets, commerce, and investments. Whilst acknowledging new housing policies that have tried to address inequities, discrimination, and homelessness, a recent United Nations report has called the state of Aotearoa New Zealand's housing a human rights crisis (United Nations General Assembly, 2021). Statistics tell us that finding an adequate affordable home has hit Māori, Pasifika people, people with disabilities, single parents, the LGBTQIAP2S+ community, and other minorities the hardest. The right to adequate housing starts with the notion that every human deserves to live in

> security, peace, and dignity and that assumptions about what type of house someone needs based on social difference are challenged (United Nations Committee on Economic, Social and Cultural Rights, 1991). A human rights response to the mistakes of the past and the current housing crisis would ensure that housing policies see homes as an entitlement rather than just a need. Human rights are also innately occupation focused and would encourage adequate housing that would give opportunities and choices for all citizens to participate in the occupations that they want, need, and are entitled to.

13.6 What can occupational therapy students and practitioners contribute to address social justice and intersectionality issues from an occupational perspective?

- *Challenge your own unconscious biases and privilege:* Question your own beliefs about others and stop to reconsider behaviours and attitudes (as more that might disadvantage or discriminate).
- *Educate yourself:* Learn about what intersectionality means and stay aware of social justice issues that affect society and people's ability to participate in meaningful and purposeful occupations.
- *Be mindful of the complexity of human beings:* When considering the patient/client holistically, be aware of the influences of all identities that they may have that affect participation.
- *Get involved:* Participate in local professional and non-professional groups that address social justice issues and support intersectional communities.
- *Amplify marginalised voices:* Seek out opportunities to promote the stories and lived experiences of marginalised communities to challenge existing narratives and inequity in health and social care.
- *Advocate for inclusion:* Advocate for policies and practices that promote equity, inclusion, and diversity in the access and receipt of health and social care services through professional and community organisations, including occupational therapy services.
- *Protect the freedom to do and be:* Advocate for individuals and groups who are being prevented from pursuing the occupations they want, need, and are expected to do. Investigate the root causes and action evidence-based solutions.
- *Prioritise dignity and occupational rights:* Ask yourself what valued occupations your clients should not be expected to give up due to discrimination and inequity.
- *Empower rights holders:* When a client or group of people is being prevented from participating in an occupation they have a right to engage in, actively look for ways of increasing occupational opportunity and choice.

13.7 Conclusion

This chapter introduces the concepts of social justice and intersectionality and associated concepts. It highlights the importance of addressing social, economic, political, and cultural injustices that hinder occupational justice. The discussion on intersectionality further deepens our understanding of how overlapping social identities shape experiences of privilege and discrimination. Recognising these complexities is essential for occupational therapists to move beyond surface-level interventions and understand the root causes of injustice. Two vignettes illustrate how public and private life are deeply intertwined through the enactment of policies rooted in hegemonic ideals, revealing the far-reaching impact of systemic injustices on occupational participation in private and public spaces. Finally, the chapter addresses the critical question of what can occupational therapy students and practitioners contribute to addressing social justice and intersectionality issues from an occupational perspective. By equipping readers with the theoretical and practical tools to recognise and challenge injustice, the chapter calls attention to the transformative role of occupational therapy in fostering equitable and inclusive participation in meaningful occupations.

13.8 Summary

- Occupational therapists must focus on social and occupational justice to promote occupational enablement and equality for individuals, families, communities, collectives, and organisations from a range of backgrounds.
- Occupational therapists have a professional and ethical responsibility to work towards building a society where occupations can be equitably realised.
- Inequality and inequity must be recognised not as a personal pathology or individual experience but as phenomena with specific causal factors that require awareness and action. Occupational therapists must examine these experiences using an intersectional lens.
- Occupational justice occurs when all people can engage in occupations that are just, health-promoting, and meaningful.

13.9 Review and reflection questions

- Define the concepts of social justice and intersectionality.
- How can the concept of intersectionality be applied to clients, families, and groups that occupational therapists engage with?
- What is the difference between social justice and occupational justice?
- Describe four strategies that occupational therapy clinicians and students can complete to address social justice and intersectionality issues.

References

Ambrosio, L., & Silva, C. R. (2022). Intersectionality: An Amefrican diasporic concept for occupational therapy. *Cadernos Brasileiros de Terapia Ocupacional, 30*, e3150. https://doi.org/10.1590/2526-8910.ctoEN241431502

Angell, A. M. (2012). Occupation-centred analysis of social difference: Contributions to a socially responsive occupational science. *Journal of Occupational Science, 21*(2), 104–116. http://doi.org/10.1080/14427591.2012.711230

Balanta-Cobo, P., Fransen-Jaïbi, H., Gonzalez, M., Henny, E., Malfitano, A. P. S., & Pollard, N. (2022). Human and social rights and occupational therapy: The need for an intersectional perspective. *Cadernos Brasileiros de Terapia Ocupacional, 30*, e30202203. https://doi.org/10.1590/2526-8910.ctoED302022032

Barker, R. L. (2013). *The social work dictionary* (6th ed.).

Bauer, G. R., Churchill, S. M., Mahendran, M., Walwyn, C., Lizotte, D., & Villa-Rueda, A. A. (2021). Intersectionality in quantitative research: A systematic review of its emergence and applications of theory and methods. *SSM – Population Health, 14*, 100798. https://doi.org/10.1016/j.ssmph.2021.100798

Boulton, A., Allport, T., Kaiwai, H., Harker, R., & Potaka Osborne., G. (2022). Māori perceptions of 'home': Māori housing needs, wellbeing and policy. *Kōtuitui: New Zealand Journal of Social Sciences Online, 17*(1), 44–55. https://doi.org/10.1080/1177083X.2021.1920984

Brittanie, E. (2023). Social work and social justice: A conceptual review. *Social Work, 68*(1), 38–46. https://doi.org/10.1093/sw/swaa049

Brookes, B. (1997). Nostalgia for 'innocent homely pleasures': The 1964 New Zealand controversy over washday at the pa. *Gender and History, 9*(2) 242–261. https://doi.org/10.1111/1468-0424.00057

De Silva, M. (2020). Intersectionality. In A. Kobayashi (Ed.), *International encyclopedia of human geography* (2nd ed., pp. 397–401). Elsevier. https://doi.org/10.1016/B978-0-08-102295-5.10197-0

Dicklitch-Nelson, S., & Rahman, I. (2022). Transgender rights are human rights: A cross-national comparison of transgender rights in 204 countries. *Journal of Human Rights, 21*(5), 525–541. https://doi.org/10.1080/14754835.2022.2100985

Emery-Whittington, I. (2021). Occupational justice – colonial business as usual? Indigenous observations from Aotearoa New Zealand. *Canadian Journal of Occupational Therapy 88*(2), 153–162. https://doi.org/10.1177/00084174211005891

Gussen, B. F. (2017). A comparative analysis of constitutional recognition of Aboriginal peoples. *Melbourne University Law Review, 40*(3), 867–867. http://law.unimelb.edu.au/__data/assets/pdf_file/0003/2340417/05-Gussen.pdf

Hall, L. (2008). *Māori and Pacific peoples' housing needs in the Auckland region: A literature review.* Auckland Regional Council.

Harris, J. (2015). What kind of movement is Black Lives Matter? The view from Twitter. *Journal of Race, Ethnicity, and Politics, 1*, 35–50. https://doi.org/10.1017/rep.2015.2

Hennecke, J., Meehan, L., Pacheco, G., & Turcu, A. (2022). *Fathers' household and childcare involvement in New Zealand: A snapshot, determinants and consequences.* New Zealand Work Research Institute.

Jakobsen, K. (2004). If work doesn't work: How to enable occupational justice. *Journal of Occupational Science, 11*(3), 125–134. https://doi.org/10.1080/14427591.2004.9686540

Jones, M., & Marks, L. A. B. (1996). Mediating rights: Children, parents and the state. *Australian Journal of Human Rights, 2*(2), 313–327. https://doi.org/10.1080/1323238X.1996.11910962

Lothian, K. (2007). Moving Blackwards: Black Power and the Aboriginal Embassy. In I. Macfarlane & M. Hannah (Eds.), *Transgressions: Critical Australian Indigenous histories* (pp. 19–32). ANU Press.

Memmott, P., Long, S., Chambers, C., & Spring, F. (2003). *Categories of Indigenous 'homeless' people and good practice responses to their needs* (AHURI Final Report No. 49). Australian Housing and Urban Research Institute. https://www.ahuri.edu.au/research/final-reports/49

Nakata, S., & Bray, D. (2023). Political representation of Aboriginal and Torres Strait Islander youth in Australia. In B. Sandin, J. Josefsson, Hanson, & S. Balagopalan (Eds.), *The politics of children's rights and representation. Studies in childhood and youth* (pp. 301–323). Palgrave Macmillan. https://doi.org/10.1007/978-3-031-04480-9_13

Nilsson, I., & Townsend, E. (2010). Occupational justice-bridging theory and practice. *Scandinavian Journal of Occupational Therapy, 17*(1), 57–63. https://doi.org/10.3109/11038120903287182

Nivette, A. E., Zahnow, R., Aguilar, R., Ahven, A., Amram, S., Ariel, B., Burbano, M. J. A., Astolfi, R., Baier, D., Bark, H. M., Beijers, J. E. H., Bergman, M., Breetzke, G., Concha-Eastman, I. A., Curtis-Ham, S., Davenport, R., Díaz, C., Fleitas, D., Gerell, M., Jang, K. H., . . . Eisner, M. P. (2021). A global analysis of the impact of COVID-19 stay-at-home restrictions on crime. *Nature Human Behaviour, 5*(7), 868–877. https://doi.org/10.1038/s41562-021-01139-z

Northern Territory Government. (2024, March 27). *Alice Springs emergency declaration.* https://nt.gov.au/__data/assets/pdf_file/0009/1364922/emergency-declaration-27-march-2024.PDF

Quan-Haase, A., & Mendes, P. D. (2021). Mapping #MeToo: A synthesis review of digital feminist research across social media platforms. *New Media & Society, 23*(6), 1700–1720. https://doi.org/10.1177/1461444820969669

School Publications Branch. (1949). *Houses to live in.* Department of Education.

Simpson, B., & Simpson, C. (1993). The use of curfews to control juvenile offending in Australia: Managing crime or wasting time? *Current Issues In Criminal Justice, 5*(2), 184–199. https://doi.org/10.1080/10345329.1993.12036604

Stadnyk, R., Townsend, E., & Wilcock, A. (2010). Occupational justice. In C. H. Christiansen & E. A. Townsend (Eds.), *Introduction to occupation: The art and science of living* (2nd ed., pp. 329–358). Pearson Education.

Statistics New Zealand. (2010). *New Zealand childcare survey 2009* (Revised 17 December 2010). Statistics New Zealand. https://www.infonews.co.nz/news.cfm?id=62243

Stubbs-Richardson, M., Gilbreath, S., Paul, M., & Reid, A. (2023). It's a global #MeToo: A cross-national comparison of social change associated with the movement. *Feminist Media Studies, 24*(2), 1330–1349. https://doi.org/10.1080/14680777.2023.2231654

United Nations General Assembly. (2021). *Visit to New Zealand: Report of the special rapporteur on adequate housing as a component of the right to an adequate standard of living and on the right to non-discrimination in this context, Leilani Farha.* A/HRC/47/43/Add.1.

Wanhalla, A. (2006). Housing un/healthy bodies: Native housing surveys and Māori health in New Zealand 1930–45. *Health and History, 8*(1), 100–120. https://doi.org/10.2307/40111531

Whiteford, G. E., & Hocking, C. (Eds.). (2012). *Occupational science: Society, inclusion, participation.* Wiley-Blackwell.

Wilcock, A., & Hocking, C. (2015). *An occupational perspective of health* (3rd ed.). Slack.

Wilding, C. (2011). Raising awareness of hegemony in occupational therapy: The value of action research for improving practice. *Australian Occupational Therapy Journal, 58*(4), 293–299. http://doi:/10.1111/j.1440-1630.2010.00910.x

Zahnow, R., & Goldsworthy, T. (2017). FactCheck: Did the Northbridge WA curfew see a 'dramatic drop' in crime? *The Conversation.* https://theconversation.com/factcheck-did-the-northbridge-wa-curfew-see-a-dramatic-drop-in-crime-87016

CHAPTER 14

Embracing social transformation

Occupational therapy in community practices

Vagner Dos Santos, Ana Paula Serrata Malfitano, and Gelya Frank

Authors' positionality statement

The authors of this chapter are advocates and scholar-activists for democratic rights. Their work aims to promote collective engagement in addressing shared social issues and emphasises ensuring democratic rights, particularly for equity-deserving groups, by advocating compassionate treatment and equitable access to public goods such as housing, education, healthcare, transportation, and work. In a dialogue between scholars from South America and North America, we believe we can highlight different perspectives to inform a more social responsive practice in the field. We are scholars, university-educated, professionally qualified, and locally economically privileged in each of our countries, dedicating our work to challenging various kinds of social oppression.

Key terms
- Social occupational therapy
- Occupational reconstruction
- Democratic participation
- Equity-seeking groups
- Social technologies

Objectives
This chapter will allow the reader to:

- Examine the role of the occupational therapy profession in promoting social transformation with collectives working toward social emancipation and equity
- Gain an overview of two theoretical frameworks – social occupational therapy and occupational reconstruction – that can underpin the advancement of socially transformative practices in the profession

DOI: 10.4324/9781003495666-16

- Identify practices (social technologies and strategies) that occupational therapists can use within these frameworks to address socially structured problems through community participation

14.1 Introduction

In recent decades, there has been a growing recognition among occupational therapists of the socially structured problems that individuals and communities face (Dos Santos, 2025; Hammell, 2020; Lopes et al., 2025; Taff et al., 2025). An emerging international movement is advocating for the occupational therapy profession to have a role in fostering community practices that include political engagement and social transformation (Dos Santos et al., 2022; Farias et al., 2016, 2025; Farias & Laliberte Rudman, 2016; Farias & Lopes, 2023; Hammell, 2023; Lopes & Malfitano, 2021). Accordingly, socially structured problems such as inequality, discrimination, and social exclusion are being seen as something more than issues or shortcomings pertaining to individuals alone. Instead, they are being recognised also as problems embedded in the broader socio-political landscape in which individual lives are lived (Das, 2006; Fassin, 2018, 2010; Kleinman & Kleinman, 1996; Marmot, 2005). Consequently, new practice frameworks are needed to facilitate occupational therapists to engage ethically and straightforwardly with issues affecting social groups and collectives. We refer especially to equity-seeking groups that are marginalised and denied meaningful participation based on socially and culturally determined factors such as gender identity, religion, ethnicity, disability, language, and economic status.

Equity-seeking groups, also referred to as equity-deserving groups, are communities that have historically, persistently, or systemically faced marginalisation and discrimination, such as Black, Brown, Indigenous, and economically disadvantaged populations, among others (Patrick, 2024). The concept of vulnerability is closely tied to these groups, as systemic inequities and exclusion increase their susceptibility to adverse outcomes in areas such as healthcare, education, and professional settings (Kapiriri & Razavi, 2022). We argue that occupational therapy, as a profession that is committed to enhancing human health, well-being, and social participation must also consider critically how people can improve their situations through social cohesion and democratic social action. We suggest that occupational therapists widen their professional lens to include an understanding of social dynamics and social structures and expand their toolkit of practices to work with collectives – that is, people as members of certain groups, communities, and populations – to enact social change.

Traditional approaches in occupational therapy reflect professional boundaries grounded predominantly in western biomedicine, with its scientific reductionism that focuses on individual rehabilitation and individual models of care (Dos Santos & Leon Spesny, 2016; Hammell, 2022). Alternatively, a critical and politically-informed approach recognises the role of social systems not only in shaping lives and ways of living, but also in creating limitations within a scientific and medicalised worldview (Dos Santos et al., 2019; Dos Santos, 2025; Dos Santos & Frank, 2024; Frank, 2022; Malfitano et al., 2021; Østergaard Madsen et al., 2024). From this critical perspective, occupational therapists' role can shift from its individualising focus to one that actively fosters community engagement and collective action. We do not suggest this shift as an abstract exercise but as a development for the profession that introduces new and arguably necessary kinds of practice. It encourages occupational therapists to work not only with individuals but also with collectives to enact and promote social transformation. Such a shift would further align practice with broader social goals and social movements that aim to dismantle systemic barriers contributing to inequality (Farias et al., 2025; Frank, 2020; Hammell, 2023; Lopes & Malfitano, 2021; Tofeti & Dos Santos, 2020; Whiteford et al., 2018).

This chapter thus introduces theoretical and practical guidance for occupational therapists to engage with such questions as: What does the profession need to understand about socially structured inequalities? What needs to be changed? What can be done to promote those changes? We reflect critically on the idea of democratic participation as a strategy for occupational therapists who work with collectives to promote equity and inclusion. Collective strategies challenge Western, biomedical, and neoliberal economic assumptions that treat socially structured problems as problems for which individuals bear sole or primary responsibility for causing, adapting to, or correcting for themselves alone. Collective strategies underlie both *social occupational therapy* and *occupational reconstruction*, two frameworks of theory and practice described in this chapter (Dos Santos & Frank, 2024; Lopes & Malfitano, 2021).

Social occupational therapy is a field within the broader occupational therapy profession that focuses on understanding and addressing social questions. It is rooted in the recognition that people's lives are deeply influenced by socially structured factors such as poverty, inequality, racism, gender, migration, and politics. *Social occupational therapy* integrates socio-political analysis and emancipatory practices so that occupational therapists can contribute to building a more equitable and inclusive society when working with collectives.

Occupational reconstruction is a theory and practice framework for a collective process of transforming social realities through shared engagement in occupations. The process begins with an intentional response by members of a group to a shared problematic situation and it proceeds by narrative alignment and experimental actions. *Occupational reconstruction* as a theory and practice framework justifies social transformation as a treatment goal consistent with the occupational therapy profession's foundational values. It further guides and supports occupational therapists to implement the theory through socially transformative strategies for practice.

In summary, this chapter's overall aim is to introduce frameworks that articulate a lexicon and demonstrate methods for how occupational therapists can: (1) define their roles when working with collectives to address shared socially structured problems; and (2) provide support to equity-seeking groups in their pursuit of goals such as justice, access to social goods and life-enhancing opportunities, and health and well-being.

14.2 Embracing democratic participation and community ties

Democracy is variously a model of governance, a political system and a philosophy of equality. It can also be viewed as a participatory framework designed to centre collective interests in political decision-making and cooperative action to accomplish shared desires and objectives. It accomplishes this through participation, inclusion, and the protection of citizen rights (i.e., right to life, freedom of expression, equality before the law, fair trial, privacy, assembly and association, education, fair work and labour conditions, freedom of religion, and housing, etc.) (Fassin, 2010; Unger, 1998). Beyond the politics of balancing individual interests with collective rights, social democracy as an ideal and a practice aims to enable more profoundly agentic forms of collective engagement and collective-driven action. In line with democratic values, Paulo Freire's concept of critical consciousness (*conscientização*) emphasises the power of democratic participation to drive change (Freire, 2000). Freire's pedagogy advocates for marginalised groups to engage in dialogue and collective action to challenge and address shared social problems. In other words, collective action is at the core of democratic participation, not only facilitating social improvements but also strengthening the social fabric.

The quest for scientific and political neutrality – typically taught as essential to objectivity and professional integrity – shows the overwhelming influence of the biomedical model on occupational therapy, emphasising standardisation, neutrality, and individualised care. Medicine and psychology dominate professional explanations and approaches to dealing with human suffering (Gusfield, 1996; Kleinman & Kleinman, 1996). Yet such individualistic approaches can be characterised as repressive, if they place all responsibility for diagnosis, treatment, and care at the individual level. In a study of incarcerated youth, for example, professionals blamed youth individually for their offenses and consequences of social inequalities they experienced (Leon Spesny & Dos Santos, 2025). A social occupational therapy or occupational reconstruction approach would focus compassionately on promoting their participation in changing the inequalities at the root of their offenses.

Under neoliberalism, the dominant form of global economy in our time, the tendency to explain social outcomes in terms of individualised responsibilities – the individualisation of life – is enforced through economic and political measures of individual accountability (Dos Santos, 2022; Farias et al., 2025; Farias & Lopes, 2023; Frank, 2022). As Frank (2022) comments in an evaluation of the contributions of science to occupational therapy, neoliberalism is a political ideology advocating free markets, privatisation, deregulation, and minimal government intervention in the economy, and reduction of public investments in education, housing, health and wellbeing. So, while biomedical knowledge and individual approaches have significantly contributed to the advancement of occupational therapy practice and professional credibility, the profession's scope and jurisdiction of practice has been limited with few exceptions to treating one individual at a time.

Only now are occupational theorists beginning to advance collective approaches to socially structured problems that impact so many patients' and clients' lives, as well as lives of others who could be helped. The principle of scientific neutrality, a gold standard in biomedical outcomes research that incidentally is aligned with neoliberal accounting methods, suggests that the occupational therapist's role should remain detached from socio-political influences and focused purely on statistically derived clinical outcomes, mainly related to individual functionality and independence (Hammell, 2022). However, this stance can obscure the systemic and structural factors that create disparities and injustices among populations with whom occupational therapists currently work or could potentially work with the tools of the profession.

The entanglement of social inequalities generates intersectional disadvantages, compounding vulnerabilities, and limiting opportunities for marginalised groups. Thus, occupational therapists are increasingly seeking to develop socially engaged practices that recognise democratic participation and rights as intertwined with dignity, access to resources, political voice, and community support. Dos Santos (2025) discusses a political project for the profession of occupational therapy aimed at identifying and challenging moral and political inequalities, emphasising that not all lives are treated equitably. These inequalities result in a division between those deemed deserving of compassion and those subjected to repression. By highlighting this disparity, professionals can challenge conventional political perspectives, underscore the inherent value of all human lives, and advocate for actions to address and reduce inequities.

Shifting from a neutrality stance to a role of engagement enables occupational therapists to foster community participation, enact changes working with collectives, and advocate for policies that promote equity and inclusion. This shift transforms the role of the occupational therapist from a detached expert to a collaborator and participant in a dynamic process to facilitate marginalised voices being heard and acted upon for such goals as: securing the right to be safe from physical violence, economic deprivation, and other harms; accessing public goods such as school, health services, and housing, and being respected regardless of characteristics such as economic status, language, ethnicity, sexuality, disability status, religion, and skin colour.

The theoretical exploration of democratic participation and community ties emphasises the importance of critically engaging with socio-political contexts and embracing socially engaged practices. By doing so, occupational therapy can contribute to broader movements for justice and equity. Importantly, this chapter does not encourage occupational therapists to act outside their scope or jurisdiction of practice (Abbott, 2014). Rather, it aims to illustrate the value of democratic participation and socio-political consciousness in enhancing occupational therapy's contribution to social participation, health and well-being. This shift aligns with a vision of a more inclusive and participatory approach, where occupational therapists actively support and act for transformative social change while remaining within their professional boundaries. The following section will delve into social occupational therapy and occupational reconstruction theory, illustrating how these frameworks support occupational therapists in promoting democratic participation, collective action, and social transformation.

14.3 Social occupational therapy: Scope and development

The emergence and development of social occupational therapy in Brazil represents a significant shift in the profession, moving beyond the traditional confines of medical and psychological paradigms to embrace a socially engaged practice (Lopes et al., 2025; Lopes & Malfitano, 2021). Influenced by the ideas of Brazilian educator and philosopher Paulo Freire (e.g. Freire, 2000), social occupational therapy prioritises social participation. At the same time, the Constitution of the Federative Republic of Brazil (Brasil, 1988) adopted in 1988 with subsequent amendments, has supported the emergence of social occupational therapy. The Constitution establishing a democratic government in Brazil was adopted after the overthrow of a 21-year-long military dictatorship lasting from 1964 to 1985. The new Constitution authorised the establishment of a democratic social welfare state in Brazil that guarantees civil, political, and social rights. Yet, preservation and development of individual and collective rights within a democratic framework remains an ongoing project.

Within this overall situation, then, social occupational therapy represents a transformative development deeply influenced by Paulo Freire's vision of education and social participation. To operationalise this kind of collective-oriented practice, which expands the scope of occupational therapy as a profession with a biomedical history that focuses on individuals, it is necessary to integrate the social question (Castel, 2003) in the professional role. If, according to Castel (2003), social structures in capitalist societies are fundamentally based on the labour-capital relationship, then social occupational therapy pays attention to the positioning of work and wages as primary vehicles for social inclusion. Social occupational therapists and other professionals can use their knowledge of Freire and other philosophers and practitioners of social transformation to mediate collective participation of the people we try to help. In this way, we and they act as agents of social transformation.

Freire's ideas, particularly those articulated in his seminal work, *Pedagogy of the Oppressed*, advocate for education as a practice of freedom, where dialogue and critical reflection are central to the learning process (Freire, 2000). Freire challenged the conventional teacher-student hierarchy, instead promoting a co-intentional approach, where both educator and learner contribute to the process of understanding and transforming reality. These principles have been instrumental in shaping social occupational therapy theory and practice, as they encourage occupational therapists to engage with groups and communities as active partners in the emancipatory process. The focus is not on addressing individuals in an individualised way, but, instead, understanding that 'the individual' results from a dialectical process between personal characteristics and the social context. This dynamic understanding of individuals – of the process of being an individual – takes into account and confronts the social, cultural, and economic factors that impact democratic participation and reduce access to citizen rights (see Box 14.1). In this context, occupational therapy becomes a professional mediating social process, aimed at dismantling the structures that perpetuate marginalisation and inequality (Lopes et al., 2011; Lopes et al., 2014). This approach recognises that factors such as poverty, discrimination, and lack of access to education are significant determinants of experience and, consequently, well-being (Lopes & Borba, 2022).

Box 14.1
Dialectical process between individual characteristics and the collective context

In an elementary school, the principal requested assistance from the occupational therapy team to support a young boy who was coming to terms with his identity as gay and experiencing depression. Through conversations with the boy, the occupational therapy team discovered that he was being bullied at school due to his sexuality. They concluded that his depression was not an inherent issue but rather a response to his interaction with the school community. To address this, the occupational therapy team decided to organise workshops, interactive activities, and projects for all students during school breaks, focusing on topics related to sexuality. These initiatives, referred to as a form of social technology in social occupational therapy (Lopes et al., 2025; Lopes & Malfitano, 2020), aimed to foster bonds, initiate dialogue, and, in this case, engage the school community in meaningful discussions about sexuality. During these workshops, students participated in shared activities, which facilitated conversations about their prejudices, fears, and personal experiences related to sexuality. Topics such as diversity and individual rights within Brazilian society were also addressed. After some time, the occupational therapy team followed up with the boy to discuss his well-being and asked if he would like specific mental health support. He responded that he was feeling fine because the school environment had changed, and he was no longer experiencing bullying. By employing this social technology, the team was able to avoid an individualised approach that might have pathologised his experience. This prevented an over-reliance on a biomedical framework, which could have misattributed the issue solely to the boy, overlooking the broader social dynamics at play.

Incorporating a social perspective into occupational therapy practice means engaging with the social, political, cultural and economic conditions that shape people's lives. Social occupational therapists seek to inform policies that reduce social inequalities and promote social inclusion. They work in diverse settings, such as health services, social and welfare institutions, schools and community, cultural centres, and justice services applying their knowledge to promote social participation of people. To accomplish this purpose, it is necessary to understand the individual needs of the person, his/her everyday life/occupations shaped by the social question – that is, their positioning about work and wages as primary vehicles for social inclusion. Depending on the situation, it can be necessary to address issues like unemployment, housing insecurity, and social exclusion, using a mediating process to try to achieve a dignified everyday life. By doing so, social occupational therapists help to build a more participatory society where citizens, not clients, can participate in the social fabric (Silva & Malfitano, 2020).

In the context of social occupational therapy, the professionals' practices are guided by social technologies. Social technologies refer to collaborative efforts built in a communitarian way with the goal of social transformation. These technologies are not clinical interventions; they are strategic actions, or political enactments, designed to support groups' and communities' emancipation build capacity, and promote social justice. They are tailored to the specific needs and contexts of the communities they serve, ensuring that interventions are relevant, viable, and impactful (Lopes et al., 2025).

One example was a community project developed in a poor area in an urban Brazilian city with a group of young people spending their days on the streets. A social occupational therapy project was started using free activities in a public square as a social technology (Lopes et al., 2025; Lopes & Malfitano, 2021). The intention was for the activities to help create social bonds making it possible to discuss topics relevant to the wellbeing of the youth and start a participatory approach to address their needs (Silva et al., 2019) The activities were implemented using maps of the cities, recognising where the young people go usually, approaching these questions: Where do they go? What kind of activities/occupations do they do every day? What kind of circulation do they have in the city? This involves analysing the process of discussing public space with young people.

Based on field notes and interviews with participants, the workshops were analysed for information about creating possible living spaces where the youth could practice equality and social interconnection, highlighting elements related to the concept of public space, such as plurality, visibility, and freedom. The aim of social occupational therapy using the city mapping strategy was to create spaces where the plurality (diversity) of the people and their visibility were discussed. Occupational therapists' fostering among the youth a conscious process about their socially vulnerable conditions and their freedom to participate in decision-making processes are important lessons about collective life and citizenship. The goal was for the youth to recognise themselves as participants in fostering public spaces where multiple social experiences could take place (Silva & Malfitano, 2020).

14.4 Occupational reconstruction theory and framework

Occupational reconstructions are observable social phenomena where individuals organise themselves into a collective to address shared problems in each situation. A situation is a shared context in which active participants introduce changes that they believe will improve a socially structured problem. These organising efforts range from local actions, such as creating a community garden in a vacant city lot or 'a community of gardens' on people's urban windowsills, to broader movements, such as protests demanding justice, legislation, and systemic change, as, for example, in response to racialised shootings by police as violations of legal and human rights. Unlike rituals, which embody cultural norms by repeating certain actions on specific occasions, occupational reconstructions are intentionally transformative and disruptive to challenge and reform social conditions. Occupational reconstructions rely on experimentation, risk, and voluntary participation, making them expressions of freedom in civil society (Frank, 2013, 2020; Frank & Muriithi, 2015; Dos Santos & Frank, 2024).

It is important to recognise that not all forms of social change qualify as occupational reconstruction. For instance, government-imposed policies or actions enforced under authoritarian regimes do not align with the values central to occupational reconstruction as theorised here. Occupational reconstruction emphasises non-violent, emancipatory practices that arise when individuals and groups voluntarily act to exercise their rights and advocate for equity and the expansion of social well-being. These are civil actions that assume the right of freedom of speech and of freedom to associate with others, whether those rights are currently legally recognised in a given country or regime. Therefore, occupational therapists wishing to use the occupational reconstruction framework must consider the risks that might be associated with various collective occupations and the professional jurisdiction of their employment.

As for the idea that collective actions of this sort are 'occupational,' we emphasise the potential of ordinary activities to bring people together in everyday life. Occupational reconstructions work with this phenomenon by guiding 'doing together' with mindfulness and professional knowledge of human capacities. The transformative power of doing activities together can be seen in the example social occupational therapy with street youth in Brazil discussed previously and with respect to building social relationships in South Africa (Motimele, 2022; Motimele & Ramugondo, 2014; Ramugondo & Kronenberg, 2015). The film *War/Dance*, portraying a culturally traditional dance programme for child refugees and former child soldiers in Uganda, conveys many examples of the transformational effect of collective occupations (see Frank, 2017).

Occupational reconstruction theory and practice exist together as a framework emphasising change driven by voluntary, community-based engagement in collective occupations aimed at addressing inequities and fostering democratic participation and justice (see Box 14.2). The framework has emerged from an ongoing creative synthesis of occupational therapy participatory practices, emancipatory social philosophies, theories and cases of social movements, and the study of other situations where ordinary people come together to confront and transform shared problematic situations. The theory identifies these core elements:

1. **Problematic Situations:** These are socially structured problems that require collective engagement. A critical analysis of the social and political context can offer a deeper, historically situated understanding of these social issues.
2. **Collective Actors and Doings:** Collective action emerges from shared desires and interdependence. This emphasises the shift from individual-centred practices to collective effort and engagement.
3. **Mind-Body Engagement:** There is an intrinsic connection between mind and body in the process of doing. The collective action is seen as a transformative experience for those involved that occupational therapists are particularly well equipped to guide.
4. **Creativity and Imagination:** Disrupting routine habits of thinking and doing is essential for addressing complex social issues. Occupational reconstruction fosters creativity and innovation to envision and engage with emancipatory experimentalism.
5. **Hope and Risk:** The process is inherently experimental and involves navigating uncertainty. Hope provides the drive for action, even in the face of risks and indeterminate outcomes.
6. **Self-Organising Desire:** The self-organising principle underscores the agency and autonomy of communities in driving change that is voluntary and arises from shared motivations enacted dramatically over time.
7. **Narrative Dimension:** Stories and narratives are integral to occupational reconstruction. They align personal and collective experiences, fostering a shared identity and purpose among participants.

Box 14.2
Understanding collective action with occupational reconstruction theory

On 15 May 2023, the Peruvian newspaper *La República* published an article titled 'Popcorn and entry for 5 bottles! Cinema promotes recycling for the best movies in Cusco' ('*¡Canchita y entrada por 5 botellas! Cine promueve el reciclaje por las mejores películas en Cusco*'), highlighting how a community collectively enacted change by integrating environmental action, cultural activities, and activism. CINERECICLAJE exemplifies a voluntary, community-driven effort to address environmental and cultural problems through innovative, collaborative action. It reimagines waste management in waterways not just as a problem but as a resource, creating new possibilities and fostering social identities. In the following, we apply Occupational Reconstruction Theory to analyse the CINERECICLAJE initiative.

What Was the Problematic Situation? The initiative addresses three socially structured issues: waste management, environmental sustainability, and limited access to cultural activities in regional areas. The absence of effective recycling systems resulted in plastic bottles being discarded into waterways, causing environmental harm. Simultaneously, the community faced limited opportunities to engage in cultural activities, highlighting a lack of accessible, meaningful leisure experiences.

Who Are the Collective Actors and Actions? CINERECICLAJE involves a range of collective actors, including bottle pickers (mostly children supervised by adults), community members, and environmental activists. Together, they engage in activities such as collecting recyclables, organising film screenings, and mobilising participation. For example, bottles picked from the waterways by children served as 'tickets' to access an improvised cinema where they could watch movies, creating a direct link between environmental cleanup and cultural participation.

How Does the Initiative Engage Mind and Body? Recycling and upcycling require both physical engagement and creative thinking, particularly due to the sacredness of the waterways for the local community. Participants are involved in meaningful activities that not only promote environmental preservation but also foster individual and social transformation through their engagement with culturally and spiritually significant spaces.

How Does CINERECICLAJE Demonstrate Creativity and Imagination? CINERECICLAJE disrupts habitual ways of addressing waste by introducing innovative practices, such as using discarded bottles as tickets for cultural events. This creative process reimagines waste management not merely as a necessity but as an opportunity to foster cultural inclusion and community engagement, reshaping how resources and cultural activities are perceived and valued.

What Role Do Hope and Risk Play? Starting and sustaining a collective initiative like CINERECICLAJE involves significant risks, including financial uncertainty, social resistance, and challenges such as improper disposal and contamination of waste. Despite these obstacles, hope for a cleaner environment, the preservation of sacred waterways, and improved access to cultural experiences motivates continued participation and experimentation, sustaining the initiative's momentum.

How Does the Initiative Reflect Self-Organising Desire? The initiative is driven by the voluntary engagement of community members, who share a collective desire to improve both their cultural opportunities and environmental conditions. This demonstrates the community's shared motivations, highlighting their collective agency and ability to self-organise around shared goals.

Was There a Narrative Dimension in CINERECICLAJE? CINERECICLAJE creates a shared narrative that integrates sustainability, access to culture in regional areas, and environmental responsibility. This initiative is embedded in stories of personal and community transformation, building a collective identity and purpose that sustains its efforts and inspires broader social change.

In summary, the occupational reconstruction framework provides a conceptual foundation for understanding the hopeful collective efforts through which groups come together and cooperate in a democratic way to address socially structured problems through shared action. Occupational reconstruction's radical edge is sharpened by bearing in mind the early pragmatist John Dewey's (1859–1952) notion of social experimentation and Brazilian political theorist Roberto Mangabeira Unger's (b. 1947) critical and emancipatory perspectives, which were influenced by Dewey's thought. Dewey's and Unger's careers combining philosophy and practice provide models to support our own advocacy for ongoing, sustainable social transformation that increases democracy and rights, legal rights and human rights, social participation, and human freedom (see Dewey, 1958; James, 2017; Unger, 1998; West, 1986).

Early-stage professionals who would like to begin working with an occupational reconstruction framework should be mindful of the following suggestions. First, the elements of occupational reconstruction are not a protocol in any sense of clinical practice under the medical model. Its rules of evidence are distinct from the principles of evidence-based practice but rather correspond in practice to methodologies based in naturalistic inquiry and its root disciplines of anthropology, sociology, public health, and psychology. The framework was developed from observing social change practices on the ground, as they occur in real life and real time. The core elements are not wholly distinct but are dynamically interrelated.

A good starting point is to think in terms of building consensual social experimentation that will occur in a three-part model of dramatic action. As the research of anthropologist and occupational science contributor Cheryl Mattingly shows, social action has an intrinsic narrative structure (Mattingly, 1998). In observing and guiding occupational reconstructions, the collective process unfolds in three phases: Introduction (Pre-Experimentalism), Emancipatory Experimentalism (Collective activities that produce emergent results or 'Happenings'), and Denouement (Post-Experimentalism). This dramatic structure allows the occupational therapist using the framework to engage and facilitate a group or community process guided by principles of collaboration, creativity, and shared storytelling. The occupational therapist's role is as an actor of social transformation, helping communities to navigate and overcome socially structured problems (see Dos Santos & Frank, 2024), as visualised graphically in Figure 14.1.

- ■ **Introduction (Pre-Experimentalism):** This phase focuses on identifying problematic situations and forming groups willing to act collectively based on a shared narrative.
- ■ **Emancipatory Experimentalism (Happenings):** This phase consists of creative and experimental actions (occupations, activities) to address the identified challenges.
- ■ **Denouement (Post-Experimentalism):** This phase involves reflecting on the outcomes and aligning narratives to consolidate learning and shared experiences.

The Occupational Reconstruction Practice Framework serves as a roadmap especially for entry-level occupational therapists to facilitate change by identifying a group or community's shared problematic situations, experimenting with innovative actions, and reflecting and attributing meaning to the process and outcomes through narrative alignment. See text for discussion of the core elements the occupational reconstruction framework.

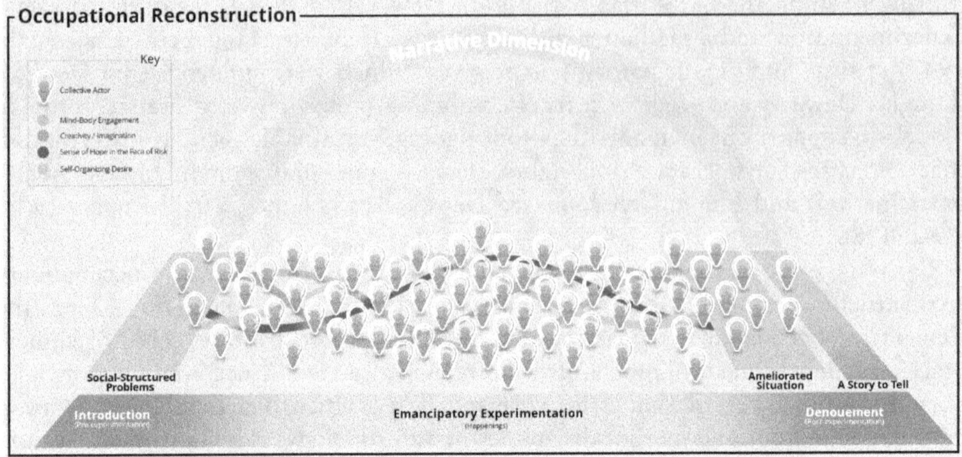

Figure 14.1 Occupational reconstruction

14.5 Conclusion

This chapter has examined the role of occupational therapy in advancing social transformation within communities, particularly when engaging with equity-seeking groups. As described in the introduction, the entanglement of social inequalities generates intersecting disadvantages, compounding vulnerabilities and limiting opportunities for marginalised groups. Thus, some occupational therapists in diverse countries, each with its own political and social histories and structures, are working to engage professionally, ethically, and legally with groups that are marginalised and denied meaningful participation based on factors like gender, religion, ethnicity, disability, language, and socio-economic status. A political project for the profession of occupational therapy would aim at identifying the experienced moral and political inequalities of such populations, recognising that not all lives are treated equitably even in constitutional democracies that recognise individual rights and social welfare. These inequalities result in a division between those deemed deserving of compassion and those subjected to repression. By highlighting this disparity, the profession underscores its commitment to the inherent value of all human lives and advocates for actions to address and reduce inequities.

14.6 Summary

- Occupational therapy is positioned as an agent of social transformation, partnering with collectives to advance emancipation and equity. A critical, politically informed stance urges therapists to facilitate social cohesion and democratic action alongside groups and communities, recognising how systems both enable and constrain everyday living.
- Theoretical frameworks such as social occupational therapy and occupational reconstruction underpin some of the various socially transformative practices emerging in the occupational therapy profession.

- Social occupational therapy emerges as a tradition dedicated to addressing social questions, leveraging collective doings and social technologies for community-driven change.
- Occupational reconstruction offers a theoretical and practical framework to guide therapists in understanding collectives occupations and supporting equity-seeking groups toward justice, access, and well-being.

14.7 Review and reflection questions

- In what ways can occupational therapists position themselves as agents of social transformation when working with groups and communities?
- How can an exploration of democratic participation and community ties inform occupational therapists' development and implementation of socially engaged practices?
- How does the emerging field of social occupational therapy differ from more traditional, individual-focused approaches, and what are 'social technologies' that it employs?
- Reflecting on the seven elements of occupational reconstruction theory, how would you define your role – and that of your community – in co-designing and implementing occupations aimed at promoting justice, access to social goods, and well-being?

References

Abbott, A. (2014). *The system of professions: An essay on the division of expert labor.* University of Chicago Press.

Brasil. (1988). *Constituição da República Federativa do Brasil de 1988.* https://www.planalto.gov.br/ccivil_03/constituicao/constituicao.htm

Castel, R. (2003). *From manual workers to wage laborers: Transformation of the social question.* Routledge.

Das, V. (2006). *Life and words: Violence and the descent into the ordinary.* University of California Press.

Dewey, J. (1958). *Experience and nature.* Dover Publications.

Dos Santos, V. (2022). Social transformation on the neoliberal university: Reconstructing an academic commitment. *Journal of Occupational Science, 29*(4), 482–486. https://doi.org/10.1080/14427591.2022.2110660

Dos Santos, V. (2025). A political project for occupational therapists. In M. Curtin, M. Egan, T. Parnell, Y. Prior, D. C. da Cruz, K. Sauvé-Schenk, & R. Galvaan (Eds.), *Occupational therapy for people experiencing illness, injury or impairment* (8th ed., p. 29). Elsevier Health Sciences.

Dos Santos, V., & Frank, G. (2024). Creativity, hope and collective emancipatory experimentation: Tools for social transformation through occupational therapy. In T. Brown, L. Gustafsson, S. Gutman, & T. Barlott (Eds.), *Human occupation: Contemporary concepts and lifespan perspectives* (1st ed.). Taylor and Francis.

Dos Santos, V., Bezerra, W. C., Godoy, A., & Terra, E. (2022). A terapia occupacional de um Brasil democrático e livre. In *Questões e práticas contemporâneas da terapia ocupacional na América do Sul* (pp. 41–52). CRV.

Dos Santos, V., & Leon Spesny, S. (2016). Questioning the concept of culture in mainstream occupational therapy. *Cadernos de Terapia Ocupacional Da UFSCar, 24*(1), 185–190. https://doi.org/10.4322/0104-4931.ctoRE0675

Dos Santos, V., Rodrigues, I. O., & Galvaan, R. (2019). "It is not what I planned for my life". Occupations of live-in domestic workers. *Cadernos Brasileiros de Terapia Ocupacional, 27*, 467–479. https://doi.org/10.4322/2526-8910.ctoAO1873

Farias, L., & Laliberte Rudman, D. (2016). A critical interpretive synthesis of the uptake of critical perspectives in occupational science. *Journal of Occupational Science, 23*(1), 33–50. https://doi.org/10.1080/14427591.2014.989893

Farias, L., Laliberte Rudman, D., & Magalhães, L. (2016). Illustrating the importance of critical epistemology to realize the promise of occupational justice. *OTJR: Occupation, Participation and Health, 36*(4), 234–243. https://doi.org/10.1177/1539449216665561

Farias, L., Lapierre, M., & Dos Santos, V. (2025). The neoliberal framing of occupational therapy practices and the rise of the health consumer. In P. Talero Cabrejo, V. Dos Santos, & N. Pollard (Eds.), *Occupational therapy in Latin America* (Chap. 8). Jessica Kingsley Publishers.

Farias, M. N., & Lopes, R. E. (2023). Terapia ocupacional e a armadilha neoliberal progressista: Desafios para uma práxis antiopressiva. *Revista de Terapia Ocupacional da Universidade de São Paulo, 33*(1), Article 1. https://doi.org/10.11606/issn.2238-6149.v33i1pe209610

Fassin, D. (2010). Ethics of survival: A democratic approach to the politics of life. *Humanity: An International Journal of Human Rights, Humanitarianism, and Development, 1*(1), 81–95. https://doi.org/10.1353/hum.2010.0000

Fassin, D. (2018). *Life: A critical user's manual* (1st ed.). Polity.

Frank, G. (2013). Twenty-first century pragmatism and social justice: Problematic situations and occupational reconstructions in post-civil war Guatemala. In M. P. Cutchin & V. A. Dickie (Eds.), *Transactional perspectives on occupation* (pp. 229–243). Springer Netherlands. https://doi.org/10.1007/978-94-007-4429-5_18

Frank, G. (2017). Collective occupations and social transformations: A mad hot curriculum. In D. Sakellariou & N. Pollard (Eds.), *Occupational therapies without borders: Integrating justice with practice* (2nd ed., pp. 596–604). Elsevier.

Frank, G. (2020). Social Transformation theory and practice: Resources for radicals in participatory art, occupational therapy and social moviments. In H. van Bruggen, S. Kantartzis, & N. Pollard (Eds.), *'And a seed was planted . . .' Occupation based approaches for social inclusion: Volume 1: Theoretical views and shifting perspectives*. Whiting & Birch Ltd.

Frank, G. (2022). Occupational science's stalled revolution and a manifesto for reconstruction. *Journal of Occupational Science, 29*(4), 455–477. https://doi.org/10.1080/14427591.2022.2110658

Frank, G., & Muriithi, B. A. K. (2015). Theorising social transformation in occupational science: The American Civil Rights Movement and South African struggle against apartheid as "occupational reconstructions." *South African Journal of Occupational Therapy, 45*(1), 11–19.

Freire, P. (2000). *Pedagogy of the oppressed* (30th anniversary ed., 1st ed.). Continuum Academic.

Gusfield, J. R. (1996). *Contested meanings: The construction of alcohol problems* (1st ed., 1st Printing). University of Wisconsin Press.

Hammell, K. W. (2020). Ações nos determinantes sociais de saúde: Avançando na equidade ocupacional e nos direitos ocupacionais. *Cadernos Brasileiros de Terapia Ocupacional, 28*(1), 387–400. https://doi.org/10.4322/2526-8910.ctoARF2052

Hammell, K. W. (2022). A call to resist occupational therapy's promotion of ableism. *Scandinavian Journal of Occupational Therapy*, 1–13. https://doi.org/10.1080/11038128.2022.2130821

Hammell, K. W. (2023). Focusing on "what matters": The occupation, capability and wellbeing framework for occupational therapy. *Cadernos Brasileiros de Terapia Ocupacional, 31*, e3509–e3509. https://doi.org/10.1590/2526-8910.ctoAO269035092

James, V. D. (2017). Pragmatism and radical social justice: Dewey, Du Bois, and Davis. In S. Dieleman, D. Rondel, & C. Voparil (Eds.), *Pragmatism and justice* (pp. 163–178). Oxford University Press. https://doi.org/10.1093/acprof:oso/9780190459239.003.0010

Kapiriri, L., & Razavi, S. D. (2022). Equity, justice, and social values in priority setting: A qualitative study of resource allocation criteria for global donor organizations working in low-income countries. *International Journal for Equity in Health*, 21(1), 17. https://doi.org/10.1186/s12939-021-01565-5

Kleinman, A., & Kleinman, J. (1996). The appeal of experience; the dismay of images: Cultural appropriations of suffering in our times. *Daedalus*, *125*, 1–24.

Leon Spesny, S., & Dos Santos, V. (2025). Between compassion and repression: State agents governing vulnerable youth in Brazil. In G. Martin & E. Pierce (Eds.), *Elgar research handbook on youth criminology*. Edward Elgar Publishing.

Lopes, R. E., & Borba, P. L. de O. (2022). A inclusão radical como diretriz para terapeutas ocupacionais na educação. *Revista Ocupación Humana*, 22(2), Article 2. https://doi.org/10.25214/25907816.1402

Lopes, R. E., Borba, P. L. de O., Trajber, N. K. de A., Silva, C. R., & Cuel, B. T. (2011). Oficinas de atividades com jovens da escola pública: Tecnologias sociais entre educação e terapia ocupacional. *Interface – Comunicação, Saúde, Educação*, *15*, 277–288. https://doi.org/10.1590/S1414-32832011000100021

Lopes, R. E., & Malfitano, A. P. S. (2020). *Social occupational therapy: Theoretical and practical designs* (1st ed.). Elsevier.

Lopes, R. E., Malfitano, A. P. S., & Borba, P. L. O. (2025). Social occupational therapy: Principles for action towards participation. In M. Curtin, M. Egan, Y. Prior, T. Parnell, R. Galvaan, K. Sauvé-Schenk, & D. C. da Cruz (Eds.), *Occupational therapy for people experiencing illness, injury or impairment: Promoting occupational participation* (8th ed., pp. 40–52). Elsevier Health Sciences.

Lopes, R. E., Malfitano, A. P. S., Silva, C. R., & Borba, P. L. de O. (2014). Recursos e tecnologias em terapia ocupacional social: Ações com jovens pobres na cidade/resources and technologies in social occupational therapy: Actions with the poor youth in town. *Cadernos Brasileiros de Terapia Ocupacional*, 22(3), Article 3. https://doi.org/10.4322/cto.2014.081

Malfitano, A. P. S., Whiteford, G., & Molineux, M. (2021). Transcending the individual: The promise and potential of collectivist approaches in occupational therapy. *Scandinavian Journal of Occupational Therapy*, 28(3), 188–200. https://doi.org/10.1080/11038128.2019.1693627

Marmot, M. (2005). Social determinants of health inequalities. *The Lancet*, *365*(9464), 1099–1104. https://doi.org/10.1016/S0140-6736(05)71146-6

Mattingly, C. (1998). *Healing dramas and clinical plots: The narrative structure of experience.* Cambridge University Press. https://doi.org/10.1017/CBO9781139167017

Motimele, M. R. (2022). Engaging with occupational reconstructions: A perspective from the Global South. *Journal of Occupational Science*, 29(4), 478–481. https://doi.org/10.1080/14427591.2022.2110659

Motimele, M. R., & Ramugondo, E. L. (2014). Violence and healing: Exploring the power of collective occupations. *International Journal of Criminology and Sociology*, *3*, 388–401. https://doi.org/10.6000/1929-4409.2014.03.33

Østergaard Madsen, J., Morrison, R., Dos Santos, V., & Barlott, T. (2024). Pragmatism: Current and future influence on occupational therapy and occupational science. In T. Brown, L. Gustafsson, & S. Gutman (Eds.), *Human occupation: Contemporary concepts and lifespan perspectives* (1st ed.). Taylor and Francis.

Patrick, K. (2024). CMAJ's commitment to equity-seeking groups. *CMAJ*, *196*(32), E1122–E1123. https://doi.org/10.1503/cmaj.241356

Ramugondo, E. L., & Kronenberg, F. (2015). Explaining collective occupations from a human relations perspective: Bridging the individual-collective dichotomy. *Journal of Occupational Science*, 22(1), 3–16. https://doi.org/10.1080/14427591.2013.781920

Silva, M. J. da, & Malfitano, A. P. S. (2020). Oficinas de atividades, dinâmicas e projetos em terapia ocupacional social como estratégia para a promoção de espaços públicos. *Interface-Comunicação, Saúde, Educação*, *25*, e200055.

Silva, M. J. da, Oliveira, M. L., & Malfitano, A. P. S. (2019). The utilization of public squares: Considerations on the action of the social occupational therapist. *Cadernos Brasileiros de Terapia Ocupacional, 27*, 438–447.

Taff, S. D., Moreno, C. E., Nuwere, E., West-Bruce, S., & Malfitano, A. P. (2025). Equity, diversity, and inclusion in occupational therapy: Small steps, slow pace, and unrealized potential. In *Equity, diversity, and inclusion in healthcare* (pp. 119–138). Elsevier. https://www.sciencedirect.com/science/article/pii/B9780443132513000065

Tofeti, A. R., & Dos Santos, V. (2020). Sustainable occupational opportunities in protected areas in Brazil. *World Federation of Occupational Therapists Bulletin, 76*(1), 40–49. https://doi.org/10.1080/14473828.2020.1758398

Unger, R. M. (1998). *Democracy realized: The progressive alternative*. Verso Books.

West, C. (1986). Between Dewey and Gramsci: Unger's emancipatory experimentalism. *Northwestern University Law Review, 81*, 941.

Whiteford, G., Jones, K., Rahal, C., & Suleman, A. (2018). The participatory occupational justice framework as a tool for change: Three contrasting case narratives. *Journal of Occupational Science, 25*(4), 497–508.

CHAPTER 15

Reimagining occupational therapy

Culturally responsive practice and First Peoples' health and well-being

Kerrie Thomsen

Acknowledgment to Country

I want to start by acknowledging our Ancestors, our Older and Young People, who have walked this land for more than 60,000 years. I pay my deep respects to Elders past, present, and emerging, for they hold the stories, the knowledge, and the Lore that guides us. I acknowledge the Traditional Owners of the land on which I write, the Gunaikurnai Peoples, and the lands on which you, the reader, now sit reading this book. This Country has been a place of learning, of healing, of ceremony, and of occupation since the first sunrise, and we must never forget that it always was, and always will be, Aboriginal land.

I acknowledge my husband, my extended family, my community 'the Wook-koo Clan on Butchulla Country', and the many First Nations peoples; clients, and friends that have been a part of my journey. They have graciously shared their stories, art, poetry, back yards, lounge rooms, cups of tea, and their strength with me over 45 years. Your truths are woven into the fabric of this chapter.

Acknowledgements

I also acknowledge my allied health colleagues and academic allies on this journey and thank them for their support particularly in the last 10 years. There are many allies in our amazing group practice team working hard in the complex health and disability systems. Then there are my Australian Catholic University (ACU) academic allies, sharing a joint vision, our brilliant ACU cultural mentors, and the bright stars of the future – our ACU students – for being on a transformational journey with us.

Key terms
- Cultural responsiveness
- Indigenous Australians
- First Nations Peoples' occupations

DOI: 10.4324/9781003495666-17

- Occupation
- Lived experience
- Indigenising occupational therapy
- Buranga approach

Objectives

This chapter will challenge the reader

- To think beyond their current 'ways' of knowing and enter a place of 'not knowing' open to new learning
- To critically examine the power imbalance inherent in the therapist-client relationship
- To privilege First Nations cultural perspectives of occupations and occupational therapy
- To journey in a non-linear way of learning
- To respond to the call to action

15.1 Introduction: a yarn in three parts

Galangoor Djali (hello). My name is Kerrie Thomsen, a woman proud of her Aboriginal and European ancestry with deep connections to my family and community. In 1982, I graduated from the University of Queensland, becoming the first identified Aboriginal occupational therapist in Australia. This chapter is a yarn, a sharing of my journey, but it's more than just my story. It's an invitation to you – the next generation of occupational therapists – to walk alongside us as we reimagine a profession that has, for too long, been a tool of colonisation.

This chapter is not written in the linear, segmented way you might be used to. It is structured to reflect our ways of knowing, being, and doing – a circular, holistic approach where the past informs the present, and our actions today create our future. We will journey through three interwoven parts:

1. **Ways of Knowing:** Understanding our shared history and the deep knowledge systems of First Peoples.
2. **Ways of Being:** Reflecting on our own position, our biases, and how we show up in our practice and our relationships.
3. **Ways of Doing:** Translating this knowledge and self-awareness into tangible, culturally responsive, and transformative action.

(Indigenous Allied Health Australia [IAHA], 2019)

15.1.1 Positioning: My standpoint and a poem

Before we go on to yarn a bit more, it's important you know who I am more deeply and where I come from. This is a fundamental part of our way – to position ourselves so that you can understand the lens through which we see the world. I am an Aboriginal woman, an other-mother, a kinship grandma, an Aunty, a cultural mentor, and an occupational therapist. My identity is not a series of hats I wear; it is a single, woven cloak. My Aboriginal frame of reference, my lived experience of navigating two worlds, informs everything I do. For over 25 years, I have worked in community settings, and for many more, I have carried the responsibility of leadership, guiding allied health professionals on their journey towards safer, more responsive practice. My work, particularly with ACU in tertiary curricula indigenisation, is about embedding these ways of knowing, thinking, feeling, and being into the very heart of how we train our future therapists.

My understanding of time itself is different. It is not a straight line marching from past to future. It is circular, interconnected. My father's daughter, Yenna Kerrie, captures this within the beauty of a poem.

Time

by Yenna Kerrie Thomsen
Time is not a linear thread,
A past that's gone, a future ahead.
It is the turning of the tide,
Where ancestors and spirits ride.
It is the whisper in the breeze,
The ancient stories in the trees.
The river's flow, a constant hum,
Of what has been, and what's to come.
The past is now, it lives in me,
My grandmother's face, I still can see.
The future is in every child's birth,
A renewal of this sacred earth.
So do not rush, do not despair,
The lessons of the past are there.
In the Dreaming, in the story, in the song,
Where all of time, and we, belong.

This poem reminds us that the historical context is not a separate, dusty chapter of a book. It is alive, today, in the experiences of our people and we have a responsibility as allies and occupational therapists when we work within the systems that continue to impact our health and well-being to first take a humanistic approach, be respectful, be humble, and be open.

15.1.2 Historical context and current state: acknowledging the scars

To understand the present, we must persevere and look at the past. The history of occupational therapy in Australia is deeply enmeshed with the history of colonisation. While the profession's philosophy speaks of enabling occupation for health and well-being, its application to First Nations peoples has often been the opposite. It has been used as a tool of assimilation, enforcing Western ideals of 'productive' and 'meaningful' occupation while systematically devaluing our own.

Our occupations: our ceremonies, our lores, our languages, our raising up of children, our family relationships, our hunting and fishing, our agriculture, our art, our songs, our storytelling, our collectivism, our protection of the environment, our custodianship, and our very connection to Country – were disrupted and dismissed as primitive or irrelevant. The institutions where many early occupational therapists worked – missions, reserves, and hospitals – were sites of immense control and trauma. Therapy was often prescriptive, aimed at making us more like the coloniser, severing our connections to culture, kin, and Country, which was 'devastation', as these are the very pillars of the social and emotional well-being model we know today (Kelly et al., 2024).

This legacy has left scars and a deep wound. It has created a profound and justified mistrust of the healthcare system. Today, this legacy manifests in the 'stubbornness of deficit discourse' (Sherwood & Geia, 2017). This is the pervasive, often unconscious, tendency for health professionals to view First Nations peoples and our communities through a lens of problems to be solved – 'poor' health outcomes, 'low' educational attainment, 'high' rates of unemployment. This language frames us as lacking rather than as a people possessing immense strength, resilience, and sophisticated systems of knowledge that have sustained us for over 60,000 years.

The challenge for contemporary occupational therapy practitioners is to actively dismantle this discourse. It means rejecting interview styles, assessment tools, and intervention models that are normed on non-Indigenous populations and that fail to capture our holistic view of health. It means challenging the reductionist nature of a healthcare system that wants to treat a person's mind in one department and their body in another. With my long-standing ally and colleague Loretta Sheppard, we dream of a health system aligned with First Nations peoples' thinking which would not be siloed. It would be a holistic, community-led, place-based system where the therapists, the doctor, the teacher, the Elders, the gardener, the artist, and the bus driver are all valued for their role in the well-being of the community.

15.1.3 A visual story: ways of knowing, thinking, being, and doing

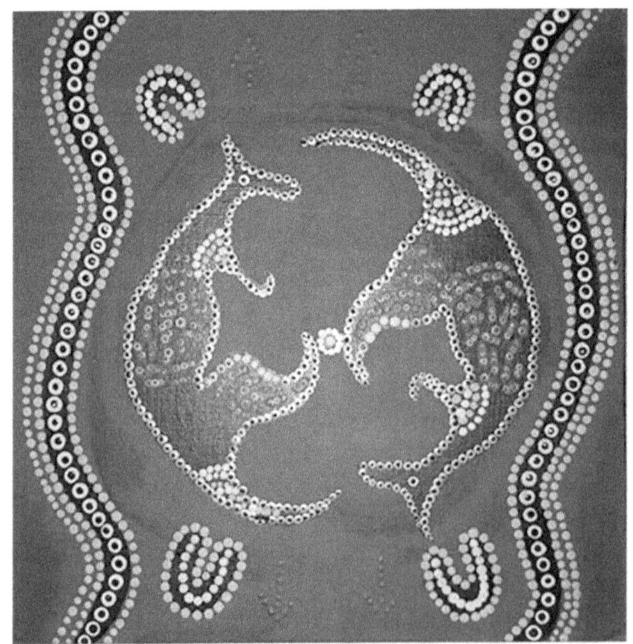

Figure 15.1 Ways of Being by Kerrie Thomsen 2013

Acrylic painting on board: My painting is circular in design, with no clear top or bottom, no linear hierarchy. In the centre is a symbol representing community and home for me. Radiating outwards are intricate pathways, footprints, and symbols for people, animals, land, and water. The colours that connect for me are earthy, with bright flashes of ochre, pink, gold, and green. The lines flow like rivers, and we (Wook-koo Aboriginal people) are river people. There are no straight edges in nature, and like in life, we flow together and thrive interconnected.

This painting is my story. It's our story. It represents our *Ways of Knowing, Thinking, Being, and Doing.*

- **The Centre (Knowing):** This represents our core – our knowledge, our Law, our Dreaming. It's the foundation that comes from our Elders and our Ancestors. It is our collective heart, deep, spiritual, and unshakable.
- **The Black Mist (Thinking):** Kerrie Thomsen's thinking is deeply based in a circular, holistic approach, reflecting First Peoples' ways of knowing, being, and doing, where the past informs the present and actions create the future. She views time as interconnected rather than linear, embracing ancestral knowledge and community to co-design better futures and challenge colonial frameworks in occupational therapy.
- **The Pathways (Doing):** These are the actions we take, the occupations we engage in. See how they connect everything? They are not isolated tasks. Tending to Country is connected to our spiritual health. Yarning with family is connected to our mental health. Creating art is connected to our cultural and economic health. This is occupation in its truest sense.
- **The Footprints (Being):** These represent our journey. They show that we are always moving, always learning. They represent our identity, our standpoint, and how we walk in this world. Notice how the footprints lead both away from and back to the centre. We may walk in the non-Indigenous world, but we always carry our knowledge with us, and we always return to our community, our source of strength.

This is one personal map for culturally responsive practice. It reminds us that everything is connected. You cannot address one part of a person's life without understanding its relationship to the whole.

15.2 Core principles of culturally responsive occupational therapy: 'Ways of knowing'

Cultural responsiveness is not a destination; it is a continuous journey of learning, unlearning, and reflecting. It is an ethical way of practice built on respect, relationship, and a commitment to redistributing power. It is grounded in a strengths-based approach that sees our culture not as a barrier but as the primary source of healing and strength. Cultural humility is emerging as a preferred approach over cultural competence in occupational therapy. While cultural competence focuses on acquiring specific knowledge about different cultures, cultural humility emphasises a lifelong learning process, self-reflection, and an awareness of power dynamics in healthcare interactions (Beagan, 2015; Agner, 2020; Nelson et al., 2023). Cultural humility involves recognising one's biases and engaging with clients in a respectful, non-superior manner, which can lead to stronger therapeutic alliances and improved client outcomes (Hook et al., 2013).

Key components include:

- **Self-Determination:** The fundamental right of First Peoples to determine our own futures. In occupational therapy practice, this means community-led and co-designed initiatives are paramount. We must move away from 'doing to or for' and towards 'walking with'. The community really does hold the solutions; our role is to help facilitate them. The theory of closing the gap has failed in many ways because it originated from governments, and this did not change until 2019.
- **Incorporating First Peoples Ways of Knowing, Thinking, Being, and Doing:** This is about more than just including an acknowledgement of Country in your email signature. It is about fundamentally reshaping our practice to align with a holistic worldview. This brings us to the social and emotional well-being (SEWB) model (Gee et al., 2014). The SEWB model is an Indigenous framework for health that is beautifully aligned with the holistic principles of occupational therapy. It recognises that well-being is derived from the harmonious interplay of multiple domains: connection to spirit and spirituality, connection to Country, connection to culture, connection to community, connection to kinship, connection to mind and emotions, and connection to body. For an occupational therapist and ally, this can be a practice roadmap. When you meet a client, you should be asking: How can we strengthen these connections?
- **Critical Self-Reflection:** Understanding your own culture, biases, and privilege is one of the essential early steps. As non-Indigenous therapists, you must ask yourselves: What is the shape and nature of my lens? How does my worldview impact my assumptions and my practice? How can I describe my position statement to my clients and colleagues? This is not about guilt; it is about responsibility.

15.3 A story of knowing

My dear friend and colleague, Loretta Sheppard, an amazing ally and very experienced occupational therapist, spent time yarning on a long car trip. We were dreaming of what an ideal system would look like. 'Imagine,' she said, 'if the funding wasn't given to a hospital, but to a community. And the community decided how to use it for their health, their education, and their well-being. Not in little buckets, but as one whole budget.'

In that yarn, we weren't just complaining about the system. We were engaging in a deeper act of *knowing*. We were drawing on 80 years of combined experience as occupational therapists, ancestral knowledge of community, of holistic living, to co-design a better future. Loretta's vision is a standout example of self-determination and a strengths-based approach. It assumes the community is capable, knowledgeable, and has the right to control its own destiny. This is the kind of 'knowing' we must bring into our professional lives. It's not just about knowing facts *about* Aboriginal or Torres Strait Islander people; it's about valuing and integrating First Peoples *ways of knowing*.

15.4 Practical application in occupational therapy practice: 'Ways of thinking and feeling' and 'ways of doing'

How do we translate this deep knowing into our everyday practice? It begins with how we think and feel, which in turn shapes what we do.

15.4.1 Building relationships and trust

Trust is the currency of our communities. It is not given; it is earned through time, consistency, humility, and genuine care. This is the most important 'doing' you will ever do.

- **Show up:** Go to community events, BBQs, art exhibitions. Be a person before you are a therapist.
- **Listen more than you talk:** Practice deep listening through *Dadirri* (Official Miriam-Rose Ungunmerr Video, 2017). Listen to understand, not just to reply. Listen to the stories, the silences, and what is not being said.
- **Be patient:** Relationships are not built in a 45-minute appointment slot. It takes time. Do not be discouraged by initial caution; it is a wise and protective response to a long history of harm.

Summary of a yarn about allyship with Yanaya Charles and Vivian Petre from the Victorian Aboriginal Health Service (VAHS)

Viv, a non-Indigenous occupational therapist, describes allyship and that it involves recognising her limitations in cultural understanding and actively seeking the guidance of Aboriginal health workers like Janaya. She emphasises that building trust within the community is paramount, often facilitated by the existing relationships and endorsements of Aboriginal colleagues. Viv highlights the importance of working in true partnership, acknowledging that her Aboriginal colleagues bring crucial cultural perspectives that she, as an outsider, might miss, especially in sensitive situations like palliative care where returning to country might be the most important goal. She also learned that clients might be more comfortable disclosing financial constraints or literacy challenges to Aboriginal health workers, underscoring the need for a collaborative approach to address these types of barriers.

Janaya, a proud Mutti Mutti woman and Team Leader of the Allied Health Section at VAHS, reinforces the idea of person-centred and community-centred care. She explains that allyship means understanding the historical traumas that make Aboriginal people wary of non-Aboriginal professionals entering their homes. Janaya stresses the importance of 'yarning,' or conversational engagement, to uncover underlying needs beyond initial requests. She and Viv prioritise immediate, small problem-solving activities to build trust, as larger issues often involve lengthy processes. Janaya also emphasises the power of word-of-mouth endorsement within the community, valuing genuine positive experiences over formal marketing. Both Viv and Janaya demonstrate that effective allyship in their field is a continuous journey of learning, adapting, and working together to meet the unique cultural and practical needs of their clients and the local Aboriginal community.

15.4.2 Storytelling is occupation

In our culture, story is everything. It is our library, our university, our therapy. The sharing of 'story' is a sacred and powerful occupation. When an Elder shares a story with you, they are giving you a precious gift. They are also engaging in a deeply meaningful occupation that reinforces their identity, their role as a knowledge keeper, and their connection to past and future generations.

As therapists, I believe we must recognise that *story is occupation*. When we take a 'case history', we must reframe it as receiving a story. This changes the power dynamic. It is not an extraction of information; it is a sacred exchange. Furthermore, we can use storytelling, or 'story re-telling', as a therapeutic tool. Helping someone reframe their story from one of deficit and trauma to one of strength and resilience is one of the most powerful interventions we can facilitate.

> **Healing in the Bush:** As a team within our allied health practice, we supported a teenage boy who had lost his foster father, a loss that left him silent and restless. He was happiest building things, and so we planned some time outdoors; we took therapy into the bush close by. Alongside other young teens, he learned to make fire safely, find water and food, read the land, and listen to the wildlife around him. These were survival skills – but also healing skills. The bush gave him space to grieve, to feel light, to laugh, and to belong. Occupation, in this space, became about reconnection – with nature, peers, and his young self.

15.4.3 Activities of daily living are 'talk in another language,' and it needs interpretation!

The activities of daily living (ADL) assessment is a cornerstone of occupational therapy. But used without a cultural lens, it can be a blunt and harmful instrument. We need to understand that ADL is another language, and it needs interpretation.

Let's take showering. A Western ADL assessment tool or checklist might ask, 'Can the client shower independently?' and tick a box. But this misses the entire cultural context. For some of us, for example, to make a point: the concept of a private, daily, hot shower is a distant one and asking about 'showering' might not only be irrelevant but also carry a hidden judgment. The occupation may be memories of swimming in the river with family, a communal and connecting activity. Our job is not to assess against a white, middle-class benchmark. Our job is to be an interpreter. We need to ask: 'What do you need to do to feel clean and good in yourself? What does that look like for you? Who helps you with that? What gets in the way?' This reframes the conversation from a test of function to a respectful exploration of a person's lived reality and occupational needs. We can support all people who are homeless with an approach like this. This example is a real person living from a wheelchair and couch surfing and often staying in a dwelling with 14 stairs which two people carry him up, or he climbs backwards up on his bottom using his arm strength.

> **Finding calm and connection;** A very shy Aboriginal man I worked with was living alone, struggling with isolation and sexual identity. He didn't smile and was sad every time I saw him. Together, we built small but meaningful routines with some support: morning walking, gym sessions, shopping for fresh ingredients, and cooking meals he was proud to share. Gradually, we added community – through shared meals. Cooking became core to his talking therapy – a way to nourish both body and spirit. Through occupation, he accepted advice from his GP and found calm, pride, and opportunities to belong.

15.5 Knowledge translation: A two-way street

In the Western academic world, 'knowledge translation' often means taking expert knowledge and giving it to laypeople. In our way, it must be a two-way process of learning and sharing. You bring your specialist occupational therapy skills, and the person and their community bring their deep, lived expertise. It is a partnership. You are translating your clinical language into plain English, and they are translating their cultural and personal world for you. True collaboration happens when both knowledge systems are valued equally.

Loretta's standpoint

Connecting to the humanity in each of us is a binding thread in occupational therapy, one which frames and guides any work we do. The human right to good health, wellbeing and valued community membership is fundamental, with different meanings for different people. My journey towards allyship became a sharp imperative when I began working with a new occupational therapy programme at ACU in 2012. I was struck by the lack of voice and awareness of the occupational rights of the oldest living culture on the planet and infuriated that my Australian education had systematically and purposely denied me political and historical truths about colonisation. I felt a profound sense of loss for us as an Australian community and an urgent need to connect with and understand the lived experience of occupational therapy in Aboriginal communities. But where to start? To build a curriculum that could honour and privilege First People's voices required partnerships. Looking to local communities with humility and reciprocity was key and trying to work out what to teach was just the beginning. The true learning comes with the deepening of relationships and trust over time to understand, respect, and value different ways of knowing. We live in a western dominant paradigm. The many cultural mentors and Elders involved with our staff and students over many years have brought diversity of perspective, humour, patience, and wisdom and nurtured collective respect and humility. An ancient saying along the lines of 'when the learner is ready, the teacher appears' might mean we need to 'allow space' for learning we might not even know we need until it arrives. And reciprocate with respect and allyship, knowing when to stand up, when to walk alongside, and when to step back.

15.6 Empowering future occupational therapy practice: Ways of knowing, thinking, feeling, and being

As you step into your careers, you are stepping into a profession at a crossroads. You have the opportunity and the responsibility to help forge a new path.

15.6.1 The importance of allyship: Buranga

In the Butchulla–English language translation, *Buranga* means:

- Buranga – Think/ing, hear, know/ing, listen
- Buranga-li-nj – Feeling
- Buranga-man – Understanding
- Buranga-mi – Knew

Being an ally is not a passive identity; it is an action verb. It is about using your privilege as a non-Indigenous person to challenge the racist and colonial structures that continue to harm culturally diverse people, families, and communities.

An ally (in the *Buranga approach*):

- **Listens** to our voices and amplifies them without speaking for us.
- **Educates** themselves and others, taking the burden of education off our shoulders.
- **Challenges** racism when they see it – in their colleagues, in their organisations, in their policies.
- **Advocates** for systemic change, like the indigenisation of university curricula or the employment of more First Peoples health professionals.
- **Accepts** that they will make mistakes, and when they are corrected, they listen humbly, learn, and do better.

Finding your place and passion in this work is your lifelong journey. It is not an add-on; it is your whole of practice.

15.7 Conclusion: Occupation is hope

I began this yarn by saying that occupational therapy has, at times, been a tool of colonisation. However, I have dedicated my life to this profession because I believe, with all my heart, that it can be a powerful tool of healing and justice.

The very core of our profession – the profound belief in the power of occupation – is our hope. Occupation is the stuff of life. It is how we express who we are, how we connect with others, how we find meaning and purpose. For First Peoples, occupation is our culture, our spirituality, our connection to Country, our survival, and our future. My definition therefore is;

Occupation:

> What gives life shape, balance, and meaning, as defined by the person (inclusive of their family and community) in their time, place, connection to self, and their culture.

My call to you is this: Be brave. Be humble. Be a listener. Challenge the systems that perpetuate inequity. See the strength, resilience, and beauty in our people and our communities. Reimagine an occupational therapy that is not just culturally aware but culturally responsive, not just non-racist but actively anti-racist, not just a service but a partnership.

Let us walk together on this journey, with respect as our guide and hope as our destination. Let us create a future where occupational therapy helps all people to engage in the occupations that make their spirit sing.

15.8 A final story: The power of connection

Years ago, I was working with a frail woman in her fifties, who had been through much. She was withdrawn, unwell, and disconnected from her community but had a large supportive family group. The medical team saw her as 'non-compliant'. I just sat with her for a while every couple of weeks. I didn't need to bring any assessment forms. I just relaxed and was myself. We yarned about her younger days, about her children, about the Country she grew up in.

One day, I brought in some picture frames and we gathered up some of her many photographs and together we put together a collage in one large frame and when it was ready hung it on the wall near her chair. She was then able to use this collage of photographs to yarn with many outsiders and professional people who visited her.

In those moments, she wasn't a client. She was 'not a compiled list of deficits'. She was a creator, a knowledge keeper, a woman connected to her culture, her ancestors, and her spirit. The photographs were just a medium. Maybe the true occupation was connection; yes, I think it might have been – what do you think of that? That is the power of what we do. That is our hope as occupational therapists. Humanity should always come first.

Kerrie Thomsen

15.9 Summary

■ Occupational therapy must be reimagined to be culturally responsive, move away from colonial thinking, and find ways of being and doing to genuinely support First Peoples' health and well-being.

■ Understanding and embracing First Peoples' 'Ways of Knowing, Thinking, Being, and Doing' is crucial for authentic and effective practice, recognising that well-being is holistic and interconnected.

■ Critical self-reflection on one's own biases, positionality, and privilege is an essential early step and ongoing journey for non-Indigenous therapists to engage respectfully and responsibly.

■ Building trust through genuine relationships, deep listening (*Dadirri*), and patience is paramount, as is understanding that 'story' is a powerful and sacred occupation.

■ Conventional assessment tools, like ADL tools, need cultural interpretation to avoid judgment and truly understand a person's lived reality and occupational needs within their own cultural context.

■ Allyship is an active commitment that involves listening, educating oneself, challenging racism, advocating for systemic change, and humbly learning from mistakes to foster truly equitable occupational therapy practice.

15.10 Review and reflection questions

■ Review Kerrie's position statement and create your own. Revisit this periodically and update as you grow personally and professionally.

■ Review the concept of allyship and set yourself a goal related to growing your capability as an ally. Create an action plan with several steps you will take to develop your thinking, knowing, being, and doing in the allyship role.

■ Reflect on an aspect of your thinking or feeling that has been changed as you've read this chapter and commit to speaking about this with a family member, friend, or colleague. Prepare a two-minute monologue to express your thoughts and feelings.

■ Reflect on your own daily life, choose one daily occupation, and describe the way you would prefer to have that assessed by an occupational therapist using words that you feel would be respectful, give you choice, and be meaningful.

References

Agner, J. (2020). Moving from cultural competence to cultural humility in occupational therapy: A paradigm shift. *American Journal of Occupational Therapy*, 74(4), 7404347010p1–7404347010p7. https://doi.org/10.5014/ajot.2020.038067

Beagan, B. L. (2015). Approaches to culture and diversity: A critical synthesis of occupational therapy literature. *Canadian Journal of Occupational Therapy*, 82(5), 272–282. https://doi.org/10.1177/0008417414567530

Emery-Whittington, I. (2025). Decoloniality in occupational therapy practice: Preparation and readiness. In S. Mahani & A. Zafran (Eds.), *Theorizing occupation: A tapestry of perspectives*. Slack Incorporated.

Gee, G., Dudgeon, P., Schultz, C., Hart, A., & Kelly, K. (2014). Aboriginal and Torres Strait Islander social and emotional wellbeing. In P. Dudgeon, H. Milroy, & R. Walker (Eds.), *Working together: Aboriginal and Torres Strait Islander mental health and wellbeing principles and practice* (2nd ed., pp. 55–68). Australian Government Department of the Prime Minister and Cabinet.

Guerzoni, M. A. (2020). *Indigenising the curriculum: Context, concepts and case studies*. University of Tasmania.

Hook, J. N., Davis, D. E., Owen, J., Worthington Jr, E. L., & Utsey, S. O. (2013). Cultural humility: Measuring openness to culturally diverse clients. *Journal of Counseling Psychology*, 60(3), 353–366. https://doi.org/10.1037/a0032595

Indigenous Allied Health Australia. (2019). *Cultural responsiveness in action: An IAHA framework* (3rd ed.). https://iaha.com.au/workforce-support/training-and-development/cultural-responsiveness-in-action-training

Kelly, M., Marriott-Statham, K., Clapham, K., Metusela, C., & Mackay, M. (2024). Understanding the cultural determinants of health: A scoping review. *First Nations Health and Wellbeing – The Lowitja Journal*. https://doi.org/10.1016/j.fnhli.2024.100036

Nelson, R., Zahl, M. L., Bell, S. A., & Bennett, J. R. (2023). Evolving beyond cultural competence and embracing cultural humility. *American Journal of Recreation Therapy*, 22(1), 1–8. https://doi.org/10.5055/ajrt.2023.0274

Official Miriam-Rose Ungunmerr Video. (2017, November 29). Dadirri [Video]. *YouTube*. https://www.youtube.com/watch?v=tow2tR_ezL8

Sherwood, J., & Geia, L. (2017). Historical and political perspectives on Indigenous health. In J. Daly, S. Speedy, & D. Jackson (Eds.), *Contexts of nursing: An introduction* (5th ed., pp. 224–241). Elsevier Australia.

Tuck, E., & Yang, K. W. (2012). Decolonization is not a metaphor. *Decolonization: Indigeneity, Education & Society*, 1(1), 1–40. https://doi.org/10.25058/20112742.n38.04

CHAPTER 16

Māori health and occupational therapy in Aotearoa New Zealand

Georgia Brown, Yasmin Sadler, Renee Fitisemanu, and Haylee Martell

Pepeha
Ki te taha o tōku Koro
Ko Mataatua te Waka
Ko Hikurangi (nō Tai Tokerau) te Maunga
Ko Kaikou te Awa
Ko Te Horo te Marae
Ko Ngāti Hine te Hapū
Ko Ngāpuhi te Iwi
Ki te taha o tōku Kui
Ko Mataatua te waka
Ko Mauao te Maunga
Ko Tauranga te Moana
Ko Oruarahi te Marae
Ko Ngāi Tamawhariua te Hapū
Ko Ngāi Te Rangi te Iwi
Ko Yasmin Sadler ahau

Ki te taha o toku Pāpā
Ko Ngatokimatawhaorua me Māhuhu Ki Te Rangi ngā waka
Ko Motatau me Whakairiora ngā maunga
Ko Taumarere me Ngunguru ngā awa
Ko Ngāti Hine, Ngātiwai, Te Waiariki ngā hapū
Ko Ōtiria me Ngunguru ngā marae
Ko Hineamaru rāua ko Kerepeti Te Peke ōku tūpuna
Ki te taha o toku māmā
Ko Māhuhu Ki Te Rangi te waka
Ko Tutamoe te maunga
Ko Kaihu te awa

DOI: 10.4324/9781003495666-18

Ko Ngāti Whātua te iwi
Ko Ngāti Hinga me Ngāti Torehina ngā hapū
Ko Ahikiwi me Taita ngā marae
Ko Netana Patuawa rāua ko Panapa Hohapata ōku tūpuna.
Ko Georgia Brown Tawhiri toku ingoa

Ki te taha o tōku Koro
Ko Rangiuri te maunga
Ko Kaituna te awa
Ko Te Arawa te waka
Ko Te Arawa te iwi
Ko Tapuika te hāpu
Ko Makahae te marae
Ki te taha o tōku Kuia
Ko Otawa te Maunga
Ko Te Rapa-rapa-a-hoe Te awa
Ko Te Arawa te waka
Ko Te Arawa te iwi
Ko Waitaha te hāpu
Ko Hei te marae
Ko Renee Fitisemanu ahau

Ki te taha o tōku Koro
Ko Taupiri te Maunga
Ko Waikato te Awa
Ko Tainui te Waka
Ko Waikato te Iwi
Ko Horahora te marae
Ko Ngāti Naho me Ngāti Pou me Ngāti Pareue ngā Hapū
Ko Horahora te Marae

Ki te taha o tōku Kuia
Ko Pirongia te Maunga
Ko Waipa te Awa
Ko Tainui te Waka
Ko Ngāti Maniapoto te Iwi
Ko Ngāti Apakura te Hapū
Ko Kahotea te Marae
Ko Haylee Martell ahau

Authors' positionality statement
In this chapter we will explore occupations through a te ao Māori lens. We touch on colonial constructs and the damage that occurred, weaving together *past* injustices with their *present*-day effects on Māori health and wellbeing, and share positive actions that can be taken to enhance our practice for the *future* of Māori health and wellbeing. Many Māori kupu/words used in this chapter are common terms that are useful to be familiar with in practice.

As Kaiwhakaora Ngangahau Māori (Māori occupational therapists) affiliated with various iwi across Aotearoa, we speak from our lived realities and not on behalf of all Māori. We are practitioners with backgrounds in both physical and mental health, engaged in both academic roles and clinical practice across public and private sectors.

We are grounded in our whakapapa, informed by mātauranga Māori, and committed to upholding the spirit and obligations of Te Tiriti o Waitangi. This positionality informs our practice, research, and advocacy for culturally responsive and equitable health outcomes. We are also dedicated to collective growth, ensuring that our efforts contribute to the advancement and well-being of Māori communities.

We are privileged to include in this chapter excerpts from tangata whenua and tangata tiriti and to have our mahi reviewed by Eru Kapa-Kingi, Roxanne Waru, and Sharon Bryant.

Key terms
- Cultural responsiveness
- Cultural safety
- He Whakaputanga
- Te Tiriti o Waitangi
- Te Whare Tapa Whā
- Tino Rangatiratanga

Objectives
This chapter will allow the reader to:

- Discuss their understanding of He Whakaputanga and Te Tiriti o Waitangi as foundational documents to inform ethical and equitable engagement with Māori
- Critically analyse the ongoing impacts of colonisation on occupational participation and wellbeing of Māori communities
- Consider Māori models of health as approaches for providing culturally responsive occupational therapy

16.1 Past

16.1.1 Te Whakaminenga and He Whakaputanga

In the early 1800s, Māori had a thriving international trade but were not recognised due to their flag being made from harakeke/flax. As a result, some of the vessels were detained (Tudor, 2016). Northern chiefs (Rangatira), alongside settlers, selected the first national flag of Aotearoa in March 1834, known as Te Kara o Te Whakaminenga o Nga Hapu o Nu Tireni (the United Tribes' flag). He Whakaputanga o te Rangatiratanga o Nu Tireni (Declaration of Independence) was signed on 28 October 1835 by 34 northern Rangatira; a further 18 signatures were obtained by 1839. He Whakaputanga was born through discussions within Te Whakaminenga (Confederation of Chiefs). It was a declaration of sovereignty by the Rangatira of the numerous hapū throughout the country and declared to the world that 'we' are the tangata whenua of this land and that law-making powers would not be given to anyone else (Mutu, 2019).

He Whakaputanga was drafted by a British official and then a translated version was completed in te reo Māori – the Māori document was signed, sovereignty was never ceded, and it consisted of four articles that asserted mana/authority and sovereign power in Aotearoa belonged fully with Māori, and that foreigners would not be allowed to make laws (Keane, 2012):

- In the first article, Rangatira declared Aotearoa a 'whenua rangatira' (independent state).
- The second article stated 'kingitanga' (sovereign power) was held collectively by the Rangatira.
- The third article stated a huihuinga (congress) would meet each autumn to make laws and decisions.
- The fourth article explained a copy of this declaration would be sent to the King of England and asked him to be a parent of the infant state.

The king of England formally acknowledged He Whakaputanga, and it has been considered the parent document to Te Tiriti o Waitangi. Both documents do not compete with one another; they have a shared whakapapa/ancestry and working relationship (Waitangi Tribunal, 2014; Kapa-Kingi, 2025).

16.1.2 Te Tiriti o Waitangi

Te Tiriti o Waitangi is considered a cornerstone document of Aotearoa's history, signed in 1840 between Māori Rangatira and the British Crown. This document came about by Māori Rangatira becoming tired of lawless settlers and how they were behaving in Aotearoa (this included substance abuse, theft, rape, and disorderly conduct) and the need for the Crown to assume responsibility to bring them to order (Mutu, 2019).

On 6 February 1840, Māori Rangatira and representatives of the Crown signed Te Tiriti o Waitangi, a treaty written in te reo Māori that affirmed the 1835 He Whakaputanga, protecting their rangatiratanga (tribal authority). The treaty included five articles.

Preamble: highlighted the Crown's promises to secure rangatiratanga and ensure Māori land ownership.

Article One: Kāwanatanga: governance by the Crown over British settlers, intended to address the request from Rangatira for recognition and respect for their full authority over their lands while unburdening them from the responsibility for the unruly behaviour of British settlers.

Article Two: Tino Rangatiratanga: Māori self-determination and authority: guaranteed tino rangatiratanga of Rangatira not only over their whenua/land, hapu, iwi, and taonga/treasures but also te reo, ways of living, and kainga/homes. It also gave the Crown exclusive rights to purchase land from Māori for settlers.

Article Three: Ōritetanga: outlined Māori would have the same rights and duties of citizenship as British settlers. This meant that any benefit that Pākeha had, Māori would have as well.

Article Four is often referred to as the 'phantom article' because it is not part of the written text; it is based on a verbal agreement made at the time of the signing, intended to guarantee religious freedom and the protection of Māori spiritual beliefs and practices.

This document was intended to establish a contractual agreement for interactions between Māori and Pākehā, but its interpretation and execution have not been honoured (Waitangi Tribunal, 2014).

16.1.3 Distinguishing between 'The Treaty' and Te Tiriti o Waitangi

Te Tiriti o Waitangi and the Treaty of Waitangi (English version) are described as two separate texts (Waitangi Tribunal, 2014). The English text could not be understood by the 39 Rangatira who signed it, and the te reo Māori text was signed by 500 Rangatira. Although the English text attempted to be an exact translation of Te Tiriti o Waitangi, it was not. Instead, it falsely suggested Māori ceded sovereignty to the British Crown. In 2014 the Waitangi Tribunal recognised that Māori could not and did not cede sovereignty (Waitangi Tribunal, 2014).

The contra proferentem rule has been applied to Te Tiriti o Waitangi to resolve ambiguities between the English and Māori text. This legal principle dictates that any unclear terms in a contract or treaty should be interpreted against the party that drafted it. The Waitangi Tribunal has consistently used this rule to honour the Māori language text and the cultural context in which the Treaty was signed, reflecting the true spirit of Te Tiriti o Waitangi (Waitangi Tribunal, 2014).

16.1.4 Māori occupations prior to colonisation

Māori occupations are intrinsically connected to the taiao/natural environment informed by pūrākau/culturally laden stories, traditions, and intergenerational practices. Māori interpreted ngā tohu o te taiao/sign in the natural environment, which helped them to navigate the world. An example is living by the maramataka/lunar calendar. The maramataka was initially a means of survival and now serves as a guide for seasonal occupations such as planting, fishing, and managing our emotional wellbeing and performance.

Māori engaged in spiritual occupations like karakia, waiata, to invoke and acknowledge atua/ancestral beings and the environment before undergoing tasks, maintaining the harmonious relationships between people and elements. Māori are communal beings, and occupations revolved around benefit for and survival of the hapū. Therefore, things were done in an intentional and inclusive manner to care for the collective and the whenua.

Māori occupations preserve the stories of tāngata whenua through the oral passing of whakapapa and mātauranga found in pūrākau/stories, waiata, and haka/dance. This was also recorded in mahi toi/arts such as raranga harakeke/flax weaving, moko/Māori tattoo, and whakairo/carving, which are often referred to as living entities that encapsulate the essence of our identity and heritage (Te Hiku Media, 2023). These occupations weave together the fabric of being Māori. Keeping these practices alive reinforces a strong sense of identity, community, and belonging within te ao Māori.

16.1.5 Occupations of Māori post colonisation

Colonisation in Aotearoa was brutal and violent, involving the taking of 'lands and lives' (Jackson, 2021), kainga, and occupations (Kapa-Kingi, 2025). Colonisation in Aotearoa continues to trickle (and occasionally flood) into our present societal structures. Colonisation is often spoken about in the past, but it is necessary to note the ongoing adverse and destructive consequences that continue to disadvantage Māori today.

British opportunists, particularly the New Zealand Company, came with the aim to possess land and undertake systematic colonisation of Aotearoa. Māori did not perceive land as a possession, instead as taonga. The differing perception of what land was and is, and a colonial sense of superiority, was the justification for Te Tiriti o Waitangi not being honoured by the Crown. No longer accessing or living on the whenua meant Māori were stripped of their ability to practice and maintain their spiritual, social, and physical wellbeing. No land meant no access to natural resources, waterways, food sources, or rongoā/remedies and traditional healing, resulting in not being able to participate in wellbeing occupations.

The Crown attempted to eradicate Māori by stripping them of their identity and connection to indigenous ways of living and thriving, forcing conformity and assimilation to western ways (Mutu, 2019), and through introducing strategic legislation intentionally disconnecting Māori from the elements that were core to their existence and wellbeing like the Native Schools Act 1867 and the Tohunga Suppression Act 1907 (Tohunga being very learned, skilled, and educated people, healers, and teachers). Legislation made it illegal for Māori to access language and traditional or spiritual means of healing and wellbeing. Consequently, generations of Māori are unable to kōrero Māori and have restricted engagement with rongoā.

16.2 Present

16.2.1 Distrust of the health system

Aotearoa's health system has evolved over generations but remains an extension of the Crown, its racist systems, and assimilation (Came et al., 2020). Māori distrust in the health system is based on continuous negative experiences and outcomes within

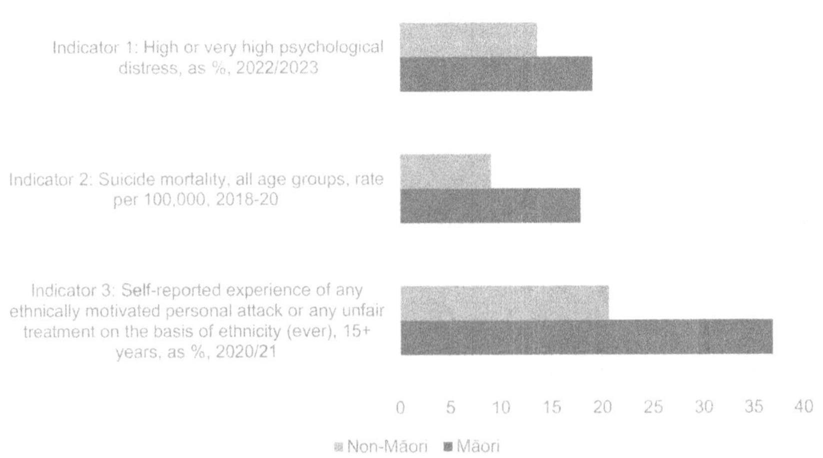

Figure 16.1 Indicators of health outcomes

government systems. Māori had their own processes and practices of health and wellbeing, and these were fractured by colonisation and the distrust that emerged in response to breaches of Te Tiriti o Waitangi (Masters-Awatere & Graham, 2019).

16.2.2 Health outcomes for Māori

After nearly two centuries of colonisation, Māori continue to face disproportionately poor health outcomes, largely due to the health system's ongoing failure to uphold Māori rights and Te Tiriti o Waitangi (see Figure 16.2). There is an urgent need for cultural reform within the health sector – one that aligns with Te Tiriti o Waitangi and places equity at the forefront (Sheridan et al. 2023, 2024, as cited in Kidd et al. 2025).

16.2.3 WAI2575 Health Services and Outcome Kaupapa Inquiry

The Waitangi Tribunal was established in 1975 to investigate breaches of Te Tiriti o Waitangi and to assist in reconciliation efforts between the Crown and Māori. Issues surrounding Māori health fall within the remit of the Waitangi Tribunal, and in 2016 the claim WAI2575 Health Services and Outcome Kaupapa Inquiry was opened to hear grievances about the Aotearoa health care system (Came et al., 2020). The inquiry found the Crown failed to deliver equitable outcomes for Māori and therefore breached Te Tiriti o Waitangi. The most significant recommendation made was to adopt Tiriti-compliant legislation and policy. To ensure equitable health outcomes, Māori not only need to be considered in policy review and development but also included and granted influence at every stage of this process, aligining with Article 2 of Te Tiriti o Waitangi. This recommendation also aligns with the Responsiveness to te Tiriti o Waitangi competency set by Te Poari Whakaora Ngangahau o Aotearoa/Occupational Therapy Board of New Zealand (OTBNZ), which all Kaiwhakaora Ngangahau must meet (OTBNZ, 2022).

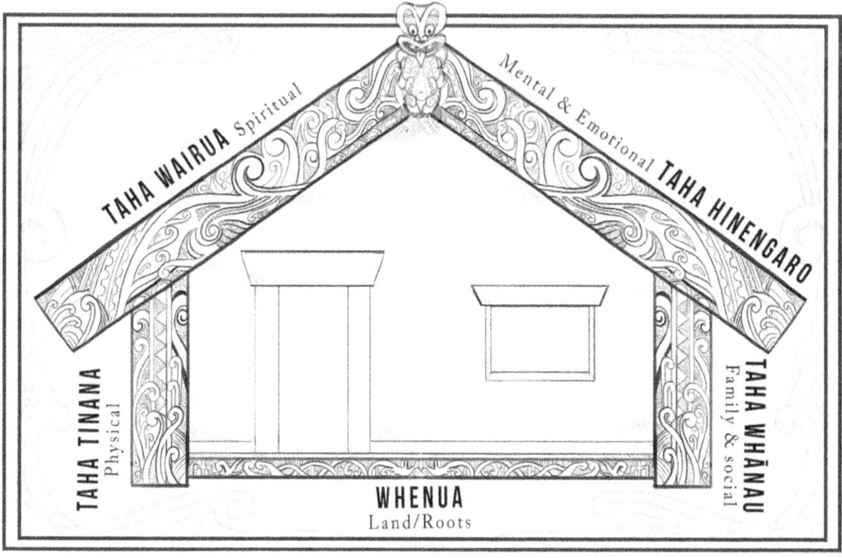

Figure 16.2 Te Whare Tapa Wha | Indicators of health outcomes

16.2.4 Revitalisation of Māori health practices

Hauora Māori encompasses spiritual and social wellbeing, as well as connection to te taiao/natural environment and a life force, known as mauri. An influential Māori health model is Te Whare Tapa Whā by Dr Mason Durie. The four-part framework consists of four walls of a whare. All domains are necessary to strengthen, stabilise, and sustain the individual – Taha Wairua/spiritual health, Taha Hinengaro/mental health, Taha Tinana/physical health, and Taha whānau/family and community wellbeing (Durie, 1998). This whare stands grounded on the whenua, highlighting the importance of identity and connection to place.

Taha Wairua considers a person's spirituality. Spirituality not only applies to the religious beliefs and practices; it considers the deep connection Māori have with te taiao, known to also hold and transfer mauri.

Taha Hinengaro is a person's capacity to communicate, think, and feel. For Māori, emotional communication is practiced more than the spoken word, which can be a foreign concept to non-Māori.

Taha Tinana refers to physical health and the capacity to grow and develop. Durie discusses the relationship between tapu/sacred and noa/ordinary and explains that certain parts of the body in te ao Māori are seen as sacred or special. Subsequently, interventions involving the upoko/head, sexual organs, hair, and nail clippings require caution and sensitivity.

Taha Whānau recognises the individual as part of a wider social system and that whānau wellness has a direct impact on the individual. This speaks to the importance of including whānau in care decisions for tangata whaiora.

Māori health frameworks such as The Hui Process (Lacey et al., 2011) and Meihana model (Pitama et al., 2014) build on the mahi of other Māori health models, such as Te Whare Tapa Whā. They share the application of specific processes health practitioners can use to enhance the clinician-Māori client relationship.

16.3 Future

16.3.1 Māori values and practices

Māori values and practices centre on connection between tangata, taiao, atua, and whakapapa. Engagement and relationship-building are fundamental when working with Māori, shaping their experiences and health outcomes.

Whakawhānaungatanga is the reciprocal process in which Māori relate to others; it is about establishing, building, and nurturing relationships. Traditionally, this includes sharing pepeha and whakapapa (Bennett, 2018). Today it can include sharing interests, values, and using icebreakers. Whakawhānaungatanga requires vulnerability to be open and share information about yourself; this is important within clinical spaces, as it humanises both parties and enables power-sharing (Komene et al., 2023). Kanohi-ki-te-kanohi/face-to-face is important, as this enriches communication, deepening connections physically and spiritually (The Putaiora Writing Group, 2010).

Māori are communal, valuing inclusion and collectively. Kotahitanga involves working together as a collective, mirroring working and functioning as a whānau, but may vary from typical whānau dynamics to include extended whānau and friends. Kotahitanga strengthens connections and builds manaaki/caring. Manaakitanga/

hospitality involves sharing food, space, and conversation, fostering harmonious and uplifting relationships.

Tikanga is essential for Māori health and wellbeing, providing practical and spiritual safeguards (Mead, 2016). It is important to recognise the diversity among Māori in terms of whakapapa, connection to Māoritanga/Māori culture, and upbringing. Cultural beliefs, values, and practices may vary, so what works for one Māori individual may not be appropriate for another. Awareness and sensitivity to the ongoing impacts of colonisation are crucial to avoid unsafe and mana-diminishing situations (Bennett, 2018).

16.3.2 Te Tiriti o Waitangi as a foundation in occupational therapy practice

Given the significance of Te Tiriti o Waitangi, it is pertinent to consider how the Articles can be integrated into daily practice as Kaiwhakaora Ngangahau. The following outlines brief examples of how to start the journey to becoming tangata Tiriti.

Preamble: assessing biases you may hold, looking inwards and exploring preconceived notions you have of Te Tiriti o Waitangi and or/Indigenous marginalised populations.

Article 1: Kawanatanga: advocacy for policies and practices that promote equity and address health disparities for Māori. Working collaboratively with Māori health providers and community leaders to ensure services are culturally safe and appropriate.

Article 2: Tino Rangatiratanga: providing treatment options to whānau and tangata whaiora, ensuring they are the key decision-makers for their own health and wellbeing. Providing clear and culturally appropriate information to Māori tangata whaiora and whānau to ensure they are at the centre of the decision-making.

Article 3: Ōritetanga: ensuring Māori patients have equitable access to occupational therapy services. Offering a high standard and quality of care for all whānau you work with; identifying and addressing barriers that may impact Māori and their whānau.

Article 4: ensuring the Māori worldview is considered; can include taking time to understand the whānau dynamics, the value of karakia, whakawhānaungatanga, and allowing tikanga to guide interactions.

16.3.3 Being Tangata Tiriti

Being 'tangata Tiriti' is both aspirational and political. It involves building relationships with Māori, understanding the historical context, acknowledging inequities, and committing to the ongoing advocacy for Māori self-sovereignty. Tangata Tiriti are encouraged to engage in antiracism work, which includes understanding and addressing institutional racism, being honest and exploring one's own privilege, structural analysis, and disrupting racist narratives (Dewes, 2022).

This approach not only benefits Māori but all of Aotearoa. Practicing tangata Tiriti/ Kaiwhakaora Ngangahau reflect in the following.

Openly reflecting about my lack of cultural competence and safety, required acknowledging and accepting that I don't know anything due to my upbringing and privilege. Initially I didn't reflect openly about this as I didn't want to seem incompetent, but during this discomfort I recognised and learnt the importance of actually identifying this and being open about it in order to move forward and start learning and unlearning things that were incorrect. . . . Through this journey I have learnt and continue to learn how to practice in a culturally mindful way, and have incorporated Māori values and practices into assessments and interventions following the guidance of Māori colleagues and experts. The interventions around Māori culture and identity, are based around tangata whaiora actually wanting to do this rather than me assuming every tangata whaiora Māori needs to do this.

(Alysha Kanongata'a – occupational therapist/tangata Tiriti)

How can we as tangata Tiriti better enact our cultural responsiveness to ensure Māori receive an equitable opportunity to thrive and succeed in their health?

- Embody a genuine, honest, and humble approach and attitude when stepping into Te Ao Māori. As tangata Tiriti we are manuhiri/guests.
- Correct pronunciation is essential; when unsure, ask for help and then practice, practice, practice.
- Prioritise whakawhānaungatanga, founded upon trust and respect with your tangata whaiora and whānau. Implement the Hui Process to guide interactions, allowing intentional and necessary time to understand, connect, and feel safe with one another.
- As tangata Tiriti our role is to walk alongside and collaborate with our kaumatua, Māori cultural advisors, and services. We have a responsibility to uphold tikanga in our workspaces.
- Never assume that because a tangata whaiora is Māori that they feel connected to their culture. But always open the conversation and be a safe place for your tangata whaiora to guide you.

(Sharayah Rice – occupational therapist/tangata Tiriti)

16.3.4 Kaiwhakaora Ngangahau Māori

There is hope that drives us to address these disparities and create meaningful change. It is grounded in who we are as Māori – 'Just be Māori. Be Māori all day, every day. We are here. We are strong,' as Kiingi Tuheitia Potatau te Wherowhero VII reminded us (E-Tangata, 2024).

We must remember who we descend from, drawing strength from our tūpuna/ancestors' experiences, stories, and attributes of resilience, determination, and courage. Their actions empower us and shape how we engage in the system as Indigenous Kaiwhakaora Ngangahau.

Echoing the strength of our tūpuna, we must remain steadfast in our purpose, paving the way and creating space for other Kaiwhakaora Ngangahau Māori. We need to continue advocating for our worldview, ensuring our culture is embedded in curriculums, work environments, and systems. By doing so, we will support, motivate, and inspire the future of our profession, ensuring they are empowered to walk this journey and advocate for their rightful place within it.

(Sénae Mitchell – Kaiwhakaora Ngangahau Māori)

Ko au te hua o te kaupapa/I am a product of Te Aho Matua/the philosophical base for Kura Kaupapa Māori education, kōhanga reo/Māori language school, and kura kaupapa Māori [Māori language immersion school]. As an uri/descendent of Ngāti Raukawa and Ngāti Maniapoto, I bring a lived understanding of mana Motuhake [governing] autonomy into my occupational therapy practice.

I see my role as a Kaiwhakaora Ngangahau not just as a clinician, but as a practitioner of occupational justice. I actively centre Māori models of health, resist deficit narratives, and advocate for tino rangatiratanga in how Māori engage in daily occupations, including healing.

As a tāne/male Kaiwhakaora Ngangahau Māori, I hold space for other tāne to reconnect with their wairua, strength, and purpose. I challenge harmful stereotypes and uplift culturally congruent pathways to recovery.

My top tohutohu/advice:

- Whakarongo/listen before you kōrero: Builds trust and respects whakapapa.
- Engage the whānau, not just the file: Healing is intergenerational and collective.
- Uphold Te Tiriti and embed kaupapa Māori/proceedings: Reflect equity and cultural authenticity.

Chaz Brown – Kaiwhakaora Ngangahau Māori

16.4 Summary

- Te Tiriti o Waitangi and He Whakapūtanga are the founding documents of Aotearoa and guide how we should be working with Māori
- Colonisation has had, and continues to have, a significant impact on the occupational health and wellbeing of Māori
- Māori face significant health disparities as a result of colonisation and displacement from land, language, and culture
- Māori models of health have been developed to address health inequities and are currently used in practice
- Tikanga, whakawhānaungatanga, and manaakitanga are essential when interacting with Māori

16.5 Review and reflection questions

- In what ways has colonisation impacted the health and occupational wellbeing of Māori?
- What are the key articles of Te Tiriti o Waitangi, and how can Kaiwhakaora Ngangahau incorporate these into their practice?
- Why are tikanga, whakawhānaungatanga, and manaakitanga essential when interacting with Māori, and how can these values be integrated into culturally safe practice?

References

Bennett, S. (2018). Transforming psychological services for Māori. In T. K. Kingi, M. Durie, H. Elder, R. Tapsell, M. Lawrence, & S. Bennet (Eds.), *Maea te toi ora: Māori health transformations* (pp. 193–222). Huia.

Came, H., O'Sullivan, D., Kidd, J., & McCreanor, T. (2020). The Waitangi Tribunal's WAI 2575 report: Implications for decolonizing health systems. *Health and Human Rights Journal, 22*(1), 209–220. https://www.hhrjournal.org/2020/06/the-waitangi-tribunals-wai-2575-report-implications-for-decolonizing-health-systems/

Cram, F. (2014). *Equity of healthcare for Māori: A framework*. Ministry of Health.

Dewes, T. K. D. (2022, February 6). What does it mean to be tangata Tiriti? *The Spinoff*. https://thespinoff.co.nz/atea/06-02-2022/what-does-it-mean-to-be-tangata-tiriti

Durie, M. (1998). *Whaiora: Māori health development* (2nd ed.). Oxford University Press.

E-Tangata. (2024, September 1). *Be Māori all day, every day*. https://e-tangata.co.nz/comment-and-analysis/be-maori-all-day-every-day/

Gibbs, R. (2021). *Te whare tapa wh*ā [Photograph]. Rebecca Gibbs Illustration. https://www.rebeccagibbsillustration.com/allresources/te-whare-tapa-wh

Husband, D. (2021, July 18). Rereata Makiha: Holding on to ancestral knowledge. *E-Tangata*. https://e-tangata.co.nz/korero/rereata-makiha-holding-on-to-ancestral-knowledge/

Jackson, M. (2021). *Decolonisation and the stories in the land*. E-tangata. https://e-tangata.co.nz/comment-and-analysis/moana-jackson-decolonisation-and-the-stories-in-the-land/

Kapa-Kingi, E. (2025, October 28). *The first declaration of Māori sovereignty and why it still matters*. The Spinoff. https://thespinoff.co.nz/atea/28-10-2025/eru-kapa-kingi-the-first-declaration-of-maori-sovereignty-and-why-it-still-matters

Keane, B. (2012). *He Whakaputanga – Declaration of independence*. Te Ara – Encyclopaedia of New Zealand. http://www.TeAra.govt.nz/en/he-whakaputanga-declaration-of-independence

Kidd, J., Tipa, Z., Arnet, H., & Rēnata, H. (2025). Hauora Māori: Aspirations of Māori health practitioners for a culturally relevant health system. *Ethnographic Edge, 8*(1), 57–76. https://ojs.aut.ac.nz/ethnographic-edge/article/view/294/271

Komene, E., Pene, B., Gerard, D., Parr, J., Aspinall, C., & Wilson, D. (2023). Whakawhānaungatanga-building trust and connections: A qualitative study Indigenous Māori patients and whānau (extended family network) hospital experiences. *Journal of Advanced Nursing, 80*(4), 1545–1558. https://doi.org/10.1111/jan.15912/v2/response1

Lacey, C., Huria, T., Becket, L., Gilles, M., & Pitama, S. (2011). The Hui process: A framework to enhance the doctor-patient relationship with Māori. *Journal of the New Zealand Medical Association, 124*(1347), 72–78. http://journal.nzma.org.nz/journal/124-1347/5003/

Masters-Awatere, B., & Graham, R. (2019). Whānau Māori explain how the Harti Hauora tool assists with better access to health services. *Australian Journal of Primary Health, 25*(5), 471–477. https://doi.org/10.1071/py19025

Mead, H. (2016). *Tikanga Māori: Living by Māori values*. Huia.

Ministry of Health. (2024). *Tatau kahukura: Māori health chart book 2024* (4th ed.). Ministry of Health.

Mutu, M. (2019). 'To honour the treaty, we must first settle colonisation' (Moana Jackson 2015): The long road from colonial devastation to balance, peace and harmony. *Journal of the Royal Society of New Zealand, 49*, 4–18. https://doi.org/10.1080/03036758.2019.1669670

The Native School Act. (1867). https://www.nzlii.org/nz/legis/hist_act/nsa185821a22v1858n65306/

Occupational Therapy Board of New Zealand. (2022). *Competencies for registration and continuing practice for occupational therapists*. https://otboard.org.nz/document/6151/7569%20OTBNZ%20%E2%80%93%20Competencies%20for%20practice%20FINAL.pdf

Pitama, S., Huria, T., & Lacey, C. (2014). Improving Māori health through clinical assessment: Waikare o te waka a meihana. *Journal of the New Zealand Medical Association, 127*(1393), 107–119.

The Putaiora Writing Group. (2010). *Te ara tika: Guidelines for Māori research ethics: A framework for researchers and ethics committee members*. HRC. https://www.hrc.govt.nz/resources/te-ara-tika-guidelines-maori-research-ethics-0

Rickard, K. (Host). (2025). *Treaty Talks Episode 3: Eru Kapa-Kingi*. YouTube. https://www.youtube.com/watch?v=My__wPF8SUc

Te Hiku Media. (2023, December 14). *Mahi toi: Rongoa in Māori art forms.* https://tehiku.nz/te-hiku-radio/tautinei/42719/mahi-toi-rongoa-in-Māori-art-forms

The Tohunga Suppression Act. (1907). https://www.nzlii.org/nz/legis/hist_act/tsa19077ev1907n13353/

Tudor, K. (2016). *Raising (issues about) the banner: A critical reflection on the New Zealand flag debate (2015–2016).* Counterfutures. https://counterfutures.nz/2/tudor.pdf

Waitangi Tribunal. (2014). *He Whakaputanga me Te Tiriti: The Declaration and the Treaty: The report on Stage 1 of the Paparahi o Te Raki Inquiry (Wai 1040).* Legislation Direct.

Waitangi Tribunal. (2023). *Hauora: Report on stage one of the health services and outcomes kaupapa inquiry (Report No. Wai 2575).* Legislation Direct.

Wilson, D., Moloney, E., Parr, J. M., Aspinall, C., & Slark, J. (2021). Creating an Indigenous Māori-centred model of relational health: A literature review of Māori models of health. *Journal of Clinical Nursing, 30,* 3539–3555. https://onlinelibrary.wiley.com/doi/epdf/10.1111/jocn.15859

CHAPTER 17

Pacific health and occupational therapy in Aotearoa New Zealand

Marina Elisara, Rachel Kapa-Vivian, Emily Glennon, Vicky Tariau, Adriana Bootten, and Ema Tokolahi

E 'Otua,

'Oku mau kolea ho'o tāpuaki mo ho'o kelesi ma'ae kau ngāue Pasifika Kaiwhakaora
*   Ngangahau kotoa pē,*
Malu'i moke fakaivia kinautolu mo 'enau ngaahi ngaue 'oku fai, ko hono tokāekina,
*   si'i ngaahi fānau moe Kainga 'oku nau fiema'u tokoni.*

O God,

We ask for your blessings and grace, bless all the Pacific Occupational Therapists,
Keep them safe and enable them to do their work with the Pacific communities they serve.
(Tongan lotu | prayer)

Authors' positionality statement

We acknowledge the diversity of perspectives within the Pacific community (those island-born and born elsewhere) and that our group could not represent all views. Four of the six authors identify as Aotearoa-born Pacific Peoples, with affiliations to Sāmoa (Elisara and Bootten) and the Cook Islands (Glennon and Tariau). Two authors identify as non-Pacific (Kapa-Vivian and Tokolahi), with professional and personal experiences of walking alongside Pacific communities. All authors are women and registered occupational therapists in Aotearoa, with clinical experiences across physical and mental health, education, private, and corporate settings. *Talanoa* presented in the chapter were the lived experiences of the authors and from occupational therapists in the broader Pacific community.

Chapter summary

This chapter presents a description of Pacific Peoples in Aotearoa and their unique history that contributed to health inequities faced today. *Talanoa* (discussion), from

DOI: 10.4324/9781003495666-19

occupational therapists working with Pacific Peoples in Aotearoa, showcase culturally responsive practices. The importance of *vā*, roles and relationships, is highlighted as central to the health and wellbeing of Pacific Peoples. Building and nurturing *vā* involves demonstrating key Pacific values like integrity, humility, respect, and reciprocity. Professional practices and models may need adaptation to be culturally safe and responsive and meet the needs of Pacific Peoples.

Key terms
- Culturally responsive practice
- Cultural safety
- Family
- Health inequities
- Talanoa
- Tuakana-Teina
- Values
- Vā

Objectives
This chapter will allow the reader to:

- Outline historical and socioeconomic factors that contribute to health inequities experienced by Pacific Peoples in Aotearoa
- Analyse the significance of *vā*, roles and relationships in Pacific cultures, and their implications for occupational therapy practice
- Identify culturally safe and responsive practices to occupational therapy models that are essential when working with Pacific Peoples

Glossary
- Talanoa: A formal or informal verbal interaction or conversation to talk about nothing and share stories; respectful and inclusive to build relationships and share knowledge (Vaioleti, 2016); a term shared by Tongans, Sāmoans, and Fijians
- Tuakana-Teina: Sibling relationship concept
- Vā: Between-ness, space that relates

17.1 Introduction

Pacific Peoples is a collective term for individuals who descend from one (or more) of over 17 island nations in the Pacific. In Aotearoa (known in colonial terms as New Zealand), the largest Pacific ethnic groups are Sāmoan, Tongan, Cook Island, Niuean, and Fijian (see Figure 17.1). Despite sharing common worldviews and values, each nation has its own ethno-specific cultural beliefs, values, traditions, language, social structure, and history. Family, reciprocity, respect, integrity, humility, and spirituality are central values – it is worth noting in this context, family is inclusive of extended family and significant others who all play a role in shaping the Pacific person's day-to-day life (see Figure 17.2 for examples of the word family in various Pacific languages). Understanding this diversity is essential for implementing culturally responsive practice that addresses Pacific Peoples' unique contributions, identities, patterns of participation,

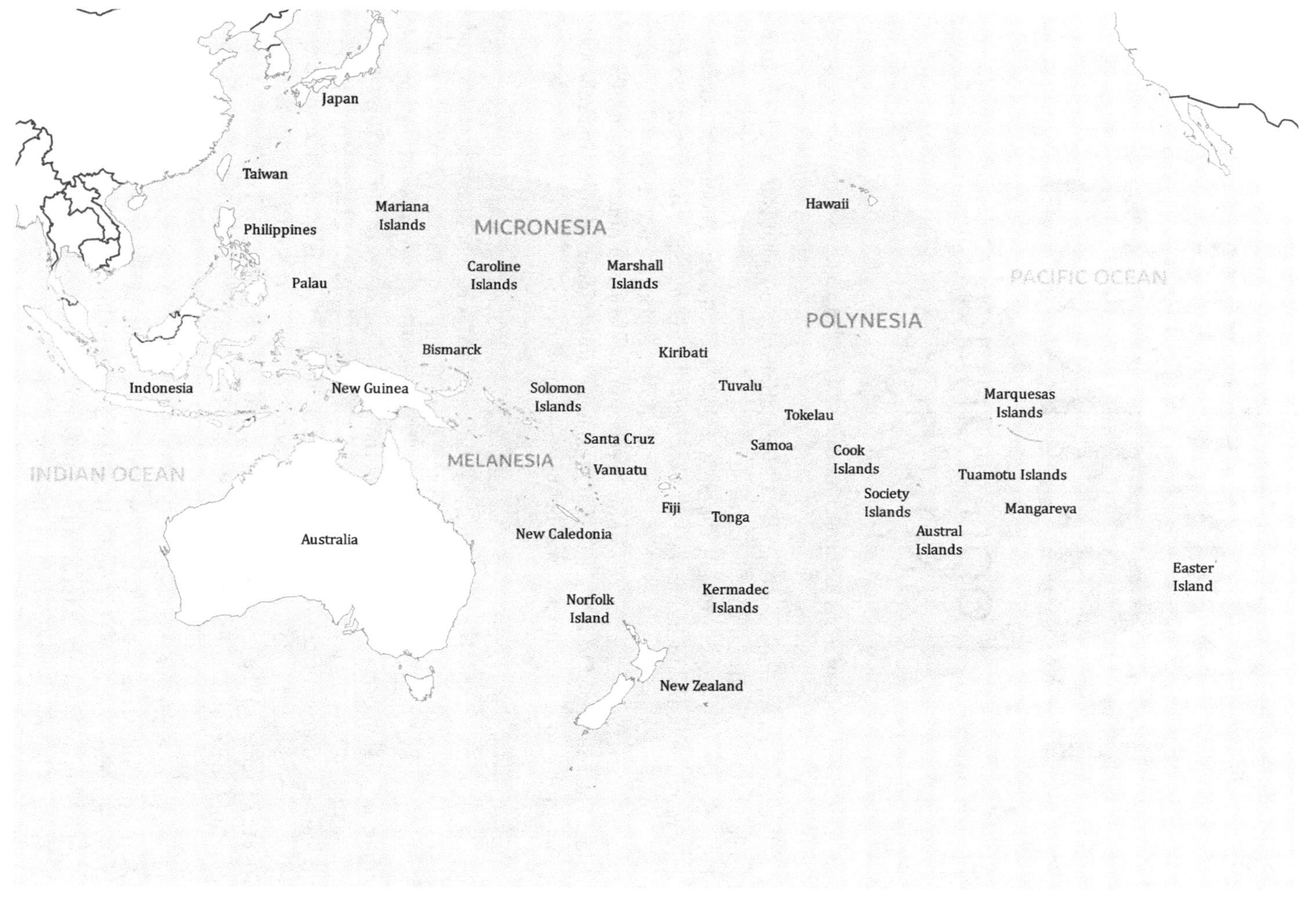

Figure 17.1 A map of the Pacific Ocean shows the Oceania continent with major islands and culture areas highlighted. 'We should not be defined by the smallness of our islands but in the greatness of our oceans. We are the sea, we are the ocean. Oceania is us.' – Hau'ofa et al. (1994)

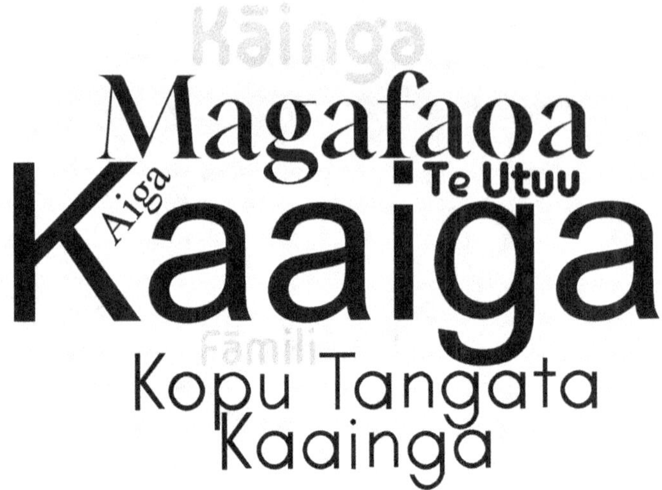

Figure 17.2 Word cloud of terms for family in various Pacific languages

and collective relationships (see Chapter 15 for elaboration on what is meant by culturally responsive and culturally safe practice).

This chapter will briefly present the unique history of Pacific Peoples in Aotearoa and the resulting health inequities faced today. *Talanoa* (discussions) from Pacific occupational therapists are shared to showcase culturally responsive occupational therapy practices, which the reader can reflect on in relation to their own practices with Pacific Peoples. The concept of *vā* is discussed alongside the importance of roles and relationships as critical to the health and wellbeing of Pacific Peoples.

17.1.1 Pacific peoples and Māori

There is shared ancestry between Pacific Peoples and Māori. The wars, protests, and loss of life endured by Māori have inadvertently contributed to Pacific Peoples having a voice in Aotearoa, leading to deep respect for Tangata Whenua (people of the land). A sibling relationship concept known as 'Tuakana-Teina' exists, where the Tuakana (older wiser sibling) provides guidance, support, and knowledge, and the Teina (younger sibling) learns and grows from that relationship. While this term is Māori and more has been written about this concept in Māori contexts, there are similar understandings across the Pacific. In the context of Aotearoa, and the signing of Te Tiriti o Waitangi, Māori hold the Tuakana role and Pacific Peoples the Teina (The Policy Project, 2022).

17.1.2 History of Pacific in Aotearoa

In Aotearoa, following World War II, growth in the manufacturing sector led employers to recruit workers from the Pacific Islands. Pacific families were provided visas and enticed by employment and educational opportunities. The economic downturn in the 1970s led the Labour government to initiate what are now known as the 'Dawn Raids', where Pacific Peoples who had overstayed their visas were targeted for deportation. Raids involved aggressive police actions conducted at dawn, late at night, often without warrants, and involved random entry of homes and workplaces to check documentation before deporting people to their country of origin. Inter-generational trauma from the Dawn Raids resulted in eroded trust and reluctance to engage with government agencies, including health services. In 2021, the Labour government formally apologised for the harm and trauma caused to Pacific Peoples by these events.

Currently, Pacific Peoples make up 9% of Aotearoa's population, expected to rise to 11% by 2043. Two-thirds of this group were born in Aotearoa, and over 40% identify with multiple Pacific ethnicities. The population is predominantly youthful, with a large concentration in Auckland, Wellington, Waikato, and Canterbury. Despite growing numbers, Pacific Peoples remain underrepresented in the health workforce: in occupational therapy, only 95 of 3,555 practitioners identified as Pacific in 2023.

17.1.3 Health inequities

Pacific Peoples in Aotearoa (and Australia) face significant health disparities, with life expectancy being 5.5 years lower than non-Pacific, higher rates of chronic conditions, co-morbidities, mental health issues, and unmet healthcare needs. The ability to self-identify as Pacific based on heritage is crucial for ensuring healthcare services are designed and funded to serve effectively. Key factors impacting timely healthcare access are variable levels of health literacy, relationships with providers, navigation of complex health systems (Neville et al., 2022a), and different views of wellness (Taafaki, 2022). Western healthcare services typically prioritise efficiency over culturally responsive practices, missing the importance of relational approaches central to Pacific customs, such as taking the time to establish trust and including extended family as part of consultations. Subsequently, Pacific Peoples report perceiving the public health system as potentially untrustworthy or threatening (Graham & Masters-Awatere, 2020), and expectations of receiving culturally unsafe care often become reality (Brewer et al., 2024; Sheehy et al., 2025).

Acknowledging this context for practice with Pacific Peoples is important when considering implications of *vā*, roles and relationships, professionalism, and the integration of occupational therapy models in practice, when serving Pacific communities (Brewer et al., 2024; Taafaki, 2022).

17.2 Negotiating spaces and *vā*

Important to most Pacific cultures is the concept of *vā* – 'a space that relates' – contrasting with the common Western notion of space that separates (Mila-Schaaf & Hudson, 2009). In professional relationships, *vā* is central to therapeutic rapport and can help overcome communication and access barriers (Neville et al., 2022b). The phrase 'we don't care what you know, until we know that you care' underscores the importance of taking time to build genuine relationships. When first meeting Pacific Peoples, ethno-specific language and customs should inform protocols for greetings, for example, greeting a Sāmoan client using 'tālofa lava' and removing shoes before entering their home. All Pacific cultures value respect, demonstrated through language use and behaviours such as humility, not speaking out of turn, and knowing one's place and one's role within the family and community (see *Talanoa* 1**).[1] Time must be given to getting to know each other; creating a safe space; finding points of difference and connection; showing interest in the person's life and not just their illness; having significant others present whom the family trust – such as kui (grandparents), head of the family, or ministers – and reinforcing cultural factors as a valuable resource; this is nurturing *vā*. Further theoretical and philosophical descriptions of *vā* are beyond the scope of this chapter.

17.2.1 Vignette 17.1 Talanoa 1

Years of anticipation built pressure on the multi-disciplinary team (MDT) and family to see a client discharged after a five-year admission. As the Pacific occupational therapist, I was asked to facilitate the discharge meeting. Although the client's father had previously agreed to the discharge plan, it became apparent during the meeting he did not agree and articulated this through his friend whom he had brought as his spokesperson*. The sudden agenda change frustrated the MDT, who had put weeks of work into discharge planning. Being Pacific, I realised if the MDT expressed their disappointment, they risked losing the family's trust, which had taken years to build. Reassuring the father that the MDT understood and respected his decision enabled everyone to reach an agreement on how to proceed, and the MDT followed my lead by not addressing the change directly**. Afterwards, I drew from occupational therapy models to shape the language used to explain my Pacific approach to the MDT, which they accepted***. The family remained engaged, and we supported the client to be discharged later on.

17.2.1.1 *The effect of questions on* vā

In Western systems, healthcare practitioners ask questions for clarification, demonstrating engagement in the person's health journey. A questioning approach can be interpreted, in many Pacific cultures, as disrespectful or confrontational. Directly asking questions may convey lack of attentiveness, leading a family to think practitioners do not genuinely care about their situation. However, not asking questions can make it challenging for healthcare practitioners to address issues in real time and may lead to misunderstandings and impact engagement in therapy and timely access to interventions. This could place an unnecessary burden on the family (who take extreme measures to follow healthcare recommendations), disengagement, or discouraging others from engaging with services. Practitioners are encouraged to invite families to tell their story and use less directive questioning to access important information.

Pacific Peoples often view healthcare practitioners as high-ranking figures of authority, knowledge, and power, resulting in a power imbalance. Subsequently, the acceptability of asking questions largely depends on the context and roles of those involved. It is important to be aware that sometimes answers provided may not fully reflect the person's lived experience. For Pacific Peoples, respecting roles is crucial to nurturing *vā*, which presses for expressions of humility and overt acceptance of roles within the collective culture, characterised by duty and obedience. This way of being works well in the context of Pacific cultures and their family networks and must be respected. Practitioners must be mindful for Pacific Peoples seeking healthcare that agreeing with plans and not asking questions of healthcare practitioners is a respectful response that honours the practitioner's status. Encouraging the person to ask questions and offering opportunities for support people to attend meetings as spokespersons means they can ask questions freely on behalf of the healthcare recipient – the spokesperson's indirect role reduces servility (see *Talanoa 1**).

17.3 Significance of roles and relationships

Healthy roles and relationships in Pacific cultures maintain safe spaces where people relate with a strong emphasis on familial ties, community relationships, ethno-specific customs, and social structures. These determine the order of events during formal gatherings, including where people may sit, when they may speak, how much time to allocate, and sometimes what food to take. For example, Sāmoa and Tonga both observe different hierarchical social structures. Involving a cultural advisor to navigate family dynamics may improve engagement with Pacific Peoples. Additionally, thinking of the Pacific person as part of the collective will help identify resources and strengths in the wider family system and influence outcomes, with interdependence given greater priority than independence for many (see *Talanoa* 2).

17.3.1 Vignette 17.2 Talanoa 2

An 11-year-old Tongan autistic boy was part of a large family who lived together in state housing. The main issue identified was school attendance, related to inadequate sleep from excessive device use. After a month of phone calls, spontaneous contact, and scheduled home visits, the child's mother responded to occupational therapy by trialling recommended solutions independent of the practitioner, signalling her readiness to engage. Working with the mother from the outset naturally drew the rest of the family into the plan. The mother felt empowered in her role as a resource for her son. The family collectively worked with the boy to be 'independent' by completing routines 'together' as a family, promoting better sleep and school attendance. This served to strengthen his role and sense of mastery and the roles of others in the family.

17.4 Professionalism when serving Pacific Peoples

Occupational therapy practice seeks to understand what is important to the client and their family, identifying enablers and barriers to participation. Occupational therapy language and concepts can be applied to navigate engagement with Pacific Peoples and their families and to articulate such taken-for-granted or overlooked cultural factors to colleagues (see *Talanoa* 1). Some key challenges to serving Pacific Peoples include managing roles and boundaries. Western cultures lean towards individualism, personal agency, independence, and autonomy. In Pacific cultures, roles are collectively determined in response to life events, such as birth, death, marriage, or sickness. The families occupational therapists serve will usually determine their role with them, informed by their intrinsic cultural knowledge.

Role formation may be influenced by many unspoken factors, such as age, gender, social connections and status, ethno-specific cultural structure, and context (historical, personal, and current). Families may allocate roles they are comfortable with, which can go beyond 'healthcare practitioner' to one of 'sister' or 'uncle' (see *Talanoa* 3). Through a Western lens, taking on a familial role may be perceived as overstepping professional boundaries. However, the role does not include familial duties. Rather, it suggests how formal to be and how to address family members and serves as a reference guide for how to nurture *vā* between family and practitioner.

When it comes to managing boundaries, offerings are an important practice in Pacific cultures and may include practitioners providing light refreshments during meetings or home visits, setting the scene for (verbal) sharing to take place (i.e. *talanoa*) and encouraging a warm and supportive environment. Furthermore, families offering gifts to demonstrate their appreciation for the healthcare received uplifts their esteem – to refuse could be perceived as disrespectful. Both practices of providing and accepting offerings can go against Western service policies and require careful negotiation to ensure practice remains culturally responsive and safe.

17.4.1 Vignette 17.3 Talanoa 3

Working with a young Sāmoan man, I found out I was the age of his younger sister, which led him to treat me with respect and transparency. He would call me 'sis' and I would call him 'bro'. I was considered a daughter in his family, so I showed respect by acknowledging his parents before him whenever they were in the same room as us.

17.4.1.1 Pacific workforce

For Pacific occupational therapists, practice is enhanced by nurturing the relationship with the family as a priority, and ensuring delivery of care is informed by Pacific values (see *Talanoa* 1). When seeking support from non-Pacific supervisors, the complex challenges faced by many Pacific Peoples can create a level of shock that overshadows problem-solving during supervision. Pacific practitioners thrive when there is a protected space that fosters opportunities for cultural supervision, Pacific networking, and *talanoa* in the workplace, a space where issues can be discussed without overwhelm, focusing on alternative solutions, in a context of cultural and emotional support to manage practice issues, difference, and racism.

Being part of a collective, Pacific Peoples typically see the value of their abilities if they are also seen as valuable by the collective. Subsequently, Pacific occupational therapists may not put themselves forward for career opportunities unless someone else notices or mentors and suggests they step up. Those in leadership roles have often been called forward and mentored by a Pacific peer, an acceptable cultural practice given the centrality of the *vā* as a place for Tuakana-Teina relationships.

17.5 Occupational therapy and pacific models

Occupational therapy models can provide structure for conveying clinical information in a meaningful way (see *Talanoa* 1***). Pacific cultures strongly value collectivism, so occupational therapy models can reflect this by framing individual factors as representing people, families, or communities etc. Knowledge of Pacific models of health, such as the Fonofale Model (Pulotu-Endermann, 2021), Te Vaka Atafaga (Kupa Kupa, 2009), and the Fonua Ola Model (Tu'itahi, cited in (Talemaitoga, 2010), guide occupational therapists to emphasise the relational and holistic aspects of health, addressing the unique needs of Pacific families. It is important to identify when there is a mismatch between Western-developed tools and Pacific values and ways of doing and being (see *Talanoa* 4). Pacific ways may look different to Western ways yet be equally effective, safe, and successful. Occupational therapists must recognise different ways of participating so they can identify limitations in our assessments and expose the implications of applying assessment criteria too rigorously.

17.5.1 Vignette 17.4 Talanoa 4

A functional assessment was undertaken with an elder Pacific woman who selected the task of mopping the floor for task analysis to determine whether she could continue to live alone. She was confident in her ability to complete the task, using rags to scrub the floor on her hands and knees, a process she had used for more than 50 years. As soon as it became evident, she could perform the task, I stepped in to finish the task for her – from my cultural lens it was inappropriate for me, as a younger person, to stand watching, without contributing, whilst the elder woman undertook household chores.

17.6 Conclusion

It is crucial to integrate Pacific cultural understanding into occupational therapy for Pacific Peoples, to reduce health inequities. The collectivist nature of Pacific cultures requires a nuanced approach that respects the concept of *vā* (relational space) and extends roles beyond Western social structures and clinical boundaries. Pacific models and occupational therapy frameworks can assist in navigating these complexities. Ultimately, culturally responsive occupational therapy enhances the therapeutic process and promotes the wellbeing of Pacific families and communities. We conclude with a Sāmoan saying that translates as giving thanks for the opportunity to discuss this important topic.

Fa'afetai mo lenei avanoa e talanoaina ai se mataupu taua.

17.7 Summary

- Pacific Peoples have a unique history in Aotearoa that contributed to health inequities
- *Talanoa* are used to showcase culturally responsive occupational therapy practices when working with Pacific Peoples
- Nurturing *vā* – the space that relates – involves demonstrating key Pacific values like integrity, humility, respect, and reciprocity
- Roles and relationships are critical to the health and wellbeing of Pacific Peoples
- Western practices may require adaptation to be culturally responsive and safe and meet the needs of Pacific Peoples

17.8 Review and reflection questions

- What historical and socioeconomic factors contribute to health inequities experienced by Pacific Peoples in Aotearoa, and how does this impact engagement with the healthcare system?
- How is *vā* defined, and what specific examples are provided to illustrate its significance in the roles and relationships relevant to providing occupational therapy to Pacific Peoples?
- What adaptations to practice are suggested to ensure occupational therapy practice reflects Pacific values and ways of doing?
- What would you consider when working with someone from a Pacific culture that is unfamiliar to you?
- How might you reconcile the advocacy role for Pacific Peoples with the need to maintain professional boundaries and avoid imposing your own values and beliefs?

Acknowledgements

Thank you to our families who have supported us to have space to write this chapter. We would like to thank those in the Pacific community who have advised on or shaped the thinking and the words in this chapter; in particular, we would like to acknowledge Dr Carolyn Simmons, Tangi Poko, Brigitta Samuela, Lucy Charles, and Arul Hamill.

Note

1 Asterisks indicate which part of the *Talanoa* is most relevant to each part of the text.

References

Brewer, K. M., Taueetia-Su'a, T., Hanchard, S., Vaka, S., Ameratunga, S., Tane, T., Newport, R., Selak, V., Grey, C., & Harwood, M. (2024). Māori and Pacific families' experiences and perspectives of cardiovascular care; A qualitative study. *Australian and New Zealand Journal of Public Health*, 48(3), 100149. https://doi.org/10.1016/j.anzjph.2024.100149

Graham, R., & Masters-Awatere, B. (2020). Experiences of Māori of Aotearoa New Zealand's public health system: A systematic review of two decades of published qualitative research. *Australian and New Zealand Journal of Public Health*, 44(3), 193–200. https://doi.org/10.1111/1753-6405.12971

Hau'ofa, E., Naidu, V., & Waddell, E. (1994). The contemporary Pacific. In *A new Oceania: Rediscovering our sea of islands* (Vol. 6, No. 1, pp. 147–161). School of Social and Economic Development, The University of the South Pacific. https://scholarspace.manoa.hawaii.edu/server/api/core/bitstreams/77265cd6-ddfd-469d-a96b-04ace31ea67c/content

Kupa Kupa. (2009). Te vaka afaga: A Tokelau assessment model for supporting holistic mental health practice with Tokelau people in Aotearoa. *Pacific Health Dialog*, 15(1), 156–163. https://www.abuseincare.org.nz/__data/assets/pdf_file/0024/28581/kupa-k-te-vaka-atafaga-a-tokelau-assessment-model-for-supporting-holistic-mental-health-practice-with-tokelau-people-in-aotearoa-new-zealand-pacific-health-dialog-151-2009.pdf

Mila-Schaaf, K., & Hudson, M. (2009). The interface between cultural understandings: Negotiating new spaces for Pacific mental health. *Pacific Health Dialog*, 15(1), 113–119. https://pubmed.ncbi.nlm.nih.gov/19585741/

Neville, S., Wrapson, W., Savila, F., Napier, S., Paterson, J., Dewes, O., Soon, H. N. W., & Tautolo, E. S. (2022a). Barriers to older Pacific peoples' participation in the health-care system in Aotearoa New Zealand. *Journal of Primary Health Care*, 14(2), 124–129. https://doi.org/10.1071/HC21146

Neville, S., Wrapson, W., Savila, F., Napier, S., Paterson, J., Dewes, O., Soon, H. N. W., & Tautolo, E. S. (2022b). Barriers to older Pacific peoples' participation in the health-care system in Aotearoa New Zealand. *Journal of Primary Health Care*, 14(2), 124–129. https://doi.org/10.1071/HC21146

The Policy Project. (2022). *YAVU – Foundations of Pacific engagement*. https://www.mpp.govt.nz/publications-resources/resources/yavu/

Pulotu-Endermann, F. K. (2021). *Fonofale model: Pacific health and wellbeing*. https://www.mpp.govt.nz/assets/Resources/Pacific-Wellbeing-Strategy/Fonofale-presentation-to-Pacific-Wellbeing-Talanoa-May-2021.pdf

Sheehy, B., Wepa, D., & Collis, J. M. (2025). Māori experiences of physical rehabilitation in Aotearoa New Zealand: A scoping review. *Disability and Rehabilitation*, 47(6), 1342–1352. https://doi.org/10.1080/09638288.2024.2374494

Taafaki, J. (2022). *The lived experiences of rural Tuvaluans navigating the Aotearoa New Zealand healthcare system*. University of Otago.

Talemaitoga, A. (2010). The health of Pacific Peoples in Aotearoa is 'everybody's business.' *Best Practice Journal*, 32, 5–9. www.bpac.org.nz

Vaioleti, T. M. (2016). Talanoa research methodology: A developing position on Pacific research. *Waikato Journal of Education*, 12(1), 21–34. https://doi.org/10.15663/wje.v12i1.296

Academic education of occupational therapists in Australia

Carol McKinstry, Lynne Adamson, Tracy Fortune, and Samantha Ashby

Authors' positionality statement

This chapter is authored by four academics of white settler backgrounds. We acknowledge that the cultural, historical, and social contexts in which we have lived shape our perspective of the world, as have our experiences as practitioners and academics. We are aware of the social and institutional privileges linked to our racial and cultural identities, and we have endeavoured to address any biases that may influence our writing based on these privileges.

We are committed to critically reflecting on our positionality and the influences on our work. In this chapter we have aimed to include a range of views related to academic education of occupational therapists in Australia. In particular we have aimed to address some historical factors that influence occupational therapy education and to develop future-looking perspectives that prioritise cultural safety and indigenous knowledge that are essential for contemporary occupational therapy practice.

Key terms
- Education
- Accreditation
- Professional identity
- Competency

Objectives
Upon completion of this chapter, readers will be able to:

- Relate the history and scope of occupational therapy education in Australia
- Describe the standards set for accreditation of educational programmes and the commitment of occupational therapy education programmes to develop culturally safe practitioners, to understand Indigenous knowledge related to practice, to

DOI: 10.4324/9781003495666-20

> address racism, and to ensure the involvement of Aboriginal and Torres Strait Islander people in design and implementation of learning opportunities
>
> ■ Highlight the importance of professional identify and the development of knowledge and skills to bridge the education to practice nexus
>
> ■ Discuss contemporary issues impacting occupational therapy education in the context of higher education in Australia

18.1 History and scope of occupational therapy education in Australia

Occupational therapy education commenced during World War II, when the need for rehabilitation of injured soldiers created a demand for the emerging profession of occupational therapy (Anderson & Bell, 1988). The value of occupational therapy had already been identified in other countries and Australian military senior personnel recognised the lack of such expertise within their ranks. Significantly, they determined that therapists working with injured soldiers should be qualified. A small number of occupational therapists, trained in the United States or Great Britain were working in Australia at the time, but the urgent need identified within military medical services meant that a training programme was required. In 1942, the first occupational therapy training programme in Australia was established in New South Wales. In 1947, a second training programme opened in Victoria (Anderson & Bell, 1988). Other states followed, with programmes in occupational therapy established in Queensland in 1950, Western Australia in 1960 and a decade later in South Australia. There are now over 35 programmes in Australia. A course commenced in Northern Territory in 2021, and the first programme in Tasmania started in 2025. Now every state and territory in Australia has at least one entry to practice occupational therapy university.

For the early training programmes or courses, a diploma level qualification was awarded after two and a half years of study. All occupational therapy curricula at the time included studies in psychiatry, psychology, anatomy, physiology, medical and surgical conditions, occupational therapy, and clinical practice. Also included were skills in arts and crafts, for example, weaving, pottery, and woodwork. The length of courses soon increased to three years; then by the early 1970s all occupational therapy entry level educational programmes in Australia changed to three and a half or four-year baccalaureate level degrees. These changes reflected a move from 'training' to 'education' in the approach to qualification of occupational therapists.

The evolution of occupational therapy education in Australia reflected changes that were occurring within the profession internationally. Coulthard (2002) argued that this was necessary because the environments in which occupational therapists were required to work were more demanding, practice decisions had to be supported by evidence and occupational therapists were required to work independently. By the beginning of the 21st century, entry-level qualifications in the United States and Canada were raised to master's level and subsequently to clinical doctorate level in some courses in the United States. Some Australian universities developed graduate-entry master's degree (GEM), as well as maintaining a bachelor's degree qualification, therefore giving prospective students greater choice to the pathway for gaining a qualification in occupational therapy.

Student occupational therapists today have a range of course choices, including location of the university, level of qualification, and the number of years they are required to study for completion of their course. Regardless of these options, all occupational therapy graduates share a common knowledge base and adhere to strict standards of practice. Occupational therapy programmes are required to be accredited by the Occupational Therapy Council of Australia Limited (OTC) and approved by the Occupational Therapy Board of Australia (OTBA), as discussed later in this chapter and in Chapter 6. All programmes are also impacted by the factors influencing universities and the context in which students participate in higher education, as will now be discussed.

18.2 Australian higher education sector

The Australian higher education sector has been undergoing significant change for over a decade. The implementation of the Bradley Review of Australian Higher Education (Bradley et al., 2008) recommendations essentially deregulated the sector by removing the caps on the number of university places subsidised by the Commonwealth government to significantly increase participation rates. There has also been an increase in the number of post graduate entry master's courses on offer. The recommendations of the recent Australian University Accord Final Report (O'Kane et al., 2024) propose significant policy reforms to increase tertiary education participation rates, particularly for equity student groups such as those living in rural areas, those from low socio-economic status, and those living with a disability. With the current health workforce shortages, including in occupational therapy, increased tertiary education enrolments in health are anticipated. Strategies such as university preparation pathways and articulations with the vocational education sector will be promoted. In recognition of 'placement poverty' associated with increased financial pressure on students while on placement, there is hope that financial support as is available to nursing and social work students through the Commonwealth Prac Payment from 2025 will be extended to other health students in coming years (O'Kane et al., 2024).

With the COVID pandemic prompting most universities to move to online learning during 2020–2021 so students could progress and graduate, there has been a shift in how higher education courses are now delivered. An increased recognition that students need to balance study with other aspects of their lives including paid work and caring responsibilities underlies a need for greater flexibility in modes of teaching and learning. Increasingly course content is accessed in 'hybrid' manners with online content such as pre-recorded lectures and on-campus classes for students to learn technical or practice related skills such as assessments or interventions (Wang et al., 2024).

The other major challenge and opportunity since the pandemic has been the increased and potential use of generative artificial intelligence in learning, teaching, and research and implications for clinical practice. Ethical use of artificial intelligence within higher education is being embraced by universities however academic integrity needs to be upheld and mechanisms to ensure that graduate competencies are met. Students may also be using generative artificial intelligence on placement where appropriate and ethical. The Australian Tertiary Education Quality and Standards Agency (TEQSA) in conjunction with universities have developed a range of resources to guide both teachers and researchers (https://www.teqsa.gov.au/guides-resources/higher-education-good-practice-hub/artificial-intelligence). Currently this is a rapidly developing area that will continue to impact students, teachers and practitioners.

18.3 Regulation of Australian occupational therapy education

While academic programmes in Australia develop their own perspectives and focus on areas of interest and expertise, all programmes leading to an entry-level qualification in occupational therapy must be accredited by the OTC and approved as a programme of study by the OTBA. Read Chapter 6 for more information about the role of OTC and OTBA.

The requirement to be accredited by OTC and approved by OTBA means that each programme is assessed against criteria, as set out in the *Accreditation Standards for Entry Level Occupational Therapy Education Programs* (OTC, 2018). These standards set out mandatory requirements for entry level occupational therapy education and are aligned with the *Australian Occupational Therapy Competency Standards* set by OTBA and the international requirements of the World Federation of Occupational Therapists (WFOT), as outlined in Chapter 6.

The WFOT Revised Minimum Standards the Education of Occupational Therapists came into effect in January 2020, and every occupational therapy programme must demonstrate adherence to these standards across five domains:

- public safety,
- academic governance and quality assurance,
- programme of study,
- the student experience, and
- assessment.

A comprehensive assessment process seeks evidence for each domain, including input from universities, academics, students, occupational therapy practitioners, and clients of occupational therapy services.

18.4 Commitment to cultural safety and Aboriginal and Torres Strait Islander knowledge

The occupational therapy profession is committed to active participation in addressing the impact of colonisation on the health of Aboriginal and Torres Strait Islander people. Education programmes are key to ensuring culturally safe and responsive occupational therapy practice. In Chapter 14 you read about the importance of decolonising occupational therapy through a strength-based framework. The OTC has developed a specific occupational therapy approach to the *Aboriginal and Torres Strait Islander Health Curriculum Framework (Commonwealth of Australia, 2014)*. Education programmes are required to demonstrate how they implement strategies to address the two key priorities to:

1. Ensure genuine and reciprocal partnerships exist with a variety of Aboriginal and Torres Strait Islander stakeholders who influence the way things are done, and
2. Ensure best practice principles regarding developing, teaching, and evaluating Aboriginal and Torres Strait Islander curricula are implemented (OTC, 2023).

18.5 Graduating *entry-to-practice* occupational therapists in Australia: Bridging the education–practice nexus

Occupational therapy has been described as both art and science (Peloquin, 1994; Wood, 1995; Zemke, 2004). Occupational therapy graduates must 'know that' and 'know how' (Tal-Saban et al., 2026) in equal measure. Exactly what students are required to learn, what they must demonstrate competence to 'do', shifts in response to a dynamic interplay of historical, social, political, and geographic factors influencing health priorities, service systems, and entities that govern and guide education and practice direction. Occupational therapy is not focussed on any one health issue, as might be argued for professions such as (for example) podiatry, prosthetics, physiotherapy, or psychology. Occupational therapy education must, by necessity, prepare graduates to work across the lifespan, across multiple service systems, and in all phases of the treatment–prevention spectrum. Professional education or fieldwork must traverse knowledge and skills to inform a graduate's beginning practice with people and settings as diverse as school children living with a physical disability; adults hospitalised due to mental illness, and older adults striving to live well in a residential aged care setting to incarcerated adults living with an acquired brain injury.

The knowledge, or the ability to generate and use knowledge, and deploy the practice behaviours required is potentially *unlimited*. A 'stuffed curriculum' is a risk that needs constant managing, particularly as educators juggle decisions about what is fundamental and enduring versus what is extracurricular (Cousin, 2006). The profession's *focus of curricula* is on understanding and enabling participation in occupation.

The curricula of entry-level occupational therapy programme prepare graduates for all areas of practice. Thus, while programmes focus on occupational therapy and occupational science concepts, they also include foundational knowledge from a broad range of disciplines. This knowledge enables occupational therapists to underpin community-based practice with understandings of public health and health promotion. In addition, enhancing occupational participation requires an understanding of a person's diagnosis and its associated clinical features. In turn, this is underpinned by biomedical knowledge including anatomy, physiology, and pharmacology. This is also underpinned by the application of developmental psychology to ensure life span demands inform practice. This is particularly important in paediatric practice, where foundational knowledge of typical development is fundamental to assessment and programme planning.

18.6 Current challenges and opportunities for occupational therapy education

The Australian and New Zealand Council of Occupational Therapy Educators (ANZCOTE) provides the opportunity for heads of programme from each university offering occupational therapy courses to come together annually and consider issues relating to the education of occupational therapy students and research. Practice and workforce issues are discussed in collaboration with Occupational Therapy Australia and the Occupational Therapy Board of Australia. Course accreditation by Occupational Therapy Council of Australia Limited is often a topic of discussion. The Australian and New Zealand Occupational Therapy Practice Education Academics (ANZOTPEA) group also meet annually to consider issues relating to fieldwork or work integrated learning. Given the increased number of new education programmes and student enrolments, there is more collaboration between universities to identify innovative placements, supervision models, and the use of simulation.

18.7 Learning and teaching approaches

Case- or scenario-based learning is a longstanding and widely used teaching and learning approach in occupational therapy entry-level education. Case-based learning reflects the diversity of occupational therapy practice and range of practice contexts. Working on case-based scenarios enhances opportunities to learn how and where to seek information and how to apply complex occupation-focused practice models to enhance interventions (Roberts et al., 2020). In addition, scenarios reinforce the profession's domains and enhance professional reasoning and professional identity. The intention of experiential learning and the practicing of skills is that they are then applied during practice-education opportunities. Case-based learning can also incorporate interprofessional simulations where students from a range of disciplines learn how to work together on cases. This reflects real-world scenarios where health care professionals are required to work as a team to enhance client outcomes. Interprofessional working and the need for role definition is one means of reinforcing professional identity (Walder et al., 2021).

Australian programmes can include up to 200 hours of case-based simulation to meet the World Federation of Occupational Therapists requirement for 1000 hours of practice education (Occupational Therapy Council (Australia & New Zealand), 2013). The range of simulation activities accepted by the Occupational Therapy Council for accredited programmes within Australia includes simulation activities involving high fidelity and case-based or real-world practice scenarios which provide students with opportunities to apply their acquired theoretical knowledge and demonstrate their practical skills, allowing them to practice the decision-making required for practice. Evidence for the use of simulation within occupational therapy programmes was supported by the findings of a randomised control trial, indicating that a two-week simulation early in the programme could develop similar skills to a two-week placement (Imms et al., 2018).

18.8 Professional practice and identity

Across the health professions, professional identity includes 'the recognition of beliefs, attitudes, values, knowledge, skills and understanding of the role, within the context of the professional group to which you belong' (Adams et al., 2006, p. 56). The development of professional identity is a dynamic process shaped by multiple factors, which include entry-level curricula content and pre-programme experiences of occupational therapy, which often influence a person's decision to enrol in a particular programme (Ashby et al., 2016). Thus, the development of case-based scenarios and other teaching strategies which develop professional identity during entry-level programmes is a key step for educators because it contributes to a successful transition from study into the workforce (Walder et al., 2021).

This is necessary because like other healthcare professions, occupational therapists face workplace challenges that place them at high risk of job-related stress and professional burnout. In turn, the development and maintenance of professional identity can act as a protective factor that sustains professional resilience and career longevity, because it allows practitioners to combat issues such as role blurring and difficulties in enacting occupation-based practices. In addition, professional identity can strengthen practitioners resolve to advocate for occupation-based practices in workplaces where the role of occupational therapy and an occupational perspective of health and wellbeing may not be well understood or validated (Ashby et al., 2015).

The use of case scenarios and embedded practice education teach student-practitioners how to use professional language unique to occupational therapy, which is another important aspect and facilitator of professional identity (Walder et al., 2021). Indeed, Ashby et al. (2016) identified that student-practitioners place value on the occupational content of the curricula and recognise the role of occupation-focused models and occupational science. However, student-practitioners considered practice education and professional socialisation the most significant programme factors that influenced their professional identity development. This reinforces the importance of practice education, which provides opportunities to observe and enact occupation-based practice.

18.9 Postgraduate and research education opportunities

As a registered health profession, there are annual continuing professional requirements to maintain registration for Australian occupational therapists. Currently registered occupational therapists are required to undertake a minimum of 20 hours over a range of continuing professional development activities that build on existing knowledge, aim to improve outcomes for patients, and are evidence based. Activities can include attending seminars and conferences, reading journal articles, practice observation, reflection, and undertaking a higher education course.

Australian occupational therapists are required to have a minimum of a four-year bachelor degree (Australian Qualifications Framework [AQF] Level 8) or graduate entry master's (AQF 9). The bachelor's degree may include an embedded individual research honours project or a group project. Individual research honours are a pathway to entry into a Doctor of Philosophy (PhD) (AQF10). If a therapist has not undertaken research honours, they can undertake a research-based masters, sometimes called a Master of Philosophy, which is usually two years full-time or four years part-time and may include some coursework subjects or units to increase research knowledge and skills. Practitioners or clinicians with practice experience of over five years but without a research Honours or Master of Research can apply to undertake a professional doctorate, which also requires coursework subjects or units to upskill the therapist sufficiently to undertake an independent research project.

Most universities offering undergraduate or graduate-entry Master of Occupational Therapy Practice also offer Masters of Research and doctoral programmes (PhD or professional doctorates). Some universities also have postgraduate courses such as a Master of Advanced Occupational Therapy Practice, which extends knowledge and allows specialisation in areas such as public health, leadership, and management and health systems. They may also undertake tertiary education in related areas such as a Master of Public Health, Master of Health Science, or a Master of Business Administration. Some universities also offer driver assessment and rehabilitation courses that are two-week equivalents and have a minimum practice experience requirement.

18.10 Conclusion

Australia has high-quality occupational therapy education programmes that utilise contemporary learning and teaching approaches, including case- or scenario-based, simulation, and experiential learning. Universities offer both bachelor and graduate entry master programmes that are accredited by the Occupational Therapy Council of Australia and meet the Australian Occupational Therapy Competency Standards. These programmes also meet the WFOT Revised Minimum Standards for the Education of Occupational Therapists, enabling Australian graduates to be eligible to work in other countries.

18.11 Summary

- Australian occupational therapy education commenced in 1942 in response to the need for occupational therapists after World War II. Initially programmes were diploma level and then became degrees at a bachelor level in the 1970s.
- Today the Occupational Therapy Council of Australia accredits four-year bachelor degrees and two-year graduate-entry master's. Programs are increasingly delivered in more flexible hybrid ways and can use simulation to prepare students for placement and substitute for up to 200 hours of the 1000 hours of placement required by the OTC and WFOT.
- Every programme is assessed against the Australian Occupational Therapy Competency Standards. They also need to ensure that genuine and reciprocal partnerships exist with a variety of Aboriginal and Torres Strait Islander stakeholders who influence the way things are done and ensure best practice principles regarding developing, teaching, and evaluating Aboriginal and Torres Strait Islander curricula are implemented.
- Programs also need to prepare graduates to work across the lifespan, across multiple service systems, and in all phases of service delivery, recognising that occupational therapy is both an art and a science.
- Occupational therapy education programmes mostly utilise case- or scenario-based learning, applying complex occupation-focused practice models and experiential learning during placements.
- The development of professional identity is an important feature of programmes that is fostered through case-based scenarios and helps protect students and graduates against the challenges of job-related stress and professional burnout.
- There is also an increasing emphasis on interprofessional education to ensure students and graduates can work effectively in teams.
- As registered health professionals, Australian occupational therapists are required to continue learning through undertaking at least 20 hours annually, and this continuing professional development may also include postgraduate study such as research master or doctoral degrees.

18.12 Review questions

- Describe the roles of the key organisations involved in the regulation of Australian occupational therapy education.
- What are the current challenges facing occupational therapy education in Australia?
- What teaching and learning approaches are appropriate for occupational therapy education?

- What postgraduate opportunities exist for Australian occupational therapists?
- How many placement hours are required by OTC and the WFOT?

References

Adams, K., Hean, S., Sturgis, P., & Clark, J. (2006). Investigating the factors influencing professional identity of first-year health and social care students. *Learning in Health and Social Care, 5*, 55–68.

Anderson, B., & Bell, J. (1988). *Occupational therapy: Its place in Australia's history.* Association of Occupational Therapists.

Ashby, S. E., Adler, J., & Herbert, L. (2016). An exploratory international study into occupational therapy students' perceptions of professional identity. *Australian Occupational Therapy Journal, 63*(4), 233–243.

Ashby, S. E., Gray, M., Ryan, S., & James, C. L. (2015). Maintaining occupation based practice in Australian mental health services: A critical stance. *British Journal of Occupational Therapy, 78*(7), 431–439. https://doi.org/10.1177/0308022614564168

Bradley, D., et al. (2008). *Review of Australian higher education. Final report.* www.deewr.gov.au/he_review_finalreport

Brandt, S. (2021). Ryle on knowing how: Some clarifications and corrections. *European Journal of Philosophy, 29*(1), 152–167.

Commonwealth of Australia. (2014). *Aboriginal and Torres Strait Islander health curriculum framework.* https://www.health.gov.au/sites/default/files/documents/2020/12/aboriginal-and-torresstrait-islander-health-curriculum-framework.pdf

Coulthard, M. (2002). Preparing occupational therapists for practice today and into the future. *Canadian Journal of Occupational Therapy, 69*(5), 253–260. https://journals.sagepub.com/doi/10.1177/000841740206900501

Cousin, G. (2006). An introduction to threshold concepts. *Planet, 17*(1), 4–5.

Imms, C., Froude, E., Chu, E. M. Y., Sheppard, L., Darzins, S., Guinea, S., . . . & Mathieu, E. (2018). Simulated versus traditional occupational therapy placements: A randomised controlled trial. *Australian Occupational Therapy Journal, 65*(6), 556–564.

Occupational Therapy Council (Australia & New Zealand). (2013). *Occupational Therapy Council accreditation standards: Explanatory guide: Use of simulation in practice education/fieldwork.*

Occupational Therapy Council (Australia & New Zealand). (2018). *Accreditation standards for entry level occupational therapy education programs.*

Occupational Therapy Council of Australia Ltd. (2023). *Aboriginal and Torres Strait Islander health curriculum implementation project – Occupational Therapy program accreditation.* https://www.otcouncil.com.au/wp-content/uploads/OTC-Aboriginal-and-Torres-Strait-Islander-Health-Curriculum-Implementation-Project-2023.1.pdf

O'Kane, M., Behrendt, L., Glover, B., Macklin, J., Nash, F., Rimmer, B., & Wikramanayake, S. (2024). *Australian universities accord.* https://www.education.gov.au/australian-universities-accord/accord-final-report

Peloquin, S. M. (1994). Occupational therapy as art and science: Should the older definition be reclaimed? *American Journal of Occupational Therapy, 48*(11), 1093–1096. https://doi.org/10.5014/ajot.48.11.1093

Roberts, M., Hooper, B., & Molineux, M. (2020). Occupational therapy entry-level education scholarships in Australia from 2000 to 2019: A systematic mapping review. *Australian Occupational Therapy Journal, 67*(4), 373–395. https://doi.org/10.1111/1440-1630.12661

Tal-Saban, M., Zaguri-Vittenberg, S., & Weintraub, N. (2024). Enhancing professional identity of first-year occupational therapy students with the community-academia student tutoring program. *British Journal of Occupational Therapy, 87*(2), 106–113. https://doi.org/10.1177/03080226231198341

Walder, K., Bissett, M., Molineux, M., & Whiteford, G. (2021). Understanding professional identity in occupational therapy: A scoping review. *Scandinavian Journal of Occupational Therapy*, 1–23. https://doi.org/10.1080/11038128.2021.1974548

Wang, X., Liu, J., Jia, S., Hou, C., Jiao, R., Yan, Y., Ma, T., Zhang, Y., Liu, Y., Wen, H., Wang, Y. F., Zhu, H., & Liu, X. Y. (2024). Hybrid teaching after COVID-19: Advantages, challenges and optimization strategies. *BMC Medical Education*, 24(1), 753. https://doi.org/10.1186/s12909-024-05745-z

Wood, W. (1995). Weaving the warp and weft of occupational therapy: An art and science for all times. *American Journal of Occupational Therapy*, 49(1), 44–52. https://doi.org/10.5014/ajot.49.1.44

Zemke, R. (2004). Time, space, and the kaleidoscopes of occupation. *American Journal of Occupational Therapy*, 58(6), 608–620. https://doi.org/10.5014/ajot.58.6.608

CHAPTER 19

Practice education of occupational therapists in Australia

Mong-Lin Yu, Anne-Maree Caine, Thomas Bevitt, and Emma Clark

Authors' positionality statement

This position statement sets out the chapter authors' collective commitment to contributing to quality, inclusive, and equitable practice education in the occupational therapy profession. The authors are academic occupational therapists teaching at (Australian) universities on the lands of Traditional Owners. All of us have extensive involvement and leadership in occupational therapy practice education design, development, delivery, and coordination. We value the significance of inclusive quality practice education in the occupational therapy profession in its development as well as in the current and future health workforce. We understand the complexity of effective practice education learning, necessitating high-level collaborative engagement and interaction among multiple collaborators who take on different responsibilities. Our (inclusive and diverse) author team is formed by members from White Australian-born settlers and Asian immigrant backgrounds working in occupational therapy programmes at four universities having campuses in metropolitan, regional, and rural areas across three different Australian states (Queensland, Australian Capital Territory, and Victoria). Each of our university courses has different distributions of domestic and international student enrolment. This brings us various experiences working with students from a range of ethnic, cultural, educational, and socioeconomic status backgrounds to contribute to this chapter (and advocate for equality and fairness in practice education).

Key terms
- Practice education
- Practice placement
- Quality
- Supervision
- Evaluation
- Roles and responsibilities

DOI: 10.4324/9781003495666-21

Objectives
This chapter will allow the reader to:

- Describe the professional standards and guidelines governing occupational therapy practice education in Australia
- Understand the contemporary context of practice education in Australia
- Explain the roles and relationships between multiple collaborators involved in practice education within Australian context
- Discuss the range of practice education forms used in Australia to assist students develop the knowledge, skills, attitudes, and behaviours necessary for professional practice
- Identify various supervision and evaluation approaches used in practice education

19.1 Introduction

Practice education is central to occupational therapy education allowing students to integrate and further develop professional knowledge, skills, and behaviours for practice. This chapter will cover key elements in occupational therapy practice education in Australia. The guidelines, contemporary context, and forms of practice education will be described. Quality practice education, relevant professional groups, multiple collaborators involved, and evaluation of student practice education performance will also be discussed. Finally, this chapter will discuss a future consideration for practice education in Australia.

19.2 Occupational therapy practice education in Australia

Practice education is compulsory and integrated into the occupational therapy curriculum at every year level, with a strong emphasis on scaffolding students' competency development (World Federation of Occupational Therapy [WFOT], 2016). Practice education is the umbrella term for several curriculum activities where a student implements part or the whole occupational therapy practice process with a person or persons. Practice education includes activities such as simulations, scenario based or problem-based learning, community engagement experiences as well as practice placements (Gustafsson et al., 2017; Occupational Therapy Council of Australia (OTCA), 2024). Practice education activities can take place in classrooms, at student-led clinics, and with external service providers.

Since the 1990s, the number of occupational therapy programmes and student enrolments in Australia has grown significantly, with universities expanding across metropolitan and rural areas. In 1991, only five bachelor-level programmes existed, whereas by 2024, 26 universities offered 52 occupational therapy programmes nationwide. This growth has increased the demand for practice education opportunities. Historically, practice education was seen as limited to clinical primary health settings, but it now placements spans both university-based and industry-based environments representative of the diversity of practice settings. Classroom-based education builds foundational skills in a structured setting, while industry-based placements provide immersive learning in diverse practice contexts, preparing students for safe and effective practice with individuals, groups, organisations, and communities, thereby achieving safe and appropriate practice.

19.3 What informs practice education in Australia?

To become an accredited occupational therapist, students in entry level educational programmes are required to complete a minimum of 1000 hours of practice education (WFOT, 2016). Practice education activities are distributed in every year of the curriculum, to assist students with integrating knowledge and skills in an applied practice context. Australian course accreditation standards permit 200 hours of practice education to be accounted for by simulated learning activities and community engagement experiences (OTCA, 2024).

Students are required to experience a variety of placement opportunities with a range of people who have different occupational needs and in different contexts, including approaches with individuals, communities/groups, and populations and people of different ages, gender and ethnicity, health conditions, and delivery settings. Both the Australian accreditation standards (Occupational Therapy Board of Australia [OTBA], 2018) and the World Federation of Occupational Therapy Revised Minimum Standards the Education of Occupational Therapists (WFOT, 2016) specify that placements need to be reflective and responsive to local professional context and practices to assist students in being prepared for local practice. Additionally, both accreditation standards also emphasise that practice is more than at the level of individuals or groups and should include working at societal levels in the areas of health promotion and community development. Practice education provides opportunities for students to integrate knowledge, professional reasoning, and professional behaviours within practice to the level of competence required as outlined in the Australian occupational therapy competency standards (OTBA, 2018).

19.4 Professional groups supporting quality practice education

Increasing demand for practice education, diverse student needs, educator expectations, and varied supervision approaches challenge the consistency and quality of practice education in Australia. Formation of professional groups at both state and a national level has occurred to mitigate some of these challenges.

Nationally, the Australian and New Zealand Occupational Therapy Practice Education Academics (ANZOTPEA) group works to ensure collaboration across universities by sharing current approaches and identifying significant issues impacting practice education. The group promotes debate, defines procedures between Australia and New Zealand, and conducts and promotes research related to practice education. Membership consists of academic staff responsible for practice education from each university. ANZOTPEA makes recommendations to the Australia and New Zealand Council of Occupational Therapy Education (ANZCOTE).

State-based groups have also formed in different ways to address more local practice education issues. These statewide collaboratives work together in varying ways to ensure a coordinated and consistent approach to tasks, which may include sourcing, distribution, allocation, and capacity building in practice education. They work together to promote innovation and sustainability in the local context, including the development of resources and training to support establishment of new practice education opportunities, and to promote quality supervision. Groups also contribute to the national agenda. Membership may include university practice education coordinators, heads of university education programmes, professional bodies, and representatives from industry. Examples include Queensland's OT Futures, the Victorian Occupational Therapy Practice Education Alliance (VOTPEA), and the Occupational Therapy Practice Education Development group (OTPED) in New South Wales.

Industry-based practice education providers sometimes form organisation-specific collaboratives or special interest groups which aim to support educators in providing high-quality practice education experiences for students. These collaboratives operate as communities of practice amongst practice educators, providing support through systems and resources which optimise the potential for, and quality of practice education opportunities. Organisation-specific groups also support students with resources which can assist them in understanding contextual factors and maximising their learning within specific practice education settings. These have had positive impacts on the willingness and confidence of practice educators to provide students with practice education experiences across services. Research funding has also been used to help representative groups collaborate to produce resources which promote high quality in practice education (e.g., ClinEdAus, https://www.clinedaus.org.au/).

19.5 Practice placement in practice education

Practice placements are a specific period of learning where the 'students spend time interpreting specific person-occupation-environment relationship and their relationship to health and well-being, establishing and evaluating therapeutic and professional relationships, implementing an occupational therapy process (or some aspect of it), demonstrating professional reasoning and behaviours, and generating or using knowledge of the context of professional practice with and for real live people' (WFOT, 2016, p. 71). Placements are often referred to as integrating theory into practice. However, placements offer an opportunity for students to learn broader workforce and employability skills such as teamwork, communication with various groups of people, critical thinking, reflective practice, problem solving, and self-management. Additionally, students learn about themselves, develop their own professional identity, and the perspectives they bring to practice and the impact of these perspectives, as well as the service users' health care journey (Penman et al., 2023). Practice placements may take place over a period of days, weeks or months and may be completed on a part-time or full-time basis depending on the course structure and learning objectives.

19.5.1 Practice placement and workforce

Industry-based placements are facilitated in partnerships with health and community organisations and are closely linked to workforce trends. The shift in healthcare funding towards community health, exemplified by the implementation of the National Disability Insurance Scheme (NDIS), has altered the distribution of the occupational therapy workforce. In 2021, more than a quarter of occupational therapists were practising in the private sector, making private practice the largest practice setting (Occupational Therapy Australia [OTA], 2023). However, there is tension between demand for placements and workforce resource shortages. Disability and paediatrics were the two fastest growing practice areas between 2013 and 2021, while rehabilitation declined the most during the same period (OTA, 2023). The top three occupational therapy practice areas have shifted from rehabilitation, paediatrics, and aged care in 2013 to paediatric, disability, and aged care in 2021 (OTA, 2023). Placements offered to universities have directly reflected these changes.

Increasing funding, such as the NDIS and My Aged Care, has significantly enhanced access to allied health services. This has led to a heightened demand for occupational therapy and expanded the scope of practice, contributing to the creation of numerous job opportunities. Over the past decade, the occupational therapy workforce has expanded by more than 80% (OTA, 2023), largely attributed to the influx of new graduates. However, the need for occupational therapy continues to exceed workforce capacity. Additionally, the trend towards a younger workforce has implications for newly graduated occupational therapists' capacity to support students during practice education placements (OTA, 2023). Establishing graduate programmes within health services has emerged as a popular strategy to attract employment and prepare new graduate occupational therapists for practice, although this approach inevitably strains the resources available for practice education placements. Universities are actively undertaking initiatives to implement various forms of practice education in workplaces, services, and locations with limited resources (e.g., regional and rural areas) aiming to develop and enable more placement opportunities.

19.5.2 Funding of practice placement

Funding for placement varies across states, universities, and organisations. The costs associated with placement are commonly shared between universities and placement providers. There has been a history of placement providers offering placements at their cost to support practice education in recognition of the value of training the future occupational therapy workforce. However, with increasing pressure on providers' resources, some states have moved to a billable placement system to increase training capacity. For example, Placeright in Victoria and South Australia provides a state-wide online platform to plan and coordinate health placements and sets maximum chargeable fees to guide public providers. Currently, no standard funding is available to provide financial support for occupational therapy students to attend placements. This lack of funding means that some placements, particularly those that incur additional travel and accommodation costs, such as community and rural placements, may not always be affordable for students.

19.5.3 Practice placement allocation

The allocation of placements is a complex process that varies among universities. Student placements are typically assigned by the university's practice education team, considering a variety of parameters relevant to, but not limited to, accreditation requirements, available placement resources, students' individual circumstances, and the existence of legal agreements between universities and placement providers. Many universities use student allocation systems, such as InPlace and SONIA, to support placement allocations.

19.5.4 Practice placement quality

High-quality practice education experiences should be a priority for all involved and each has a role to play (Isbel et al., 2021). Many researchers have studied the key features of a high-quality placement, from varying perspectives. Universities play a role in providing educator training regarding expectations, evaluation of student performance, and structuring of learning and support (Rodger et al., 2011). Placement practice educators ensure high quality by preparing and planning well, facilitating a range of scaffolded learning opportunities individualised to the student, and providing feedback that is regular and balanced (Grenier, 2015; Rodger et al., 2011). It is important that practice educators are approachable, have strong communication skills, provide realistic expectations, and ensure the workplace is appropriately resourced to provide a safe learning environment (Grenier, 2015; Lalor et al., 2019; Rodger et al., 2011).

Students contribute to high quality in practice education in many ways too. Being an active participant who is prepared and able to take initiative and drive learning is critical, along with the ability to receive and respond to feedback, and reflect critically on performance (Lalor et al., 2019). Various frameworks have been developed to support reflection and planning regarding quality in practice education, such as the Improving Quality in Practice Education (IQIPP-AH) Guides (The University of Queensland [UQ], 2012) and the Australian Collaborative Education Network's Institutional Quality Assurance of Work Integrated Learning Framework (Campbell et al., 2019).

19.6 Collaborators in practice placement

Learning on practice placement occurs through interactive and dynamic interactions between several collaborators, where all collaborators are learning with and from each other. Those involved include university staff, university students, practice educators and their organisations, and consumers of occupational therapy services. Collaborators play wide and varying roles throughout the range of processes necessary for a successful practice education experience. Key collaborators and their roles and responsibilities are described in the following.

19.6.1 Universities

Key university staff establish partnerships with industry which focus on building capacity for high-quality practice education opportunities within varied practice settings. This involves ensuring that experiences meet accreditation standards regarding practice education, course learning objectives, and legal and ethical compliance. Universities coordinate the sourcing and allocation of practice education experiences to eligible students, and prepare and support organisations, educators, and students before, during and after placements. This includes development and negotiation of reasonable adjustments for students with identified learning or other needs, such as additional time for complex tasks. University academic staff are responsible for determining final outcomes for students, based on educator assessment and feedback.

19.6.2 Practice educators and organisations

Practice educators and their employer organisations are responsible for identifying opportunities and capacity to host students and work with universities to negotiate legal agreements and appropriate resourcing for practice education. They develop orientation materials and other resources specific to the placement context to ensure the provision of scaffolded learning opportunities, timely reflection and high-quality feedback. Practice educators and organisations also collaborate with universities and students to develop learning plans and to complete fair and equitable assessment of student performance. Participation in practice educator training is a vital step in establishing and maintaining high-quality practice education.

19.6.3 Students

Students start preparing for practice education as soon as they commence their studies, with a key component of this the completion of a range of requirements such as vaccinations, licences and certificates, online training, and site-specific modules which contribute to what is known as 'fitness to practice'. These mandatory requirements are based on the needs of government, placement organisations and universities, and students are responsible for completing them to maximise health and safety for all. During practice education, students participate in learning using a variety of approaches such as observation, graded service provision, reflection, feedback, peer-assisted learning etc. They are expected to drive their own learning to develop and demonstrate professional competencies that are transferable across all practice areas. This requires the creation of collaborative relationships with educators and consumers to support learning.

19.7.4 Consumers

Increasingly within occupational therapy education, consumers are being recognised as being an essential contributor in student learning both in the university classroom and in practice placements (OTCA, 2024; WFOT, 2016). During placements, students and practice educators are required to seek informed consent from consumers for student service provision. While consumers are the experts on their own wellbeing and their contribution to student learning is invaluable, consumer care must never be compromised by the need to provide learning experiences for students. Consumers should be encouraged to consider providing feedback to students and/or educators to promote learning or contribute to student performance evaluation.

19.7 Forms of practice placement used in Australia

Various forms of practice placements are used in Australia, accompanied by a variety of terms that attempt to categorise them. Commonly used terms include direct service provision placement, project placement, university-supervised placement, short or sessional placement, and simulation (Isbel et al., 2023). No consistency in terminology currently exists, so terms described in the following may differ across contexts.

Some practice placements focus on students' direct involvement in interaction, observation, intervention, and service evaluation with individuals or collectives and can be arranged in any practice setting where the roles and responsibilities of occupational therapists are defined (sometimes termed *direct service provision placements*). Other practice placements can have a project focus involving quality assurance, service development, capacity building, community development, and project management activities. Students can use their problem-solving skills, creativity, and initiative, as well as building skills in professional reasoning, client-centred practice, and professional and personal development during these placements (Overton et al., 2009). This form of practice education is often referred to as a *project placement*, which brings additional benefits to address health and well-being service gaps but also the potential to develop a wider, more current, employment base, and new practice niches for graduates of occupational therapy programmes.

Many forms of practice placement may include a project component. Practice placements may also occur in new or emerging occupational therapy practice areas that have limited capacity to provide supervision. They take place in organisations, facilities, or services without occupational therapists. Supervision is provided by university-employed supervisor/s, hence these are often called *university-supervised placements* or *role emerging placements*. Some *short or sessional practice placements* are designed to allow students to apply early theoretical principles (e.g. an occupational perspective) or to experience a specific workplace, service, or population. These can occur through once-off or regular visits or volunteering.

However, placement forms do vary and can involve elements from each form defined previously. Two placement examples are provided subsequently that integrate various learning opportunities.

19.7.1 Example 19.1

Aaron is a first-year graduate entry student who has completed simulated activities at university to practice initial interviews and explaining occupational therapy. Aaron then visits a community mental health service with a small group of occupational therapy student peers for two hours to learn about the role of occupational therapy in that setting. Across the following three weeks Aaron and his student peers visit a different setting each week to continue to develop an understanding of occupational therapy scope of practice. After the service visits, Aaron and his peers then complete a reflection activity at university focused on professional competencies they observed or experienced as part of an assessment item for the unit of study.

19.7.2 Example 19.2

Jas is a third-year undergraduate occupational therapy student currently completing an eight-week placement at a local primary school. Before starting this placement, Jas completed a problem-based learning activity at university (simulation) to enhance their communication skills for interacting with children and families during basic information gathering. Throughout their placement at the school, Jas receives supervision from a paediatric occupational therapist employed by the university (university-supervised placement) which includes weekly face-to-face meetings and regular support via email and telephone. Jas works closely with several children identified by their teachers as needing occupational therapy support, completing observation, assessment, and intervention (direct service provision component). Additionally, as part of their placement, Jas dedicates four hours per week to a small project, developing a social skills activity booklet for the primary school (project component). Jas's performance is evaluated by the practice educator, with contributions from school staff and children, using the Student Practice Evaluation Form – Revised 2nd Edition (SPEF-R2) (The University of Queensland, 2020).

19.8 Supervision approaches

Practice educators employ a range of supervision approaches based on the diversity of those involved and the practice setting. Supervision in practice education is no longer confined to the approach of one-on-one student-therapist supervision, where a supervisor provides a student with discipline-specific and individualised feedback in a structured format. Other common supervision approaches include team, group, joint, peer, and real-time supervision (Isbel et al., 2023). Team-based supervision is becoming increasingly common in practice education, including occupational therapy. The educational, supportive, and administrative functions that are essential for effective supervision are divided and shared among various educators (Hylton & Manit, 2020). The educators involved in team-based supervision are not limited to occupational therapists; they can also include other health professionals. Group supervision involves supervision of two or more students at a time, facilitating robust discussions that enhance the learning experience. Joint supervision refers to two or more educators sharing a specific educational role and responsibility. Peer supervision enables students at the same or similar learning stages and experience levels to offer mutual support for each other's educational development. Real-time supervision is informal and occurs as opportunities arise. These supervisory methods can be conducted in person or remotely and are often used in combination during a practice education placement.

19.8 Example 19.3: Team supervision approach

Emma attends final placement at a NDIS organisation with her peer Hannah. Emma's supervisory team includes:

- Lia (psychologist and manager) who liaises with the multidisciplinary team to arrange and monitor placement learning opportunities and completes the orientation, induction, and occupational health and safety procedures with students using group supervision.
- Jane (primary practice educator) and Sean are occupational therapists who jointly provide supervision four days a week using a mix of onsite and online modes. They give Emma and Hannah weekly individualised and group occupational therapy–specific feedback, feedback from the other supervising professionals, and real-time feedback on the days they are responsible for supervision. Jane and Sean are responsible for completing Emma's performance evaluation. They discuss their perspectives regarding Emma's performance and consider feedback from other supervisory team members when completing the SPEF-R2. Jane and Sean meet with Emma to provide the SPEF-R2 evaluation results and feedback.
- Kim (speech pathologist) provides supervision on Wednesdays to develop knowledge and skills for multidisciplinary practice and advance communication skills and professional behaviours necessary for working in a multidisciplinary team.
- Cathy (speech pathologist and student coordinator) supervises Emma and Hannah's project, runs interprofessional training sessions and student case conferences, and provides individual learning support.

Emma also has daily peer supervision time with Hannah to support each other. A new graduate occupational therapist mentor, Riley, also provides a safe and non-evaluative near-peer support for Emma to ask questions or advice (see Table 19.1).

Table 19.1 Emma's supervision timetable

	Monday	*Tuesday*	*Wednesday*	*Thursday*	*Friday*
AM	Jane (OT)	Jane (OT)	Kim (SP)	Sean (OT)	Sean (OT, online)
PM	Jane (OT)	Cathy (SP, project)	Kim (SP)	Sean (OT)	Cathy (SP, IPE training and case conference, individual support)
3:30–4:30pm	Hannah (peer supervision)				
As needed	Lia (manager)				
	Riley (new graduate OT)				

19.9 Evaluation of practice placement performance

Student evaluation is a core component of the practice education experience. It is an important part of students developing and demonstrating necessary skills, behaviours, and attitudes for professional practice. Multiple varied forms of evaluation exist for practice placements and can be determined by course requirements and practice education contexts. Evaluation of student performance primarily involves both student and practice educator input; however, feedback from other key collaborators is valued for ongoing learning.

The Student Practice Evaluation Form – Revised (Second Edition) (SPEF-R2©) is an important tool used by all Australian universities to evaluate occupational therapy student practice education performance. Mapped to the Australian occupational therapy competency standards (OTBA, 2018), the SPEF-R2 supports both formative and summative feedback for students undertaking practice education across contemporary practice contexts (Caine et al., 2021). The SPEF-R2 evaluates core occupational therapy competencies related to professional behaviour, self-management, communication, documentation, information gathering, documentation, service provision, and service evaluation/reflection (The University of Queensland, 2020).

Predominantly used by the practice educator to evaluate performance and provide feedback at the midway and final points of the placement, the SPEF-R2 can be a valuable tool for discussions during supervision sessions to clarify expectations. Students can also use the SPEF-R2 to reflect and prepare for supervision. Other forms of evaluation related to practice education can include self-reflection, portfolio development, review of learning plans, and other academic tasks.

19.10 A future consideration of occupational therapy practice education in Australia

An important consideration for the future of occupational therapy practice education is artificial intelligence (AI). AI has rapidly expanded its applications and transformed the ways people work, live, and interact. Healthcare professionals, including occupational therapists, have begun to utilise AI to enhance service efficiency and improve client experiences. In occupational therapy practice, AI has been employed to analyse data for guiding evaluation and interventions, drafting documentation, searching for relevant research articles, scoring assessments, motivating clients, and assisting with administration and client communication (American Occupational Therapy Association [AOTA], 2024).

AI has also been used as a teaching tool to provide simulated practice education, allowing students to practice client interactions, information gathering, and professional reasoning for developing treatment plans. AI undoubtedly holds vast potential for occupational therapy practice education, and AI education is recommended to be incorporated into future occupational therapy education curricula (AOTA, 2024). The pressing questions for practice educators are: How can AI be used to enhance practice education in occupational therapy? How can we establish boundaries in practice education to cultivate future occupational therapists who ethically embrace AI without relying on it or being replaced by it, particularly when making professional judgments, decisions, and developing knowledge? Furthermore, we must consider whether and how AI will alter competency requirements for the profession and the expectations of student performance necessary to be deemed competent.

19.11 Conclusion

This chapter has presented an overview of contemporary practice education for occupational therapy students in Australia. Practice education occurs in various forms and across a multitude of different settings and contexts. In Australia, students are required to complete 1000 hours of practice education and meet national and international standards. Practice education equips students with diverse skills to be practice ready in a growing range of positions and settings. Quality practice education occurs through a complex and highly interactive process that requires a partnership among students, practice educators/organisations, clients, and universities through pre-, during-, and post-placement phases and is influenced by multiple contextual factors. Technological advancements in healthcare and education will continue to impact practice education. All collaborators have a role to play in ensuring that practice education continues to contribute to quality occupational therapy education.

19.12 Summary

- There are a range of guidelines that inform the structure of practice education in Australia.
- Multiple collaborators play unique and important roles in the provision of quality practice education.
- Practice education occurs in a range of forms and across a variety of classroom and industry contexts.
- Various supervision approaches exist to meet the needs of diverse practice educators, students, course learning objectives, and practice contexts.
- Evaluation is a core component of the practice education experience.

19.13 Review and reflection questions

- What professional guidelines inform occupational therapy practice education in Australia?

- Who are the key collaborators contributing to quality practice placement and their role?
- What are the forms of practice placement used in Australia that contribute to 1000 hours in addition to the classroom-based practice education?
- What supervision approaches are integrated in occupational therapy practice placement Australia?
- What role can you as a student play to optimise your learning through practice education?
- As a student, what are some ethical considerations relevant to your participation in practice education?

References

American Occupational Therapy Association (AOTA). (2024). *Artificial intelligence's role in occupational therapy: The innovation and instability.* https://www.aota.org/publications/student-articles/career-advice/ai-innovation-instability

Caine, A.-M., Copley, J., Turpin, M., Fleming, J., & Herd, C. (2021). Development of the Student Practice Evaluation Form-Revised (second edition) (SPEF-R2): The first action research cycle. *Australian Occupational Therapy Journal, 68*(1), 21–31. https://doi.org/10.1111/1440-1630.12702

Campbell, M., Russell, L., Smith, L., McAllister, L., Tunny, R., Thomson, K., & Barrett, M. (2019). *A framework for the institutional quality assurance of work integrated learning.* Queensland University of Technology, RMIT University & the University of Sydney. https://acen.edu.au/resources/institutional-quality-assurance-of-wil/

Grenier, M. L. (2015). Facilitators and barriers to learning in occupational therapy fieldwork education: Student perspectives. *American Journal of Occupational Therapy, 69*(Supp 2), 6912185070p1–6912185070p9. https://doi.org/10.5014/ajot.2015.015180

Gustafsson, L., Brown, T., McKinstry, C., & Caine, A. (2017). Practice education: A snapshot from Australian university programmes. *Australian Occupational Therapy Journal, 64*(2), 159–169. https://doi.org/10.1111/1440-1630.12337

Hylton, M., & Manit, J. (2020). Multi-layered supervision: The role of team-based approaches in field education. *Fieldwork Educator, 10*(1), 1–7. https://fieldeducator.simmons.edu/article/multi-layered-supervision-the-role-of-team-based-approaches-in-field-education/

Isbel, S., Bevitt, T., Yu, M., & Brown, T. (2023). Leadership, supervision, and management skills for practice. In E. Duncan (Ed.), *Skills for practice in occupational therapy* (2nd ed., pp. 209–219). Elsevier.

Isbel, S., Brown, T., Yu, M., Bevitt, T., Greber, C., & Caine, A.-M. (2021). Practice education in occupational therapy: Current trends and practices. In D. Nestel, G. Reedy, L. McKenna, & S. Gough (Eds.), *Clinical education for the health professions: Theory and practice* (pp. 209–219). Springer. https://doi.org/10.1007/978-981-13-6106-7

Lalor, A., Yu, M. L., Brown, T., & Thyer, L. (2019). Occupational therapy international undergraduate students' perspectives on the purpose of practice education and what contributes to successful practice learning experiences. *British Journal of Occupational Therapy, 82*(6), 367–375. https://doi.org/10.1177/0308022618823659

Occupational Therapy Australia (OTA). (2023). *Occupational therapy national workforce data report.* https://drive.google.com/drive/u/1/folders/1r7oP9zxhff3UQBcXcdJmThbsam9nu_4i

Occupational Therapy Board of Australia (OTBA). (2018). *Australian occupational therapy competency standards.* https://otaus.com.au/publicassets/e15160a1-f1e5-ec11-9452-005056be13b5/Occupational-Therapy-Board---Standards---Australian-occupational-therapy-competency-standards-2018%20%201.pdf

Occupational Therapy Council of Australia (OTCA). (2024). *Guidelines and evidence guide for the accreditation of Australian entry-level occupational therapy programs* (Version 3).

https://www.otcouncil.com.au/wp-content/uploads/Accred-guidelines-and-evidence-guide-Update-February-2024-V3.pdf

Overton, A., Clark, M., & Thomas, Y. (2009). A review of non-traditional occupational therapy practice placement education: A focus on role-emerging and project placements. *British Journal of Occupational Therapy*, 72(7), 294–301. https://doi.org/10.1177/030802260907200704

Penman, M., Raymond, J., Kumar, A., Liang, R. Y. R., Sundar, K., & Thomas, Y. (2023). Allied health professions accreditation standards for work integrated learning: A document analysis. *International Journal of Environmental Research and Public Health*, 20(15), 6478. https://doi.org/10.3390/ijerph20156478

Rodger, S., Fitzgerald, C., Davila, W., Millar, F., & Allison, H. (2011). What makes a quality occupational therapy practice placement? Students' and practice educators' perspectives. *Australian Occupational Therapy Journal*, 58(3), 195–202. https://doi.org/10.1111/j.1440-1630.2010.00903.x

The University of Queensland. (2012). *iQIPP-AH – Improving quality in practice placements guides – Allied health*. The University of Queensland.

The University of Queensland. (2020). *Student practice evaluation form – revised 2nd edition (SPEF-R2)*. https://spef-r.shrs.uq.edu.au/

World Federation of Occupational Therapy (WFOT). (2016). *Minimum standards for the education of occupational therapy*. https://wfot.org/resources/new-minimum-standards-for-the-education-of-occupational-therapists-2016-e-copy

CHAPTER 20

Occupational therapy academic and practice education in Aotearoa New Zealand

Heleen Reid, Penelope Kinney, Narinder Verma, Zainab Badat, Huhana Whautere, and Tiffany Brooke

Authors' positionality statements

Heleen Reid – first-generation Dutch immigrant living in Aotearoa New Zealand for 40+ years. Educated in NZ with both positivist and humanist perspectives. I acknowledge my privilege in education, nationality, gender/sexual orientation, multilingualism, and limited disabilities and that these have shaped this writing to some extent.

Huhana Whautere – identify as Māori with whakapapa connections to Ngāpuhi iwi and Dutch heritage. My perspective is shaped and reflects the positioning of myself in two different worlds.

Zainab Badat – First-generation Indian South African immigrant living in Aotearoa New Zealand since 2016. My perspective is shaped by my multicultural background and diverse educational and practice experiences across both countries.

Narinder Verma – British-trained occupational therapist and educator; my perspective reflects my Western, English-speaking, Global North background. I acknowledge the biases and privileges of my positionality, including being university educated in predominantly white institutions. As a woman of colour, my experiences of both privilege and marginalisation heighten my awareness of systemic inequities, shaping my commitment to social justice, anti-racism, and inclusion.

Penelope Kinney – fifth-generation New Zealander from Irish/Scottish immigrants. Born and educated in Aotearoa New Zealand, including university education. I identify as part of the LGBTQIA+ community. I acknowledge my privilege in education, nationality, and minimal disabilities. These, along with my insights into marginalisation, have shaped my writing to some degree.

Tiffany Brooke – fourth-generation New Zealander. Aotearoa New Zealand–trained occupational therapist. I acknowledge my privilege in education and practice from a western perspective.

DOI: 10.4324/9781003495666-22

Key terms
- Occupational therapy education
- Practice education
- Kaupapa māori practice education
- Supervision models
- Role-emerging practice education
- Accreditation
- Supervision models

Objectives
This chapter will allow the reader to:

- Detail the progression and extent of occupational therapy training programmes in Aotearoa New Zealand
- Summarise the key accreditation standards and educational requirements for entry-level occupational therapy programmes in Aotearoa New Zealand
- Explore the value of dynamic and culturally responsive practice education in occupational therapy, including the implementation of Kaupapa Māori practice placements and novel supervision frameworks
- Identify and discuss the key contemporary issues that impact practice education in Aotearoa New Zealand

20.1 Introduction

This chapter explores the evolution, history, current programmes, and future prospects of occupational therapy education in Aotearoa New Zealand, including practice education. The accreditation of the programmes is discussed, linking to Te Poari Whakaora Ngangahau Occupational Therapy Board of New Zealand (OTBNZ) and the World Federation of Occupational Therapists (WFOT) standards as well as other key stakeholders in the education of occupational therapists. Practice education forms a third of the bachelor's degrees and is a crucial part of the development of skills, knowledge, and attitudes. The chapter explores student-focused aspects like reflection, supervision models, and diverse practice education settings, including kaupapa Māori placements.

20.2 History of occupational therapy education in Aotearoa New Zealand

The first occupational therapists to be trained in New Zealand completed a six-month course at Auckland Mental Hospital in 1940 (Gordon et al., 2009). Over the last 85 years, there have been many changes in occupational therapy education, reflecting the growing recognition of the essential role of occupational therapy across a wide range of practice areas. By 1971, Occupational therapy education moved from hospital training to the Central Institute of Technology (CIT) as the sole provider of formal and structured occupational therapy education (Pollock, 2024). During its tenure, CIT was recognised for its specialised health education programmes and contributed significantly to the professional development of occupational therapists in New Zealand.

A review of the CIT occupational therapy programme was ordered by OTBNZ and the Occupational Therapy Association and funded by the Ministry of Education and

Health Board. In 1987 a six-week nationwide travelling review took place to engage with professionals and stakeholders, which led to the recommendation to the Minister of Health (Hnr Helen Clarke) and Minister of Education (Hnr Phil Goff) to disestablish the CIT school and create two new schools.

In May 1988, the decision was made to collocate occupational therapy/whakaora ngangahau education with the medical schools in Ōtepoti Dunedin and Tamaki Makau Rau Auckland. This resulted in the suspension of intake for a year. However, an extensive RV/radio advertising campaign called 'it takes a special person' ensured the new schools enrolled students. CIT's last occupational-therapy student graduated with a diploma in occupational therapy in 1992 (Central Institute of Technology, n.d.), and from 1991 occupational therapists have been educated through the now Auckland University of Technology (AUT) and Otago Polytechnic.

The development of these two new educational programmes with different curricula ensured that all occupational therapists were not cut from the same cookie cutter and were able to offer different skills to the country. The two programmes collaborate frequently on matters related to the impact of wider system issues and the impact this could have on teaching and practice education.

20.3 Current education programmes in Aotearoa New Zealand

20.3.1 Auckland University of Technology

The Department of Occupational Science and Therapy at the AUT has offered undergraduate education for occupational therapists since 1991. The first intake of 50 occupational therapy/whakaora ngangahau students to Auckland Institute of Technology's (AIT) Diploma of Occupational Therapy was chosen from 500 applicants. A high proportion of Māori students were accepted thanks to Titiwhai Harawira's influence and advocacy through the Māori Health Clinic at Carrington Hospital.

The first three student cohorts completed a Diploma in Occupational Therapy programme. A degree bridging programme, which ran as a summer school from 1993 to 1996, allowed previous diploma students to complete additional study and graduate with a Bachelor of Health Science (Occupational Therapy). The first intake to the three-year baccalaureate degree was in 1994. During this period academic staff established an occupational therapy department, designed and developed three programmes (diploma, degree completion, degree), and taught rapidly increasing student cohorts whilst completing their own advanced studies (C. Hocking & V. Wright-St.Clair, personal communication, November 10, 2020).

In 2002, planning for a new curriculum began at the renamed AUT, involving input from New Zealand registered occupational therapists, international experts, practitioners of other disciplines, service managers, and fund holders, as well as academic staff. In 2006 a new curriculum for the Bachelor of Health Science (Occupational Therapy) was implemented, and the first cohort from this curriculum graduated in December 2008. This programme was based on theoretical understanding and practice competence relating to the link between people, their occupations, and participation within their environments. The curriculum stood the test of time with little change over the decades it has been taught and is a testament to the planning and approach taken in its design. A revised baccalaureate curriculum will be delivered from 2026/2027 with a focus on occupation, innovation, equity, and social justice. Additionally, a graduate entry master's programme (Master of Occupational Therapy Practice) will offer an accelerated two-year path to registration. AUT also extensive post-graduate courses and opportunities to progress to PhD-level studies.

20.3.2 Otago Polytechnic

Te Kura Whakaora Ngangahau | The School of Occupational Therapy has offered undergraduate education since 1991. In preparation for that first intake, the government funded a new building to house the school (Dougherty, 2016). The school continues to operate out of this building today.

In October 1990, Dr Linda H Wilson was employed as the inaugural head of school along with several other staff to develop a quality programme that was ready to deliver to the first intake. Initially a Diploma in Occupational Therapy was offered, but they quickly moved to develop a three-year Bachelor of Occupational Therapy, which was first delivered in 1995, with the first graduates in December 1997 (Dougherty, 2016). A degree bridging programme was offered for a limited time. The bachelor's programme is reviewed every five years to ensure the programme is meeting the needs of the people kaiwhakaora ngangahau/occupational therapists work with and aligns with current research.

In the early 2000s a third occupational therapy school at WINTEC, Waikato, was proposed. Concern and opposition were indicated by both Otago and AUT based on programme viability and impact on sourcing clinical placements. The institutions resolved the situation when Otago collaborated with WINTEC to deliver the Otago Bachelor of Occupational Therapy from WINTEC in 2009.

The school has had a continued focus on Te Tiriti o Waitangi responsiveness. Ākonga study te Ao Māori (Māori worldview) and importantly attend noho marae (overnight marae experience). The school and kaimahi (staff) who work within it are committed to a journey towards te Tiriti responsiveness in the design and delivery of its programmes.

A work-augmented model of delivery has been developed to create pathways for ākonga in Te Tai Tokerau | Northland to study the bachelor's degree and to 'earn while they learn'. The model enables ākonga to continue meeting their existing commitments and boost the numbers of regionally and culturally relevant occupational therapists.

The focus now is on developing a graduate-entry-masters (GEMs) programme which offers an accelerated two-year programme to registration as an occupational therapist.

20.4 Occupational therapy education accreditation and stakeholders

In New Zealand occupational therapy programmes are accredited by the OTBNZ, with a reaccreditation process every five years to ensure continued compliance with the standards and criteria necessary for producing competent and ethical occupational therapists and eligibility to apply for registration in New Zealand (Occupational Therapy Board of New Zealand, 2022). Occupational therapy programmes are also approved by the WFOT against the WFOT Revised Minimum Standards for the Education of Occupational Therapists, giving graduates international recognition (World Federation of Occupational Therapists, 2016). OTBNZ accreditation standards for education programmes in New Zealand and Australia are similar and focus on public safety, academic governance and quality assurance, programme of study, student experience, and assessment (see Chapter 6).

Programmes must also meet the requirements of their respective educational institutions and the expectations of government-level authorities. The New Zealand Qualifications Authority focuses on the quality assurance of qualifications at Otago, while the Universities New Zealand does the same for AUT, and the Tertiary Education Commission handles the funding and performance monitoring of all tertiary education providers. Furthermore, the public and profession's needs and outlook influence what is taught within the programmes.

20.5 Practice education

Practice education (PE) embodies the use of experiential learning and provides students with the opportunity to develop professional competencies and apply learned skills and theories in various practice settings. Its purpose is to facilitate the transition from student to practitioner through work-based learning and socialisation in a professional environment (Taylor, 2024). With a range of PE experiences across the three years of study, mentorship, education, and feedback practice education ensure students acquire the competencies needed to meet societal demands for employability (Christensen et al., 2017) and align their skills with the evolving demands of healthcare (Isbel et al., 2020). The skills developed through PE experiences are highly transferable and provide employability in a wide range of future careers.

Registered occupational therapists provide supervision to students with support from the PE team at the school, who remain in contact via telephone, e-mail, online meetings, and the learning management system. The PE team create the interface between student education and professional practice, have unique insights into factors that are shaping the profession (O'Shea & McGrath, 2018), and provide support to both students and supervising occupational therapists. To remain relevant in a dynamic work environment, occupational therapy educators must ensure PE adapts to changing practices (Isbel et al., 2020).

A significant development in occupational therapy has been the introduction of role-emerging placements, where students work in settings without established occupational therapy services and receive long-arm supervision (Tokolahi & Robinson, 2021). These placements promote the profession in new contexts and help students develop a clearer understanding of occupational therapy's unique contributions (Thew et al., 2023). These placements can help demonstrate the benefit of the profession within these settings, with the potential of generating occupational therapy roles in future.

20.6 Student engagement in practice education

Prior to PE, preparation is conducted face to face with all students and includes self-care and stress management while away on placement. Students are expected to prepare for placements by researching and reviewing their learning relevant to the placement. Practice education is offered in settings throughout Aotearoa/New Zealand and selected to meet students' individual learning needs. Students need their own resources to travel and meet additional accommodation expenses to undertake PE.

Assessment of PE requires both that student meet the learning outcomes and performance indicators aligned to the placement and they achieve the required number of hours on placement. Practice education hours are defined by the WFOT (2016) as 'the time each student spends implementing an occupational therapy process, or an aspect of an occupational therapy process with or for a real live person' (p. 24). The curricula ensure that students achieve additional hours, exceeding the 1,000 hours of PE required by WFOT (2016). This surplus accommodates absences due to illness or other circumstances, ensuring students meet the minimum requirement.

The WFOT's Revised Minimum Standards for the Education of Occupational Therapists (2016) also mandate a range of experiences across various parameters, including diversity in personal factors (e.g., gender and ethnicity), individual and group approaches, health conditions, delivery systems, and emerging services. The curricula models ensure students gain balanced PE experiences, include working with individuals across age groups; addressing recent and long-standing health needs; and focusing on interventions that consider the person, occupation, and environment (WFOT, 2016).

20.7 Kaupapa Māori practice education

In Aotearoa New Zealand, kaupapa Māori services are becoming increasingly common and occupational therapy as a profession utilised more frequently in these spaces. Kaupapa Māori services follow a te Ao Māori perspective and focus on delivery by Māori kaimahi (staff) for Māori whai ora (service users seeking health). Non-Māori can access these services if they want to be in a service which follows tikanga (customary practices) Māori. Practice education in kaupapa Māori services allow ākonga to work closely with Māori communities to improve health inequities, immersion into Māori tikanga and the regular use of te reo Māori (Māori language), and increase their knowledge of cultural safety. For ākonga who identify as Māori, these experiences can grow their sense of identity and connection to their whakapapa (link to ancestors and ancestral lands). Integrating kaupapa Māori perspectives within the broader PE context is essential, as it enriches learning through indigenous knowledge systems, fosters inclusive and holistic practice, and supports the development of culturally responsive practitioners. These experiences reflect a meaningful commitment to upholding Te Tiriti o Waitangi through partnership, participation, and protection in education and practice.

20.8 Supervision in practice education

Students are expected to engage in at least one hour each week of formal supervision with a registered occupational therapist during their placement. Supervisors play a key role in facilitating reflective practice with students through informal and scheduled supervision (Isbel et al., 2020). Supervision includes monitoring student progress, discussing documentation, and caseload planning. Additionally, supervision allows students to explore and connect workplace learning opportunities to their academic and professional development, ensuring a comprehensive educational experience. Supervision is scaffolded across the three years and changes from being more student-led rather than supervisor-led as students progress in their learning.

To encourage reflective practice during PE experiences, students keep reflective journals, merging theoretical knowledge with clinical practice, deepening understanding, self-awareness, professional reasoning, and decision making (Guy et al., 2020).

Journaling fosters self-awareness and professional identity by reflecting on strengths, weaknesses, and emotional responses (Bassot, 2023). It also builds resilience and emotional regulation, crucial for sustainable healthcare practice (Au et al., 2025).

20.9 Different supervision models

There are a range of supervision model in practice education in Aotearoa New Zealand. Educators, students and therapists have utilised at least 14 types of supervision arrangements (Beveridge & Pentland, 2020; Pope et al., 2023), for example, 2:1, group supervision, interprofessional education (IPE), and role emerging. The 2:1 or group model, where two or more students are with one supervisor, can provide opportunity for peer-to-peer learning, critical thinking, problem solving, and reflection between students (Beveridge & Pentland, 2020; Price & Whiteside, 2016). IPE programmes have been developed (Pelham et al., 2016) in Aotearoa to address rural health needs. These programmes involve students from multiple disciplines working collaboratively and learning from, with, and about each other (Flood et al., 2021). Graduates who have experienced these programmes may be more likely to take up employment in rural communities that typically struggle to attract healthcare workers, benefiting these areas significantly.

20.10 Practice education issues

Occupational therapy practice has evolved in response to changing healthcare demands, technological advancements, and shifting social and political contexts (Taylor, 2024). As a result, therapists are embracing a growing scope of practice, where roles and responsibilities impact not just individuals but entire communities and systems. This presents exciting opportunities for the future of the profession, and together educational institutions and students navigate and adapt to the complexities and opportunities of contemporary practice. Therefore, the curricula and types of PE experiences must align with current and emerging practice trends. By doing so, students gain not only foundational theoretical concepts but also contemporary insights to enhance their practical skills, fostering a cohesive and engaging learning environment that prepares them for real-world practice.

Securing diverse PE placements demands extensive networking and collaboration between educational institutions and PE providers (Karp, 2020). Active partnerships between occupational therapy schools and the OTBNZ are essential for developing clear guidelines that ensure meaningful PE experiences for both students and clinical educators. This collaboration has led to initiatives such as workshops, resource sharing, and enhancing training. A recent survey by OTBNZ found that of 3005 occupational therapist completing annual practising certification renewal, only 21% had supervised a student for PE (OTBNZ, 2022). The main barriers identified to hosting students were unsuitable roles (33%), being short-staffed, lacking employer support, conditions on scope of practice, and impacts of maternity leave, common in Aotearoa's female-dominated professions (OTBNZ, 2022). This information highlights the need to address structural issues within the profession and academic institutions, working collaboratively with OTBNZ to generate support for PE while identifying emerging challenges and solutions.

From a student perspective, several factors may hinder the PE experience. These include financial costs associated with travel, accommodation, and working 40 hours a week unpaid. As well as, clinical educators' varied expectations and teaching styles and placement shortages may limit exposure to areas of interest (Grenier, 2015). Students with extenuating circumstances or health and disability needs often require specific accommodations that may not be feasible given the limited availability of placement options and/or extensive clinical support. This can exacerbate existing inequities in access to practical learning experiences. By addressing these barriers, a more equitable and supportive environment can be created for all students, enriching the future of occupational therapy practice.

20.11 Conclusion

This chapter explored occupational therapy education in Aotearoa New Zealand, including practice education and supervision. An overview of the historical developments, current programmes, and future foci is provided. The chapter demonstrates that occupational therapy education is dynamic, evolving, and cutting edge with responsiveness to Te Tiriti o Waitangi as a unique feature of occupational therapy education in Aotearoa ensuring graduates are culturally safe and competent on graduation. Exploring diverse ways of delivering occupational education that is accessible to a wide range of future practitioners continues, with practice education a central part to this.

20.12 Summary

- Both AUT and Otago Polytechnic have developed their own unique curricula, ensuring that graduates have diverse skills and knowledge to offer the profession.
- Occupational therapy programmes in New Zealand are accredited by the Occupational Therapy Board of New Zealand (OTBNZ) and approved by the World Federation of Occupational Therapists (WFOT), ensuring international recognition.
- Practice education is a crucial part of occupational therapy education, allowing students to apply their classroom learning in real-world settings.
- Kaupapa Māori practice education provides opportunities for students to work closely with Māori communities, improving health equity and increasing cultural competence.

20.13 Reflective questions

- How has the history of occupational therapy education in Aotearoa New Zealand influenced current educational practices and standards?
- What are the benefits and challenges of incorporating kaupapa Māori placements into occupational therapy education?
- In what ways can different supervision models enhance or hinder the learning experience of occupational therapy students?
- How do role-emerging placements contribute to the development of the occupational therapy profession, and what skills are essential for success in these settings?

- Reflect on a recent practice education experience: How did it help you integrate theoretical knowledge with practical skills, and what areas do you feel need further development?

References

Au, M., Knelson, J., Grinde, G., & Chen, S. P. (2025). The role of reflective activities for occupational therapy education: Key elements from a student perspective. *Occupational Therapy in Health Care*, 1–22. https://doi.org/10.1080/07380577.2025.2450712

Bassot, B. (2023). *The reflective practice guide: An interdisciplinary approach to critical reflection* (2nd ed.). Routledge.

Beveridge, J., & Pentland, D. (2020). A mapping review of models of practice education in allied health and social care professions. *British Journal of Occupational Therapy*, 83(8), 488–513. https://doi.org/10.1177/0308022620904325

Central Institute of Technology. (n.d.). *History*. UHCL Recollect. Retrieved August 26, 2024, from https://uhcl.recollect.co.nz/nodes/view/23955

Christensen, M. K., Henriksen, J., Thomsen, K. R., Lund, O., & Mørcke, A. M. (2017). Positioning health professional identity: On-campus training and work-based learning. *Higher Education, Skills and Work-Based Learning*, 7(3), 275–289. https://doi.org/10.1108/HESWBL-01-2017-0004

Dougherty, I. (2016). *Continuing education of quality: A history of Otago Polytechnic and its predecessors 1870–2006*. Otago Polytechnic.

Flood, B., Smythe, L., Hocking, C., & Jones, M. (2021). Interprofessional practice: The path toward openness. *Journal of Interprofessional Care*, 36(5), 635–642. https://doi.org/10.1080/13561820.2021.1981264

Gordon, B., Riordan, S., Scaletti, R., & Creighton, N. (Eds.). (2009). *Legacy of occupation: Stories of occupational therapy in New Zealand 1940–1072*. Bush Press Wellington.

Grenier, M. L. (2015). Facilitators and barriers to learning in occupational therapy practice education: Student perspectives. *American Journal of Occupational Therapy*, 69(2), 6912185070p1–6912185070p9. https://doi.org/10.5014/ajot.2015.015180

Guy, L., Cranwell, K., Hitch, D., & McKinstry, C. (2020). Reflective practice facilitation within occupational therapy supervision processes: A mixed method study. *Australian Occupational Therapy Journal*, 67(4), 320–329. https://doi.org/10.1111/1440-1630.12660

Isbel, S., Bevitt, T., Yu, M., & Brown, T. (2023). Leadership, supervision, and management skills for practice. In E. Duncan (Ed.), *Skills for practice in occupational therapy* (2nd ed., pp. 209–219). Elsevier.

Isbel, S., Brown, T., Yu, M. L., Bevitt, T., Greber, C., & Caine, A. M. (2021). Practice education in occupational therapy: Current trends and practices. In D. Nestel, G. Reedy, L. McKenna, & S. Gough (Eds.), *Clinical education for the health professions* (pp. 2–22). Springer. https://doi.org/10.1007/978-981-13-6106-7_137-1

Karp, P. (2020). Occupational therapy student readiness for transition to the practice education environment: A pilot case study. *The Open Journal of Occupational Therapy*, 8(4), 1–14. https://doi.org/10.15453/2168-6408.1719

Occupational Therapy Board of New Zealand. (2022). *Accreditation standards for occupational therapy education programmes*. https://otboard.org.nz/document/4909/OTBNZ%20Accreditation%20Standards%202022.pdf

O'Connor, A., Cahill, M., & McKay, E. A. (2012). Revisiting 1:1 and 2:1 clinical placement models: Student and clinical educator perspectives. *Australian Occupational Therapy Journal*, 59(4), 276–283. https://doi.org/10.1111/j.1440-1630.2012.01025.x

O'Shea, J., & McGrath, S. (2018). Contemporary factors shaping the professional identity of occupational therapy lecturers. *British Journal of Occupational Therapy*, 82(3), 186–194. https://doi.org/10.1177/0308022618796777

Pelham, K., Skinner, M. A., McHugh, P., & Pullon, S. (2016). Interprofessional education in a rural community: The perspectives of the clinical workplace providers. *Journal of Primary Health Care, 8*(3), 210–219. https://doi.org/10.1071/HC16010

Pollock, K. (2024). *Courses: Occupational therapy, Central Institute of Technology, 1971.* Te Ara – the Encyclopedia of New Zealand. Retrieved August 19, 2024, from https://teara.govt.nz/en/photograph/34421/courses-occupational-therapy-central-institute-of-technology-1971

Pope, K., Barclay, L., Dixon, K., & Kent, F. (2023). Models of pre-registration student supervision in allied health: A scoping review. *Focus on Health Professional Education: A Multi-Professional Journal, 24*(2), 27–62. https://doi.org/10.11157/fohpe.v24i2.559

Price, D., & Whiteside, M. (2016). Implementing the 2:1 student placement model in occupational therapy: Strategies for practice. *Australian Occupational Therapy Journal, 63*(2), 123–129. https://doi.org/10.1111/1440-1630.12257

Taylor, L. (2024). Practice-based placement learning and innovation: Essential for the professional identities of tomorrow's occupational therapist and the future of the occupational therapy profession. *British Journal of Occupational Therapy, 87*(1), 3–5. https://doi.org/10.1177/03080226231197313

Thew, M., Cezar da Cruz, D., & Thomas, Y. (2023). Comparing and measuring the practice-based performance and competence of occupational therapy students between traditional and role emerging placements: A retrospective cohort study. *Brazilian Journal of Occupational Therapy/Cadernos Brasileiros de Terapia Ocupacional, 31,* 1–16. https://doi.org/10.1590/2526-8910.ctoao265734672

Tokolahi, E., & Robinson, R. (2021). A scoping review of role-emerging, school-based fieldwork placements in occupational therapy education. *New Zealand Journal of Occupational Therapy, 68*(2), 26–33.

World Federation of Occupational Therapists (WFOT). (2016). *Minimum standards for the education of occupational therapists: Revised 2016.* https://www.wfot.org/assets/resources/COPYRIGHTEDWorld-Federation-of-Occupational-Therapists-Minimum-Standards-for-the-Education-ofOccupational-Therapists-2016a.pdf

CHAPTER 21

Occupational science in Australia and Aotearoa New Zealand

Mandy Stanley, Shoba Nayar, and Matthew Molineux

Authors' positionality statement

The authors of this chapter write from the position of identifying as occupational scientists, having been involved in the development of occupational science in Australia and Aotearoa New Zealand as well as internationally for a sustained period of time. Mandy worked alongside of Ann Wilcock and was involved in the *Journal of Occupational Science* for almost 30 years as well as holding leadership positions with occupational science. Shoba was introduced to occupational science during her masters degree in 2003 by Clare Hocking, a student of Ann Wilcock. Since then, she has worked with the *Journal of Occupational Science* for 20 years and has supported graduate students in Aotearoa New Zealand and India who have undertaken research using an occupational science lens. Matthew was a key figure in the development of occupational science in the United Kingdom (UK), where he established occupationUK and Ireland, as well as the UK occupational science symposia. He developed two entry-level programmes, one in the UK and one in Australia, which enacted occupational science in occupational therapy education, and the first masters in occupational science in the UK.

Although we have experiences of being members of marginalised groups, we acknowledge the Western influence that has shaped our coming to and understanding of occupational science, as well as the privileged position from which we write. Further, given our positionality, a First Nations (Australian) or Tangata Whenua (Māori, Aotearoa New Zealand) author was sought; however, a partnership was unable to be developed given time and other commitments.

Key terms
- Occupational science
- Occupational balance
- Occupational deprivation
- Occupational adaptation
- Occupational justice

DOI: 10.4324/9781003495666-23

Objectives

This chapter will allow the reader to:

- Define occupational science
- Describe the history of occupational science in Australia and Aotearoa New Zealand
- Identify key concepts within occupational science
- Describe the relationship between occupational science and occupational therapy

21.1 Introduction

This chapter introduces the reader to the discipline of occupational science as it has developed within Australia and New Zealand from the 1990s onwards. As a discipline, occupational science provides the foundational knowledge about humans as occupational beings that informs occupational therapy practice. Thus, there is an inherent link between the discipline of occupational science and the profession of occupational therapy. Following an overview of the origins of occupational science, the next section in the chapter unpacks some of the foundational knowledge about humans as occupational beings by exploring four key concepts – occupational balance, occupational justice, occupational deprivation, and occupational adaptation. Next, the story of Felicity an occupational therapist working in aged care is shared with the intention to help readers understand how these aspects of foundational knowledge – occupational science – can be translated to occupational therapy practice. Finally, the future of occupational science and areas for further research and development are put forth.

21.2 Occupational science: A brief history

The initial development of occupational science as a discipline is formally acknowledged as occurring at the University of Southern California (USC) under the stewardship of Elizabeth Yerxa and, subsequently, Florence Clark. Occupational science was defined as the study of humans as occupational beings (Yerxa et al., 1989) and the first occupational science doctoral programme, for which Clark was the inaugural chair (Pierce, 2014), commenced at USC in 1989 with seven students. Students recall the experience as an exciting time of exploration with a strong sense of creating a science of occupation (Pierce, 2014).

The 1990s was a period of intensive scholarly development as occupational therapists began to nurture the growth of occupational science. One of the collaborations driving that development was between Elizabeth Yerxa and Ann Wilcock, who were both interested in understanding the rich, situated, and complex nature of occupation. Indeed, when Elizabeth and Ann met for the first time at the World Federation of Occupational Therapists congress in Melbourne in 1990, they immediately recognised the synchronicity of their work. Subsequently, Ann developed and taught the first post-graduate course in occupational science in Australia at the University of South Australia in 1992 and in 1988 published her groundbreaking text *An Occupational Perspective of Health*.

Many of the leaders in occupational science in Australasia, including Gail Whiteford, Mandy Stanley, and Clare Hocking, were students in those early classes. They were exposed to a vast array of readings (e.g., works by humanists Bronowski and Marx) and were encouraged to develop their ideas on how to understand the complex phenomenon called *occupation*. All the students had occupational therapy backgrounds and found that the richness of the area for scholarship fuelled their interest and passion for occupation as a phenomenon of interest. Building on this passion, Hocking championed the development of occupational science in Aotearoa New Zealand, initiating a post-graduate course in occupational science at Auckland University of Technology and encouraging master's and doctoral thesis students to incorporate an occupational science perspective into their research.

In 1993, Wilcock launched the *Journal of Occupational Science* with the aim of publishing research related to the occupational nature of human beings. Her vision for the journal was to bring together the work of people from a range of backgrounds including, but not exclusively, occupational therapy, as well as human geography, anthropology, sociology, public health, and organisational psychology, who had a common interest in what people do and intersections with health and well-being.

From those early days, the *Journal of Occupational Science* has gone on to make a significant contribution to the development of the corpus of research on occupation internationally. The journal had its editorial office based at the University of South Australia for over 20 years before signing with the publishing house Taylor and Francis, reflecting the growth in the journal in that time. It remains the only journal in occupational science, and with an impact factor of 2.4 and Q1–impact factor best quartile, it is held in high regard. The journal receives submissions from all around the world and has a reputation for publishing high-quality articles. Although the journal has an international editorial and advisory board, Australians and New Zealanders have had significant input to the development of the journal. The contribution of Aotearoa New Zealand academic Professor Clare Hocking as executive editor of the journal through the developments over time cannot be overstated.

Australian and Aotearoa New Zealand occupational scientists have also made significant contributions to the development of occupational science internationally through their involvement in establishing the Australasian Society of Occupational Scientists (ASOS) and the International Society for Occupational Science (ISOS), particularly Dr Alison Wicks, who has held leadership positions in both organisations. For a full description of the development and impact of ASOS and ISOS, we recommend readers review Wicks' chapter in Whiteford and Hocking's (2012) book, *Occupational Science: Society, Inclusion, Participation.*

21.3 Occupational science key concepts: A brief review

In this section we begin with an overview of the occupational nature of humans and consider three key concepts within occupational science: occupational balance, occupational justice, and occupational deprivation. We also present the concept of occupational adaptation, drawing on an example of loneliness and older people. The concepts we have chosen to focus on in this chapter are commonly discussed in the occupational science literature; however, there are others that have emerged as occupational science scholarship has developed, for example, occupational apartheid (Morrison et al., 2024), occupational possibilities (Opland Stenersen et al., 2015), and occupational consciousness (Ramugondo, 2024), to name a few. We encourage readers to review these concepts as discussed in the *Journal of Occupational Science.*

21.3.1 The occupational nature of humans

One of the most significant Australian contributions to occupational science has been Ann Wilcock's original work on the occupational nature of humans and the occupational brain. Wilcock (1993) and Wilcock and Hocking (2015) drew on literature from evolutionary science and anthropology to propose the idea that engagement in occupation was the mechanism for people to fulfil their basic needs and thus survive. Further, occupational engagement enabled people to achieve health and well-being and the ability to reach their potential and thrive. Wilcock argued that because of the advanced evolution of the human brain and its ability to integrate and adapt, humans have an innate need to engage in occupations that are shaped by the socio-cultural context in which they are performed.

21.3.2 Occupational balance

One of the more developed concepts within occupational science is that of occupational balance (Wagman & Håkansson, 2018). The notion of occupational balance was part of the very beginnings of the occupational therapy profession posited by Adolf Myer (1922, 1977), based on his extensive observations of patients in long-term institutional environments. Early ideas of occupational balance were that individuals needed to achieve a balance of work, rest, and play to have a balanced lifestyle and thus health and well-being. This fairly simplistic conceptualisation can be questioned by thinking about people who are healthy who do not have a balance of work, sleep, and leisure, such as those retired from paid employment. There has been considerable theoretical development of the concept, with Matuska and Christiansen (2008) arguing that the balance is between desired and actual patterns of occupation to meet basic needs as well as having satisfactory social relationships and occupations that give meaning, challenge, and contribute to a sense of self. Recent research has explored how occupational balance reveals itself among a range of specific populations, including, for example, gender diverse populations (Morrison et al., 2024; Reid & Way, 2025). However, development of the concept with regard to moving beyond individuals in western societies, as well as understanding how to effectively measure occupational balance (Park & Lee, 2023), is still needed.

21.3.3 Occupational justice

Linking to the concept of social justice, occupational justice is 'the right of every individual to be able to meet basic needs and to have equal opportunities and life chances to reach toward her or his potential but specific to the individual's engagement in diverse and meaningful occupation' (Wilcock & Townsend, 2009, p. 193). It is centred on the understanding that circumstances and occupational needs of individuals and collectives are different; yet, regardless of age, ability, gender, social class, or other differences, everyone has the right to engage in everyday occupation. That said, occupational scientists also recognise that where privilege and power exist, inequitable opportunities are likely to hinder the attainment of occupational justice (George & Stanley, 2018; Zafran, 2025). In such instances, where occupational justice does not occur, potential outcomes are occupational imbalance, marginalisation, alienation, or deprivation.

Again, these outcomes may be at an individual or collective level. More recently, scholars have argued for an understanding of intergenerational occupational justice as, globally, societies tackle issues such as climate change which has resulted from people's engagement in certain occupations and potentially impacts future occupational choices (Drolet et al., 2020).

21.3.4 Occupational deprivation

As a concept, occupational deprivation has gained traction internationally as consideration is given to the many forces that can prevent people – individuals, families, and communities – from engaging in occupations. Drawing on Wilcock's (1993) earlier work, Whiteford (2004) defined occupational deprivation as 'a state of prolonged preclusion from engagement in occupations of necessity and/or meaning due to factors which stand outside the control of the individual' (p. 305). Whiteford (2005) went on to examine how occupational deprivation was experienced by people who have gone through refugee processes and, most recently, worked with Aakifah Suleman in extrapolating occupational deprivation to understandings of the impacts of forced migration (Suleman & Whiteford, 2013). In a future which clearly has many challenges, including climate change, pandemics, workplace reforms, labour shifting, and increasing numbers of people in forced migration around the globe, there is a lot of scope (and arguably a moral argument) to continue investigating occupational deprivation and its impacts on health and well-being.

21.3.5 Occupational adaptation

Occupational adaptation is the overcoming of occupational challenges presented by occupational disruption or transition and a response to opportunities across the lifespan which involve reconstruction of one's occupational identity and mastery of the environment and is negotiated through engagement in occupation (Nayar & Stanley, 2015). To understand occupational adaptation as a concept, consider the story of Mary and loneliness:

> Mary, 88 years old, was recently hospitalised for several weeks following major surgery and subsequent complications. This episode of ill health followed closely the death of her long-term partner. Her children live interstate and out of concern for Mary convinced her to move to a smaller unit after coming out of hospital rather than return to her large family home. Mary says she is feeling very lonely. She is not as mobile as she used to be, has moved away from her friends and neighbours, and has not made new connections in her community. She has experienced a number of major changes in the last six months. She is reluctant to reveal to her family that she feels lonely, as she does not want to be a burden.

Mary's change of environment no longer supports her capacity to engage in social occupations and thereby address her loneliness. Mary decides to ask her neighbours to her unit for a coffee and discovers that she shares an interest in the same football team as one of her neighbours. She also rings an old friend and asks if they would pick her up and take her to the church service they used to attend together weekly. Through re-connecting and building relationships with others, Mary is able to use occupation to adapt to her situation over time. In doing so, she is also better positioned to face future challenges or changes in her life.

Mary's story reveals that occupational adaptation is necessary after a change such as bereavement, loss, or ill health. Other occupational transitions that might precipitate the need for occupational adaptation include becoming a parent for the first time, migrating to a new country, or acquiring a disability such as stroke (c.f., Delaisse & Huot, 2020; Williams & Murray, 2013). A conceptual analysis of occupational adaptation concluded that conceptually it is not fully mature which limits the clinical utility (Walder et al., 2019). Occupational scientists need to rise to the challenge of better defining and theoretically developing the concept.

21.4 Relationship between occupational science and occupational therapy practice

While occupational science originated from within occupational therapy, the relationship between them is neither generally well understood nor well communicated. This scenario is fuelled by the lack of agreement internationally about what the relationship *should* be (Molineux, 2010). For instance, some authors argued that the research efforts within occupational science would reduce available research funding to establish the effectiveness of occupational therapy interventions (Morley et al., 2011), thereby undermining the profession. Currently, differing views are held regarding the relationship between occupational science and occupational therapy. Many occupational therapists believe that occupational science is the unique domain of occupational therapists and that the two are so closely related they cannot be separated. Still others (including Wilcock, 1993) have argued that all occupational therapists should be occupational scientists but that occupational science is open to and enriched by multidisciplinary contributors.

In some countries – such as the United States – there are PhD and masters programmes in occupational science. In Australia and Aotearoa New Zealand, however, there are no programmes of study leading to a formal qualification in occupational science. Some academic occupational therapy departments include occupational science in the title, but generally occupational science knowledge is incorporated within the entry-level occupational therapy curriculum. Few programmes offer specific courses in occupational science, and in this respect occupational science and occupational therapy have continued to inform each other. Whether this is problematic may be a matter of some conjecture, but, as Pierce (2014) cogently suggested: 'It is no longer necessary to argue why one vision of occupational science may be better than another. Clearly, occupational science has multiple intents' (p. 7).

Our view, which has, admittedly, been heavily influenced by Wilcock, is that knowledge generated within occupational science provides the knowledge base that informs occupational therapy practice. Clearly, this is important if occupational therapists are to claim their domain *as* occupation and their expertise *in* occupation.

21.5 Occupational science translated into occupational therapy

In the following story, readers are introduced to Felicity, an experienced occupational therapist who has recently changed jobs. In her new environment she quickly identifies the need to expand occupational therapy interventions to support her clients' well-being. As you read the story, consider how the four concepts discussed previously – occupational balance, occupational justice, occupational deprivation, and occupational adaptation – feature and how you might respond to each of these aspects if you were employed in Felicity's role.

Felicity has over 15 years working in general hospital wards, with the majority of her clients aged 65 years or older. With a passion for working with older people and a desire to do more than rapid discharge planning, she recently took a job at a residential aged care setting. Her workload includes assessment of individual residents and working with nursing staff and care workers on developing care plans which support residents in their daily living tasks. In the six months that Felicity has been working at the residential aged care facility, she has become concerned that residents are at risk of reduced opportunities for occupational engagement with only group programmes for seating exercise, bingo, and a singalong available. Felicity is the first occupational therapist to be employed by the facility, and previous lifestyle coordinators were constrained in what they were able to offer in the time available. Felicity believes that residents could easily become bored and disinterested with little to engage them for large parts of the day and little connection between residents. She has also observed that many of the residents have few visitors and it is likely that they experience loneliness, particularly those who are frail but do not have dementia. As the majority of residents are experiencing some degree of cognitive decline, Felicity understands that occupations need to be stimulating and at a level that supports engagement from people with cognitive challenges.

To begin, Felicity compiles an occupational profile for each resident to gain a comprehensive understanding of both their current and past occupational interests. The process involves talking to family and friends and staff. She makes sure that the occupational profile is easily accessible for staff in the resident's room so they can draw on the information in their interactions with residents while also keeping it as a living document for family and staff to add to over time. In compiling the profiles, Felicity could see that some residents had common interests that could be incorporated into activity programmes and facilitate connections between residents. She also became aware of occupations that residents were no longer able to participate in, which prompted further thinking and problem solving. Felicity was able to draw on the resources of family and volunteers to enable re-engagement in some occupations or, at a minimum, reminiscence about the engagement experiences in the past.

Felicity was also intrigued by recent publicity about intergenerational programmes within residential aged care and the clear occupational features of those programmes. With the support of the site manager, she put together a discussion paper and presented to the board of management. They supported Felicity to forge ahead with her idea of bringing a local play group into the complex which would provide opportunities for the residents to form reciprocal relationships with young children and their parents through engaging in occupations. It would bring a wider range of occupations, including art, craft, and music, and the noise of young people in the facility could help brighten the lives of residents who otherwise did not have the chance to interact with young people. The idea was not without obstacles such as hygiene, exposure of residents to coughs and colds, and that some might find it too noisy. However, with the support of staff and the local play group association, Felicity went ahead and implemented the idea. As anticipated, Felicity encountered some of the identified obstacles, but, overall, the implementation was successful.

21.6 The future of occupational science

As occupational science has matured, it has grown in depth and scope of scholarship. Pierce (2014) pointed to studies that found that occupational science publications quadrupled between 1990 and 2000 and that between 1996 and 2006 not only did the numbers of articles increase dramatically, but the research approaches used and the foci of the research also diversified significantly. A more recent review of occupational science publications highlighted the global interest in occupational science with authors spanning 40 countries contributing to occupational science publications (Li et al., 2025).

Despite the increase in publications numerically, a deeper analysis shows that the origin of the authors is largely from Western countries and tends to reflect the cultural, philosophical, and linguistic traditions of those countries. To be of the greatest value and relevance, there needs to be a greater diversity of perspectives reflected in the literature (Hocking, 2012; Kinsella, 2012). Excellent examples of this in recent times are represented by the work of Shetty and Nayar (2023), who considered the erosion of tribal occupations in India as an ongoing result of oppressive socio-political structures, and Simaan (2021), who has drawn attention to the plight of olive farmers in Palestine and the ongoing occupational apartheid that they experience.

Such research has a great deal of salience. For occupational science to fulfil its potential, then, there also needs to be continued movement from the focus on individual engagement in occupation – an orientation arguably influenced by occupational therapy's relationship to biomedicine – to consideration of occupational engagement by collectives, communities, and populations. Additionally, there is the need for greater consideration of how changing environments due to the current climate crisis and changes in ecology have the potential to impact human occupations. These avenues very possibly herald in yet another stage in the genesis of a discipline whose potential has yet to be realised fully.

21.7 Conclusion

Australia and Aotearoa New Zealand have made a significant contribution to the development of occupational science over time and have been leaders in the advancement of the discipline. The contribution of scholars who have variously provided important inputs on conceptual, philosophical, and pragmatic issues has furthered understandings of the important relationship between occupational science and occupational therapy. A number of key occupational science concepts, as discussed in this chapter, as well as other significant concepts, such as occupational consciousness (Ramugondo, 2024) and occupational apartheid (Morrison et al., 2024), have been developed through a range of research approaches in a variety of contexts. Further development and debate are needed to extended understandings of these concepts. For example, some may argue that occupational apartheid is unique to the South African experience; nevertheless, the concept has been used in global contexts and offers a different lens through which to understand occupational participation. As occupational science continues to evolve in Australasia and internationally, such research will only continue to contribute to the richness and diversity of understanding humans as occupational beings.

21.8 Summary

- Occupational science is the study of occupation as a complex, situated phenomenon.
- Occupational science and occupational therapy have an important relationship, as understanding occupation is requisite to enabling engagement in occupation.
- Australasian scholars, led by Ann Wilcock, have made a unique and important contribution to the development over time.
- Key concepts contributing to the foundational knowledge of humans as occupational beings include occupational balance, occupational justice, occupational deprivation, and occupational balance.
- Occupational science will be strengthened by greater diversity of researchers globally and a more pluralistic epistemic foundation.

21.9 Review and reflection questions

- How have Australia and Aotearoa New Zealand influenced the development of occupational science locally and internationally? Who have been the key players?
- How would you describe the relationship between occupational science and occupational therapy?
- What are some of the key concepts discussed in occupational science?
- Where are the areas in which occupational science scholarship can continue to grow?
- How would you define the concepts occupational adaptation and occupational balance? What was important for you to consider in developing these definitions?
- Using the definition provided, consider the ways in which occupational deprivation, other than that discussed in the chapter, may appear in the areas in which you live and practice. What action would you take to counter occupational deprivation?

References

Delaisse, A. C., & Huot, S. (2020). Using theory to inform understandings of occupation in a migration context. *Journal of Occupational Science, 27*(3), 359–375. https://doi.org/10.1080/14427591.2020.1734961

Drolet, M. J., Désormeaux-Moreau, M., Soubeyran, M., & Thiébaut, S. (2020). Intergenerational occupational justice: Ethically reflecting on climate crisis. *Journal of Occupational Science, 27*(3), 417–431. https://doi.org/10.1080/14427591.2020.1776148

George, E., & Stanley, M. (2018). Exploring the occupational injustices of human trafficking. *Journal of Occupational Science, 26*(3), 394–407. https://doi.org/10.1080/14427591.2018.1515104

Hocking, C. (2012). Occupations through the looking glass: Reflecting on occupational scientists' ontological assumptions. In G. Whiteford & C. Hocking (Eds.), *Occupational science: Society, inclusion, participation* (pp. 54–66). Wiley-Blackwell.

Kinsella, E. A. (2012). Knowledge paradigms in occupational science: Pluralistic perspectives. In G. Whiteford & C. Hocking (Eds.), *Occupational science: Society, inclusion, participation* (pp. 67–85). Wiley-Blackwell.

Li, Z., Vaughn, R. M., Kawabata, S., Syu, Y. C., & Bagatell, N. (2025). A descriptive review of occupational science publications in English since 2007: Key trends and challenges. *Journal of Occupational Science, 32*(1), 124–141. https://doi.org/10.1080/14427591.2024.2394852

Matuska, K., & Christiansen, C (2008). A proposed model of lifestyle balance. *Journal of Occupational Science, 15*(1), 9–19. https://doi.org/10.1080/14427591.2008.9686602

Meyer, A. (1922). The philosophy of occupation therapy. *Archives of Occupational Therapy, 1*(1), 1–10.

Meyer, A. (1977). The philosophy of occupation therapy (Original work published 1922). *American Journal of Occupational Therapy, 31*(10), 639–642.

Molineux, M. (2010). Occupational science and occupational therapy: Occupation at center stage. In C. Christiansen & E. Townsend (Eds.), *Introduction to occupation: The art and science of living* (2nd ed., pp. 337–362). Prentice Hall.

Morley, M., Atwal, A., & Spiliotopoulou, G. (2011). Has occupational science taken away the occupational therapy evidence base? A debate. *British Journal of Occupational Therapy, 74*(10), 494–497. https://doi.org/10.4276/030802211X13182481842065

Morrison, R., Cirineu, C. T., Lagos-Cerón, D., & Cantero-Garlito, P. (2024). LGBTQ+ parenting: An interpretative review of Latin American literature from an occupational science perspective. *Journal of Occupational Science*, 1–18. https://doi.org/10.1080/14427591.2024.2415292

Nayar, S., & Stanley, M. (2015). Occupational adaptation as a social process in everyday life. *Journal of Occupational Science, 22*(1), 26–38. https://doi.org/10.1080/14427591.2014.882251

Opland Stenersen, A., Laliberte Rudman, D., & Raanaas, R. K. (2015). Shaping occupational possibilities for Norwegian immigrant children: A critical discourse analysis. *Journal of Occupational Science, 23*(1), 17–32. https://doi.org/10.1080/14427591.2015.1070783

Park, S., & Lee, C. D. (2023). Psychometric properties of self-reported instruments for occupational balance: A COSMIN-based systematic review. *Journal of Occupational Science, 31*(2), 371–385. https://doi.org/10.1080/14427591.2023.2243281

Pierce, D. (2014). *Occupational science for occupational therapy.* SLACK.

Ramugondo, E. L. (2024). Occupational consciousness: Theorising to dismantle systemic racism and dehumanisation. *Journal of Occupational Science*, 1–17. https://doi.org/10.1080/14427591.2024.2429681

Reid, H., & Way, K. (2025). Defying the deficit: Imagining intersections of occupation, gender euphoria, and trans joy. *Journal of Occupational Science*, 1–16. https://doi.org/10.1080/14427591.2024.2437773

Shetty, R., & Nayar, S. (2023). How are marginalized communities represented in the Indian Journal of Occupational Therapy? A scoping review. *Indian Journal of Occupational Therapy, 55*(1), 23–28. https://doi.org/10.4103/ijoth.ijoth_87_22

Simaan, J. (2021). Occupational apartheid in Palestine, global racism, and transnational solidarity: Update on Simaan (2017). *Journal of Occupational Science, 28*(3), 435–440. https://doi.org/10.1080/14427591.2021.1880265

Suleman, A., & Whiteford, G. (2013). Understanding occupational transitions in forced migration: The importance of life skills in early refugee resettlement. *Journal of Occupational Science, 20*(2), 201–210. https://doi.org/10.1080/14427591.2012.755908

Wagman, P., & Håkansson, C. (2018). Occupational balance from the interpersonal perspective: A scoping review. *Journal of Occupational Science, 26*(4), 537–545. https://doi.org/10.1080/14427591.2018.1512007

Walder, K., Molineux, M., Bissett, M., & Whiteford, G. (2021). Occupational adaptation – analysing the maturity and understanding of the concept through concept analysis. *Scandinavian Journal of Occupational Therapy, 28*(1), 26–40. https://doi.org/10.1080/11038128.2019.1695931

Whiteford, G. (2004). When people cannot participate. In C. Christiansen & E. Townsend (Eds.), *Occupation: The art and science of living* (pp. 303–328). Prentice Hall.

Whiteford, G. (2005). Understanding the occupational deprivation of refugees: Case study from Kosovo. *Canadian Journal of Occupational Therapy*, 72(2), 78–87. https://doi.org/10.1177/000841740507200202

Wicks, A. (2012). The International Society for Occupational Science: A critique of its role in facilitating the development of occupational science through international networks and intercultural dialogue. In G. Whiteford & C. Hocking (Eds.), *Occupational science: Society, inclusion, participation* (pp. 163–183). Wiley-Blackwell.

Wilcock, A. A. (1993). A theory of the human need for occupation. *Journal of Occupational Science: Australia*, 1(1), 17–24. https://doi.org/10.1080/14427591.1993.9686375

Wilcock, A. A., & Hocking, C. (2015). *An occupational perspective of health* (3rd ed.). SLACK.

Wilcock, A. A., & Townsend, E. A. (2009). Occupational justice. In E. B. Crepeau, E. S. Cohn & B. A. Boyt Schell (Eds.), *Willard & Spackman's occupational therapy* (11th ed., pp. 192–199). Lippincott Williams & Wilkins.

Williams, S., & Murray, C. (2013). The experience of engaging in occupation following stroke: A qualitative meta-synthesis. *British Journal of Occupational Therapy*, 76(8), 370–378. https://doi.org/10.4276/030802213X13757040168351

Yerxa, E. J., Clark, F., Frank, G., Jackson, J., Parham, D., Pierce, D., Stein, C., & Zemke, R. (1989). Introduction to occupational science, a foundation for occupational therapy in the 21st century. *Occupational Therapy in Health Care*, 6(4), 1–17. https://doi.org/1080/j003v06n04_04PMID23931133

Zafran, H. (2025). (Im)possibilities: The occupation of storytelling injustice. *Journal of Occupational Science*, 1–17. https://doi.org/10.1080/14427591.2025.24852167

CHAPTER 22

Research in occupational therapy

Helen Bourke-Taylor, Ted Brown, Lisa O'Brien, and Michael Curtin

Authors' positionality statement
We are Western, higher educated occupational therapists working in leadership positions in Australia. We are white, cisgender, able-bodied, English-speaking Australian citizens. We acknowledge our white privilege and support decolonisation; racial and all equality; and honour diversity, cultural sensitivity, and social and occupational justice. We uphold gender-affirmative, inclusive, and culturally safe and responsive health care and education.

Key terms
- Research
- Evidence-based practice
- Qualitative
- Quantitative
- Mixed-methods
- Occupational therapy

Objectives
This chapter will allow the reader to:

- Understand the importance of becoming an informed and skilled research *consumer* occupational therapy student and professional
- Describe how research underpins and justifies occupational therapy practice
- Explain contemporary research approaches to occupational therapy research and practice
- *Ask* and *acquire* relevant research evidence to answer a clinical question

22.1 Introduction
Research evidence underpins contemporary occupational therapy practice, safeguarding the future of the profession. Competency in practice is maintained through lifelong

DOI: 10.4324/9781003495666-24

learning, professional development activities, and contributing to the development and evaluation of services (Occupational Therapy Australia, 2018). The occupational therapy regulatory boards in Australia and New Zealand aim to protect members of the public from ineffective, harmful, incompetent, or unethical practice and therefore mandate that occupational therapists must keep up to date with research evidence and deliver evidence-based interventions.

22.2 Research and ethics in occupational therapy

Occupational therapy research often involves people from marginalised or minority groups, including those adversely affected by their environment or living with health differences or acquired disability. Accordingly, occupational therapy research must adhere to the ethical principles that guide all human research in Australia and New Zealand, ensuring the careful and judicious consideration of the rights of all. Occupational therapists conducting research with First Nations Peoples in Australia have obligations and responsibilities under the National Health Medical and Research Council (NHMRC) to adhere to a set of principles that ensures research is safe, respectful, responsible, high quality, and of benefit to First Nations People. Similarly, in New Zealand, research with First Nations peoples is guided by the Te Ara Tika Guidelines for Māori Research Ethics.

Harm is more than injuring a person. It results from unethical research and practice, poor risk management, provision of interventions with low value or no evidence, wasting the time, resources, and money of clients (Moyers, 2010). Harm can also occur when occupational therapists make decisions on behalf of clients that may be based on evidence but without agreement from clients. Involving clients in discussions about intervention options and effectiveness (for whom, when, in what amounts or circumstances) is a necessary step in service provision. Denying clients the autonomy to make decisions about intervention options also prevents collaborative and person-centred practice.

22.3 Evidence based practice in occupational therapy

Evidence-based practice (EBP) is fundamental to occupational therapy practice and is defined as: 'the conscientious, explicit, and judicious use of current best evidence in making decisions about the care of individual patients' (Sackett et al., 1996, p. 71). Classically, EBP upholds three pillars: the scientific research-based knowledge; individual practitioner knowledge to provide the most effective, client-centred health care; and the client's wants, needs, and perspectives. Being an evidence-based practitioner ensures that clients are receiving the best intervention at the right time, in the right amount, at the right cost, and that the client was actively involved in decision making around their own needs (Hoffmann et al., 2023).

Cusick et al. (2024) identified the different roles occupational therapists assume to make valuable research contributions to the profession:

- research *producer*, actively engaging in research that produces new knowledge for the field and beyond;
- research *collaborator*, being an adviser, co-investigator, provider of intervention or evaluation, data collector, or co-author;

- research *consumer*, implementing evidence-based practice with clients; and
- research *advocate*, actively identifying knowledge gaps, generating research questions, and lobbying for the investigation or evaluation of an issue that is known to be underserved and under-researched.

Occupational therapy as a profession has moved into a phase where many clinicians conduct, produce, and consume research, with some becoming expert *clinician/practitioner researchers*.

22.4 Building occupational therapy knowledge and scholarship

There are many ways for research *consumers* to stay current, including perusing scientific journals, attending special interest groups and/or national conferences that provide opportunities to listen to and interact with researchers, or joining workplace or online research groups. Scientific literature may be accessed via libraries using scientific databases, public databases such as Google Scholar or research social media such as ResearchGate. Occupational therapy research *collaborators* are in many universities and workplaces. Occupational therapy students can be research *producers* by conducting research in honours programmes and through higher degrees.

The World Federation of Occupational Therapists (WFOT) conducted a Delphi study to identify, rate, and rank global research priorities (WFOT et al., 2017). The resulting eight research priorities have been adopted internationally, guiding occupational therapy researchers to build the profession's evidence base in key contemporary areas of practice (see Table 22.1). Each priority area has an underlying rationale. For example, the rationale for including technology and occupational therapy (Priority 7) is 'Technology is growing and affecting all aspects of everyday life, therefore, occupational therapists need to explore how technology can facilitate participation in occupations, or if it has detrimental effects on some aspects of participation' (WFOT et al., 2017, p. 79). See Table 22.2 for examples of occupational therapy research classified by WFOT priorities.

Whether at an international, national, or local level, occupational therapists are working to build the evidence base of the profession which, in turn, builds the reputation and effectiveness of the profession.

22.5 Research approaches in occupational therapy

As a result of the breadth and complexity of professional practice, 'occupational therapy research can range from exploring individuals' and collectives' experiences of participating in meaningful occupations to evaluating the effectiveness of occupational therapy interventions' (Mackenzie et al., 2024, p. 303). Research can take many forms depending on the context and research questions posed and may draw on a range of paradigms and methods (Bennett & Mottram, 2024; Mackenzie et al., 2024).

A research paradigm is a theoretical framework that underpins the assumptions, concepts, and propositions that guide 'the intent, motivation and expectations for the research' (Mackenzie & Knipe, 2006, p. 194). A research *producer* should be clear on their research paradigm as this will guide the research design. Mackenzie and Knipe (2006) suggest that the most used research paradigms are:

Table 22.1 World Federation of Occupational Therapy Research Priority Areas in rank order, definition, and scope of associated research (WFOT et al., 2017)

World Federation of Occupational Therapy research priority	Definition of the research priority area
Research priority 1: Effectiveness of occupational therapy interventions	Research that establishes and demonstrates the impact (health, wellbeing, cost effectiveness, and social inclusion) of occupational therapy services across the scope of practice.
Research priority 2: Evidence-based practice and knowledge translation	Research in the area of development, use, and integration of scientific evidence by occupational therapy practitioners and ways in which the practice-research interactions shape and inform practice.
Research priority 3: Participation in everyday life	Research which explores the ways in which occupation enables participation in everyday life, shapes identity, and influences individual, community, and public health outcomes.
Research priority 4: Healthy aging	Research about the health and wellbeing of older adults, including determinants of social inclusion/exclusion, poverty, environmental barriers and facilitators, and occupational choice.
Research priority 5: Occupational therapy and chronic conditions	Research about the role and impact of occupational therapy services for individuals and collectives experiencing chronic health conditions across the lifespan.
Research priority 6: Sustainable community development and population-based occupational therapy interventions	Research that investigates the role of occupation in building and sustaining wellness, effective access to rights, and civic participation.
Research priority 7: Technology and occupational therapy	Research that investigates the design, development, deployment, use, usability, and technology acceptance of everyday as well as assistive technologies in relation to occupation.
Research priority 8: Occupational therapy professional issues	Research that explores the education of occupational therapists and continued learning and interdisciplinary initiatives impacting the profession.

- *Positive/postpositive* – scientific research that tests a hypothesis or theory using observations and measurements to predict and control various factors. This paradigm is commonly aligned with quantitative methods of data collection and analysis. As outlined in Table 22.2, quantitative methods of umbrella review, systematic review, randomised control trial, cohort study, and single-subject experimental design belong to this paradigm.
- *Interpretive/constructivist* – research that relies on the views and experiences of participants about the incident/phenomena being studied. This paradigm is commonly aligned with qualitative methods of data collection and analysis. In Table 22.2 the qualitative methods of grounded theory, phenomenology, ethnography, and narrative belong to this paradigm.

- *Transformative* – developed to address social justice issues. Researchers using this paradigm often use a mixed methods approach as this can provide a fuller understanding of the multiple perspectives that underpin the diversity of values and positions of individuals and collectives (Creswell & Plano Clark, 2018). In Table 22.2, participatory action research (PAR) belongs to this paradigm.
- *Pragmatism* – uses methods of data collection and analysis that fit the research question and has no loyalty to any specific paradigm. This could include quantitative, qualitative, or mixed-methods approaches to data collection and analysis.

The following is a brief overview of quantitative, qualitative, and mixed-methods designs. Common research designs for each method listed are in Table 22.2.

- *Quantitative methods* involve the collection and analysis of numerical data to identify patterns, relationships, and causal effects between different variables using statistical analyses. In occupational therapy these methods are commonly used to measure the clinical impact of interventions or the incidence and prevalence of factors that may impact the occupational participation of individuals and collectives (Bennett & Mottram, 2024). Measures of quality and credibility of quantitative studies are validity, reliability, biases, and replicability (MacDermid & Law, 2024).
- *Qualitative methods* are grounded in real-world practice and focus on understanding the lived experiences, behaviours, perceptions, and contexts of individuals and collectives. Data are commonly gathered using, but not limited to, interviews, observations, research self-reflection, and document analysis. Qualitative methods align to occupational therapy practice as occupational therapists work in a collaborative relationship-focused manner, focusing on exploring and understanding the lived experiences of occupational participation of people (Pepin, 2018). Measures of quality and trustworthiness of a qualitative research are thick description, triangulation, member-checking, collaboration, transferability, and reflexivity (Curtin & Fossey, 2007).
- *Mixed-methods* collects both qualitative and quantitative data to answer a research question or explore a topic in more depth. Creswell and Plano Clark (2018) proposed three mixed-methods research designs:
  - *Sequential explanatory design* involves the initial collection of quantitative data, followed by the collection of qualitative data that is used to explain the quantitative data. After both phases of data collection are completed, data are interpreted.
  - *Sequential exploratory design* involves the initial collection of qualitative data to explore the topic under investigation. Then, based on the qualitative findings, a quantitative project is developed that may, for example, gather data from a larger number of participants. The final step is the integration and explanation of the two data sets.
  - *Convergent design* is when both qualitative and quantitative data are collected simultaneously. Each data set is analysed separately and then compared and combined to identify new information/interpretations.

Traditionally, research *producers* and organisations defined research priorities. Now, an essential aspect of contemporary health research involves genuine consumer

Table 22.2 Research methods, examples of occupational therapy research and findings and World Federation of Occupational Therapy research priority areas

Research method	Brief definition	Example of occupational therapy research	Summary of study
Quantitative			
Umbrella review	Represents one of the highest levels of evidence, gathering evidence from several existing systematic reviews, and allowing easy comparison between them. They address broader questions and may compare interventions and develop practice guidelines.	Giummarra et al. (2022). Interventions for social and community participation for adults with intellectual disability, psychosocial disability or on the autism spectrum: An umbrella systematic review. *Frontiers in Rehabilitation Sciences*, 3, 935473. https://doi.org/10.3389/fresc.2022.935473	Data from 522 studies in 57 eligible systematic reviews (pooled sample = 28,154 study participants) were extracted for narrative synthesis. **Findings:** Social and community participation requires purposeful strategies with meaningful participation preferences with support to build capacity or enable ongoing participation. **WFOT Priority areas 1, 2, 3 and 5**
Systematic review	A critical assessment and combined evaluation of the available evidence (usually RCTs or clinically controlled studies) on a particular assessment or intervention. It is usually focused on a clinical question, and aims to identify, appraise, select, and synthesise all high-quality research evidence relevant to that question.	Bennett, S., et al. (2019). Occupational therapy for people with dementia and their family carers provided at home: A systematic review and meta-analysis. *BMJ open*, 9(11), e026308. https://doi.org/10.1136/bmjopen-2018-026308	Data from 15 clinical trials (pooled sample = 2063 study participants) were extracted for important outcomes including ADL performance and number of behavioural and psychological symptoms (after occupational therapy intervention and at follow-up). **Findings:** Home-based occupational therapy may improve a range of important outcomes for people with dementia and their family carers. **WFOT Priority areas 1, 2, 3, 4 and 5**

(Continued)

Table 22.2 (Continued)

Research method	Brief definition	Example of occupational therapy research	Summary of study
Randomised control trial (RCT)	A planned experiment comparing the effectiveness of an intervention compared to a 'control'. Participants are randomly allocated with groups comparable at baseline. Thus, differences in outcomes after treatment can be attributed to the true effects of the treatment that the experimental group received.	Lockwood, K. J., et al. (2019). Predischarge home visits after hip fracture: A randomized controlled trial. *Clinical Rehabilitation, 33*(4), 681–692. https://doi.org/10.1177/02692155 18823256	This trial randomised 77 adults aged >50 recovering from hip fracture to either pre-discharge home assessment visit vs no visit. **Findings:** Home visits by occupational therapists reduced the number of hospital readmissions, increased functional independence at six months, and potentially reduced the risk of falls in the first 30 days post-discharge. **WFOT Priority areas 1, 2, 3, 5 and 8**
Cohort study	Any group of people who are similar in some way (e.g., have the same condition/ were treated with same therapy) and followed over time. Researchers measure outcomes in a group that were exposed to a specific variable compared to a similar group that has not been exposed. They can be prospective (the researcher collects data at a future date after exposure) or retrospective (the researcher collects data from past records to see if an outcome happened).	Harper, K. J., et al. (2022). An observational cohort study to determine the impact of research capacity building strategies implemented in an Australian metropolitan hospital occupational therapy department. *Australian Occupational Therapy Journal, 69*(2), 190–204. https://doi.org/10.1111/1440-1630.12782	This observational pre–post-cohort study was conducted with hospital occupational therapists to evaluate outcomes of research capacity building toolkit implementation. **Findings:** Improvements at the organisation and team levels; none at an individual level. **WFOT Priority areas 1, 2, 3 and 5**

(*Continued*)

Table 22.2 (Continued)

Research method	Brief definition	Example of occupational therapy research	Summary of study
Single-subject experimental design (SCED)	One participant (or unit, e.g., hospital ward) is studied in an experiment in which the person (or unit) acts as their own control. Measurement of the outcome variables is repeated at different times, to determine whether the outcome has been affected by the intervention.	Tate, R. L., et al. (2020). Evaluating an intervention to increase meaningful activity after severe traumatic brain injury: A single-case experimental design with direct inter-subject and systematic replications. *Neuropsychological Rehabilitation*, 30(4), 641–672. https://doi.org/ 10.1080/09602011.2018 .1488746	This study used a multiple-baseline design to evaluate the Programme for Engagement, Participation and Activities (PEPA) with seven participants with severe traumatic brain injury (impairments: apathy, inability to work, limited leisure/ social activities). **Findings:** PEPA shows promise as an effective intervention to increase non-vocational activity and improve mental health outcomes in this population. **WFOT Priority areas 1, 2, 3 and 5**
Qualitative Grounded theory	Theory is constructed through the analysis of data. Data are the stories told through in-depth interviewing and other collected data. This inductive methodology requires a systematic and objective analysis of peoples' experiences to derive a theoretical framework or model.	White, C., et al. (2020). 'I know what I am doing': A grounded theory investigation into the activities and occupations of adults living with chronic conditions. *Scandinavian Journal of Occupational Therapy*, 27(1), 56–65. https://doi.org/10.1080/1 1038128.2019.1624818	This study investigated the activities and occupations of 16 adults living with chronic conditions. **Findings:** Three two-dimensional categories of meaning from the data: (i) connecting/ reconnecting and disconnecting, (ii) caring and harming, and (iii) contributing and detracting. **WFOT Priority areas 1, 3 and 5**

(Continued)

Table 22.2 (Continued)

Research method	Brief definition	Example of occupational therapy research	Summary of study
Phenomenology	Focus on the way people experience their world, and how best to understand their experiences.	Hoffmann, M., et al. (2022). Exploring stroke survivors' experiences and understandings of occupational therapy. *Scandinavian Journal of Occupational Therapy*, 29(2), 165–174. https://doi.org/10.1080/11038128.2020.1831060	This study explored the experience and understanding of occupational therapy with nine stroke survivors. **Findings:** Both impairment-based and occupation-based therapy were considered valuable. **WFOT Priority areas 1, 2, 3, 4, and 5**
Ethnography	A method for constructing knowledge and understanding about the shared culture and experience of a group of people called 'key informants'.	Haines, C. et al. (2010). Participation in the risk-taking occupation of skateboarding. *Journal of Occupational Science*, 17(4), 239–245. https://doi.org/10.1080/14427591.2010.9686701	This study used in-depth interviews with seven active skateboarders to describe the values, behaviours, beliefs, and attitudes to injury to understand the meaning and identity derived. **Findings:** Core values of freedom and striving to achieve one's best outweigh the risk of injury inherent to skateboarding. **WFOT Priority area 3**
Narrative	Takes the form of an account, over time, of an event or action experienced by a person/group. It draws on multiple data sources and may be a collection of stories that compare lived experience or may shed light on some aspect of the person or identity of the person participating.	Ong, M., Baker, A., Aguilar, A., & Stanley, M. (2019). The meanings attributed to community gardening: A qualitative study. *Health & Place*, 59, 102190. https://doi.org/10.1016/j.healthplace.2019.102190	This narrative inquiry study aimed to understand the meanings attributed to community gardening from an occupational science perspective with eight metropolitan community gardeners. **Findings:** Meanings included community, sharing, growth, therapeutic place, and eco-systems. **WFOT Priority areas 3 and 5**

(Continued)

Table 22.2 (Continued)

Research method	Brief definition	Example of occupational therapy research	Summary of study
Participatory action research (PAR)	PAR involves researchers reflecting on everyday problems, identifying key issues, and forming improvement strategies. They implement these, evaluate changes after some time, and may repeat the cycle for deeper knowledge and evolved practice.	Bennett, S., et al. (2016). Building capacity for knowledge translation in occupational therapy: Learning through participatory action research. *BMC Medical Education*, 16, 1–11. https://doi.org/10.1186/s12909-016-0771-5	This study engaged occupational therapists as co-researchers in a cyclical PAR process to identify barriers and enablers to knowledge translation and implement strategies to build clinicians' capacity. **Findings:** Participants continue to be actively involved in learning and shaping the knowledge translation programme across the department and within their specific clinical areas. **WFOT Priority area 8**

engagement which means that the research is carried out in collaboration with, or by, consumers and is not done to, for, or about them (Cox et al., 2021; Martin & Ward, 2024). Consumer engagement is considered an ethical and moral right and contributes to more relevant and acceptable research, enhancing the quality, integrity, and accountability of research design and findings and better translation and implementation of research findings into practice (Cox et al., 2021; Liddle et al., 2024).

Critiques of the profession by First Nations occupational therapists challenge the profession to decolonise and recognise cultural, historical, and political contexts in which research is conducted (Emery-Whittington, 2025; Gibson, 2020). Thomas et al. (2011) stated that 'for non-Indigenous researchers and occupational therapists, the effects of colonisation in terms of the undermining of Indigenous knowledge are ingrained and unconscious' (p. 12). Research *producers, collaborators, consumers,* and *advocates* are encouraged to take a critical stance and consider how knowledge is produced and how this shapes practice. Taking a critical stance 'can support openness to diverse worldviews [and] avoid enacting colonial agendas that maintain the dominant social order' (Farias, 2025, p. 25).

22.6 Finding the best evidence to answer your occupational therapy practice question

Evidence-based practice (EBP) allows occupational therapists to link research to practice improving care quality, reduce costs, minimise potential harm, increase the satisfaction of clients and families, and increase efficiency (Valera-Gran et al., 2024). Locating and synthesising the scientific evidence requires mastery of a five-step process summarised as ask, acquire, appraise, apply, and assess (Hoffman et al., 2023). The first two steps, ask and acquire, are explained in detail in the following to help students and practitioners to answer occupational therapy questions with precision, conceptual clarity, accuracy, and efficiency.

22.6.1 Finding the best evidence to answer your practice question: ask and acquire

As a practicing therapist, you may also be asked by clients, their families, other professionals, or funding bodies to provide specific evidence of the effectiveness of interventions (Hoffman et al., 2023). Therefore, it is essential that you use the best evidence to answer your question. Evidence can take several forms including your own clinical and professional reasoning, policy documents published by governments, published dissertations and theses, and scientific publications in reputable journals.

22.6.2 Finding the best research evidence: The PICO approach

Considerable skills are required to ask a searchable clinical question that will yield appropriate studies for appraisal. The PICO approach enables you to find the most relevant evidence efficiently and effectively (Eriksen & Frandsen, 2018). PICO is a helpful tool for formulating clinical questions, informing a database search strategy, and guiding evidence-based searches (Schiavenato & Chu, 2021).

Specifically, PICO refers to:

- Patient/Population/Problem: Who are the patients and what are their characteristics, conditions, or diagnoses?
- Intervention/Issue: What intervention, treatment, or clinical issue are you investigating?
- Comparison: If applicable, what alternative intervention or comparison group are you considering? It should be noted that inclusion of the Comparison component of your PICO approach is optional.
- Outcome: What outcomes or findings are you looking for? What is the measurable impact?

22.6.3 The PICO process in action

22.6.3.1 Step 1: Formulate your PICO question

A four-year-old boy who attends the kindergarten programme was recently diagnosed with autism and is presenting with social, fine motor, and sensory processing challenges was referred to you by a local paediatrician. The kindergarten is using a play-based curriculum and has asked that your occupational therapy interventions be provided using this approach if appropriate. Using the PICO format, you construct the following question:

> P: In a 4-year-old boy with autism . . . I: does using a play-based approach to therapy intervention . . . C: compared to traditional Ayres Sensory Intervention methods . . . O: . . . lead to improvements in social, fine motor, and sensory processing skills?

22.6.3.2 Step 2: Plan your search strategy
Plan your search strategy by identifying relevant terms for each of the **P I C O** elements. Now that you have a clear question, it is time to plan your search strategy:

- **Databases:** Determine which databases (e.g., CINAHL, ERIC, PsycInfo, Embase, Scopus, Cochrane, Web of Science) to search.
- **Terms:** Identify relevant terms related to each PICO element. Translate natural language terms into subject descriptors, like medical subject headings (MeSH) or synonyms.
- **Search:** Look for primary sources (original studies), secondary sources (systematic reviews, guidelines), and reviews of research on specific topics (meta-analyses). Grey literature, such as theses, may also be relevant.

22.6.3.3 Step 3: Search for the relevant best evidence
Execute your search using the terms you have identified and the databases you have selected. You will retrieve articles that help you answer the question about utilising play-based approaches for children with autism in kindergarten settings using rigorous evidence.

22.6.3.4 Step 4: Evaluate your search outcomes and implementation outcomes
You may need to revise your PICO question, modify your terms, as you acquire studies, appraise them and apply findings to your clinical question. It is common to refine your search strategy as you sharpen the focus of the research yield.

22.7 Conclusion

This chapter provided an overview of research in the occupational therapy profession, an ever-growing body of evidence that improves the profession's capacity to effectively support individuals and collectives to participate in meaningful and necessary occupations. In this chapter, the global priority research areas that guide our evidence-based profession into the future were presented, and the philosophical underpinnings to contemporary research methods and designs were described and illustrated. Finally, readers were introduced to evidence-based practice principles for *asking* searchable questions and *acquiring* research evidence.

22.8 Summary

- All occupational therapy students and practitioners must be informed research consumers, able to competently appraise evidence and apply it to practice.
- Occupational therapy is an evidence-based profession that generates research knowledge relevant to individuals and populations in practice contexts.
- Occupational therapists often undertake quantitative, qualitative, and mixed methods research that incorporate consumer perspectives, with co-design an increasingly essential element to contemporary research design and dissemination.

22.9 Review and reflection questions

- Explain three ways that qualitative research differs from quantitative research and justify the need for both types of research in the occupational therapy profession.
- What type of research provides occupational therapists with knowledge about lived experience and informs client-centred practice?
- Do new graduate occupational therapists need to be able to evaluate the strengths and limitations of published research that relates to their clients? Explain and justify your answer.

References

Bennett, C., & Mottram, A. (2024). Research priority 6: How can occupational therapy services be more inclusive of mental and physical health. *British Journal of Occupational Therapy*, 87(6), 331–333. https://doi.org/10.1177/0308022623119

Cox, R., Kendall, M., Molineux, M., Miller, E., & Tanner, B. (2021). Consumer engagement in occupational therapy health-related research: A scoping review of the *Australian Occupational Therapy Journal* and a call to action. *Australian Occupational Therapy Journal*, 68(2), 180–192. https://doi.org/10.1111/1440-1630.12704

Creswell, J. W., & Plano Clark, V. L. (2018). *Designing and collecting mixed methods research* (3rd ed.). Sage.

Curtin, M., & Fossey, E. (2007). Appraising the trustworthiness of qualitative studies: Guidelines for occupational therapists. *Australian Occupational Therapy Journal*, 54, 88–94. https://doi.org/10.1111/j.1440-1630.2007.00661.x

Cusick, A., Taylor, R. R., & Kielhofner, G. (2024). Professional responsibility and roles in research. In R. R. Taylor (Ed.), *Kielhofner's research in occupational therapy: Methods of inquiry for enhancing practice* (3rd ed., pp. 92–100). F. A. Davis.

Emery-Whittington, I. (2025). Decoloniality in occupational therapy practice: Preparation and readiness. In M. Curtin, M. Egan, Y. Prior, T. Parnell, R. Galvaan, K. Sauvé-Schenk, & D. Cezar Da Cruz (Eds.), *Occupational therapy for people experiencing illness, injury or impairment: Promoting occupational participation* (8th ed., pp. 2–17). Elsevier.

Eriksen, M. B., & Frandsen, T. F. (2018). The impact of patient, intervention, comparison, outcome (PICO) as a search strategy tool on literature search quality: A systematic review. *Journal of the Medical Library Association: JMLA*, 106(4), 420–431. https://doi.org/10.5195/jmla.2018.345

Farias, L. (2025). Critical perspectives in occupational therapy: Problematising practice to address the socio-political shaping of occupation. In M. Curtin, M. Egan, Y. Prior, T. Parnell, R. Galvaan, K. Sauvé-Schenk, & D. Cezar Da Cruz (Eds.), *Occupational therapy for people experiencing illness, injury or impairment: Promoting occupational participation* (8th ed., pp. 18–28). Elsevier.

Gibson, C. (2020). When the river runs dry: Leadership, decolonisation and healing in occupational therapy. *New Zealand Journal of Occupational Therapy*, 67(1), 11–20. https://doi.org/10.3316/informit.162982618221927

Hoffman, T., Bennett, S., & Del Mar, C. (2023). *Evidence-based practice across the health professions* (4th ed.). Elsevier.

Liddle, J., Redman, B., Frost, D., Worthy, P., Jamieson, P., & Wallace, S. (2024). Inclusive research: Making more impact through accessibility and collaboration. *Australian Occupational Therapy Journal*, 71(5), 641–643. https://doi.org/10.1111/1440-1630.12990

MacDermid, J., & Law, M. (2024). Evaluating the evidence. In M. Law & J. MacDermid (Eds.), *Evidence-based rehabilitation: A guide to practice* (3rd ed., pp. 129–156). Routledge.

Mackenzie, L., Lexén, A., Kaelin, V. C., Hynes, P., Roosen, I., Tam, E., Huang, L.-J., Ye, C.-W., & World Federation of Occupational Therapists (2024). An international study of diversity in occupational therapy research – A bibliographic review of English research literature. *Australian Occupational Therapy Journal, 71*(2), 302–312. https://doi.org/10.1111/1440-1630.12928

Mackenzie, N., & Knipe, S. (2006). Research dilemmas: Paradigms, methods and methodology. *Issues in Educational Research, 16*(2), 193 –205. http://www.iier.org.au/iier16/mackenzie.html

Martin, A. K., & Ward, G. (2024). Refocusing research: A mixed methods study to evaluate utilisation of the top 10 priorities for occupational therapy research in the United Kingdom. *British Journal of Occupational Therapy, 87*(5), 270–280. https://doi.org/10.1177/03080226241228098

Moyers, P. A. (2010). Competence and professional development. In K. Sladyk, K. Jacobs, & N. MacRae (Eds.), *Occupational therapy essentials for clinical competence* (pp. 749–764). Slack Inc.

Occupational Therapy Australia. (2018). *Australian minimum competency standards for new graduate occupational therapists*. Australian Occupational Therapy Board of Australia. https://www.occupationaltherapyboard.gov.au/Codes-Guidelines/Competencies.aspx

Pepin, G. (2018). Reporting rigorous qualitative results: Moving beyond small sample sizes. *Australian Occupational Therapy Journal, 65*(2), 77–78. https://doi.org/10.1111/1440-1630.12475

Sackett, D. L., Rosenberg, W. M., Gray, J. A., Haynes, R. B., & Richardson, W. S. (1996). Evidence-based medicine: What it is and what it isn't. *British Medical Journal, 312*, 71–72. https://doi.org/10.1136/bmj.312.7023.71

Schiavenato, M., & Chu, F. (2021). PICO: What it is and what it is not. *Nurse Education in Practice, 56*, 103194. https://doi.org/10.1016/j.nepr.2021.103194

Taylor, R. (2024). *Kielhofner's Research in occupational therapy: Methods of inquiry for enhancing practice*. Davis.

Thomas, Y., Gray, M., & McGinty, S. (2011). Occupational therapy at the 'cultural interface': Lessons from research with Aboriginal and Torres Strait Islander Australians. *Australian Occupational Therapy Journal, 58*(1), 11–16. https://doi.org/10.1111/j.1440-1630.2010.00917.x

Valera-Gran, D., Campos-Sánchez, I., Prieto-Botella, D., Fernández-Pires, P., Hurtado-Pomares, M., Juárez-Leal, I., & Navarrete-Muñoz, E. M. (2024). Enhancing evidence-based practice into healthcare: Exploring the role of scientific skills in occupational therapists. *Scandinavian Journal of Occupational Therapy, 31*(1), 1–11. https://doi.org/10.1080/11038128.2024.2323205

World Federation of Occupational Therapists, Mackenzie, L., Coppola, S., Alvarez, L., Cibule, L., Maltsev, S., Loh, S. Y., Mlambo, T., Ikiugu, M. N., Pihlar, Z., Sriphetcharawut, S., Baptiste, S., & Ledgerd, R. (2017). International occupational therapy research priorities. *OTJR: Occupation, Participation and Health, 37*(2), 72–81. https://doi.org/10.1177/1539449216687528

Evidence-based practice, knowledge translation, and implementation science in occupational therapy

Liana S. Cahill, Emma J. Schneider, Laura Jolliffe, Anna Joy, and Lauren J. Christie

Authors' positionality statement

As authors of this chapter, we acknowledge our shared positionality as five female, white Australian occupational therapists. Our perspectives are shaped by professional and cultural experiences in Australian healthcare and academic systems, influencing our views of evidence-based practice, knowledge translation, and implementation science. We recognise our backgrounds bring inherent biases and may not reflect the diversity of global occupational therapy. We acknowledge the importance of Indigenous knowledge systems, experiential knowledge, and non-Western frameworks that may not align with traditional evidence hierarchies.

Key terms
- Evidence-based practice
- Evidence appraisal
- Knowledge translation
- Implementation science
- Barriers and enablers
- Behaviour change

Objectives
This chapter will allow the reader to:

- Understand the process of appraising evidence in the context of knowledge translation
- Define key terms related to knowledge translation, being aware of international differences
- Recognise common barriers and facilitators to knowledge translation and their impact on practice

DOI: 10.4324/9781003495666-25

- Describe implementation science theories and implementation strategies used in occupational therapy practice
- Understand the concept of de-implementation and explain its importance in reducing ineffective practices in occupational therapy

23.1 Introduction

One of the greatest challenges for the occupational therapy profession is integrating evidence into practice. When evidence isn't used, clients are at risk of receiving outdated or ineffective therapy, which can slow their progress and negatively impact outcomes. Evidence-based practice (EBP) is a problem-based framework that uses best available research to guide collaborative decision-making between occupational therapists and clients (Hoffman et al., 2023). EBP brings together four components, outlined in Figure 23.1.

As highlighted in the previous chapter, EBP involves not only locating research evidence but also valuing and using education, skills, and experience to apply that evidence (Hoffman et al., 2023). This chapter focuses on the last three steps of EBP, appraise, apply, and assess. Once a clinical question is posed and relevant evidence located, the quality, relevance, and usefulness of that evidence needs to be determined. This stage of evidence appraisal is important, as it determines the next step of active knowledge translation, underpinned by implementation science.

Unfortunately, research evidence is often not used in practice, and there are widespread evidence-practice gaps in occupational therapy and healthcare more broadly. An evidence-practice gap is the difference (or divide) between what research recommends and how healthcare is currently delivered. The time taken to narrow these gaps

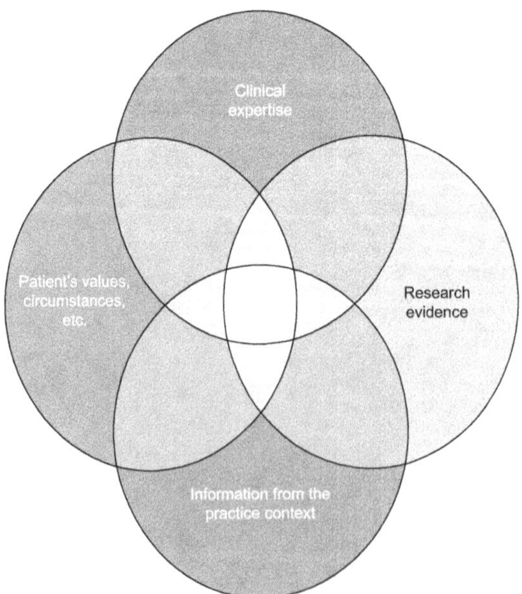

Figure 23.1 The four contributing sources of evidence-based practice

(Hoffman et al., 2023)

is significant, with research suggesting it takes 17–20 years for new research to change client care (Morris et al., 2011).

The relationship between EBP and knowledge translation is intertwined and complementary. The concept of 'bridging the gap' is often used in knowledge translation and this metaphor also emphasises a two-way interaction; while evidence flows from research to practice, feedback from occupational therapists and clients guides future research. EBP relies on active processes of knowledge translation to ensure evidence reaches therapists and is used with clients. In this way EBP provides a framework for applying evidence while knowledge translation is the vehicle that drives this practice change.

This chapter describes the evidence-appraisal stage of EBP, explores knowledge translation and implementation science and demonstrates how knowledge translation theory applies to real-world occupational therapy practice.

23.2 Appraising evidence for implementation

Occupational therapists are professionally responsible for providing safe, effective healthcare informed by high-quality research that is applicable to the client population or organisation (Occupational Therapy Australia, 2018). As new evidence emerges, occupational therapists must continuously adapt their practice in response. But how do you know if the research is 'the best available' or the 'most suitable' for your client, programme, population, or organisation? From the available research, you must decide what is relevant to you as the therapist (your own knowledge, skills, experience, and context), the client (goals, preferences, and expectations) as well as the strength or quality of the research design and methods to determine if the findings may guide clinical care (Hoffman et al., 2023). This evaluative process is a core element of EBP and is referred to as critically appraising research evidence.

23.2.1 Importance and criteria for critically appraising research

Critically appraising research is the systematic process of examining the trustworthiness (internal validity) and relevance (applicability) of published work to determine its strengths and weaknesses (Hoffman et al., 2023). This process involves careful consideration of the results (findings and what they mean) and how they apply to a particular context or setting (impact) (Hoffman et al., 2023; OT Australia, 2018).

Not all evidence is created equally. Differences in study design, methodology, and potential biases affect the strength and applicability of study findings (See Chapter 22, 'Research in Occupational Therapy'). For example, a qualitative study describing the lived experience of returning to work after stroke cannot explain the cause of perceived challenges, nor will the findings be applicable to people with hip replacements. The study findings, however, are still valuable, as they can inform evidence-based practice, with a particular emphasis on the experiences clients may face in their return to work after stroke. While this process may seem subjective, evaluating research quality involves asking: (1) Is the methodology appropriate for the research question, and do I trust the findings (e.g. study design and risk of bias)? (2) Do I have confidence in the results and their meaning (e.g. appropriate outcome measures, significance and clinical relevance of the findings)? And (3) Do I believe the study conclusions, implications, and limitations, and are they reasonable given the method and sample size?

These study elements are considered collectively to select high-quality research based on three criteria: internal validity, impact, and applicability. *Internal validity* assesses the trustworthiness of the research, determining whether findings are credible. *Impact* examines the significance and importance of the results, while *applicability* considers the relevance and practical use of research in real-world contexts.

23.3 Tools and frameworks for evaluating evidence

There are several tools and frameworks available for evaluating evidence that can be used by occupational therapists. See Table 23.1 for examples. The selection of tools or frameworks is determined by the study design, for example, risk of bias (RoB) tools for randomised trials. If the evidence source doesn't align with these research methods, for example a professional education session or conversation with a colleague, appraisal is still necessary and the EBP framework outlined by Hoffman and colleagues (2023) can guide this process.

23.4 The role and value of clinical practice guidelines

Clinical practice guidelines synthesise evidence to support informed decision-making between occupational therapists and clients. Guidelines exist for common health conditions such as cancer, hip fracture, dementia and traumatic brain injury and the Guidelines International Network (https://g-i-n.net/) provides a searchable global

Table 23.1 Resources for appraising evidence

Name of resource	Source	Description
Critical Appraisal Skills Programme (CASP)	CASP Website https://casp-uk.net/	■ Provides free critical appraisal checklists you can use when reading different types of studies (e.g. systematic reviews, randomised trials, or qualitative studies)
Cochrane Risk of Bias Tool (RoB 2)	Cochrane Library https://methods.cochrane. org/risk-bias-2	■ A specific resource to measure the risk of bias in randomised trials
Grading of Recommendations, Assessment, Development and Evaluations (GRADE)	GRADE Working Group https://www.gradeworking group.org/	■ A guide to assess the certainty of evidence and strength of recommendations in systematic reviews and practice guidelines
A MeaSurement Tool to Assess Systematic Reviews (AMSTAR 2)	AMSTAR Website https://amstar.ca/	■ Includes an online checklist with a guide to evaluate the quality of the methods used in a systematic review
Consensus-based Standards for the selection of health Measurement Instruments (COSMIN)	COSMIN Website https://www.cosmin.nl/	■ Provides tools to evaluate the quality of studies on measurement properties of patient-reported outcomes

Table 23.2 Resources for translating knowledge to practice

Name of resource	Source	Description
Theory Comparison and Selection Tool (T-CAST)	T-CAST website https://impsci.tracs.unc.edu/tcast/	■ A site to help choose the most appropriate theoretical approach to use for your knowledge translation project
United States National Institute of Health (NIH) Resources for Implementation Science Researchers	NIH website https://www.fic.nih.gov/About/center-global-health-studies/neuroscience-implementation-toolkit/Pages/resources.aspx	■ A curated collection of tools, training modules, and frameworks to support the use of implementation science methods and approaches
National Centre of Implementation Science (NCOIS)	NCOIS website https://ncois.org.au/resources/	■ An expansive suite of resources to support implementation including tools, guides, webinars, publications, and factsheets
Maridulu Budyari Gumal; Sydney Partnership for Health, Education, Research and Enterprise (SPHERE)	SPHERE website https://www.thesphere.com.au/platforms/implementation-science/	■ An Implementation Science Collaborative connecting implementation scientists, clinicians, and leaders to promote knowledge exchange and provide tools to integrate evidence into practice
The University of Washington Implementation Science Resource Hub	Resource Hub Website https://impsciuw.org/	■ A hub for educational resources for implementation science (articles, videos, guides) and research support (step-by-step pathways for designing research)

registry. A key benefit of guidelines is reducing the workload of busy clinicians and/or clinicians who are still developing evidence appraisal skills. While guidelines may not always reflect the latest research, some guidelines, such as the 'Living' Stroke Guidelines in Australia and New Zealand (Stroke Foundation, 2025), are continuously updated. Additionally, some guidelines provide accompanying toolkits for translating guidelines to practice, such as those for dementia (https://cdpc.sydney.edu.au/research/clinical-guidelines-for-dementia/). These translation toolkits can be adapted for use in other practice areas.

23.5 Applying evidence: knowledge translation

Knowledge translation (KT) is a dynamic and iterative process of using and integrating research to accelerate improvements in the health outcomes of clients, health services, and systems (CIHR, 2015). Knowledge translation seeks to reduce the time lag in the application of evidence to everyday practice, ensuring clients receive the most appropriate, effective, and up-to-date care (Graham et al., 2006).

23.5.1 Terms used in knowledge translation

There are many terms used internationally to describe the process of translating knowledge to practice (research utilisation, knowledge exchange, diffusion and dissemination), and all have slightly different meanings. In Canada, Australia, and New Zealand, the terms knowledge translation or research translation are preferred, while knowledge transfer or dissemination are often used in the United States. Knowledge translation can be conceptualised on a diffusion-dissemination-implementation continuum (Graham et al., 2006).

- **Diffusion**
  Diffusion is the passive, unplanned dispersal of new practices that is unlikely to achieve knowledge translation in isolation.
- **Dissemination**
  Dissemination is the targeted distribution of new practices to key stakeholders (e.g. decision-makers, policymakers and healthcare consumers) using methods such as workshops, social media, and publications. The approach differs depending on the target audience.
- **Implementation**
  Implementation is the active integration of research in clinical practice, requiring behaviour change at individual therapist, organisation, and policy levels. Behaviour change is the key intention of knowledge translation, and this approach increases the likelihood of sustained evidence-based practice compared to passive approaches.

A useful introductory guide for knowledge translation is the Knowledge-to-Action (KTA) Framework (Graham et al., 2006) (Figure 23.2). This framework provides a structured yet flexible approach with two components: *knowledge creation*, represented by a central funnel, and an *action cycle*, represented by outer circular steps. The bidirectional arrows highlight the iterative nature of the process. The framework emphasises the importance of understanding and addressing barriers and facilitators for use of research in practice.

See Table 23.2 for freely available sources to guide knowledge translation.

23.6 Barriers and facilitators to knowledge translation in occupational therapy

Barriers and facilitators (sometimes called enablers) are important determinants of practice and can influence the success of knowledge translation. Barriers are obstacles that may prevent the adoption of evidence, while facilitators support and advance knowledge translation, enabling a smoother translation of evidence to practice. By identifying these factors, occupational therapists are better positioned to address the gap between research and practice. Though they vary by context, common barriers and facilitators, at individual, organisational, and health system levels, have been identified (Kinney et al., 2023).

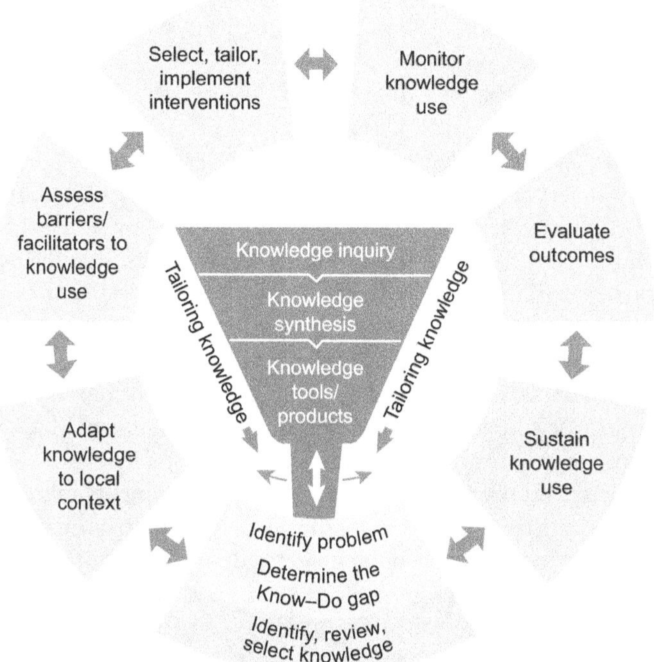

Figure 23.2 The Knowledge-to-Action Framework
(Graham et al., 2006)

Barriers to knowledge translation can include:

- Lack of therapist knowledge or skill related to evidence-based therapy
- Lack of equipment or resources to provide therapy
- Competing demands of healthcare professionals
- High staff turnover disrupting continuity of practice change
- Resistance from senior staff or managers to change established work practices

Facilitators to knowledge translation can include:

- Mentorship from experienced evidence-based therapists
- Peer encouragement and role modelling from colleagues (clinical champions)
- Organisational support for accessing high-quality research materials

Effective knowledge translation depends on identifying and addressing barriers and facilitators and drawing on principles of implementation science to promote practice change. The science of Implementation will be discussed in the following.

23.7 An introduction to implementation science

Implementation science is defined as 'the study of methods to promote the systematic uptake of research findings and other evidence-based practices into routine practice, and, hence, to improve the quality and effectiveness of health services and care' (Eccles

& Mittman, 2006, p. 1). At its core, implementation science aims to understand and address factors that influence adoption and integration of evidence-based practices within complex healthcare systems.

Unlike traditional approaches that often relied on the ISLAGIATT principle: 'it seemed like a good idea at the time' (Michie et al., 2014, p. 14), modern implementation science emphasises the importance of diagnosing barriers to change. Implementation efforts based on intuition or trial-and-error often fail by overlooking critical contextual factors or root causes of issues (May et al., 2016). By contrast, diagnosing an implementation problem involves identifying underlying factors, such as organisational readiness, resource availability, or staff attitudes. A crucial element of implementation science is its pragmatic nature, it recognises that context is critical and discourages a one-size-fits-all or formulaic approach. Every healthcare setting is different in terms of resources, staff expertise, culture, and patient populations, making it essential to tailor strategies to local circumstances. Addressing these contextual factors increases the likelihood of successful, sustainable practice change.

Theories, models, and frameworks are foundational elements in implementation science. They add structure and rigour to the field by underpinning the methods and approaches used to systematically implement evidence-based practices. However, the terminology itself, often used interchangeably, can add complexity, making it difficult to navigate the nuances between theories, models, and frameworks (Nilsen, 2015).

The challenge of selecting a theory, model, or framework to inform your implementation approach is compounded by the sheer number of options. In healthcare alone, there are over 140 different frameworks and models available (Wang et al., 2023), making it difficult to determine which approach is most relevant for a specific problem or context. Despite this overwhelming variety, these theories, models, and frameworks can generally be grouped into five broad categories: those that *guide* the implementation process, *identify* barriers and enablers, *develop* tailored implementation strategies, *assess* the impact and fidelity of implementation efforts, and *sustain* long-term outcomes.

1. **Guiding the Implementation Process:** Frameworks like the Knowledge-to-Action (KTA) Framework (Figure 23.2) or Normalisation Process Theory (NPT) outline a structured series of steps to plan, implement, and sustain change. These provide a roadmap for integrating evidence-based practices into routine practice, ensuring a systematic and organised approach.

2. **Identifying Barriers and Enablers:** Models such as the Capability, Opportunity, Motivation-Behaviour (COM-B) Model (West & Michie, 2020), the Theoretical Domains Framework (TDF) (Cane et al., 2012), and the Consolidated Framework for Implementation Research (CFIR) (Damschroder et al., 2022) help diagnose factors that affect implementation. These are used to identify key barriers and facilitators, whether they are related to individual behaviours, organisational culture, or broader system (or fiscal) constraints.

3. **Developing Implementation Strategies:** Frameworks like the Behaviour Change Wheel (BCW) (Michie et al., 2011) and the Affordability, Practicability, Effectiveness, Acceptability, Side-effects, and Equity (APEASE) criteria (Michie et al., 2011) and resources like the Expert Recommendations for Implementing

Change (ERIC) (Powell et al., 2015) assist in designing targeted strategies to address identified barriers. They offer structured guidance and reasoning on selecting implementation strategies that are relevant for the specific context, enhancing the likelihood of successful implementation. For example, The Care of People with dementia in their Environments (COPE) programme, delivered by occupational therapists and nurses, was implemented in Australia using the Behaviour Change Wheel to address barriers and enablers (Clemson et al., 2021).

4. **Assessing and Evaluating Implementation:** Evaluation frameworks, such as RE-AIM (https://re-aim.org/) focus on measuring different aspects of implementation, including reach to the target population, effectiveness of the intervention, adoption of the intervention by staff and systems into practice, implementation costs, consistency of delivery and adaptations made to the intervention, and long-term maintenance. These frameworks ensure that implementation efforts are evaluated comprehensively, providing insights into both the immediate impact and the sustainability of changes over time. For example, the RE-AIM framework was used to evaluate the implementation of an interdisciplinary goal-setting package in rehabilitation services in Queensland, Australia (Baker et al., 2024).

5. **Sustaining Implementation:** Sustainability frameworks emphasise the importance of ensuring that evidence-based practices remain effective and embedded over time. The Dynamic Sustainability Framework (DSF) (Chambers et al., 2013) highlights continuous learning and adaptation, advocating for interventions to evolve with changes in the environment, organisational structures, and stakeholder needs. Similarly, the Iowa Implementation for Sustainability Framework (Cullen et al., 2022) outlines practical strategies to integrate practices by aligning interventions with organisational priorities, engaging stakeholders, and building capacity through resources and training.

Selecting an appropriate model, theory or framework can be challenging, but practical tools like the Theory Comparison and Selection Tool (T-CaST) (Birken et al., 2018) and online resources can help (refer to Table 23.2). While theories, models, and frameworks guide all stages of implementation, from planning to sustaining outcomes, this section focuses on implementation interventions and strategies, which are the most practical and actionable for therapists.

An implementation intervention involves specific actions to promote the adoption of evidence-based practices. Examples include education and training sessions, audit and feedback, the use of clinical champions to drive change, and use of reminder systems to reinforce new behaviours. Intervention should be tailored to the unique context and challenges of the setting or population, guided by frameworks mentioned earlier. This ensures that the intervention addresses the specific barriers and leverages the enablers present in the environment.

An implementation strategy is a coordinated approach that combines multiple interventions to work synergistically. Whilst there is conflicting evidence regarding the effectiveness of using single component versus multifaceted interventions (Squires et al., 2014), strategies focused on action, education, and monitoring of behaviour are more likely to be successful than passive methods, such as one-off education or simple dissemination (such as sharing of clinical guidelines) alone (Johnson & May, 2015).

For example, pairing educational sessions with audit and feedback, or engaging clinical champions alongside reminders, may drive more substantial and sustained behaviour change (Goorts et al., 2021).

Selecting appropriate interventions for a cohesive implementation strategy should be systematically guided by a framework. For instance, the Behaviour Change Wheel (BCW) and the APEASE criteria provide structured ways to design and justify intervention choices. Additionally, the Cochrane Effective Practice and Organisation of Care (EPOC) taxonomy offers a comprehensive framework of strategies to improve healthcare delivery (Cochrane Effective Practice and Organisation of Care (EPOC), 2015), helping therapists identify effective strategies based on specific goals. For example, in settings with significant knowledge gaps, educational workshops, or feedback mechanisms may be prioritised to standardise practices.

Similarly, the Expert Recommendations for Implementing Change (ERIC) offers a list of 73 strategies developed through expert consensus (Powell et al., 2015). ERIC provides a practical toolkit for addressing barriers, suggesting interventions such as conducting needs assessments, engaging key stakeholders, and providing ongoing support to maintain change. ERIC can be used alongside the EPOC taxonomy, allowing for a tailored and refined approach that fits the particular needs of the organisation or population.

Different healthcare settings face distinct challenges, influenced by factors like resource availability, staff capacity, and population characteristics. For example, a training programme that succeeds in a well-resourced urban hospital may not be effective in a rural clinic with limited resources. Tailoring strategies to the local environment ensures that interventions are culturally relevant, practically achievable, and more likely to be sustained over time. For example, Stepping On, a community-based falls prevention programme developed by Australian occupational therapists was adapted for implementation in the USA (Mahoney et al., 2020), with changes to group leader training and fidelity monitoring.

Another developing area of implementation science is de-implementation. De-implementation is the abandonment or discontinuation of practices that have been found to be ineffective or harmful (Prasad & Ioannidis, 2014). De-implementation of low-value practices is important, given that health resources are finite. Discontinuing practices that are ineffective or harmful can free up therapist time and valuable resources to deliver evidence-based interventions and contribute to improved patient outcomes.

23.8 Evaluation and sustaining implementation efforts

Evaluation and sustainability are essential components of implementation science, ensuring that evidence-based practices are not only adopted but also maintained effectively over time. Evaluation provides a systematic way to measure the success of implementation efforts, while sustainability frameworks ensure that these efforts remain integrated into routine practice and continue to deliver intended outcomes.

Evaluation focuses on three broad aspects: readiness, fidelity, and outcomes. Assessing readiness for change is a foundational step in implementation, helping organisations understand their capacity to adopt new practices. Tools like the Organisational Readiness for Change Assessment (ORCA) evaluate leadership support, staff engagement, and resource availability, providing a clear picture of preparedness (Helfrich et al., 2009). Fidelity may be assessed through process evaluation, which examines whether the intervention is delivered as it was intended while outcome evaluation measures the intervention's impact on predefined goals, such as client outcomes, staff behaviours, or system efficiency. Frameworks like RE-AIM (https://re-aim.org/) support comprehensive evaluation across these domains.

Sustaining change over time is inherently challenging, and evidence on the most effective strategies for achieving sustainability in healthcare continues to evolve. Currently, sustainment of evidence-based interventions is often inconsistently defined and reported (Hailemariam et al., 2019). Successful sustainability requires a proactive approach that adapts to evolving organisational needs and environments. Frameworks like the Dynamic Sustainability Framework (DSF) (Chambers et al., 2013) and Iowa Implementation for Sustainability Framework (Cullen et al., 2022) emphasise continuous learning, stakeholder engagement, and capacity building through ongoing support and training (see Box 23.1). Strategies to sustain evidence-based interventions include continued training for new staff to maintain skills, booster training sessions for existing staff, supervision, feedback, and ongoing organisational leadership support (Hailemariam et al., 2019).

Box 23.1

Applying research appraisal, knowledge translation, and implementation science in occupational therapy

Setting: You are a new graduate occupational therapist in a regional community rehabilitation service. You are working with Lee, a 43-year-old recovering from a left middle cerebral artery stroke. While Lee has achieved some of their goals for transition home, they are now focused on improving their upper limb activity to return to work as a carpenter. After several weekly 45–60-minute outpatient sessions with Lee, you notice slower-than-expected progress and begin questioning the amount of therapy needed to impact occupational performance.

Step 1. Identify the problem and investigate the evidence

You suspect that having only one weekly therapy session may be limiting Lee's progress, prompting critical appraisal of the evidence. Using the Knowledge-to-Action (KTA) Framework (Figure 23.2), you consult the Australian and New Zealand Guidelines for Stroke Management (https://informme.org.au/guidelines/living-clinical-guidelines-for-stroke-management), which recommend maximising scheduled therapy and using circuit class therapy (Stroke Foundation, 2025). Additional guidance includes a weak recommendation and a good practice statement supporting use of homework (self-practice), involvement of family and friends (semi-supervised practice), and aiming for a minimum of three hours of daily practice (Stroke Foundation, 2025). You critically appraise these recommendations by considering:

- The strength of the evidence (e.g., systematic reviews and randomised trials that underpin this guideline recommendation).
- Relevance to Lee's case (e.g., their stage of recovery and occupational goals).
- Feasibility in your practice setting (e.g., available time, resources, and equipment).

You reflect on the evidence and discuss this with Lee to explore how the recommendations align with their goals, preferences, and current circumstances. Lee expresses motivation and willingness to attend more therapy sessions if available.

You then meet with your clinical supervisor to address the identified 'know-do' gap and explore how additional therapy could fit within your caseload and workplace arrangements. Your supervisor notes that other stroke survivors may also be receiving insufficient upper limb therapy. Together, you conduct a spot audit of medical records of the last 20 stroke survivors, revealing consistent one-hour sessions with unclear practice intensity and no self-practice programmes (homework). You also gather feedback from stroke survivors about their therapy experiences and outcomes.

A decision is made, with Lee and with your supervisor, to focus a knowledge translation project on increasing therapy intensity.

Step 2. Identify barriers and facilitators

Using the COM-B model and the Theoretical Domains Framework (TDF), you assess barriers and facilitators through a structured discussion and brief survey in a therapy department meeting. You find:

- Your colleagues feel they lack time to deliver more than one therapy session per week with clients (Barrier – Lack of time; COM-B Opportunity – Physical)
- There are limited rehabilitation resources, such as specialised equipment or standardised protocols (Barrier – Lack of resources; COM-B Opportunity – Physical)
- Your colleagues value evidence-based practice and are motivated to provide high-quality care (Enabler – Supportive culture; COM-B Motivation – Reflective)
- Clients of the service are generally highly engaged and mostly committed to achieving their occupational goals (Enabler – Client attitudes, COM-B Motivation – Reflective)

Step 3. Develop tailored implementation strategies

Using the Theoretical Domains Framework and Behaviour Change Wheel, you design a multi-faceted implementation plan tailored to your regional context and considering barriers and enablers:

1. Education and Training
   A workshop is planned for occupational therapists, physiotherapists, and allied health assistants on evidence-based stroke rehabilitation, intensity principles, and structuring task-specific group and self-practice programmes. Interactive methods such as case discussions, role-playing, and problem-solving activities are designed. Lee is invited and wants to participate.
2. Environment Restructuring
   A small community grant is sought to purchase affordable therapy equipment. Due to the distances stroke survivors need to travel to attend therapy, an online group class is introduced to run alternatively with in-person therapy. A therapy manual is developed with occupation-based upper limb tasks and independent practice activities.

3. Audit and Feedback
   With Lee's involvement, a record sheet is created to track each stroke survivor's therapy time and independent practice, with feedback provided to stroke survivors, therapists, and allied health assistants.

Step 4. Implement the strategies

You implement the strategies from Step 3. and conduct a Plan-Do-Study-Act (PDSA) cycle.

Plan: You outline objectives, timelines, and responsibilities, for example, scheduling the workshop, developing therapy manuals, and identifying equipment needs.
Do: Execute the plan, beginning with interactive workshops and introducing self-practice templates to clients like Lee.
Study: Gather feedback from therapists and clients to assess feasibility and acceptability of strategies.
Act: Refine interventions based on feedback received.

Step 5. Measure and evaluate change

You assess the impact and fidelity of implementation efforts using elements of the RE-AIM framework (https://re-aim.org/). A repeat audit is conducted at three months to track progress. You measure Reach, the proportion of suitable clients completing an independent upper limb practice programme; Adoption, the number of upper limb groups run; and Efficacy, changes in client outcomes.

To sustain practice change, the team plan to remain open to new evidence and set a date to review the policy. They consider how to maintain: knowledge (i.e. runing an education session every six months to accommodate new staff), resources (i.e. allocating staff to equipment audits and monitoring monthly), and skills (i.e. through supervision and nomination of clinical champions).

23.9 Conclusion

Translating evidence to practice is an active process that can improve client outcomes. Translating evidence into real-world practice settings is not easy; however, using a structured knowledge translation process can increase the effectiveness of practice change efforts. Implementation science supports this process by offering theoretical frameworks and strategies to understand the complexities of changing behaviour at individual, team, and organisational levels. Evidence-based practice is not a once-off event but an ongoing commitment to improve the quality of care for and with clients. Using evidence-based approaches and actively using knowledge translation strategies not only advances the occupational therapy profession but, most importantly, improves the lives of the clients we work with.

23.10 Summary

This chapter has introduced the interconnected concepts of evidence-based practice, knowledge translation, and implementation science, highlighting their relevance to occupational therapy. The chapter outlined how evidence-based practice involves integrating research evidence with clinical expertise and client values. Knowledge translation was presented as the dynamic, context-specific process of moving evidence into everyday practice. Implementation science was highlighted as offering structured methods and theory to support the adoption and sustainability of evidence-informed interventions in real-world settings.

As a summary of this chapter, Box 23.2 provides key tips to support knowledge translation in practice.

Box 23.2
Top 10 tips for implementing knowledge to practice in occupational therapy

1. **Understand the Evidence and Gap**
   Begin by thoroughly understanding the evidence and identify the size of the evidence-practice gap through audits, observations, and team and client discussions.

2. **Be Guided by Theory**
   In knowledge translation, theories are practical and useful. Consider approaches like the Knowledge-to-Action (KTA) Framework or Theoretical Domains Framework (TDF) to guide your process.

3. **Identify Barriers and Facilitators**
   Explore barriers and facilitators to change using tools like surveys, team discussions, or observations. This minimises the risk on wasted efforts on ineffective strategies.

4. **Tailor to your Context**
   Adapt and change interventions to fit your unique context, client demographics and available resources.

5. **Engage Stakeholders**
   Collaborate with key people, clients, colleagues, and managers, early and often. Their input and support are crucial for successful implementation.

6. **Use Practical Tools**
   Use freely available tools such as Expert Recommendations for Implementing Change (ERIC) or the Behaviour Change Wheel to design and support your strategies.

7. **Measure Process and Outcomes**
   Track both the implementation process (e.g. fidelity to the intervention) and its outcomes (e.g. effectiveness) to ensure your efforts have impact.

8. **Use Feedback Loops**
   Incorporate regular points of feedback to identify what's working, address challenges, and refine your approach over time.

9. **Support Sustainability**
   Advocate for policies, procedures, and practices that embed the new practice into routine work for long-term impact.

10. **Reflect and Develop**
    Reflect on your experiences in implementation, what worked and what didn't, to strengthen your knowledge translation skills and inform future efforts.

23.11 Review and reflection questions

- What are two tools that can help you evaluate the credibility and applicability of a research study's results to your clinical practice?
- What are some common barriers to effective knowledge translation in occupational therapy, and how can they be addressed?
- Reflecting on a recent clinical experience or case study, how could the Knowledge-to-Action framework have been used to enhance client outcomes?
- What is de-implementation, and why is it an important concept for occupational therapists striving to provide evidence-based care?

References

Baker, A., Cornwell, P., Gustafsson, L., & Lannin, N. A. (2024). Implementing a tailored, co-designed goal-setting implementation package in rehabilitation services: A process evaluation. *Disability and Rehabilitation, 46*(14), 3116–3127. https://doi.org/10.1080/096 38288.2023.2243589

Birken, S. A., Rohweder, C. L., Powell, B. J., Shea, C. M., Scott, J., Leeman, J., Grewe, M. E., Kirk, M. A., Damschroder, L., Aldridge, W. A., Haines, E. R., Straus, S., & Presseau, J. (2018). T-CaST: An implementation theory comparison and selection tool. *Implementation Science, 13*(143). https://doi.org/10.1186/s13012-018-0836-4

Canadian Institutes of Health Research. (2015). *Guide to knowledge translation planning at CIHR: Integrated and end-of-grant approaches.* CIHR, Government of Canada. https:// cihr-irsc.gc.ca/e/45321.html

Cane, J., O'Connor, D., & Michie, S. (2012). Validation of the theoretical domains framework for use in behaviour change and implementation research. *Implementation Science, 7*(1). https://doi.org/10.1186/1748-5908-7-37

Chambers, D. A., Glasgow, R. E., & Stange, K. C. (2013). The dynamic sustainability framework: Addressing the paradox of sustainment amid ongoing change. *Implementation Science, 8*(117). https://doi.org/10.1186/1748-5908-8-117

Clemson, L., Laver, K., Rahja, M., Culph, J., Scanlan, J. N., Day, S., Comans, T., Jeon, Y. H., Low, L. F., Crotty, M., Kurrle, S., Cations, M., Piersol, C. V., & Gitlin, L. N. (2021). Implementing a reablement intervention, 'Care of People with Dementia in their Environments (COPE)': A hybrid implementation-effectiveness study. *The Gerontologist, 61*(6), 965–976. https://doi.org/10.1093/geront/gnaa105

Cochrane Effective Practice and Organisation of Care (EPOC). (2015). *EPOC taxonomy.* Retrieved December 18, 2024, from epoc.cochrane.org/epoc-taxonomy

Cullen, L., Hanrahan, K., Edmonds, S. W., Reisinger, H. S., & Wagner, M. (2022). Iowa implementation for sustainability framework. *Implementation Science, 17*(1). https://doi. org/10.1186/s13012-021-01157-5

Damschroder, L. J., Reardon, C. M., Widerquist, M. A. O., et al. (2022). The updated consolidated framework for implementation research based on user feedback. *Implementation Science, 17*(75). https://doi.org/10.1186/s13012-022-01245-0

Eccles, M. P., & Mittman, B. S. (2006). Welcome to implementation science. *Implementation Science, 1*(1). https://doi.org/10.1186/1748-5908-1-1

Goorts, K., Dizon, J., & Milanese, S. (2021). The effectiveness of implementation strategies for promoting evidence informed interventions in allied healthcare: A systematic review. *BMC Health Services Research, 21*(1), 241. https://doi.org/10.1186/s12913-021-06190-0

Graham, I. D., Logan, J., Harrison, M. B., Straus, S. E., Tetroe, J., Caswell, W., & Robinson, N. (2006). Lost in knowledge translation: Time for a map? *The Journal of Continuing Education in the Health Professions, 26*(1), 13–24. https://doi.org/10.1002/ chp.47

Hailemariam, M., Bustos, T., Montgomery, B., Barajas, R., Evans, L. B., & Drahota, A. (2019). Evidence-based intervention sustainability strategies: A systematic review. *Implementation Science, 14*(57). https://doi.org/10.1186/s13012-019-0910-6

Helfrich, C. D., Li, Y.-F., Sharp, N. D., & Sales, A. E. (2009). Organizational readiness to change assessment (ORCA): Development of an instrument based on the Promoting Action on Research in Health Services (PARIHS) framework. *Implementation Science, 4*(38). https://doi.org/10.1186/1748-5908-4-38

Hoffman, T., Bennett, S., & Del Mar, C. (2023). Introduction to evidence-based practice. In T. Hoffman, S. Bennett, & C. Del Mar (Eds.), *Evidence based practice across the health professions* (4th ed., pp. 1–13). Elsevier Health Sciences.

Johnson, M. J., & May, C. R. (2015). Promoting professional behaviour change in healthcare: What interventions work, and why? A theory-led overview of systematic reviews. *BMJ Open, 5*(9), e008592. https://doi.org/10.1136/bmjopen-2015-008592

Kinney, A. R., Stearns-Yoder, K. A., Hoffberg, A. S., Middleton, A., Weaver, J. A., Roseen, E. J., & Brenner, L. A. (2023). Barriers and facilitators to the adoption of evidence-based interventions for adults within occupational and physical therapy practice settings: A systematic review. *Archives of Physical Medicine and Rehabilitation, 104*(7), 1132–1151. https://doi.org/10.1016/j.apmr.2023.03.005

Mahoney, J. E., Gangnon, R., Clemson, L., Jaros, L., Cech, S., & Renken, J. (2020). Outcomes associated with scale-up of the Stepping On falls prevention program: A case study in redesigning for dissemination. *Journal of Clinical and Translational Science, 4*(3), 250–259. https://doi.org/10.1017/cts.2020.17

May, C. R., Johnson, M., & Finch, T. (2016). Implementation, context and complexity. *Implementation Science, 11*(141). https://doi.org/10.1186/s13012-016-0506-3

Michie, S., Atkins, L., & West, R. (2014). The behaviour change wheel. In *A guide to designing interventions*. Silveback Publishing.

Michie, S., van Stralen, M. M., & West, R. (2011). The behaviour change wheel: A new method for characterising and designing behaviour change interventions. *Implementation Science, 6*(42). https://doi.org/10.1186/1748-5908-6-42

Morris, Z. S., Wooding, S., & Grant, J. (2011). The answer is 17 years, what is the question: Understanding time lags in translational research. *Journal of the Royal Society of Medicine, 104*(12), 510–520. https://doi.org/10.1258/jrsm.2011.110180

Nilsen, P. (2015). Making sense of implementation theories, models and frameworks. *Implementation Science, 10*(1), 53. https://doi.org/10.1186/s13012-015-0242-0

Occupational Therapy Australia. (2018). *Evidence-based practice position statement.* ebpposition statement.pdf

Powell, B. J., Waltz, T. J., Chinman, M. J., Damschroder, L. J., Smith, J. L., Matthieu, M. M., Proctor, E. K., & Kirchner, J. E. (2015). A refined compilation of implementation strategies: Results from the Expert Recommendations for Implementing Change (ERIC) project. *Implementation Science, 10*, 21. https://doi.org/10.1186/s13012-015-0209-1

Prasad, V., & Ioannidis, J. P. (2014). Evidence-based de-implementation for contradicted, unproven, and aspiring healthcare practices. *Implementation Science, 9*(1). https://doi.org/10.1186/1748-5908-9-1

Squires, J. E., Sullivan, K., Eccles, M. P., Worswick, J., & Grimshaw, J. M. (2014). Are multifaceted interventions more effective than single-component interventions in changing health-care professionals' behaviours? An overview of systematic reviews. *Implementation Science, 9*, 1–22.

Stroke Foundation. (2025). *Australian and New Zealand living clinical guidelines for stroke management (living guidelines).* Stroke Foundation.

Wang, Y., Wong, E. L. Y., Nilsen, P., Chung, V. C. H., Tian, Y., & Yeoh, E. K. (2023). A scoping review of implementation science theories, models, and frameworks – an appraisal of purpose, characteristics, usability, applicability, and testability. *Implementation Science, 18*(1), 43.

West, R., & Michie, S. (2020). *A brief introduction to the COM-B Model of behaviour and the PRIME Theory of motivation* [v1]. Qeios, Article WW04E6. https://doi.org/10.32388/WW04E6

CHAPTER 24

Professional and clinical reasoning in occupational therapy practice

Justin Scanlan, Jennie Brentnall, Carolyn Unsworth, and Helen Jeffery

Authors' positionality statement

The author team consists of three women and one man. All authors are of European background, work as occupational therapy academics in higher education institutions in Australia and New Zealand/Aotearoa, and have been educated through Western teaching institutions. CU has a strong focus on educating occupational therapy students for practise in rural areas. HJ has interest and involvement in enabling cultural diversity in content and the lens through which occupational therapy education is offered. JS has an interest in supporting occupational therapy students to develop skills to work collaboratively towards person-led service delivery. JB has an interest in guiding occupational therapy students' development in practice education, from foundations in theory, process, and reasoning to work readiness.

Key terms
- Professional reasoning
- Clinical reasoning
- Practice reasoning
- Decision-making
- Client-centred practice
- Person-centred practice
- Novice practitioner
- Expert practitioner
- Reflection
- Intuition
- Worldview

DOI: 10.4324/9781003495666-26

Objectives

This chapter will allow the reader to:

- Describe processes of professional and clinical reasoning in occupational therapy practice
- Identify five aspects of professional and clinical reasoning in occupational therapy and influences on professional and clinical reasoning
- Describe how these aspects of and influences on professional and clinical reasoning can be applied to support the occupational therapy process

24.1 Introduction

Professional and clinical reasoning in occupational therapy involve complex processes. Although often described as 'tacit' (understood without necessarily being able to be expressed), this chapter sets out considerations that support novice occupational therapists to develop skills in applying professional and clinical reasoning in their practice. Novice occupational therapists are encouraged to consider a range of factors essential to supporting people's attainment of optimal occupational performance and participation and their desired occupational identities. Over time, with practice and critical self-reflection, the novice occupational therapist will develop more nuanced skills to support professional and clinical reasoning, and these processes will become more flexible, efficient, and integrated into their professional identity.

Occupational therapists assist people to move towards the occupational futures they want. This is achieved through focus on the inter-relationship between people, occupations, and contexts (including environments, broader geography, practice settings, social determinants of health, and cultural contexts). Professional and clinical reasoning are about considering how the best occupational outcomes can be achieved – whether through changes in people, contexts, or occupations or through enabling engagement with people, occupations, and environments/contexts that are healthful and enabling.

Professional and clinical reasoning informs not only what occupational therapists do but how and where they do it. Good practice decisions rely on occupational therapists understanding not only what people/clients want to achieve but also the influences of culture. Keeping culture front of mind – culture of the client and their community, the practice setting, and therapist themselves – will all contribute to culturally safe decisions. Additionally, decisions need to be possible in terms of resourcing, within the scope of the service, and evidence based.

In this chapter, we use the terms 'professional reasoning' and 'clinical reasoning' interchangeably. While 'clinical reasoning' is the dominant term used in medical and many health science disciplines, 'professional reasoning' has gained prominence in occupational therapy as our practice extends well beyond typical 'clinical' contexts. Other terms such as 'practice reasoning' and 'therapeutic reasoning' have also been used in the literature. While each has slight differences, the overarching themes and considerations are similar.

In addition to considering the different terms for professional and clinical reasoning, it is also important to consider other terms that describe occupational therapy practice and the people who engage with occupational therapy services. In this chapter, the terms 'clients' or 'person/people' are used to refer to the people, families, groups, or communities with whom occupational therapists work. This focus acknowledges that occupational therapists frequently work in contexts that extend beyond traditional one-to-one therapeutic interactions and that these relationships often seek to be equal rather than traditional hierarchical relationship that may be seen in other contexts. The term 'situations' will be used to refer to health conditions, impairments, circumstances, or environmental conditions that may influence clients' occupational performance. This term is used to highlight the many scenarios where factors that influence optimal occupational performance are not related to impairments or health conditions.

Given the complex interplay of factors that influence professional and clinical reasoning, this chapter breaks down and describes key aspects of professional and clinical reasoning and influences on professional and clinical reasoning that should be considered. However, before exploring these elements, there are two critically important overarching concepts that must be understood. These are worldview and shared decision-making.

24.1.1 Worldview

Wolters' (1989) seminal review described 'worldview' as encompassing individuals' assumptions about life and reality. It is formed through cultural experience and includes values, beliefs and attitudes, motivation, faith, and spirituality (Unsworth, 2004). It acts as a lens through which people view and understand the world. The worldview of every therapist and client is unique, bound by individual's experiences, family, and societal and cultural factors. Each occupational therapist's worldview shapes their thinking, including professional and clinical reasoning. Becoming a professional is to encompass the worldview of that profession – how occupational therapists consider a situation will differ from other health professionals because of the specific occupational therapy lens. Worldview affects our reasoning, often without our awareness. However, with experience and reflexive thinking, therapists can recognise and adjust for their worldview and their understanding of other worldviews: a crucial element of culturally safe reasoning and practice.

24.1.2 Shared decision-making

Practice decisions are rarely formed in isolation. Therapists take responsibility for their final decision, but how it is reached is generally a collaborative process involving the client (individuals and groups). Client perspectives, expertise, experiences, and resources inform practice decisions, which should be made in partnership (as detailed in Chapters 10, 11, and 12). This collaborative approach will empower people to engage fully in their healthcare and have benefits beyond ensuring the decisions are a good fit with them. For many Indigenous communities the client *is* the family or community group, and professional reasoning requires awareness of collective needs and understanding that assessment and intervention processes may include family members and will impact the group. Equally, in many practice settings, therapists collaborate with colleagues and teams, often working as a multidisciplinary team in a shared reasoning process. Some therapists are naturally drawn to this shared decision-making if it is a good fit with their worldview, such as Indigenous therapists from collectivist cultures.

24.2 Aspects of professional and clinical reasoning

Each client-occupational therapist collaboration is unique. The context in which both clients and therapists are situated provides parameters within which the practice must fit. Occupational therapists must ascertain the occupational challenges that have initiated clients accessing the service, their worldviews, and unique sets of skills, values, interests, roles, habits, strengths, and resources. Additionally, each therapist is unique in terms of worldview, knowledge, skill, experience, and personality. Professional reasoning is about forming decisions regarding practice that are right for client(s), occupational therapists, and the broader context.

How decisions are formed varies between people and situations. This chapter introduces five aspects of professional reasoning that are commonly employed – sometimes consciously in isolation but more often each in conjunction with the others. While by no means the only aspects of reasoning, they do provide the novice with ways to structure thinking that will enhance their ability to question and think both broadly and deeply. Overlayed across all aspects of reasoning is the concept of ethical practice – novices are encouraged to use a framework to guide their consideration of ethics in managing ethical dilemmas and in ensuring ethical practice decisions (see Chapter 8).

Occupational therapists also use an array of information sources when making practice decisions (Jeffery et al., 2024). These include research and literature (see Chapter 22), the client and family (detailed in Chapter 10), the context (of the person, community, culture, and service) and the expertise of others who have more experience and knowledge, such as colleagues or supervisors. The strongest influence on reasoning is the therapist themselves, requiring self-awareness that is enhanced through reflective practice and through reflexivity – awareness of personal biases and of one's own world view.

24.2.1 Narrative reasoning

The first aspect, 'narrative reasoning' focuses on people's occupational stories (Bonsall, 2012; Mattingly, 1991) and allows exploration of how people have made sense of their situation and the impact on their every-day life, desired roles, and occupations. This process of making sense of experiences (Christiansen, 1999) is important to consider in planning assessment, goal setting, and intervention. Through understanding the situation in the context of the person's unfolding life story, the occupational therapists can focus on elements of the story that speak to the most important aspect of practice: occupational performance and participation (Bonsall, 2012; Mattingly, 1991; Mattingly, 1998; Neistadt, 1996). Appreciating the impact of the situation on occupation enables the exploration of people's values, their beliefs in their abilities, and what is important to them and to the people and communities around them.

The process of occupational story-making (creating a picture of people's desired occupational futures) can support clients and therapists to take action in the therapeutic process (Bonsall, 2012). The story can guide practice decisions about intervention focus – therapy may be about recovery and return to the storyline or creating a different future story that is occupationally satisfying. The shared story can also guide decisions about who the occupational therapist might include in practice processes (person, family, wider community), specific occupations to focus on, and the importance of the contexts to access or adapt, thereby supporting both the client's cultural identity and the therapist's role identity. All these factors are critical in making decisions that are supportive of clients achieving their desired occupational futures.

Examples of questions aligned with narrative reasoning:

- What is the person's storyline from past to present and future?
- What have been their valued and meaningful roles and occupations in the past, and how are these impacted by their current situation?
- Can they see/what do they want for an occupational future (e.g., to return to previous occupations; do they wish or believe they need to engage in new occupations?)

24.2.2 Interactive reasoning

The second aspect, 'interactive reasoning' (Mattingly & Fleming, 1994b), holds the relationship between therapist and client foremost, with the interactions being an integral part of reasoning. People are considered in the context of their social situation (e.g. community, family, and friends), relationships with their occupational therapist, health care and support services, and others. The occupational therapist focuses on maximising the quality of therapeutic relationships so that they get to know the person as an individual and form a relationship that includes shared purpose for occupational therapy. They also identify how clients' current and previous interactions with health or social services may influence their current therapeutic interactions and consider how much and what type of informal supports they receive (Schwartzberg, 2001). This aspect of reasoning therefore guides the therapist in ascertaining who they need to be interacting with and adjusting their interactions to form and maintain the most effective relationship.

Interactive reasoning helps occupational therapists understand potential barriers or enablers to optimal engagement with the therapeutic process and what supports might be available to people. This process considers the perspectives of families and other supports, cultural considerations, and how these influence professional and clinical reasoning processes.

Examples of questions aligned with interactive reasoning

- Who else is with the client and you on the decision-making journey (e.g. family and communities, members of the multidisciplinary team, other service providers)? What are their perspectives on the best approaches and how could this influence decision-making?
- What is the best way to interact with this person?
- What experiences has the person had with other service providers in the past and how might this influence their current relationships with service providers (e.g., power, trust, autonomy)?

24.2.3 Procedural reasoning

The third aspect, 'procedural reasoning' (Fleming, 1991a), is the process whereby occupational therapists consider the most suitable services or approaches to achieve the desired outcomes, given the client's situation. In other disciplines, procedural reasoning might be referred to as *diagnostic reasoning*, *scientific reasoning*, or *hypothetico-deductive reasoning*, although these approaches can be narrow in focus and only consider diagnosis rather than the more complex interactions between people, occupations, and contexts considered by occupational therapists. Procedural reasoning supports occupational therapists to consider various intervention options and develop a 'short list' of potentially effective approaches.

Procedural reasoning is arguably the most concrete aspect of clinical reasoning. Consequently, it is often the first aspect considered by novice occupational therapists. While process is important, it is critical to avoid a *one-size-fits-all* approach. Considering the variety of factors involved in professional and clinical reasoning together, as presented in this chapter, occupational therapists account for the variety of factors important to clients' situations, avoiding an exclusive focus on diagnoses or impairments.

Examples of questions aligned with procedural reasoning:

- Is there evidence-based practice guidance that can be used in this situation?
- What approaches do other colleagues (e.g., senior occupational therapists, colleagues, or other members of the multidisciplinary team) use when working with people in similar situations?
- What are the cultural perspectives of the person, and how could these influence the selection of the most helpful approach?
- What are the potential impacts of the person's current situation on their daily functioning?
- Is the person's situation likely to remain stable, improve, or deteriorate over time, how does this influence supports required (if any)?

24.2.4 Conditional reasoning

The fourth aspect, conditional reasoning (Fleming, 1991a), considers which intervention approach is likely to be most acceptable and have the best outcomes for this client, with these specific values, needs, desires, and hopes for the future, in this specific context. At this point, occupational therapists consider what interventions or approaches are most suitable for their clients 'in a perfect world', rather than considering what is *practical* or *feasible* (Scanlan & Hancock, 2010). While practicality and feasibility are important (and are considered in pragmatic reasoning), if consideration is not first given to what would be optimal, important intervention options may be overlooked.

Examples of questions aligned with conditional reasoning:

- What is the person's current situation and potential future situation?
- Does the person have specific cultural needs or desires that should be incorporated into the final approach?
- What is the best approach for the person, their family, and context considering their abilities to complete the required activities or achieve changes in environments?

24.2.5 Pragmatic reasoning

The fifth aspect, 'pragmatic reasoning', is concerned with what is possible to achieve given the practical constraints and opportunities in the context (Unsworth, 2004; Unsworth & Baker, 2016). Pragmatic reasoning includes the thinking the therapist undertakes when considering the local practice culture, funding and reimbursement issues, access to equipment and resources, and issues around time (e.g. number of clients to see, client length of stay, and needing to treat individual clients simultaneously; Schell & Cervero, 1993; Unsworth, 2004). This extends to considering community, culture, and any culturally oriented services or approaches available within the context. When reasoning pragmatically, it is important that the therapist hold the client's priorities and desires uppermost in their mind and guard against making decisions based only on 'what is easiest' or 'what is always done here'.

Pragmatic reasoning supports occupational therapists to consider *best fit* intervention approaches for people they are working with, given limitations of systems in which their services are offered (da Silva Araujo et al., 2022). These limitations might include funding availability, access to community supports/accommodation, or the length of time available for therapeutic interventions. While these factors exert a significant influence on the reasoning process, therapists must also maintain an ethical approach to practice. If essential resources are not available, occupational therapists may need to take on advocacy roles to support their clients to access such resources.

Examples of questions aligned with pragmatic reasoning:

- What human and non-human resources are available and accessible for service provision? How do these align with community and cultural expectations?
- Are there limitations imposed by the service setting or funding arrangement, in terms of what services people can be offered or length of engagement with the service, which may impact delivering the 'optimal' approach?
- Are there 'trade-offs' that clients are willing to make?
- Given these limitations, what interventions can be delivered that will still support good outcomes for people?

24.3 Influences on professional and clinical reasoning

In addition to the key aspects of worldview and shared decision-making described previously, there are also two other important influences on professional and clinical reasoning that should be considered. These are 'intuition' and 'reflection', which are described subsequently.

24.3.1 Intuition

Intuition may be defined as immediate and 'whole' (as opposed to fragmented) knowledge, that is, without conscious reasoning (Chaffey et al., 2012; Unsworth, 2017, 2020), commonly described as 'gut instinct'. Gut instinct is apt, as we often have a visceral response to a situation that can be helpful in guiding our professional and clinical reasoning. While expert therapists appear more comfortable with trusting and acting upon their intuition, novice therapists can benefit from discussing intuition to begin accessing, understanding, and building their own intuition. Discussing and understanding our intuition is important, as it is shaped by our worldview, so while it may be guiding us 'right' within our own family and societal culture, it may not be 'right' for the client. Regular supervision, reflections, and discussions with other occupational therapists can help us question intuition and other tacit knowledge, ensuring the therapy provided is evidence-based, feels 'right', and is culturally appropriate.

24.3.2 Reflection

Reflection involves thinking critically about events, encounters, and responses – whether about past experiences (reflection on action), in the present (reflection in action), or looking forward in anticipation (reflection for action). Schön's (1983) seminal work described reflection as a bridge between theory and practice. It is thereby a key enabler of professional reasoning as thinking about therapeutic encounters and their success, as well as how they could be improved, assists novice therapists to hone practice and attain expert status faster. Reflective practice also enhances our practice more broadly. Reflecting by ourselves, or with others, about approaches that were successful, approaches that were not successful, or ethical dilemmas can help to develop our own professional identity, self-awareness, emotional intelligence and capacity to learn from feedback.

The importance of reflective practice is demonstrated by its inclusion in occupational therapy practice guidelines and standards internationally (Occupational Therapy Board of Australia, 2018; Occupational Therapy Board of New Zealand, 2022; World Federation of Occupational Therapists, 2016). Most occupational therapy students learn about reflective practice in their education programme and have time for reflective journal writing embedded in fieldwork education placements (Craig-Duchesne et al., 2018; Wong et al., 2016). While there is high interest and engagement across the profession in reflective practice, a key barrier is lack of time (Knightbridge, 2019). Students are therefore encouraged to routinely build time into their schedule to create opportunities for both group and individual reflection.

24.4 Bringing it all together

The overall process of professional and clinical reasoning in occupational therapy is complex (Fleming, 1991b; Unsworth, 2017; Unsworth & Baker, 2016). Specifically, it requires the consideration of clients' current and future occupational functioning; their connection to family, community, and culture; and how they engage and relate to others and their contexts. Without this broad focus, intervention plans are likely to be misaligned with clients' needs and goals and may not optimise the contribution of support systems. An overview of the professional reasoning process is provided in Figure 24.1.

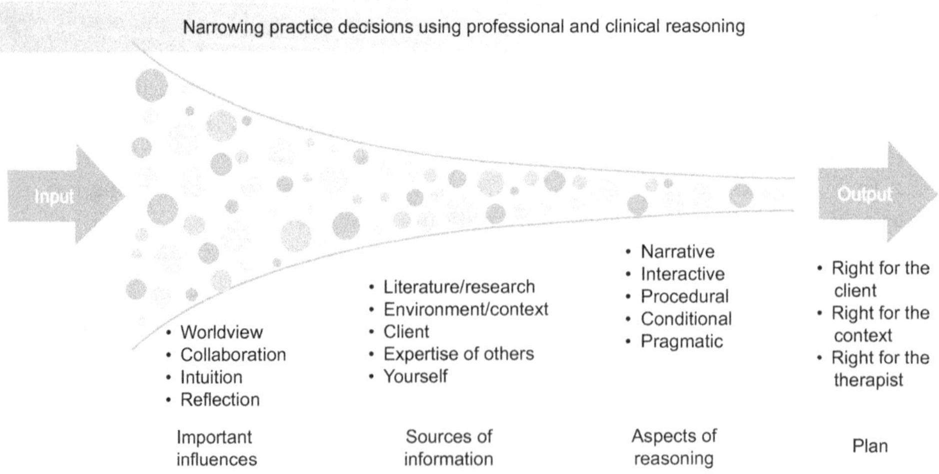

Figure 24.1 Overview of the professional and clinical reasoning process

Regular monitoring should occur throughout the occupational therapy process that provide feedback into the clinical reasoning process and may result in changes to practice decisions. Consequently, professional and clinical reasoning processes are cyclical. With each cycle of continuing assessment and evaluation, the understanding of clients' unique situations becomes more comprehensive, and the overall quality of reasoning is improved (Higgs & Jones, 2000). If outcomes are not as expected, it is important to revisit professional and clinical reasoning processes to explore factors that may have been overlooked and that may be interfering with optimal outcomes.

24.5 Developing from a novice to an expert practitioner

Over time and with experience, reasoning processes become more embedded in everyday thinking and go from very conscious processes to more *tacit* (semi-automatic) processes (Fleming, 1991a; Gibson et al., 2000; Mattingly & Fleming, 1994a; Unsworth, 2001). Although often not easily distinguished, the phases of development of expertise have been described as novice, advanced beginner, competent, proficient, and expert (Unsworth, 2001). It is also important to consider that not all therapists will reach expert status in their career, and that time and experience, while supporting expert practice, are not synonymous with being an expert occupational therapist. Students and novice occupational therapists often experience clinical reasoning as time consuming and effortful (Gibson et al., 2000). It can be disconcerting to watch more experienced therapists articulate well-reasoned intervention plans quickly, and difficult to see and explain the process of determining those plans. Often experts appear to make inexplicable leaps in their reasoning, reflecting the increased efficiency of the clinical reasoning process.

The process of development from novice to more expert practitioner takes experience and well-developed reflective skills (Craig-Duchesne et al., 2018; Gibson et al., 2000; Wong et al., 2016). Students can benefit from working with peers, to review each other's clinical reasoning processes, and challenge one another to ensure important factors are recognised and considered when creating plans that are best aligned to clients' needs and desires. Critical reflection on reasoning with supervisors, peers, and senior clinicians, particularly during fieldwork placements and in practice after graduation, assists in refining reasoning skills.

With ongoing, careful consideration and reflection, expertise develops over time. Even expert practitioners need to continue reflecting on their practice and reasoning processes (Creek, 2007), to avoid practice decisions becoming too automated and maybe failing to consider the unique situations and needs of each person. Other factors that influence the development of professional reasoning skills include organisational factors (e.g. how much employers value continuing professional development and support the provision of high-quality supervision), the service setting, and individual therapists' commitment to ongoing professional development (Jeffery et al., 2021, 2024).

24.6 Conclusion

Professional reasoning skills develop as therapists gain experience in practice settings and become intentional in what guides their thinking. Professional reasoning provides the basis for professional decision-making and day-to-day problem solving and draws from several sources of evidence to inform the decision. Different types of professional reasoning are used depending on contextual influences such as the client and family/ social situation, requirements of the practice setting, and the strengths of the therapist. It is important for students to be cognisant of the different types of clinical reasoning, and factors that may influence reasoning such as the therapist's worldview, intuition, and ability to reflect, so that they can start to implement them during their practice education placements.

24.7 Summary

- Professional and clinical reasoning in occupational therapy requires simultaneous consideration of varied factors to support optimal, collaborative decision-making with clients and consider the guiding principles of ethical practice.
- Five aspects of clinical reasoning have been presented as essential in the occupational therapy process: narrative, interactive, procedural, conditional, and pragmatic reasoning.
- In an optimal occupational therapy process, narrative, interactive, procedural, and conditional reasoning are all considered, and then a selection of intervention options identified and reviewed in terms of what is practical and feasible given situational limitations, as well as what is just and fair.
- Although initially complex and time consuming, with practice and reflection, the reasoning of novice occupational therapists becomes more flexible, integrated, and efficient.

24.8 Review questions

- Describe the five aspects of clinical reasoning and how each supports the development of optimal intervention plans.
- Describe considerations in your clinical reasoning when working with a client who has previously had negative interactions with health services, does not recognise or prioritise the need for support to meet occupational needs, and has limited or no family or community supports (particularly consider interactive, conditional, pragmatic, and ethical reasoning).
- Using narrative and conditional reasoning, describe how working with a client to identify a 'desired occupational future' can help to drive therapeutic action.
- How can you effectively include families and other important supports in your reasoning processes and ensure important cultural factors are not overlooked?
- In occupational therapy, it is not possible to determine an intervention plan based only on the client's diagnosis or current limitations. Provide some of your clinical reasoning to explain why this isn't possible.

References

Bonsall, A. (2012). An examination of the pairing between narrative and occupational science. *Scandinavian Journal of Occupational Therapy, 19*(1), 92–103. https://doi.org/10.3109/110 38128.2011.552119

Chaffey, L., Unsworth, C., & Fossey, E. (2012). The relationship of intuition and emotional intelligence among occupational therapists in mental health practice. *American Journal of Occupational Therapy, 66*(1), 88–96. https://doi.org/10.5014/ajot.2012.001693

Christiansen, C. H. (1999). Defining lives: Occupation as identity: An essay on competence, coherence, and the creation of meaning. *American Journal of Occupational Therapy*, *53*(6), 547–558. https://doi.org/10.5014/ajot.53.6.547

Craig-Duchesne, C., Rochette, A., Scurti, S., Beaulieu, J., & Vachon, B. (2018). Occupational therapy students' experience with using a journal in fieldwork and factors influencing its use. *Reflective Practice*, *19*(5), 609–622. https://doi.org/10.1080/14623943.2018.1538953

Creek, J. (2007). The thinking therapist. In J. Creek & A. Lawson-Porter (Eds.), *Contemporary issues in occupational therapy: Reasoning and reflection* (pp. 1–22). John Wiley & Sons.

da Silva Araujo, A., Anne Kinsella, E., Thomas, A., Demonari Gomes, L., & Quevedo Marcolino, T. (2022). Clinical reasoning in occupational therapy practice: A scoping review of qualitative and conceptual peer-reviewed literature. *American Journal of Occupational Therapy*, *76*(3), 7603205070. https://doi.org/10.5014/ajot.2022.048074

Fleming, M. H. (1991a). The therapist with the three-track mind. *American Journal of Occupational Therapy*, *45*(11), 1007–1014. https://doi.org/10.5014/ajot.45.11.1007

Fleming, M. H. (1991b). Clinical reasoning in medicine compared with clinical reasoning in occupational therapy. *American Journal of Occupational Therapy*, *45*(11), 988–996. https://doi.org/10.5014/ajot.45.11.988

Gibson, D., Velde, B., Hoff, T., Kvashay, D., Manross, P. L., & Moreau, V. (2000). Clinical reasoning of a novice versus an experienced occupational therapist: A qualitative study. *Occupational Therapy in Health Care*, *12*(4), 15–31. https://doi.org/10.1080/J003v12n04_02

Higgs, J., & Jones, M. (2000). *Clinical reasoning in the health professions*. Butterworth-Heinemann.

Jeffery, H., Robertson, L., & Reay, K. L. (2021). Sources of evidence for professional decision-making in novice occupational therapy practitioners: Clinicians' perspectives. *British Journal of Occupational Therapy*, *84*(6), 346–354. https://doi.org/10.1177/0308022620941390

Jeffery, H., Robertson, L., Roodt, H., & Ryan, S. (2024). *Professional reasoning in healthcare: Navigating uncertainty using the Five Finger Framework*. Wiley Blackwell.

Knightbridge, L. (2019). Reflection-in-practice: A survey of Australian occupational therapists. *Australian Occupational Therapy Journal*, *66*(3), 337–346. https://doi.org/10.1111/1440-1630.12559

Mattingly, C. (1991). The narrative nature of clinical reasoning. *American Journal of Occupational Therapy*, *45*(11), 998–1005. https://doi.org/10.5014/ajot.45.11.998

Mattingly, C. (1998). In search of the good: Narrative reasoning in clinical practice. *Medical Anthropology Quarterly*, *12*(3), 273–297. https://doi.org/10.1525/maq.1998.12.3.273

Mattingly, C., & Fleming, M. H. (1994a). *Clinical reasoning: Forms of inquiry in therapeutic practice*. F. A. Davis Co.

Mattingly, C., & Fleming, M. H. (1994b). Interactive reasoning: Collaborating with the person. In C. Mattingly & M. H. Fleming (Eds.), *Clinical reasoning: Forms of inquiry in therapeutic practice* (pp. 178–196). F. A. Davis.

Neistadt, M. E. (1996). Teaching strategies for the development of clinical reasoning. *American Journal of Occupational Therapy*, *50*(8), 676–684. https://doi.org/10.5014/ajot.50.8.676

Occupational Therapy Board of Australia. (2018). *Australian occupational therapy competency standards 2018*. https://www.occupationaltherapyboard.gov.au/Codes-Guidelines/Competencies.aspx

Occupational Therapy Board of New Zealand. (2022). *Competencies for registration and continuing practice for occupational therapists 2022*. https://www.otboard.org.nz/site/ces/competencies?nav=sidebar

Scanlan, J. N., & Hancock, N. (2010). Online discussions develop students' clinical reasoning skills during fieldwork. *Australian Occupational Therapy Journal*, *57*(6), 401–408. https://doi.org/10.1111/j.1440-1630.2010.00883.x

Schell, B. A. B., & Cervero, R. M. (1993). Clinical reasoning in occupational therapy: An integrative review. *American Journal of Occupational Therapy*, *47*(7), 605–610. https://doi.org/10.5014/ajot.47.7.605

Schön, D. A. (1983). *The reflective practitioner: How professionals think in action*. Basic.

Schwartzberg, S. (2001). *Interactive reasoning in the practice of occupational therapy*. Pearson.

Unsworth, C. A. (2001). The clinical reasoning of novice and expert occupational therapists. *Scandinavian Journal of Occupational Therapy*, 8(4), 163–173. https://doi.org/10.1080/110381201317166522

Unsworth, C. A. (2004). Clinical reasoning: How do pragmatic reasoning, worldview and client-centredness fit? *British Journal of Occupational Therapy*, 67(1), 10–19. https://doi.org/10.1177/030802260406700103

Unsworth, C. A. (2017). An overview of professional reasoning within occupational therapy practice. In M. Curtin, M. Egan, & J. Adams (Eds.), *Occupational therapy for people experiencing illness, injury or impairment* (7th ed., pp. 90–104). Elsevier.

Unsworth, C. A. (2020). The evolving theory of clinical reasoning. In E. A. S. Duncan (Ed.), *Foundations for practice in occupational therapy* (6th ed.). Elsevier.

Unsworth, C. A., & Baker, A. (2016). A systematic review of professional reasoning literature in occupational therapy. *British Journal of Occupational Therapy*, 79(1), 5–16. https://doi.org/10.1177/0308022615599994

Wolters, A. M. (1989). On the idea of worldview and its relationship to philosophy. In P. A. Marshall, S. Griffioen, & R. Mouw (Eds.), *Stained glass: Worldviews and social science* (pp. 14–25). University Press of America.

Wong, K. Y., Whitcombe, S., & Boniface, G. (2016). Teaching and learning the esoteric: An insight into how reflection may be internalised with reference to the occupational therapy profession. *Reflective Practice*, 17(4), 472–482. https://doi.org/10.1080/14623943.2016.1175341

World Federation of Occupational Therapists. (2016). *Minimum standards for the education of occupational therapists (Revised 2016)*. https://www.wfot.org/assets/resources/COPYRIGHTED-World-Federation-of-Occupational-Therapists-Minimum-Standards-for-the-Education-of-Occupational-Therapists-2016a.pdf

CHAPTER 25

Occupational therapy practice models

Merrill J. Turpin and Chloe Bryant

Authors' positionality statement

Merrill J. Turpin is a white, English-speaking Australian woman who has been an occupational therapy academic at the University of Queensland in Australia for over three decades. As an occupational therapist, she is passionate about creating societies in which people can participate equitably. She combines her advantaged educational background, which has afforded her with knowledge of how societal structures are premised on and reinforce power imbalances and inequities in participation and an awareness of her own social privilege, with her experiences of living with a chronic illness in a world largely designed for able-bodied people. While this provides her with a particular perspective, she is aware that there are many aspects of intersectionality that she has no experience of.

Chloe Bryant is a white, Australian, cisgender female occupational therapist who lives with a chronic health condition. Chloe completed a Bachelor of Occupational Therapy (Honours) in 2017 as well as a Doctor of Philosophy in 2023 at the University of Queensland. She recognises her immense privilege in having access to tertiary education, public healthcare, and affordable housing and is passionate about creating inclusive communities that recognise all individuals as equal regardless of their personal factors.

Key terms
- Occupational therapy theory and practice
- Occupational Performance Model Australia (Australia)
- Model of Human Occupation
- Person-Environment-Occupation-Performance Model
- Kawa Model
- Canadian Model of Occupational Participation
- Person-Environment-Occupation
- Canadian Model of Occupational Performance and Engagement

DOI: 10.4324/9781003495666-27

Objectives
This chapter will allow the reader to:

- Consider the role of occupational therapy models in linking theory and practice
- Describe seven internationally recognised, discipline-specific occupational therapy models
- Develop an enhanced understanding of how contextual factors, such as cultural contexts and economic environments, have shaped the creation of dominant occupational therapy theory
- Reflect on how available models represent the progression of dominant discourses and concepts in occupational therapy theory

25.1 Introduction

In any given practice situation, occupational therapists make decisions about action. They decide what to *do* with specific clients. This is a complex process, in part due to the diversity of needs and circumstances of individuals, groups, and populations. Occupational therapists must combine disparate information, sometimes contradictory, and formulate an appropriate plan of action. They combine knowledge and action.

Occupational therapy uses the terms theory and practice to refer to knowledge and action, respectively. Without theory, practitioners are akin to technicians. Without practice, theory has no grounding in the world. To guide using theory in practice, occupational therapy has a well-developed collection of discipline-specific models of practice (models). Models guide practice by:

- making explicit the values and assumptions of the profession;
- providing frameworks for organising knowledge (both generalised knowledge and client-related knowledge e.g. assessment results and narrative information); and
- outlining a systematic and comprehensive approach to practice (Turpin et al., 2024).

This chapter overviews seven of the most influential occupational therapy models of practice in Australia, the United States, and Canada (see Figure 25.1 for publication timeline). These are the Occupational Performance Model (Australia) (OPMA), Model of Human Occupation (MOHO), Person–Environment–Occupation-Performance Model (PEOP), Kawa Model, and the Canadian Model of Occupational Participation (CanMOP), with its precursors: Person–Environment–Occupation (PEO) and Canadian Model of Occupational Performance and Engagement (CMOP-E).

25.2 Occupational Performance Model (Australia)

The OPM(A) is widely used in Australia, although it does not represent an official position of Occupational Therapy Australia. It was first published as a monograph in 1997 (Chapparo & Ranka, 1997) and has a comprehensive website (http://www.occupationalperformance.com). While the OPM(A) was developed in Australia, it also provides an excellent starting point for understanding the development of models of practice in

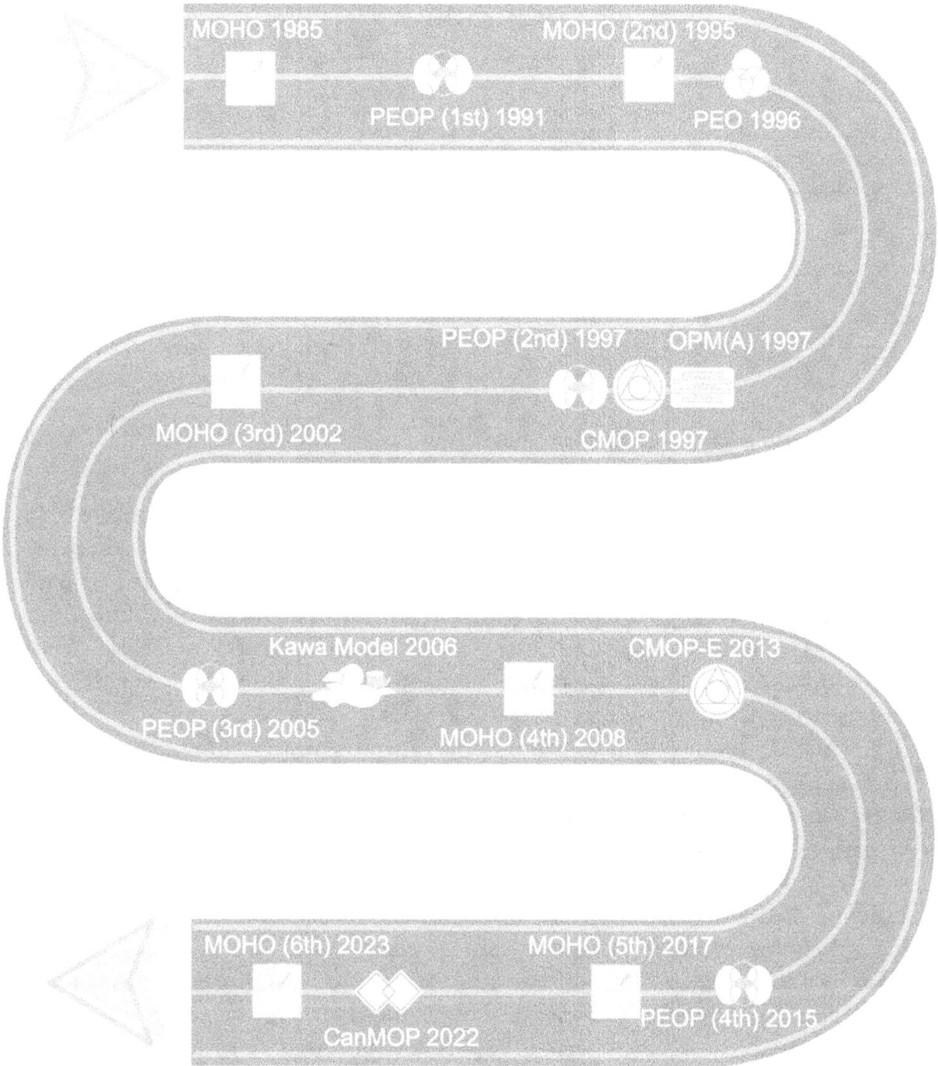

Figure 25.1 Publication timeline

occupational therapy more broadly. While its structure encompasses the original occupational performance (OP) models, its philosophy and goals differ. The earlier models OP guided occupational therapists to identify where occupational performance was breaking down by analysing its components. Influenced by the mechanistic paradigm, these models focused on internal mechanisms such as sensorimotor, cognitive and perceptual, and intra- and inter-personal skills and abilities. Interventions were generally directed towards these performance components, and this process is often referred to as a bottom-up approach (Fisher & Marterella, 2019).

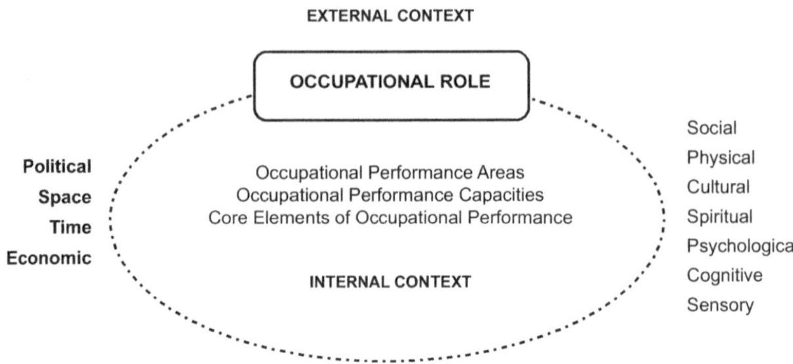

Figure 25.2 Occupational Performance Model (Australia)

In contrast to these early occupational performance models, and developed several decades later, the OPM(A) presents an ecological approach to occupational performance, recognising the importance of understanding the person and their occupational performance *in context* (see Figure 25.2). The OPM(A) defines *occupational performance* as 'the ability to perceive, desire, recall, plan and carry out roles, routines, tasks and subtasks for the purpose of self-maintenance, productivity, leisure and rest in response to demands of the internal and/or external context' (Chapparo et al., 2017, p. 137). This definition emphasises the importance of understanding the purposes of occupation in people's lives. Unlike many occupational therapy models that distinguish between person and environment, the OPM(A) overcomes this separation by using the language of internal and external contexts. Both fuse when the external context is internalised and embodied as people interpret what a situation requires and affords. This is combined with their internal considerations of what they are able and want to do and externalised through occupational engagement.

The *internal context* has four levels: occupational roles; performance areas; performance capacities; and the core elements of body, mind, and spirit. The primary concern is the performance of *occupational roles*, and all occupational therapy interventions should work towards these (see Figure 25.2). Occupational roles are the site of intersection between internal and external contexts. They are influenced by internal and external expectations of what is required, and they change over time as abilities and circumstances alter. Occupational roles have three dimensions – knowing, doing, and being. Knowing refers to understanding desired or expected occupational roles, doing refers to carrying out those roles, and being refers to the satisfaction or fulfilment a person might obtain from them.

Performance areas and *performance capacities* follow the classic dimensions of OP models. In the OPM(A), the performance areas are self-maintenance, rest, leisure, and productivity. The model emphasises that classification of specific occupations into these areas should be made by the performer (e.g., an occupation might be work for one person and leisure for another). The five performance capacities are motor, sensory, cognitive, intrapersonal, and interpersonal (see Figure 25.2). Each is presented in terms of both the perspective of the performer and the demands of the task. The final internal level consists of the *core elements* of body, mind, and spirit. These three core elements cannot be separated but are considered inter-related aspects of people – their physical nature, conscious and unconscious intellect, and their notions of meaning, hope and connectedness.

The *external context* is the context surrounding the internal context and has nine interconnected elements – physical, sensory, cognitive, psychological, social, cultural, spiritual, political, and economic. The external context shapes occupational performance by exerting press and affordance. As Chaparro et al. (2017) explained,

> An affordance is when the performance context enables opportunities for optimum performance. For example, a handle affords pulling, a quiet room affords reading, and a slippery surface affords balance reactions. Press has to do with the level of demand placed on performance and presents barriers, risks and restrictions to performance.
>
> (p. 144)

In every situation, the external elements will combine in different ways and various elements will make greater or lesser contributions to the overall pull or affordance of the external context.

Two additional constructs form part of the external context-space and time. Both have physical and felt dimensions (see Figure 25.2). Physical space includes the wider physical world, objects, and body structures. Felt space is the subjective experience of space. For example, the same space might feel safe to some people and unsafe to others or claustrophobic to some and comfortable to others. Regarding time, physical time refers to chronological time, while felt time is the subjective experience of time, such as feeling that there is ample time or insufficient time for certain occupations.

25.3 Model of Human Occupation

The MOHO was developed in the USA, has been published for over four decades and in six book editions (1985, 1995, 2002, 2008, 2017, 2023), and is the most widely used occupational therapy model (Forsyth & Brown, 2024). It was first published when the alternatives in occupational therapy were the OP models, but it represents a major departure from that way of thinking. The MOHO is structured according to systems theory, in particular dynamical systems theory. It addresses how occupation is a) chosen, b) patterned, and c) performed in the contexts in which people live and act. It assumes a close association between person and environment and outlines three interacting elements of the person – *volition, habituation*, and *performance capacity* (see Figure 25.3).

Volition is the motivation for choosing occupation and has the following three components. Personal causation refers to a person's thoughts and feelings about his or her ability to perform everyday activities effectively (sense of agency). Values are 'beliefs and commitments about what is good, right and important to do' (Forsyth & Brown, 2024, p. 556). Interests develop over time according to what a person finds enjoyable and satisfying. Whether or not particular occupations remain in a person's occupational

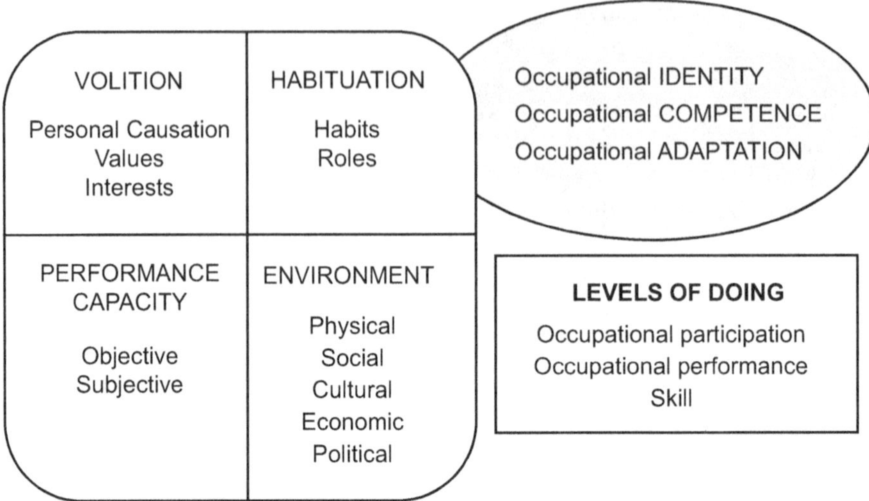

Figure 25.3 Model of Human Occupation

repertoire depends on their experiences. The process of volition changes over time as people experience, interpret, anticipate, and choose occupations (Yeasir et al., 2023).

Habituation relates to the patterns and routines into which people organise their occupations, and habits and roles are its main components. Habits develop when familiar things are done in stable environments and can involve learned ways of undertaking tasks and the enactment of regular routines. Roles have social expectations and responsibilities, as well as implications for identity. People internalise role expectations through their interactions with others and people develop an identity associated with these roles.

Performance capacity is 'a person's underlying mental and physical abilities and how those abilities are used and experienced in occupational performance' (Forsyth & Brown, 2024, p. 557). It has both objective and subjective components. Objective capacities can be observed, measured, and modified using a range of different frameworks such as motor control, cognitive, and sensory approaches. The subjective experience of performance capacity includes how people experience abilities and impairments and how they perceive the world.

Human occupation occurs within and is influenced by the environment, which has physical, social, cultural, economic, and political features (see Figure 25.3). The physical environment includes spaces and objects. The social environment includes both social groups and tasks. Both the social and cultural environments contribute to the expectations of and opportunities available to people and shape their views regarding valuable and worthwhile occupations. The economic and political environments determine the resources and occupational roles available.

The MOHO identifies three 'levels' of human occupation, referred to as levels of doing (Bowyer et al., 2023), with each embedded within the broader one above and all being influenced by volition, habituation, personal capacity, and environmental conditions. The broadest level is occupational participation or taking part in society.

This occurs through work, play, and activities of daily living. Performance capacities, habituation, volition, and environmental conditions all influence occupational participation (see Figure 25.3). Next is occupational performance, the actual performing of occupation. The final dimension of doing is skill. Skills are grouped into motor skills (those relating to moving self and objects), process skills (those required to logically sequence actions over time), and communication and interaction skills (those required for conveying need, intentions, and acting with others).

Finally, human occupation results in occupational identity, competence, and adaptation. Over the course of people's lives, they build an occupational identity, that is, a sense of themselves as occupational beings. People's occupational identities are shaped by their awareness of what they are good at and capable of, what they find interesting and satisfying to do, the roles they have, what they feel obliged to do, and their perceptions of the demands and supports of the environment. People have occupational competence when they can sustain a pattern of occupational participation that reflects their occupational identity. While occupational identity relates to subjective experience, occupational competence is about creating action from that identity. Both contribute to a person's occupational adaptation over time.

The complex interaction between people and their environment shapes human occupation. When the capacities of people correspond to the demands of the environment and available resources, occupational performance is facilitated. When people perform well, they are likely to feel good about themselves and their abilities and pursue opportunities for repeating such experiences. When the fit is poor and occupational performance is reduced, a change in either performance capacity or the environment, or both, may be required to increase the fit. For example, reduced access to resources from the political and economic environment can limit opportunities to increase the fit between the environmental demands and the person's abilities.

25.4 Person–Environment–Occupation–Performance Model

The PEOP was also developed in the USA and is in its fourth edition (1991, 1997, 2005, 2015). The model has undergone significant conceptual development over time, and each version of the model differs substantially from previous ones. Baum et al. (2015) referred to the PEOP as 'an ecological-transactional systems model' (p. 49), meaning that it centres on people in the environmental systems in which they live. As with all occupational therapy ecological models, the main concepts in the PEOP are *person, environment,* and *occupation,* to which it adds a fourth concept – *narrative* (see Figure 25.4).

Occupations are performed by people in the context of their environments. Baum et al. (2020) explained that the following three domains of knowledge 'interact to support the occupational performance of individuals, groups or populations':

> (1) the person, group or population factors (previously identified as intrinsic factors); (2) the environmental factors that include the situation and context, and relevant cultural, physical, social, policy and technological environments (previously identified as the extrinsic factors); and (3) the occupations of importance to the clients' well-being (activities, tasks and roles).
>
> *(p. 87)*

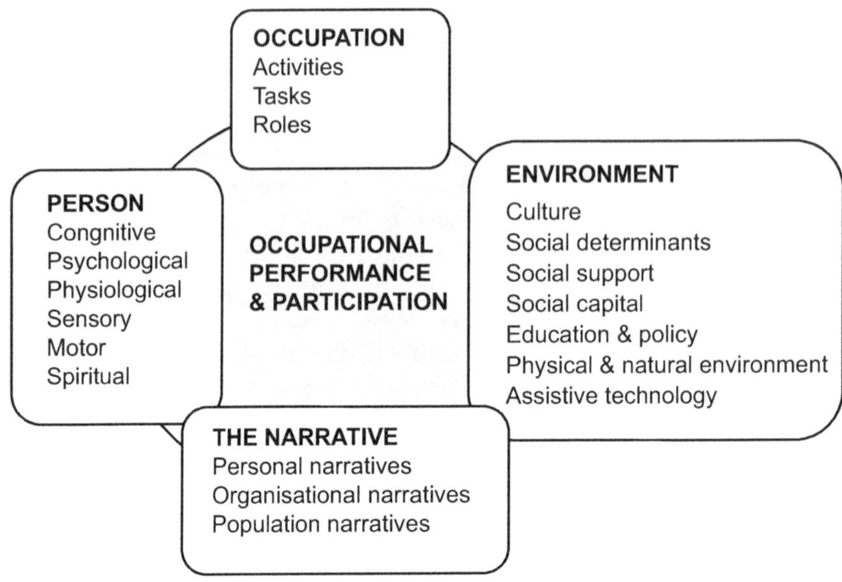

Figure 25.4 Person–Environment–Occupation–Performance Model

Narratives help to understand needs and goals in a temporal context of past, present and future. They can be at the level of individuals, organisations, and populations.

When considering occupation, the notion of occupational performance, that is, the doing of occupation, is 'front and centre' (Bass et al., 2017, p. 170) in the model, with participation and well-being being the reasons why people engage in and perform occupation. They participate in valued roles and life goals and experience a sense of well-being when they have positive perceptions of their self-esteem, confidence, physical and mental health, and social connectedness. Occupation comprises activities, tasks, and roles. The PEOP model provides detailed elements of person, environment, and narrative. The elements related to the person are cognitive, psychological, physiological, sensory, motor, and spiritual (see Figure 25.4). In discussing the psychological elements of the person, Baum et al. (2015) emphasised the importance of understanding 'the roles, activities and goals of the client' (p. 53), as these provide the motivation for occupational performance.

The environment includes culture, social determinants, social support and social capital, education and policy, the physical and natural environment, and assistive technology. Elements of the narrative are as follows: Personal narratives include perception and meaning, choices and responsibilities, attitudes and motivation, and needs and goals; organisational narratives include mission and history, focus and priorities, stakeholders and values, and needs and goals; and population narratives include environments and behaviours, demographics and disparities, incidence and prevalence, and needs and goals (see Figure 25.4). These narratives provide a framework for combining information gained from a diversity of sources, imbuing meaning and significance that supports prioritisation and goal setting.

25.5 Kawa Model

The book *Kawa Model: Culturally Relevant Occupational Therapy* was published in 2006 (Iwama, 2006). The Kawa Model was developed in collaboration with Japanese academics who found that existing occupational therapy models were not appropriate to the Japanese culture and worldview. At the time of its publication, Iwama wrote that the degree to which occupational therapy was culturally bound was largely unrecognised. Consequently, prior to presenting the Kawa Model, a substantial portion of the book is devoted to explaining aspects of the Japanese culture and worldview. The model uniquely explores the notion of occupation from a collectivist perspective, in which a 'decentralised self' requires reordering of the accepted Doing, Being, and Becoming framework (Wilcock, 1998) to Belonging, Being, and then Doing. Iwama (2006) challenged occupational therapy 'to make its ideas, ideology, theory and the practices that follow, relevant to many, many groups of people' (p. 50). In a later reflection, Nelson et al. (2017) stated that, in occupational therapy, recognition of 'occupation and health as culturally bound constructs' had increased in focus over the previous decade (p. 73). Their use of the Kawa Model with Australian Aboriginals and Torres Strait Islanders, provides an excellent example of responding to Iwama's call to use the model with a variety of peoples.

Kawa is the Japanese word for river. Just as a river flows from its source to the ocean, metaphorically, a person's life 'flows' from birth to death. The water flowing through the river represents the life energy, or life flow (see Figure 25.5). In the model, the life flow could refer that of a person or family or to the life of an organisation.

The river metaphor aptly represents the aim in collectivist cultures of creating harmony with one's surroundings. A river is shaped by the unique geography over which it courses, following valleys, flowing over and around rocks and falling in waterfalls. Similarly, the flow of the water itself can etch into the landscape, creating new channels (see Figure 25.5). As Iwama (2006) explained, 'Collectively oriented people tend to place enormous value on the *self* embedded in relationships. There is greater value in 'belonging' and 'interdependence', than a unilateral agency and in individual determinism' (p. 145, italics in original). Therefore, the meaning and purpose of occupation is most strongly shaped by the person's social context.

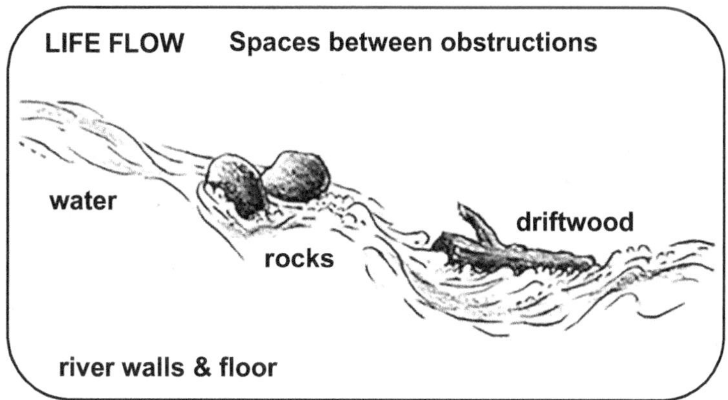

Figure 25.5 Kawa Model

Cross-sections depicting river elements can reveal the state of a person's river (life flow) at different times in their life. The elements are as follows:

- Water (*Mizu*) represents life flow. As a fluid, water will easily take on the shape of a container and fill the spaces completely. However, the power of its flow gives it the capacity to carve new channels. So too, people can conform to the demands of their surroundings, while also influencing them.
- The surroundings (social and physical environments) are represented by the river walls and floor (*Kawa no Soku-Heki* and *Kawa no Zoko*, respectively). In collectivist cultures, these are important factors in determining a person's life flow because the environmental culture is instrumental in determining how people experience 'self' and the meanings they ascribe to their actions.
- Rocks (*Iwa*, large rocks or crags) represent circumstances that impede the life flow and are considered by the person to be problematic and difficult to remove. Potential rocks include impairments to body structures and functions, difficulties with activities of daily living, lack of money and difficult social relations.
- Driftwood (*Ryuboku*) represents personal attributes and resources, which could relate to personal characteristics and abilities (e.g., values, personality, skills) as well as material assets (e.g., wealth, special equipment) and living situation (e.g., rural and urban, shared accommodation). These can affect circumstances and life flow in positive and negative ways. Compared to rocks, driftwood is less permanent and more amenable to the flow of the river. The spaces between obstructions (*Sukima*) represent places in a person's life where life energy and life flow are still occurring (the Kawa Model uses a strengths-based approach, seeking to identify strengths rather than problems). Identification of *sukima* enables an occupational therapist to work by strategically building on opportunities to maximise life flow (see Figure 25.5).

By paying particular attention to the concept of spaces between elements, rather than focusing on the elements themselves, emphasises the strength-based nature of the Kawa Model. Attention is drawn to the life flow and finding opportunities to enhance that in the context of a person, family, or organisation.

25.6 Canadian Model of Occupational Participation

The Canadian Model of Occupational Participation was published by the Canadian Association of Occupational Therapy (CAOT) in 2022 in the book entitled *Promoting Occupational Participation: Collaborative Relation-Focused Occupational Therapy* (Egan & Restall, 2022). Pervading the CanMOP are principles from the Truth & Reconciliation Commission of Canada (2007–2015), which emphasised the need to acknowledge the harms and injustices done to the Indigenous peoples of Canada and commit to the development of relationships of mutual recognition and respect. The model emphasises that occupational therapists work collaboratively with individuals and collectives such as families, groups, and populations.

The CanMOP centres on *occupational participation*, defined as 'having access to, initiating, and sustaining valued occupations within meaningful relationships and contexts' (Egan & Restall, 2022, p. 75). While earlier Canadian models

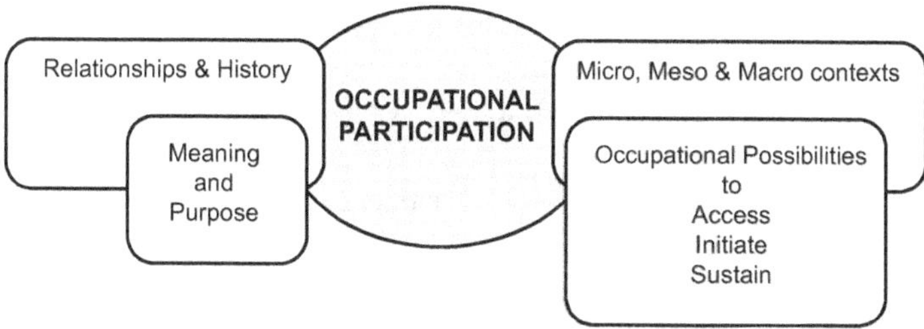

Figure 25.6 Canadian Model of Occupational Participation (CanMOP)

focused on occupational performance, the expanded notion of occupational participation attends to the meaning and purpose of occupations for both individuals and collectives.

The diagram associated with the CanMOP has two diamond shapes placed side-by-side with the two central corners overlapping behind a circle representing occupational performance (see Figure 25.6). Each diamond has a central consideration with its influences. On the left-hand diamond, the central consideration is meaning and purpose (for individuals and collectives), which is influenced by relationships and history. On the right-hand diamond, the central consideration is occupational possibilities, which is shaped by micro, meso, and macro contexts (see Figure 25.6).

Understanding meaning and purpose should be determined from the perspectives of those individuals and collectives with whom occupational therapists are working. Occupational therapists are urged to be aware of their own perspectives and those of the dominant culture, as well as how their own privileges and oppressions might be shaping their interpretations. They are cautioned not to let these interfere with listening deeply to the perspectives of the clients. When considering the purpose of occupational participation, Egan and Restall (2022) identified four basic needs that occupation can address. These are: survival and safety, autonomy, relatedness, and competence (see Figure 25.6). They emphasised that, for example, from the perspective of Indigenous peoples, the survival and safety needs of an individual are intertwined with the physical, emotional, cognitive, and spiritual needs of the community. Therefore, understanding any individual's needs will require appreciation of their obligations to the community. Understanding autonomy, relatedness, and competence means seeing people as able to act in accordance with their own values and community standards, being connected to and supported by others, and feeling they are effective in occupations that are important them.

Relationships and history provide the context for the development of the meaning and purpose of occupation for individuals and collectives. Relationships are central to determining the purpose of occupation in that engagement in occupation might fulfil obligations to others, strengthen relationships with others, or offer a reprieve from commitments to and participation with others. Time and relationships shape the meanings individuals and collectives give to occupation. As Egan and Restall (2022) stated, 'past, present, and future hoped-for occupational participation always involves specific others, even when those others are present only in memory and imagination' (p. 79).

In terms of history, CanMOP shows how occupation is influenced at both individual and collective levels. It uses a Life Course perspective to understand the temporal context of individual's lives. The Life Course perspective assumes that:

- life unfolds over time and that past experiences influence the present
- historical time and geographical contexts (i.e., when and where they live) shape people's experiences
- the timing of events in a person's life matters, in that earlier events (both positive and negative) affect later experiences
- people exist within a network of relationships; that is, their lives are linked with those of others
- people have agency in their lives in that they can take action within the opportunities and constraints they encounter in their various situations.

At a collective level, community history can shed light on the experiences of groups of people who have a shared identity. Egan and Restall (2022) explained that these can include 'historic experiences of cohesion and thriving, as well as experiences of trauma' (p. 80). Community histories can help occupational therapists understand the challenges the community has encountered, and the meaning of various occupations have for them.

The essential consideration in the diamond on the right-hand side of the diagram is occupational possibilities to access, initiate, and sustain occupational participation, with the background to this being the micro, meso, and macro levels of context. The term occupational possibilities refers to those ways and types of doing that are perceived as possible and valued within a specific socio-historical context and are, therefore, promoted and made available (Laliberte Rudman, 2010). It is important to consider how powerfully context 'determines expectations, barriers, and affordances regarding occupational participation' (Turpin et al., 2024, p. 139). Egan and Restall (2022) presented occupational therapists as experts in expanding occupational possibilities through addressing underlying assumptions about what people with certain conditions can and should do and working collaboratively with people to identify and support changes needed to the micro, meso, and macro environments.

Making explicit the three levels of context at which occupational therapists can work provides guidance about where to target intervention. The micro context refers to the level of people's direct interactions with others and the environment. Depending on their roles, this might include interactions with family members, friends, teachers, and peers at school; co-workers; and providers of health and social services, as well as with the non-human context. The meso level of context refers to social systems such as organisations and their respective programmes and community infrastructure. Examples include eligibility for and obligations to services, availability and cost of travel, and accessibility of the built environment. In general, decisions made at this level of context are beyond the control of many individuals and collectives and intervention requires advocacy. The broadest level of context is the macro level, which denotes the socio-economic and political context, including the socio-cultural values and beliefs that are embedded in policy and legislation. This level regulates the meso level by determining what is funded or allowed and shapes what is developed and provided by public and private services and organisations.

These three levels of context shape the degree to which people can access, initiate, and sustain occupational participation. In terms of access to occupational participation, context can determine who has access to which occupations and who does not. Even if people have access to occupation, they need to be able to initiate engagement. Barriers to initiating occupation might include social attitudes, cost, level of skill, the built environment, infrastructure, and the organisation of work and education. In addition, people need to be able to sustain occupational participation over time. The three levels of context can combine to support or inhibit sustained occupational participation. For example, not all buses might be accessible. Or, even if they have ramps for physical access, sustained use of them can depend on the attitudes of bus drivers and good training. Occupational therapists can be involved in advocating for accessible transport policies, training of relevant staff and increasing skills required for using accessible transport.

The last two models presented in this chapter are Canadian and show the development in thinking in occupational therapy over the past three decades. First, the PEO, which took an ecological approach to the concepts of person, environment, and occupation through the notion of the 'PEO Fit', is described. Second, the CMOP-E, which emphasised the Canadian focus on client-centredness, is presented.

25.7 Person–Environment–Occupation Model

The PEO Model was published in 1996 (Law et al., 1996) and no further revisions have been undertaken. The model is concerned with the relationship among *person, environment* and *occupation* and its contribution to occupational performance through the 'person–environment–occupation fit' (Law et al., 1996, p. 17) (*PEO fit*). Greater or lesser PEO fit leads to enhanced or reduced occupational performance.

The model differs from many other models at the time, in that it uses an ecological framework and describes a 'transactive' (as distinct from interactive) relationship among people, what they do, and their environments. In an interactive approach, person and environment are conceived as separate entities that interact and can be studied separately. In a transactive approach, a person's occupational performance cannot be separated from the context in which it occurs. Therefore, occupational performance is context-, person-, and occupation-specific. It results from specific people doing specific things in specific places and specific circumstances.

In a transactive relationship, a change in any of person, environment and occupation will change the others in ways that cannot be controlled or predicted. Therefore, the unit of study and analysis is an event, rather than the separate components of person, environment and occupation. By exploring the event as a whole, attention centres on the way PEO fit changes with a change to any components. Changes in PEO fit are also evident when taking a lifespan perspective, in that PEO fit is assumed to change over time and with different circumstances. This lifespan perspective is presented diagrammatically using a cylinder that can be transected at different places to represent the PEO fit at different times in a person's life.

In the PEO Model publication, each component is also discussed. The person is 'a dynamic, motivated and ever-developing being, constantly interacting with the environment' (Law et al., 1996, p. 17). The model takes a lifespan perspective, whereby people change over time, as they grow and develop and move through their life stages.

However, they also change in response to alterations in the environment surrounding them. Their attributes, characteristics, abilities and skills change, as well as how they think and feel about themselves, their sense of identity and their sense of what they are capable of doing and achieving. As occupational performance can be measured both objectively and subjectively, the model advocates that people's capacities should be measured (e.g. through objective assessment) and their experiences and perceptions also should be explored (e.g., through self-report).

The environment is inseparable from the person. It is defined broadly, understood as shaping and being shaped by people, and has five aspects: cultural, socio-economic, institutional, physical and social. Some or all of these five aspects will combine to shape occupational performance. Environments also change over the course of people's lives. People might relocate geographically, find themselves in altered circumstances, or their environments might change because they have changed their roles, routines and habits. Changes in environments rarely relate to only one environmental aspect. For example, a change in the physical environment might have implications for the social environment. To illustrate how people and environments are intertwined, internalised cultural views shape what people want and need to do and socio-economic circumstances will shape what opportunities they have for doing and the resources available to them. Finally, occupation is what people do in their contexts. Occupation is considered in terms of three aspects of human action – activity, task and occupation, which are considered 'nested within each other' (Law et al., 1996, p. 16).

25.8 Canadian Model of Occupational Performance and Engagement

The CMOP-E was published in *Enabling Occupation II: Advancing an Occupational Therapy Vision for Health, Well-being and Justice through Occupation* (Townsend & Polatajko, 2013) by the Canadian Association of Occupational Therapists (CAOT) (along with the Canadian Practice Process Framework and the Canadian Model of Client-Centred Enablement). The three main components of the CMOP-E are *person*, *occupation*, and *environment*.

CMOP-E still retains the essential structure of the original CMOP, published in 1997, however emphasises the ability to engage in occupation without performing it. Like OPM(A), the influence of the occupational performance models is evident in its inclusion of both performance components and performance areas. The person is presented as having three performance components – affective, cognitive, and physical, as well as a central core of spirituality. The performance areas of ADL/self-maintenance, work/productive activities, and play/leisure provide the framework for categorising occupation.

Occupation is the core domain of occupational therapy and the 'bridge' that connects person and environment. It is defined as 'groups of activities and tasks of everyday life, named, organised, and given value and meaning by individuals and a culture. Occupation is everything people do to occupy themselves, including looking after themselves (self-care), enjoying life (leisure), and contributing to the social and economic fabric of their communities (productivity)' (definition of occupation retained from the first edition of Enabling Occupation – CAOT 1997 cited in Townsend and Polatajko (2007, p. 17)). The environment has four aspects – physical, institutional, cultural, and social – and surrounds the person, emphasising that each person lives in a specific environmental context that affords (and constrains) possibilities for occupation.

Enablement through occupation is conceptualised as the core of occupational therapy. While occupational performance is an enduring component of the model, the concept of engagement was added to the second edition to emphasise that people can engage in occupation without necessarily performing it. As an exemplar, Townsend and Polatajko (2013) described a father and his severely disabled son who undertook extreme sporting events together such as marathons, triathlons and ironman events. The son engaged in these (but did not perform them), while being pushed in a wheelchair, pulled in a dinghy or pulled behind his father's bicycle.

Occupational therapy *enables* the following: a) engagement in everyday life, b) performance of occupation, and c) the creation of a just society in which people can participate. Therefore, occupational therapy practice can target both individual and societal levels. Accordingly, CMOP-E identifies six categories of client – individuals, families, groups, communities, organisations (e.g., government, non-government and corporate agencies; clubs and associations) and populations.

In CMOP-E, *client-centred practice* is also considered fundamental to occupational therapy. It involves collaboration and power sharing, working *with* people rather than doing to or for them, and prioritising client goals and outcomes. Townsend and Polatajko (2013) explained that both client-centred practice and engagement can be encountered at the level of the client and therapist or at the broader systems surrounding them. For example, factors influencing the personal level might include the client's culture and level of education, the therapist's capacity to recognise the client's expertise and to share power. Factors influencing the broader level could include management policy and practice or government philosophy and the equity of resource distribution.

25.9 Conclusion

This brief description of influential Western occupational therapy models shows the progression of some important concepts in occupational therapy thinking. Occupational performance models were the predominant models until the 1980s and were strongly influenced by the mechanistic paradigm. The OPM(A) demonstrates a later ecological development of these concepts in the 1990s, with an emphasis on understanding occupational performance *in context*. Other models that demonstrate this ecological turn are the PEOP, CMOP-E, and PEO. MOHO represents an early departure from the structure of the OP models, instead being premised on systems theory, in particular, dynamical systems theory. Other models also drawing upon systems theory are the PEOP and OPM(A). The Kawa Model emphasises the cultural relevance of occupational therapy concepts, particularly the perspectives of collectivist cultures. It contrasts the individualised self with the decentralised self. Since the model's publication, more attention has been provided in occupational therapy to cultural relevance. Finally, the most recently developed model, the CanMOP, makes explicit the inequalities that exist in contemporary Western societies that influence whether people have access to and can sustain occupational participation. It particularly acknowledges the enduring effects of the harms and injustices done to the Indigenous peoples of Canada through colonisation. Reflecting on the seven models together, it appears that there is a growing awareness in occupational therapy of the need to develop beyond hegemonic Western conceptions of occupation towards a greater awareness of diverse experiences and perspectives.

25.10 Summary

- There are a range of well-respected and internationally recognised, discipline-specific models that are available to guide practice.
- Models enshrine occupational therapy values and assumptions.
- By being familiar with a broad range of models, occupational therapists have expanded choice when considering which models best suit their practice context.
- It is important to understand the historical and contextual factors that inform the development of occupational therapy models.
- Occupational therapy models continue to evolve and develop as professional concepts change.

25.11 Review and reflection questions

25.11.1 Review questions

- Discuss how the OPM(A) differs from the original OP models and describe its structure and components.
- Identify the theoretical basis for the MOHO and describe its structure and components.
- Describe how the components of the PEOP are related in an 'ecological' way.
- Describe the metaphor and the structure and components of the KAWA Model and discuss the concepts it emphasises.
- Discuss the context in which the CanMOP was developed and describe its structure and elements.

25.11.2 Reflection questions

- How is the notion of occupation represented differently in the various occupational therapy models and what does this tell us about how it has changed over time?
- Choose one of the key models discussed in this chapter that you believe may be most useful for guiding your clinical practice then provide an in-depth reflection of why the chosen model may be helpful.

References

Bass, J., Baum, C. M., & Christiansen, C. H. (2017). Person-environment-occupation-performance model. In J. Hinojoa, P. Kramer, & C. Royeen (Eds.), *Perspectives on human occupation: Theories underlying practice* (2nd ed., pp. 161–182). F. A. Davis Company.

Baum, C. M., Bass, J., & Christiansen, C. (2020). The person-environment-occupation-performance model. In E. A. S. Duncan (Ed.), *Foundations for practice in occupational therapy* (6th ed., pp. 87–95). Elsevier.

Baum, C. M., Christiansen, C. H., & Bass, J. D. (2015). The person-environment-occupation-performance (PEOP) model. In C. H. Christiansen, C. M. Baum, & J. D. Bass (Eds.), *Occupational therapy: Performance, participation, and well-being* (pp. 49–56). SLACK Inc.

Bowyer, P., Wolske, J., Cabrera, J. P., & Fisher, G. (2023). Dimensions of doing. In R. Taylor, P. Bowyer, & G. Fisher (Eds.), *Kielhofner's Model of Human Occupation* (6th ed., pp. 110–121). Lippincott Williams & Wilkins.

Chapparo, C., & Ranka, J. (1997). *OPM: Occupational Performance Model (Australia)*. Occupational Performance Network.

Chapparo, C., Ranka, J., & Nott, M. (2017). Occupational Performance Model (Australia): A description of constructs, structure and propositions. In M. Curtin, M. Egan, & J. Adams

(Eds.), *Occupational therapy for people experiencing illness, injury or impairment: Promoting occupation and participation* (7th ed., pp. 134–147). Elsevier.

Egan, M., & Restall, G. (2022). The Canadian model of occupational participation. In M. Egan & G. Restall (Eds.), *Promoting occupational participation: Collaborative relationship focused occupational therapy* (pp. 73–95). CAOT.

Fisher, A. G., & Marterella, A. (2019). *Powerful practice: A model for authentic occupational therapy.* Centre for Innovative OT Solutions.

Forsyth, K., & Brown, C. (2024). The model of human occupation. In G. Gillen & C. Brown (Eds.), *Willard & Spackman's occupational therapy* (14th ed., pp. 555–573). Wolters Kluwer.

Iwama, M. K. (2006). *The Kawa model: Culturally relevant occupational therapy.* Churchill Livingstone.

Laliberte Rudman, D. (2010). Occupational terminology: Occupational possibilities. *Journal of Occupational Science, 17*(1), 55–59. https://doi.org/10.1080/14427591.2010.9686673

Law, M., Cooper, B., Strong, S., Stewart, D., Rigby, P., & Letts, L. (1996). The Person-Environment-Occupation Model: A transactive approach to occupational performance. *Canadian Journal of Occupational Therapy, 63*(1), 9–23. https://doi.org/10.1177/000841749606300103

Nelson, A., McLaren, C., Lewis, T., & Iwama, M. (2017). Cultural influences and occupation-centred practice with children and families. In S. Rodger & A. Kennedy-Behr (Eds.), *Occupation-centred practice with children: A practical guide for occupational therapists* (pp. 73–90). John Wiley & Sons.

Townsend, E., & Polatajko, H. (2007). *Enabling occupation II: Advancing an occupational therapy vision for health, well-being, & justice through occupation.* CAOT Publications ACE.

Townsend, E., & Polatajko, H. (2013). *Enabling occupation II: Advancing an occupational therapy vision for health, well-being, & justice through occupation* (2nd ed.). CAOT Publications ACE.

Turpin, M., Garcia, J., & Iwama, M. K. (2024). *Using occupational therapy models in practice: A fieldguide* (2nd ed.). Elsevier.

Wilcock, A. A. (1998). Reflections on doing, being and becoming. *Canadian Journal of Occupational Therapy, 65*(5), 248–256. https://doi.org/10.1177/000841749806500501

Yeasir, A. A., Martin, M., Yamada, T., & Taylor, R. R. (2023). The person-specific concept of human occupation. In R. Taylor, P. Bowyer, & G. Fisher (Eds.), *Kielhofner's Model of Human Occupation* (6th ed., pp. 9–22). Lippincott Williams & Wilkins.

Practice issues

CHAPTER 26

Fundamentals of occupational therapy I

Occupation-centred practice

Louise Gustafsson, Jessica Holding, Lachlan Pascoe, and Kaitlyn Spalding

Authors' positionality statement

All authors are occupational therapy academics from a western background, who recognise their privilege as white, educated professionals. They all work within one academic programme that is strongly centred in an occupational perspective and the promotion of occupational justice for all peoples. Three authors have recently transitioned to academia from clinical roles, and all authors engage in research with a focus on occupation-centred practice.

Key terms
- Occupation
- Occupational perspective
- Occupation-centred
- Occupation-based
- Occupation-focused

Objectives
This chapter will allow the reader to:

- Define and describe occupation-centred practice
- Understand occupation-based and occupation-focused practice as two important but distinct elements of occupation-centred practice
- Consider how therapists can remain occupation centred when working in a variety of practice contexts
- Consider how therapists can remain occupation centred when working with individuals and collectives

DOI: 10.4324/9781003495666-29

26.1 Introduction

Occupations include the things individuals and collectives need, want, and are expected to do to occupy time and bring meaning and purpose to life (World Federation of Occupational Therapy, 2012). There are several characteristics that illustrate the complexity of occupation which are often not captured in simple definitions (Molineux, 2024). All occupations are uniquely human, have purpose, are contextual, have meaning that is unique and dynamic, and require active engagement (Molineux, 2009). A contemporary view of occupational therapy highlights the importance of occupation to health and well-being, focuses on occupational challenges, and uses occupation to improve health status (Kielhofner, 2009).

This occupational perspective of humans and health is what makes the occupational therapy profession unique. The contemporary paradigm urges occupational therapists to maintain this perspective throughout all stages of the occupational therapy process when working with individuals and collectives (Kielhofner, 2009; Molineux, 2024). Occupational therapy practice that is occupation centred ensures clients benefit from the profession's unique perspective. In this chapter, key terms are defined and explored. Examples of occupation-centred, occupation-based, and occupation-focused practice when working with individuals and collectives are described in different practice contexts, including those which have been identified to present challenges in maintaining an occupational perspective.

26.2 Occupation-centred practice

In this chapter we adopt the definition of *occupation-centred practice* proposed by Fisher (2014). Occupational therapy practice is occupation centred when we hold occupation at the centre of our professional reasoning. That is, we apply an occupational perspective to understand individuals are occupational beings and highlight the power of occupation within their lives including as an agent of change. Four characteristics of occupation-centred practice have been developed (Ford et al., 2022). (See Table 26.1). The characteristics build on the definition from Fisher (2014) and provide a foundation for occupational therapists to further understand, identify, and operationalise occupation-centred practice. Occupation-based and occupation-focused practice are elements of occupation-centred practice, which help to maintain an occupational perspective throughout all stages of the occupational therapy process.

Occupation-based practice is the act of using occupation as the therapeutic agent, making use of a person's engagement in occupation as the method for evaluation and intervention (Fisher & Marterella, 2019). Occupation-based evaluations include performance and task analysis during the performance of chosen daily life tasks. It is important that these are allowed to unfold in contexts in which they ordinarily do in the person's life, for example, completing an analysis of community access by observing engagement in catching a bus to the local shopping centre. Occupation-based interventions are those where the occupational therapist uses engagement in occupation as the therapeutic agent of change (Fisher & Marterella, 2019), for example, whole task practise of cooking a meal at home when addressing meal preparation goals post-stroke.

Occupation-focused practice describes assessment, intervention, and evaluation strategies that have an immediate focus on occupation, referred to as the proximal focus (Fisher & Marterella, 2019). Occupation-focused practice is evident when assessments

Table 26.1 Characteristics of occupation-centred practice (Ford et al., 2022)

Characteristic	*Illustrative example/s*
Grounded in theory and philosophy, recognising the importance of occupation to health and well-being.	• The importance of occupation for health and well-being is prominent when you introduce yourself and occupational therapy, or when talking with individuals or collectives about the importance of occupation.
Occupation and occupational terminology prominent in verbal and written communication.	• Use occupational language when talking with others while making links to support their initial understanding. • The heading 'Occupation' and/or 'Occupational Issues' is prominent in documentation and discussions to describe the person as an occupational being and outline the presenting occupations of importance to the individual; person-related factors (impairments) are reported based on their contribution to occupational issues.
Contextual aspects and their influence on occupations are considered, including cultural, social, temporal, physical, political, and institutional environments.	• Contextual aspects and their contributions to occupational participation are explored, understood, and clearly articulated. • Evaluation and practice are best situated within the individual's real environment/s but when not feasible, the environment is adapted to approximate the person's environment/s as near as possible.
Occupation at the core of goal setting, evaluation (information gathering and assessment), and intervention.	• Occupational goals are collaboratively identified early in the occupational therapy process and continuously refined. • Evaluation explicitly addresses occupation. • Occupation is the base and/or focus of therapeutic approaches.

and evaluations directly gather information about the individual's occupational performance, experience, or participation. For example, developing an occupational history, identifying occupational concerns with the Canadian Occupational Performance Measure (Law et al., 2014), or conducting an occupation analysis. Interventions are occupation focused when occupation holds the proximal focus and a change in occupational performance, occupational experience, or participation is the immediate outcome. Examples include learning to catch a bus with a focus on getting better at catching the bus or improving the occupational experience and discussions that explore how a person can change the way that they are dressing so that they can do so without the assistance of others.

It is important to recognise that our practice can be occupation based without being occupation focused. For example, a person may be engaged in practice that is based in an occupation like baking a cake, but the focus of the therapist is on how the individual is using meta-cognitive strategies to follow the recipe. In this example the focus in on person factors and the practice is occupation based and person focused. Equally, practice can be occupation focused and not occupation based. An example is when education is provided about how to adapt an occupation without doing the occupation. Practice can be both occupation based and focused and an example is engagement in catching public transport with the sole focus of improving that person's occupational participation.

Fisher and Marterella (2019) refer to a 'sliding scale' of occupation-based and occupation-focused practice to support the dynamic interplay of promoting occupational participation and addressing individual performance components (person) or contextual barriers (environment). Table 26.2 defines the two 'ends' of the continuous sliding scale. Neither end is wrong or right, and they may both be present within one occupational therapy session. However, it is important to remember that the profession's unique occupational perspective should remain the prominent feature of our practice.

A vignette of an occupational therapist working in hand therapy is provided in Box 26.1 with notations to further illustrate this 'sliding scale' of practice.

Table 26.2 Occupation, Person or Environment?

Base = What is the action?	
Occupation-based practice involves the active doing of occupation in assessment and treatment.	**Person-based** practice involves assessment and treatment of performance components, for example, range of motion assessment or memory strategy training.
	Environment-based practice involves assessment and intervention to address environmental barriers, including assistive technology, for example, measurement to determine turning spaces for a wheelchair.
Focus = Where is the attention?	
Occupation-focused practice has an immediate focus on occupation.	**Person-focused** practice has an immediate focus on the performance components such as focus on building strength in grasp.
	Environment-focused practice has an immediate focus on the environment, for example, discussions about the assistive equipment required following a total hip replacement operation.

Box 26.1
Occupation-centred practice in a hand therapy clinic

Amira was referred to a hand therapy clinic following a right distal radius fracture. The referral from the surgeon requested oedema management, fabrication of a wrist orthosis, and active range of motion exercises. At the first therapy appointment, the occupational therapist *gathers information about Amira's occupational history,*[a] learning Amira is primarily concerned about the pain she is experiencing following her surgery and an increase in oedema over her fingers and hand. The occupational therapist *applies a cohesive bandage 'glove' to reduce oedema and fabricates a custom-made thermoplastic orthosis to protect the fracture*[b] during 'at risk' occupations.

LEGEND
a Occupation-focused
b Person-based and person-focused
c Occupation-based and between person- and occupation-focused
d Moving between occupation-focused and person-focused
e Occupation-based and occupation-focused
f Environment-based and environment-focused

The occupational therapist educates Amira regarding fracture healing and suggests that the increase in *oedema may be exacerbated by performance of occupations that require her hand to be in a dependent position such as typing. The occupational therapist encourages Amira to elevate her hand and demonstrates active range of motion exercises that will promote lymphatic drainage and tendon gliding and improve finger, wrist, and forearm joint range of motion.*[b] Amira reports difficulty completing self-care occupations with only the use of her uninjured upper limb. She has been trying to keep on top of her work emails whilst on sick leave but is having trouble typing and operating the mouse due to pain, reduced strength, and impaired coordination and control of finger movements. Together, the occupational therapist and Amira *problem solve and then practise how she can safely use her injured hand in self-care occupations.*[c] The occupational therapist *advises Amira to modify the occupation of typing so that regular rest breaks are included,d* allowing time for elevation and the completion of prescribed exercises

Amira attends weekly occupational therapy appointments for six weeks. Sessions focus *on improving range of motion, reducing oedema, and promoting scar pliability.*[b] The occupational therapist and Amira *continue to discuss challenges experienced when engaging in occupations and identify solutions to these.a* When adequate stability of the fracture fixation is confirmed by the treating surgeon, Amira is encouraged to continue to complete self-care and *practices how to conduct other light occupations such as folding laundry and simple meal preparation without the protection of the thermoplastic orthosis.*[e] Additionally, the occupational therapist *visits Amira's workplace, trialling modifications to her workstation which will enable her to type and operate the mouse with less pain and improved accuracy.*[a,f]

26.3 Illustrative vignettes of occupation-centred practice

The remainder of this chapter provides examples of occupation-centred practice across a range of practice settings.

26.3.1 Working with individuals in residential aged care

Literature is beginning to emerge that illustrate factors that may contribute to challenges in being occupation-centred clinicians when working in residential aged care facilities (RACF) (Calderone et al., 2022a, 2022b; Rooney et al., 2024). The following vignette illustrates how occupation-centred practice can improve health and well-being of people living in a RACF.

Denise had recently moved into a RACF and spent most of her time withdrawn in her room with staff reporting she now required physical assistance during self-care. The facility was also concerned that Denise was not coming to the arts and craft activities held by the lifestyle team, despite her family reporting she was interested in art. Using the Canadian Model of Occupational Participation (CanMOP; Egan & Restall, 2022) and Mountain and Craig's (2006) Activity Pebbles during the initial interview created the conditions for Denise to share stories, desires, and priorities regarding occupational participation (Restall et al., 2022). Denise identified art critiquing, reading, and gardening as occupational concerns. Denise shared that she wasn't interested in the arts and crafts activities, stating she preferred to write about art and was previously an art critic. Denise did not report participating in self-care independently as a priority;

however, the occupational therapist noted similar barriers to participation that could be addressed by focusing on Denise's priority occupational concerns.

Occupation-focused goals and an occupation-based intervention plan were developed using the Canadian Occupational Performance Measure (COPM; Law et al., 2014) and a goal planning worksheet (Mountain & Craig, 2006). Subsequent, bi-weekly sessions through the site's rehabilitation programme included:

- A walk to the facility library to find a new book. Denise would point out artwork and sculptures for the therapist to photograph. Denise was able to rest at intervals that decreased in frequency with each trip.
- The therapist would print the photographs of the artwork and sculpture for Denise to critique and develop a portfolio.
- Introduced Denise to an area of the garden that had a raised garden bed.
- Denise would tidy up the facility garden and interact with her co-residents with the graded assistance of the therapist.

At the conclusion of the twelve-week programme, Denise's self-perceived performance and satisfaction had increased for all occupational concerns, she had an art portfolio she shared with her family and was tending to the garden between sessions (she was yet to decide on a book but still appreciated the library trips). Denise was also attending bingo and meals with a resident she met in the garden, and although no specific goals or intervention plans were made in relation to the original referral, Denise no longer required physical assistance for showering.

26.3.2 Occupation-centred groups in a hospital setting

Occupation-centred groups occur across a variety of inpatient rehabilitation settings, often addressing complex occupations such as home management and community living (Spalding et al., 2020; Wall et al., 2024a). Such groups have demonstrated a positive impact on patient outcomes of occupational performance, satisfaction, and confidence post-discharge (Spalding et al., 2022a; Wall et al., 2024b). A practice example of an occupation-based group set in an inpatient general rehabilitation ward setting has been outlined subsequently from a process evaluation study (Spalding et al., 2023).

Group name: The LifeSkills Group

Objective: To enhance recovery of chosen home-based occupation performance through occupation-based practice.

Participants: General rehabilitation inpatients (variety of neurological conditions including stroke and mild traumatic brain injury and non-neurological conditions including orthopaedic fractures and general reconditioning after a medical illness).

Facilitators: Student occupational therapists under the guidance of the treating therapist.

Group structure: Ratio of two student occupational therapists to four patients. Runs four days per week for an hour.

<u>Group process:</u>

- Eligible participants referred to group by treating occupational therapist.
- Individual goals identified and set (on average four occupations per person).
- All participants would meet as an entire group before splitting to work individually on an occupational goal either sharing a mutual space or occupation focus with others.

<u>Underlying principles:</u>

- Occupation-centred goals: Practice related to individual goals which were made explicit during the session with clear links to the tasks.
- Occupation-based and focused practice: Using tailored, occupation-centred practice in an environment that fostered a realism to home. Meaningful practise encouraged, including offering participant choice and control over the details of the tasks, such as choosing to cook a certain meal.
- Encouraging motivation and engagement with peers (Cole, 2012): Socialising with other participants, sharing a common recipe and steps during a meal preparation. Consistency in facilitators and member ratios: consistent facilitator interactions and enabling shared experience between participants enabled feelings of value and self-worth.
- Motor learning with a focus on intensity of practise and feedback loop: (Muratori et al., 2013): Participants were observed to discuss and compare results from previous sessions with the facilitators, identifying new strategies for occupation-based practice.

26.3.3 Occupation-centred practice with collectives

This vignette provides an example of an occupational therapist working in partnership with a local primary school to identify and address a collective occupational concern. In this vignette, soccer was identified as an occupation valued by many of the students at the school. Children across all age groups played in their lunch and recess breaks but this required significant oversight and supervision from teachers during break times. The occupational therapist expressed curiosity around soccer as a collective occupation to teachers and students and came to understand that there were occupational concerns. Adopting an occupation-centred approach, occupation analyses were completed across different days and with different cohorts of students, supervised by different teaching staff. The occupational concern was further explored from the perspective of teachers and students using focus groups.

Identified enablers were:

- Soccer enjoyed by many children, across all age groups within the school.
- Other lunchtime clubs, which are co-created and co-led by students, identified as a potential framework to be applied to soccer.

Identified barriers were:
- Inequitable use of playing time, with more time for older students when compared to younger students.
- Only one soccer field available.
- Frequent disagreements between students regarding rules.

Following the period of consultation, occupation-centred goals were established, and the following intervention strategies implemented:

- School staff educated about benefits of soccer from an occupational perspective, including the value of student's being autonomous in their play.
- Teaching staff empowered to facilitate a session with student representatives to establish expectations for fair play.
- Program established where senior students refereed each other's games and the games of their younger peers.
- Referee training initially conducted by physical education teacher but then 'train-the trainer' model used so that graduating students would induct their peers on an annual basis.

The occupational therapist visited the school three months later. It was noted that the referee programme was running successfully with less conflict between students during games and less teacher resources required for supervision. Older students valued the opportunity for leadership and there was greater interaction between students from different age groups during break times.

26.4 Promoting and maintaining occupation-centred practice

Occupational therapists often work in contexts that view humans and their health from a biomedical or biopsychosocial perspective. However, there are some straightforward ways that we can ensure that we promote and maintain an occupational perspective (Gustafsson & Molineux, 2024).

1. Engage in continuing professional education to maintain your knowledge and understanding of the relationship between human health and occupation and be able to articulate how an occupational perspective guides your practice, for example, reading (or re-reading) literature, attending educational opportunities, seeking out people with expertise to discuss your practice.
2. Prioritise occupation-centred practice within your practice setting. Managers and supervisors play an important role by supporting attendance at professional development, prioritising occupation-centred practice in supervision sessions and team discussions, including occupation-centred practice in the mission statement or vision.
3. Adopt practices that support an occupational perspective. Approaches to goal setting, evaluation, and intervention that are occupation centred should be standard practice.
4. Prioritise occupational language and terminology. Use our language in documentation or discussions, for example, occupation rather than activities of daily living and take opportunities to link understanding for others.

26.5 Conclusion

An occupational perspective and occupation-centred practice are unique to occupational therapy. This chapter equips occupational therapists with the foundational knowledge and understanding of what it means to be occupation centred, occupation based, and occupation focused in our practice. The vignettes provide practice examples that demonstrate occupation-centred practice in action and illustrate how positive occupational participation and health outcomes can be achieved. The vignettes illustrate individual-based approaches, group-based approaches and working with a collective. Adapted from real-life scenarios, the vignettes provide a foundational understanding of how our practice can remain occupation centred across a range of contemporary practice contexts. The reader is encouraged to use the references to further explore and enrich their understanding and how to enact occupation-centred practice.

26.6 Summary

- *Occupations* are the things individuals and collectives need, want and are expected to do to occupy time and bring meaning and purpose to life.
- An *occupational perspective* highlights the importance of occupation to health and well-being, focuses on occupational challenges and guides therapy to use occupation to improve health status.
- Occupational therapy practice is *occupation centred* when it holds occupation at the centre of professional reasoning and is influenced by an occupational perspective.
- *Occupation-based* practice is the act of using occupation as the therapeutic agent.
- *Occupation-focused* practice describes assessment, intervention and evaluation strategies that have a proximal focus on occupation.
- It is the responsibility of all occupational therapists to ensure individuals and collectives benefit from the profession's unique perspective regardless of the practice context.

26.7 Review and reflection questions

- Create a diagram that conceptualises occupation-centred, occupation-focused, and occupation-based practice. For example, a flow chart or a series of labelled pictures.
- At an MDT meeting, another health discipline is concerned you may not be addressing impairments listed in a recent referral. Prepare a response that educates the team on the importance of being occupation centred as an occupational therapist.
- List the four characteristics of occupation-centred practice and identify ways that you demonstrate these in your practice.
- The Canadian Occupational Performance Measure has been identified in this chapter as an occupation-focused assessment tool. Create a list of additional occupation-centred assessment tools.
- Reflect on and write down why occupation-centred practice is important to you.

References

Calderone, L., Bissett, M., & Molineux, M. (2022a). Occupational therapy in Australian residential aged care facilities: A systematic mapping review. *Australian Occupational Therapy Journal, 69*(5), 625–636. https://doi.org/10.1111/1440-1630.12824

Calderone, L., Bissett, M., & Molineux, M. (2022b). Understanding occupational therapy practice in residential aged care facilities under the Aged Care Funding Instrument: A qualitative study. *Australian Occupational Therapy Journal*, 69(4), 447–455. https://doi.org/10.1111/1440-1630.12805

Cole, M. B. (2012). *Group dynamics in occupational therapy: The theoretical basis and practice application of group intervention* (4th ed.). SLACK Incorporated.

Egan, M., & Restall, G. (2022). The Canadian Model of Occupational Participation. In M. Egan & G. Restall (Eds.), *Promoting occupational participation: Collaborative relationship-focused occupational therapy* (pp. 73–95). Canadian Association of Occupational Therapists.

Fisher, A. G. (2014). Occupation-centred, occupation-based, occupation-focused: Same, same or different? *Scandinavian Journal of Occupational Therapy*, 21(Supp 1), 96–107. https://doi.org/10.3109/11038128.2014.952912

Fisher, A. G., & Marterella, A. (2019). *Powerful practice: A model for authentic occupational therapy*. Centre for Innovative OT Solutions Inc.

Ford, E., Di Tommaso, A., Molineux, M., & Gustafsson, L. (2022). Identifying the characteristics of occupation-centred practice: A Delphi study. *Australian Occupational Therapy Journal*, 69(1), 25–37. https://doi.org/10.1111/1440-1630.12765

Gustafsson, L., & Molineux, M. (2024). An overview of occupation-centered practice. In T. Brown, S. Isbel, L. Gustafsson, S. Gutman, D. Powers Dirette, B. Collins, & T. Barlott (Eds.), *Human occupation* (1st ed., pp. 29–46). Routledge. https://doi.org/10.4324/9781003504610

Kielhofner, G. (2009). *Conceptual foundations of occupational therapy practice* (4th ed.). F.A. Davis.

Law, M., Baptiste, S., Carswell, M., McColl, M., Polatajko, H., & Pollock, N. (2014). *Canadian Occupational Performance Measure* (5th ed.). CAOT Publications ACE.

Molineux, M. (2009). The nature of occupation. In M. Curtin, M. Molineux, & J. Supyk-Mellson (Eds.), *Occupational therapy and physical dysfunction: Enabling occupation* (6th ed., pp. 17–26). Elsevier.

Molineux, M. (2024). Overview of human occupation: Concepts and principles. In T. Brown, S. Isbel, L. Gustafsson, S. Gutman, D. Powers Dirette, B. Collins, & T. Barlott (Eds.), *Human occupation* (1st ed., pp. 29–46). Routledge. https://doi.org/10.4324/9781003504610

Mountain, G., & Craig, C. (2006). *Lifestyle matters: An occupational approach to healthy ageing* (1st ed.). Routledge. https://doi.org/10.4324/9781003416449

Muratori, L. M., Lamberg, E. M., Quinn, L., & Duff, S. V. (2013). Applying principles of motor learning and control to upper extremity rehabilitation. *Journal of Hand Therapy*, 26(2), 94–103. https://doi.org/10.1016/j.jht.2012.12.007

Restall, G., Egan, M., Valavaara, K., Phenix, A., & Sack, C. (2022). Canadian Occupational Therapy Inter-Relational Practice Process Framework. In M. Egan & G. Restall (Eds.), *Promoting occupational participation: Collaborative relationship-focused occupational therapy* (pp. 119–150). Canadian Association of Occupational Therapists.

Rooney, D., Aplin, T., Bennett, S., Gui, D. S., & Scott, T. (2024). Exploring occupational therapy practice in Australian residential aged care facilities: A cross-sectional survey. *Australian Occupational Therapy Journal*, 71(4), 578–592. https://doi.org/10.1111/1440-1630.12943

Spalding, K., Gustafsson, L., & Di Tommaso, A. (2022a). Occupation-based group programs in the inpatient hospital rehabilitation setting: A scoping review. *Disability and Rehabilitation*, 44(10), 2138–2148. https://doi.org/10.1080/09638288.2020.1813818

Spalding, K., Gustafsson, L., & Di Tommaso, A. (2022b). Exploring patient outcomes after participation in an inpatient occupation-based group: A longitudinal observational cohort study. *American Journal of Occupational Therapy*, 76(5), 7605205140. https://doi.org/10.5014/ajot.2022.049241

Spalding, K., Gustafsson, L., & Di Tommaso, A. (2023). Evaluation of an inpatient occupation-based group program using a process evaluation framework. *Australian Occupational Therapy Journal*, 70(1), 32–42. https://doi.org/10.1111/1440-1630.12829

Wall, G., Isbel, S., Gustafsson, L., & Pearce, C. (2024a). Occupation-based interventions to improve occupational performance and participation in the hospital setting: A systematic

review. *Disability and Rehabilitation*, 46(13), 2747–2768. https://doi.org/10.1080/0963828
8.2023.2236021

Wall, G., Isbel, S., Gustafsson, L., & Pearce, C. (2024b) Impact of occupation-based groups
on occupational performance and satisfaction outcomes: Pilot study. *OTJR: Occupation,
Participation and Health*, 15394492241300606. Advance online publication. https://doi.
org/10.1177/15394492241300606

World Federation of Occupational Therapy. (2012). *About occupational therapy*. https://wfot.
org/about/about-occupational-therapy

CHAPTER 27

Fundamentals of occupational therapy II

Understanding the environment

Tammy Aplin, Kathryn Martin, and Emma Crawford

Authors' positionality statement

The authors of this chapter are Australian occupational therapists who have worked with individuals, groups, and communities in clinical, education, and research work roles. We are English speaking and live and work on the lands of the Turrbal and Jagera Peoples in Meanjin (Brisbane). Kathryn Martin is a Murri (Queensland Aboriginal) woman, as well as being of Dutch and other European heritage. Emma Crawford and Tammy Aplin are White Australians and acknowledge the privilege brought about through many aspects of their social positioning. Professionally, we aim to think critically about social structures and work for and with people impacted by prejudice, discrimination, and injustice. This chapter draws from our knowledges, experiences, contexts, and life histories.

In this chapter, we have brought together ideas about environment and occupational therapy from an Australian perspective. We seek to honour Aboriginal and Torres Islander Peoples' Knowledges and perspectives; however, the profession's historical starting point for understanding the environment, much of the included literature, and two authors' perspectives are non-Indigenous. Aboriginal Knowledges and perspectives on the environment are vast – spanning over 60,000 years of history from over 250 distinct language and cultural groups. In this chapter we draw from a pool of Aboriginal and Torres Strait islander literature that is limited due to historical inopportunity for the creation of this literature and the perspectives of one Aboriginal occupational therapist authoring this chapter. This author acknowledges the influence of her Western training on her perspective, is on her own cultural learning journey, and recognises the need to continually decolonise her thinking. Therefore, we draw from *some* Australian Aboriginal and Torres Strait Islander Knowledges and perspectives on environment and occupational therapy with a goal of balancing respect, place, and humility with a push for deeper understanding through dialogue. This chapter does not represent all viewpoints and Māori and Aotearoa New Zealand voices are missing. We invite readers to critically consider the content as part of ongoing knowledge development, seek alternative viewpoints, and to continuously question and re-build understandings of environment.

Keywords
- Theory
- Models
- History
- Context
- Determinants
- Social
- Political
- Aboriginal and Torres Strait Islander Peoples' perspectives

Objectives

This chapter will allow the reader to:

- Understand the importance and influence of the environment in shaping people's lives including occupational participation
- Be familiar with a range of knowledges, terminology, and frameworks used to describe the environment
- Understand the environment as a pluralistic construct, which is understood in a range of ways based on historical and socio-political influences
- Explain the transactional nature of person, environment, and occupation
- Consider and understand the environment, with reference to nine dimensions
- Understand each dimension of the environment's influence on occupational participation and its relevance to occupational therapy practice

27.1 Introduction

Environment and occupation are inextricably linked. The environment influences when and how occupations happen; simultaneously, occupations shape the environments where they happen (Law et al., 1996). Understandings of environment depend on context, which means multiple understandings of the environment exist at once. Each occupational therapist's understanding of environment is one of many and one which may be very different to the people they work with.

This chapter critically considers conceptualisations of the environment in occupational therapy. Occupational therapy increasingly recognises historical and socio-political contexts including how they contribute to issues of occupational injustice and human rights. Indigenous knowledges and collectivist viewpoints have contributed to these changes, bringing critical and diverse perspectives. In this chapter we focus on *some* Aboriginal and Torres Strait Islander Knowledges and perspectives from Australia in relation to concepts related to the environment and occupational therapy. We first discuss different conceptualisations of the environment beginning with introductory ideas on Aboriginal and Torres Strait Islander Peoples' perspectives on the environment, followed by other concepts which have influenced the professions understandings – including the transactional nature of the environment, the Bioecological Model of Human Development, and our growing understanding of the socio-political environment. Nine dimensions of the environment are then introduced as a framework for the profession's growing understanding of the environment.

When considering occupational therapy's understandings of the environment, it is important to consider that Western perspectives have dominated occupational therapy's epistemology and discourse since the beginning of the profession in the United States of America. This differs significantly from Aboriginal and Torres Strait Islander Knowledges and relationship to the environment, with at least tens of thousands of years history. Colonialism has been a dominating force on occupational therapy's knowledge and learning (Emery-Whittington, 2025). Indigenous scholars, however, have challenged the profession to consider its coloniality and in doing so have and will continue to enrich and change the profession's understanding of the environment.

27.2 Conceptualisations of the environment

27.2.1 Aboriginal and Torres Strait Islander Peoples' perspectives on the environment

Belonging to Country and *caring for Country* are central principles in Aboriginal and Torres Strait Islander cultures. *Country* is the land, skies and waters as well as all the living things that are part of a geographic and spiritual area of deep connection to a specific group or nation of Aboriginal and Torres Strait Islander People. Each nation or tribe belongs to and has responsibilities to care for their Country, with Knowledges and Lores on how to do this having been handed down for tens of thousands of years. Reciprocally, Country cares for and sustains a people (Moreton-Robinson, 2015). As such, connection to Country is a central component of health and wellbeing for Aboriginal and Torres Strait Islander Peoples (Gee et al., 2014).

This deep and complex relationship is described in *The Aboriginal and Torres Strait Islander Social and Emotional Wellbeing (SEWB) Framework* (Gee et al., 2014). In the framework social and emotional well-being is considered from an Aboriginal and Torres Strait Islander perspective, as a multi-dimensional construct which includes important concepts related to the environment. These include connecting to Country and land, culture and community, family and kinship, and spirituality and ancestors. Historical, political, cultural, and social determinants are described as broader contexts that influence this holistic understanding of health and wellbeing. The model, while not using the term occupations identifies that culturally meaningful occupations are impacted by these determinants. For example, a community's history of colonisation, resistance, and opportunities for self-determination and sovereignty impact its historic and contemporary prospects for occupational engagement, health, and wellbeing.

The psychosocial benefits of being on Country and caring for County can differ between regions and from person-to-person but can include benefits to identity; sense of belonging; recovery from physical and mental illness; and empowerment and community cohesiveness (Trzepacz et al., 2014). Conversely, damage to Country that has resulted through colonisation, such as through mining and development creates immeasurable poor health and well-being outcomes (Trzepacz et al., 2014). For example, the destruction of Juukan Gorge resulted in irreparable loss for the Puutu Kunti Kurrama and Pinikura Peoples whose connection to the site had been maintained ongoingly for over 46,000 years (PKKP Aboriginal Corporation, 2020). Government policies which support mining and other acts that commercially benefit from the environment while ignoring or only showing token consideration of Aboriginal land and water management practices have profound negative impacts on the health and wellbeing of Aboriginal Peoples (Gibson, 2020).

Colonisation has had different impacts in different nations or regions on the way in which Aboriginal and Torres Strait Islander Peoples have been able to remain connected to their Country, and the level of self-determination and sovereignty they have in caring for it. For example, through government policies some people have been removed from Country to missions; whilst carrying Knowledges of their Country. Others have been stockmen on their Country or lived on a mission on or off their Country (Moreton-Robinson, 2015). And for many Aboriginal and Torres Strait Islander people with severe disability, there can be a need to choose between remaining on Country with family and community; or accessing suitable housing and services away from community and Country (Avery & First Peoples Disability Network, 2018).

Aboriginal and Torres Strait Islander nations or regions have maintained strong connection to Country, language and culture despite colonisation. Many nations are revitalising languages and cultural practices that have been threatened by forced removals and missions where language and culture was generally forbidden. Some Aboriginal and Torres Strait Islander People are Stolen Generations or descendants of those forcibly removed, with some people not knowing their mob or connections. Organisations like state-based LinkUp programmes (LinkUp (Qld), 2025) provide essential identity and connection support for Stolen Generations and descendants. There continue to be Stolen Generations, with more children now being removed from Aboriginal and Torres Strait Islander families than ever before (National Family Matters Leadership Group et al., 2024).

These examples convey the influence of colonisation and related environmental factors on the health and well-being of Aboriginal and Torres Strait Islander Peoples. Yet, despite the challenges posed by colonisation, many Aboriginal and Torres Strait Islander Peoples continue to care for Country and advocate for Country including their land, waters, and skies. For example, Ranger programmes which continue cultural caring for country practices have been found to improve health and wellbeing (Matthews et al., 2023), and many Torres Strait Islander communities are advocating for change at the forefront of climate action to protect their futures, which have been affected by rising sea levels. It is estimated that some islands may be uninhabitable by 2050, forcing Peoples to leave their Country (HEAL Network & CRE-STRIDE, 2021).

The intertwining of person and environment, as inseparable and co-dependent entities is well understood by Aboriginal and Torres Strait Islander cultures, and this knowledge is shared in many ways across generations including through storytelling, songs, and dance ceremonies (Matthews et al., 2023). Within occupational therapy, the more contemporary models have begun to consider the relationship between people and their environment.

27.2.2 Transactional nature of the environment

A key concept which considers this relationship and that has influenced occupational therapy theory is the broad concept of the transactional nature of the environment. The transactional nature of the environment recognises that while we are shaped by the environment, we also shape the environment. This concept, which is evident in occupational therapy models such as the PEO model and CanMOP, was founded on the concept of person-environment transaction described in the work of philosophers, environmental psychologists and gerontologists (Bunting, 2016). In the last decade of occupational therapy theory, it has been suggested that the concept of occupation has moved further towards this transactional understanding, where the environment cannot be seen as separate to the person (or their occupations); rather, the environment, person, and occupation are co-constitutive (Aldrich et al., 2025; Turpin et al., 2024). They are intertwined and constantly influencing each other and therefore cannot be understood in isolation (Bunting, 2016; Fisher & Marterella, 2019).

27.2.3 Nested layers of the environment: the Bioecological Model of Human Development

Reflecting a transactional perspective, Bronfenbrenner's Bioecological Model of Human Development (2001/2005) has strongly influenced occupational therapy theory. First conceptualised in 1979 as the Ecological Systems Theory, the model visualises nested layers of the environment that interact, with the person at the centre indicating the bi-directional relationship between an individual and their environment (Bronfenbrenner & Morris, 2006). In the model four concentric circles of the environmental context are described, the micro, meso, exo, and macro system. The inner microsystem includes the person's family, friends, school, neighbours, and home and represents the people, places and organisations that the person directly interacts with most. The next layer is the mesosystem, describing the interconnections between microsystems, for example, interactions between a school and parents for a child. The next layer is the exosystem. This includes aspects of the community which indirectly impact the person, for example, local government or disability organisational policies. The outer layer, the macrosystem, includes overarching culture, ideology, and structures of the society in which the person lives (Bronfenbrenner & Morris, 2006), for example, economic systems, and national policies on immigration, disability, education, housing, and health.

27.2.4 Growing understanding of socio-political environment

Socio-political inequities in the environment which impact occupational participation have been described for refugees and asylum seekers, people who are homeless, older adults, people with disabilities, people who experience abuse, children in foster-care, people with diverse gender identities and/or sexual orientations, people who have been incarcerated, and Indigenous Peoples (Kantartzis, 2019; Malfitano et al., 2019). The coining of the term *occupational justice* (Townsend & Wilcock, 2004) prompted consideration of these inequalities. Defined as equal opportunities to engage in meaningful life activities due to equitable societal conditions that facilitate participation, the concept of occupational justice required occupational therapists to consider occupational participation through a systemic lens (Kantartzis, 2019).

Through this systemic lens occupational therapists can understand that socio-political structures within the environment including citizenship, economics, politics, culture, language, institutional systems and organisations, societal attitudes, and media representations (Crawford et al., 2016) result in the exclusion of many people from meaningful occupations (Kantartzis, 2019). Considering an intersectional lens (see Chapter 13), these factors have also been conceptualised as social and environmental determinants of occupations (SEDOs) that interact with each other to contribute to a continuum of access to participation in culturally meaningful occupations (Smith, 2024). The broad range of contextual aspects captured in the socio-political environment includes elements of the social, temporal and historical, cultural, economic, political, and institutional dimensions described subsequently.

In the Australian context, socio-political structures of colonisation have resulted in the historical and ongoing oppression, prejudice and discrimination of Aboriginal and Torres Strait Islander opportunities to engage in meaningful occupations including cultural occupations. A decolonising and strengths-based approach to occupational therapy is proposed as a way for all occupational therapists to engage in practice that contributes to reconciliation (Ryall et al., 2021).

27.3 Understandings of environment in occupational therapy models

An understanding of the environment and its complexity has been foundational to the profession, as it is critical to occupational therapists' clinical reasoning. Table 27.1 provides an overview of how the environment is conceptualised in common occupational therapy models. When supporting goal setting, assessment, selecting intervention approaches, and evaluating outcomes the environment is a key consideration when working with individuals, families, communities, and at a societal or political level. One of the most recent conceptualisations of the environment in an occupational therapy model is in the Canadian Model of Occupational Participation (CanMOP), which explains that occupational participation occurs within layers of *micro, meso, and macro* environment (Egan & Restall, 2022).

In the CanMOP, micro context describes the direct interactions with the physical environment and the relationships and interactions with family, friends, teachers, health professionals, and co-workers. The meso context refers to system structures such as health and social care organisations, and the macro context is defined as the wider socio-economic and political context. Multi-level responsiveness describes the way occupational therapists can interweave their practice skills to address these different aspects of the environment at micro, meso, and macro levels (Crawford et al., 2022).

27.4 Dimensions of the environment

In this chapter we have drawn from a range of knowledge, models, and frameworks to discuss nine dimensions of the environment. Categorising the environment in this way is a Western approach and may overlook complexity. We have chosen to present these dimensions to support initial understandings of environment. While we take a transactional perspective to these dimensions that they are overlapping, inter-related, and co-constitutive, it is important for readers to reflect on complexities and develop more integrated ways of understanding environment as their knowledge and experience builds.

27.4.1 Social

The social environment describes relationships and interactions with, and the attitudes and expectations of others (Law et al., 1996; Fisher & Marterella, 2019). Relationships incorporate close personal connections such as family, friends and pets, communities, neighbours, workplace, school, and religious and other group connections. Relationships with others at this micro level influence the purpose and meaning of occupation (Egan & Restall, 2022). The expectations and attitudes within the social environment also influence occupational participation. The social nature of events and spaces influence our day-to-day lives and participation (American Occupational Therapy Association [AOTA], 2020). For example, a busy, noisy restaurant may make it difficult for some people with sensory differences to easily participate.

Beyond immediate close relationships, the social environment also includes broader communities and societal attitudes. Norms and attitudes influence what occupations are seen as health promoting or acceptable and valued in society (Kiepek et al., 2025); for example, paid employment is highly valued in western societies. These attitudes and norms in community and societies are the underlying drivers of the oppression of different groups of people, including experiences of colonialism, racism, ableism, sexism, ageism, classism, heterosexism, and cisgenderism. For example, societal attitudes that dehumanised people with disability meant institutional living was acceptable and expected for most of Australia's colonised history. Only in the last few decades have societal attitudes shifted to embrace a more rights-based approach to housing and support for people with disability.

Table 27.1 Conceptualisation of the environment in occupational therapy models

Occupational Therapy Model	Conceptualisation of the environment	Relationship between person, environment, and occupation	Individual and/or collective focus
Canadian Model of Occupational Participation (CanMOP) (Egan & Restall, 2022)	• Micro • Meso • Macro • Relationships and history	• The micro, meso, and macro contexts afford opportunities to access, initiate, and sustain participation in occupation. • The purpose and meaning of occupational participation derives from individual's or collective's needs, relationships, and history. • Individuals relate to each other, physical environments, ancestors, cultures, knowledges, social, political, economic structures, and the natural world.	Individual and collectives
Transactional Model of Occupation (Fisher & Marterella, 2019)	• Temporal • Sociocultural • Geopolitical • Environmental (social and physical)	• Situational elements (including the aspects adjacent, as well as client and task elements) are intertwined with occupation forming a relational whole. • The person and environment are co-constitutive, not separate.	Individual and collectives
Model of Human Occupation (MOHO) (Taylor, 2017)	• Physical • Social • Occupational	• The environment supports, constrains, and gives meaning to occupational and participation. • Environment seen as influencing and being influenced by the person. • Cultural, political, and economic components of context as well as the physical, social, and occupational, impact upon the motivation, organisation, and performance of occupation.	Individual

(Continued)

Table 27.1 (Continued)

Occupational Therapy Model	Conceptualisation of the environment	Relationship between person, environment, and occupation	Individual and/or collective focus
Canadian Model of Occupational Performance and Engagement (CMOP-E) (Canadian Association of Occupational Therapists, 1997; Townsend & Polatajko, 2007)	• Cultural • Institutional • Physical • Social	• The environment is considered external to the person and that it affords occupational possibilities and is unique for each individual. • Occupation is considered the bridge between person and environment where people influence their environment by participating in occupations. • This bridge of occupation conveys that interactions between the person, environment and occupation are dynamic and bi-directional.	Individual and collectives
The Kawa Model (Iwama, 2006)	• Physical and social context (river walls and floor • Circumstances – personal and environmental (rocks) • Temporal aspects (life flow of river at different points along the river's path)	• A metaphorical model using a river to represent life flow – the riverbed (physical and social context) and rocks – can impede the flow of the water (life flow) or create room for the water to flow freely (life flow, which may include occupational engagement). • Self is an inseparable part of nature and context.	Individual and collectives
Occupational Performance Model – Australia (Chapparo & Ranka, 1997)	• Cultural • Social • Physical • Sensory • Political • Economic	• Environment is considered external to the person. • Occupational participation is influenced by the external environment and is embedded in space and time.	Individual
The Person-Environment-Occupation Model (PEO) (Law et al., 1996)	• Physical • Cultural • Socio-economic • Institutional • Social • Temporal	• Environment dictates behaviour and is influenced by the person. • This two-way influence of person and environment is considered as a 'transaction'. • The environment is the context within which occupational performance occurs and is considered to have constraining and enabling effects on occupational performance.	Individual

27.4.2 Temporal and historical

The temporal environment reflects time and that lives and the world we live in are not static. From a western perspective, there are two main elements of the temporal environment, cyclical, and linear time (Werner et al., 1985). Non-western perspectives on the temporal environment differ and encompass wider understandings of temporality. These perspectives of time can be challenging for people who have grown up with linear perspectives on time. Time for Aboriginal Peoples is often described by the 'Everywhen', which is tied to and part of the Dreaming (Gosper, 2023). Within this understanding of time '"the eternal is always present" and "the ancient past that lives in the present determines everything"' (Gosper, 2023, p. 7). These conceptualisations of time are a starting point to learn more about some Australian Indigenous concepts of temporality. This information is presented here to prompt readers to think beyond their own perspectives on time and remember that people accessing occupational therapy may (or may not) see time differently to their therapists.

Cyclical time refers to the routines and patterns of our lives, daily, weekly, seasonally, and yearly occurrences that are influenced by culture and the naturally occurring rhythms of life (Fisher & Marterella, 2019). Linear time refers to the past, present, and future, thinking about the influence of history and our lifespan (Law et al., 1996; Werner et al., 1985). This historical dimension of the environment has recently garnered further attention in occupational therapy with more collective perspectives influencing theory. The CanMOP, for example, draws on life course theory principles in considering the relationship between history and the purpose and meaning of occupation for individuals and collectives (Egan & Restall, 2022).

27.4.3 Cultural

Culture is the confluence of beliefs, values, knowledge, perspectives, attitudes, norms, and customs that stem from people belonging to a society or group (Hammell, 2013). All groups have their own unique culture including groups based on ethnicity, gender, religion, sexuality, age, profession, ability, and socio-economic status. Culture is complex, however, because it evolves over time, there is within-group diversity, and we all have multiple and intersecting cultural identities (Agner, 2020). Behaviours and beliefs can seem to be common sense or 'right' when in fact they are reflections of culture (Hammell, 2013) and may not be the most appropriate, effective, or meaningful ways for people from other groups. Cultural humility as an occupational therapist is therefore critical to practice and is discussed more in chapter. Culture influences all aspects of occupational participation, as it is an overarching influence on all other dimensions of the environment. Consider, for example, what you did today and what elements of your culture or the dominant culture where you live influenced your occupational choices and participation.

27.4.4 Economic

The economic environment describes factors influencing the allocation of resources, including production and distribution of goods and services. It can be considered a matter of equity, access, and occupational justice, as it influences people's participation and life activities (Galvaan, 2012; Sofo & Wicks, 2017). In economics the terms personal-, micro-, and macro-economics are used to describe different levels of the economic environment – however, it should be noted these terms are used differently to occupational therapy and other models discussed in this chapter.

The personal-economic environment is most visible when considering occupational participation. This is the financial situation of each individual, family, or community, which influences participation in occupations. What we choose to do in life is influenced by resource availability (Galvaan, 2012), with people living in poverty more likely to experience barriers to occupational participation (Townsend & Wilcock, 2004). For example, an inability to access resources or services may limit participation or a need to work more to gain income might impact occupational balance.

The micro-economic environment is concerned with supply and demand in individual markets for goods and services, and the impacts are often considered in terms of how businesses run and pricing of goods and services, which can have a flow on effect for occupational participation, for example, the price of, supply of, and purchasing method for books or a computer for school, a four-wheeled-walker for community access, or food for mealtimes in remote communities.

The macro-economic environment describes the overarching influences such as inflation and gross domestic product (GDP) on industry, businesses, and public sector (government) expenditure. The impacts of these macro-economic influences are seen in institutions, flowing on to impact occupational engagement.

27.4.5 Political

While there are many ways of understanding politics and how politics shape everyday life, Rudman (2005) offers a clearly theorised and understandable perspective. She explains that power-holders use technologies of governments to enact governance and maximise their power. Governmental technologies include legislation, policy, strategies, consultations, inquiries, system reform, funding criteria, and media content. These technologies are how authorities practice their political ideologies, for example, liberalism, democracy, conservatism, religion-based ideologies, socialism, populism, Indigenous political thought, feminism, and ecologism (Baradat & Phillips, 2020)

Technologies of government influence human conduct, needs, and desires and affect different groups in inequitable ways. Shaping occupational participation and can create occupational injustices (Rudman, 2005). For example, in Australia, Aboriginal and Torres Strait Islander Peoples' opportunity to continue cultural responsibility for their traditional lands is severely impacted by the political dimension of the environment. Effectively, Aboriginal and Torres Strait Islander Peoples are legally 'trespassers' in our own lands (Moreton-Robinson, 2015, p. 18) until proving native title through exceedingly lengthy Western law court processes.

Crawford et al. (2016) provides another illustrative example of politics impacting occupational participation for asylum seekers. Multiple governments have considered asylum seekers requesting protection in Australia illegal maritime arrivals. This has resulted in their incarceration in immigration detention centres, removal of many basic human rights, and occupational deprivation while they await their refugee visa determination under Australian migration policy.

27.4.6 Institutional

People's lives occur within a web of services, systems, organisations, and policies which impact occupational participation. This web is the institutional environment. This includes welfare, social, health, disability, aged care, education, employment and housing services and organisations, utilities, telephone and internet communications platforms and providers, consumer goods, architectural and building services, transport, civil and legal protection, associations, organisations, businesses, media, and political activity (World Health Organization, 2001).

Institutions contribute to the structure of society, such as how and when health and therapy services might be accessed and the distribution of power and resources, including funding for services, equipment, and support (Townsend & Polatajko, 2013). While occupational therapists tend to be highly aware of health, disability, and aged care institutions because this is their working context, it is vital that occupational therapists also consider institutional environments beyond health and therapy services.

Occupational participation is influenced, but not completely determined, by the expectations and requirements of these institutions (Kantartzis & Molineux, 2011); both structure and agency play a role, where institutional structures and personal characteristics interact to determine occupational participation (Crawford et al., 2016).

27.4.7 Physical

The physical environment includes things that we can touch, see, smell, and hear. This includes the natural and built environment, structures, objects, layout, space, location, and ambient conditions (AOTA, 2020; Aplin & Tanner, 2019; Fisher & Marterella, 2019; Law et al., 1996). The natural environment includes everything living and non-living in our natural world, for example, trees, animals, mountains and rivers (AOTA, 2020). The built environment describes built structures and objects (AOTA, 2020). Objects include furniture, products, devices, and equipment, such as mobile phones and assistive technology. How the structures and objects are placed or arranged creates the layout of our environments and influences our space (Sanford & Bruce, 2010). The space in our environment can be understood as the areas in between the natural and built environment, for example, how much space there is in a living room, parking space, or personal space.

Another important aspect to the physical environment is location; this includes consideration of the geographic region and its influence on other dimensions, for example, political and institutional systems. Geographic locations can have deep personal, emotional, and spiritual connections. For example, Country, while not purely physical, enables a place-based connection for Aboriginal and Torres Strait Islander Peoples from that geographical area.

Location considerations also include the topography or lay of the land, which refers to how steep or flat the land is, as well as distances from family and friends, schools, shops, and other services or facilities such as transport (Aplin & Tanner, 2019; Fisher & Marterella, 2019). Ambient conditions include lighting, airflow, breezes, shade, the weather and temperature, along with noise and odour (Aplin & Tanner, 2019). The climate and weather are increasingly important considerations, with climate change impacts leading to more frequent weather events such as floods, fires, and cyclones.

27.4.8 Virtual

Being able to access and navigate the virtual environment is considered a necessity for daily life and a human right. Computers and smart devices, connected to the internet, provide access to education, health and government services, shopping, banking, entertainment, information systems, social networks, and storage of personal documents (Jaeger, 2011). These technologies provide enormous benefits connecting people globally and enabling employment, healthcare, leisure, and social occupations, along with advocacy and awareness raising. For example, Aboriginal and Torres Strait Islander Peoples use Facebook as a cultural occupation to advocate to 'change the date' of Australia Day (Ryan et al., 2020).

27.4.9 Personal

The personal dimension includes our emotional and spiritual relationships to all dimensions. This includes deep connections and spirituality linked to meaningful places, responses to the physical and social environments, relationships to the historical context, and relationship and emotional responses to socio-political factors such as government bodies. To consider this dimension further, consider how you feel when at home, visiting someone you care about at hospital, walking down a new street, in a natural location, or in a place of meaning to your community. All these places will bring about feelings/emotions and reactions in us that are experienced subjectively from an individual or collective perspective. This subjective understanding of the personal dimension draws from CanMOP's broad understanding of relationships, where relationships influence the purpose and meaning of occupation, and the SEWB Framework in relation to environment and its relationships to personal and community health and well-being.

The earlier examples point to physical places and how they are experienced, but the interdependent relationship between person and environment encapsulated in this dimension can be considered further when thinking about other dimensions. For example, government policies (political dimension) to damage Country have emotional and spiritual effects which result in profound health and well-being outcomes for Aboriginal and Torres Strait Islander Peoples. Government housing policies (political dimension) that result in unaffordable housing can result in feelings of insecurity, fear, worry, anger, and vulnerability for many. In contrast, government funding of modifications (political and institutional dimensions) that improve the accessibility of the physical dimension can create feelings of freedom, privacy, and independence at home (Aplin et al., 2015).

27.5 Conclusion

The profession's understanding of the environment continues to evolve and grow. However, there is still learning and work to be done for diverse perspectives on the environment to make equitable contributions to the development of our theoretical understandings of the environment and more broadly our theory and practice. In this chapter we highlighted that the concept of the environment is pluralistic, with a small selection of conceptualisations and models presented. We introduced some Aboriginal and Torres Strait Islander Peoples' perspectives to work towards enriching and further developing the professions understanding of the environment. We acknowledge that that this is a small step towards decolonising the profession's knowledge and discourse, and we envision a responsive and inclusive future, including iterations of this chapter enriched by ongoing connections, reflections, and critical thinking. The nine dimensions of the environment provided an initial framework to conceptualise and understand the complex nature of the environment from a historically Western perspective, and some critical considerations have been suggested. We encourage readers to take on a learning mindset, build relationships based on genuine connection, and be curious to allow occupational therapists to think in the ways in which they have been trained while also creating space and openness to listen and respond creatively to clients' world views and understandings of their environments.

27.7 Summary

- The environment is a pluralistic construct which is understood in a range of ways based on historical and socio-political influences.
- Aboriginal and Torres Strait Islander Peoples' Knowledge and perspectives in relation to environment are vast and the profession has much to learn from these Knowledges and perspectives.
- Connection to Country is a central component of health and wellbeing for Aboriginal and Torres Strait Islander Peoples.
- The environment is complex and multi-dimensional and shapes people's lives, including their occupational participation.
- The historical and socio-political environment are critical in understanding how the environment creates and hinders opportunities for occupational participation and occupational justice outcomes.
- A transactional understanding of the environment means that people, the environment, and occupation are interdependent or co-constitutional.

27.8 Review and reflection questions

- Describe the socio-political environment in your own words.
- Describe the relationship between Country and the health and well-being of Aboriginal and Torres Strait Islander Peoples.
- Choose three dimensions of the environment and describe how it has in the past or currently influences your occupational participation as a student or occupational therapist.

References

Agner, J. (2020). Moving from cultural competence to cultural humility in occupational therapy: A paradigm shift. *American Journal of Occupational Therapy*, 74(4), 7404347010p1–7404347010p7. https://doi.org/10.5014/ajot.2020.038067

Aldrich, R. M., Farias, L., Galvaan, R., & Rudman, D. L. (2025). The situated nature of human occupation. In T. Brown, S. Isbel, L. Gustafsson, S. Gutman, D. Powers Dirette, B. Cllins, & T. Barlott (Eds.), *Human occupation: Contemporary concepts and lifespan perspectives* (pp. 157–170). Routledge.

American Occupational Therapy Association. (2020). Occupational Therapy Practice Framework: Domain and process – fourth edition. *American Journal of Occupational Therapy*, 74(Supp 2), 7412410010p1–7412410010p87. https://doi.org/10.5014/ajot.2020.74S2001

Aplin, T., de Jonge, D., & Gustafsson, L. (2015). Understanding home modifications impact on clients and their family's experience of home: A qualitative study. *Australian Occupational Therapy Journal*, 62(2), 123–131. https://doi.org/10.1111/1440-1630.12156

Aplin, T., & Tanner, B. (2019). The home environment. In E. Ainsworth & D. de Jonge (Eds.), *An occupational therapists guide to home modification practice* (2nd ed., pp. 1–16). Slack Incorporated.

Avery, S., & First Peoples Disability Network. (2018). *Culture is inclusion: A narrative of Aboriginal and Torres Strait Islander people with disability.* First Peoples Disability Network Australia.

Baradat, L. P., & Phillips, J. A. (2020). *Political ideologies: Their origins and impact* (13th ed.). Routledge. https://doi.org/10.4324/9780429355042

Bronfenbrenner, U. (2005). *Making human beings human: Bioecological perspectives on human development.* Sage Publications Ltd.

Bronfenbrenner, U., & Morris, P. A. (2006). The bioecological model of human development. In R. M. Lerner & W. Damon (Eds.), *Handbook of child psychology: Theoretical models of human development* (6th ed., pp. 793–828). John Wiley & Sons, Inc.

Bunting, K. L. (2016). A transactional perspective on occupation: A critical reflection. *Scandinavian Journal of Occupational Therapy, 23*(5), 327–336. https://doi.org/10.3109/11038128.2016.1174294

Canadian Association of Occupational Therapists. (1997). *Enabling occupation: An occupational therapy perspective.* CAOT Publications ACE.

Chapparo, C., & Ranka, J. (Eds.). (1997). *Occupational performance model (Australia): Monograph 1* (pp. 66–82). Occupational Performance Network. www.occupationalperformance.com/opm-book

Crawford, E., Barlott, T., Begg, H., Mitchelson, K., Teo, A., & Turpin, M. (2022). Occupational multi-level responsiveness: Describing the skills used by occupational therapists working with children seeking asylum in Australia. *Scandinavian Journal of Occupational Therapy, 30*(3), 357–373. https://doi.org/10.1080/11038128.2022.2072384

Crawford, E., Turpin, M., & Nayar, S., Steel, E., & Durand, J-L. (2016). The structural-personal interaction: Occupational deprivation and asylum seekers in Australia. *Journal of Occupational Science, 23*(3), 1–18. https://doi.org/10.1080/14427591.2016.1153510

Egan, M., & Restall, G. (2022). The Canadian Model of Occupational Participation. In M. Egan & G. Restall (Eds.), *Promoting occupational participation: Collaborative relationship-focused occupational therapy* (pp. 73–96). Canadian Association of Occupational Therapists.

Emery-Whittington, I. G. (2025). Undoing coloniality: An indigenous occupation-based perspective. In T. Brown, S. Isbel, L. Gustafsson, S. Gutman, D. Powers Dirette, B. Collins, & T. Barlott (Eds.), *Human occupation: Contemporary concepts and lifespan perspectives* (pp. 191–208). Routledge.

Fisher, A. G., & Marterella, A. (2019). *Powerful practice: A model for authentic occupational therapy.* Center for Innovative OT Solutions.

Galvaan, R. (2012). Occupational choice: The significance of socio-economic and political factors. In G. E. Whiteford & C. Hocking (Eds.), *Occupational science: Society, inclusion and participation* (pp. 152–162). Wiley-Blackwell. https://doi.org/10.1002/9781118281581.ch11

Gee, G., Dudgeon, P., Schultz, C. Hart, A., & Kelly, K. (2014). Aboriginal and Torres Strait Islander social and emotional wellbeing. In P. Dudgeon, H. Milroy, & R. Walker (Eds.), *Working together: Aboriginal and Torres Strait Islander mental health and wellbeing principles and practice* (2nd ed., pp. 55–68). Commonwealth of Australia.

Gibson, C. (2020). When the river runs dry: Leadership, decolonisation and healing in occupational therapy. *New Zealand Journal of Occupational Therapy, 67*(1), 11–20. https://link.gale.com/apps/doc/A628283412/AONE?u=anon~69163f67&sid=googleScholar&xid=1c3af92f

Gosper, B. (2023). *Collapsing time: Indigenous storytellers and the 'Everywhen'* [Master's thesis, Columbia University]. Oral History Works. https://www.oralhistoryworks.org/collapsing-time/

Hammell, K. (2013). Occupation, well-being, and culture: Theory and cultural humility. *Canadian Journal of Occupational Therapy, 80*(4), 224–234. https://doi.org/10.1177/0008417413500465

Healthy Environments and Lives (HEAL) Network, & Centre for Research Excellence in Strengthening Systems for Indigenous Health Care Equity (CRE-STRIDE). (2021). *Climate change and Aboriginal and Torres Strait Islander Health, Discussion Paper*. Lowitja Institute, Melbourne. https://www.lowitja.org.au/wp-content/uploads/2023/12/Lowitja_ClimateChangeHealth_1021_D10.pdf

Iwama, M. K. (2006). *The Kawa model: Culturally relevant occupational therapy*. Elsevier Health Sciences.

Jaeger, P. T. (2011). *Disability and the internet: Confronting a digital divide*. Lynne Rienner Publishers.

Kantartzis, S. (2019). The Dr Elizabeth Casson memorial lecture 2019: Shifting our focus. Fostering the potential of occupation and occupational therapy in a complex world. *British Journal of Occupational Therapy, 82*(9), 553–566. https://doi.org/10.1177/0308022619864893

Kantartzis, S., & Molineux, M. (2011). The influence of Western society's construction of a healthy daily life on the conceptualisation of occupation. *Journal of Occupational Science, 18*(1), 62–80. https://doi.org/10.1080/14427591.2011.566917

Kiepek, N., Valderrama Núñez, C. M., Benjamin-Thomas, T. E., Palapal Sy, M., & Nazabal Amores, M. (2025). Occupation and social sanctioning. In T. Brown, S. Isbel, L. Gustafsson, S. Gutman, D. Powers Dirette, B. Cllins, & T. Barlott (Eds.), *Human occupation: Contemporary concepts and lifespan perspectives* (pp. 229–248). Routledge.

Law, M., Cooper, B., Strong, S., Stewart, D., Rigby, P., & Letts, L. (1996). The Person-Environment-Occupation Model: A transactive approach to occupational performance. *Canadian Journal of Occupational Therapy, 63*(1), 9–23. https://doi.org/10.1177/000841749906600304

Link-Up (Qld). (2025). *Link-up (Qld): Still bringing them home*. https://www.link-upqld.org.au/

Malfitano, A. P. S., de Souza, R. G. da M., Townsend, E. A., & Lopes, R. E. (2019). Do occupational justice concepts inform occupational therapists' practice? A scoping review. *Canadian Journal of Occupational Therapy, 86*(4), 299–312. https://doi.org/10.1177/0008417419833409

Matthews, V., Vine, K., Atkinson, A.-R., Longman, J., Lee, G. W., Vardoulakis, S., & Mohamed, J. (2023). Justice, culture, and relationships: Australian Indigenous prescription for planetary health. *Science, 381*, 636–641. https://doi.org/10.1126/science.adh9949

Moreton-Robinson, A. (2015). *The white possessive: Property, power, and Indigenous sovereignty* (1st ed.). University of Minnesota Press.

National Family Matters Leadership Group, Liddle, C., Gray, P., Secretariat of National Aboriginal and Islander Child Care (SNAICC), & Corrales, T. (2024). *Family matters report 2024*. Secretariat of National Aboriginal and Islander Child Care Inc. https://www.snaicc.org.au/our-work/child-and-family-wellbeing/family-matters/

PKKP Aboriginal Corporation. (2020, May 25). *Ancient deep-time rock shelters believed destroyed in Pilbara mining blast, calls for greater flexibility to retain sites* [Press release]. https://pkkp.org.au/wp-content/uploads/2020/06/PKKP-20200525-FINAL-Media-Release-Rio-Tinto-Juukan-Gorge-blasts.pdf

Rudman, D. L. (2005). Understanding political Influences on occupational possibilities: An analysis of newspaper constructions of retirement. *Journal of Occupational Science, 12*(3), 149–160. https://doi.org/10.1080/14427591.2005.9686558

Ryall, J., Ritchie, T., Butler, C., Ryan, A., & Gibson, C. (2021). Decolonising occupational therapy through a strengths-based approach. In T. Brown, H. M. Bourke-Taylor, S. Isbel, R. Cordier, & L. Gustafsson (Eds.), *Occupational therapy in Australia* (2nd ed., pp. 130–142). Routledge. https://doi.org/10.4324/9781003150732-13

Ryan, A., Gilroy, J., & Gibson, C. (2020). #Changethedate: Advocacy as an on-line and decolonising occupation. *Journal of Occupational Science, 27*(3), 405–416. https://doi.org/10.1080/14427591.2020.1759448

Sanford, J., & Bruce, C. (2010). Measuring the impact of the physical environment. In T. Oakland & E. Mpofu (Eds.), *Rehabilitation and health assessment* (pp. 207–228). Springer.

Smith, D. L. (2024). Social and environmental determinants of occupation: An intersectional concept focused on occupational justice and participation. *Journal of Occupational Science, 31*(2), 209–215. https://doi.org/10.1080/14427591.2023.2212676

Sofo, F., & Wicks, A. (2017). An occupational perspective of poverty and poverty reduction. *Journal of Occupational Science, 24*(2), 244–249. https://doi.org/10.1080/14427591.2017.1314223

Taylor, R. R. (2017). *Kielhofner's Model of Human Occupation: Theory and application* (5th ed.). Wolters Kluwer.

Townsend, E. A., & Polatajko, H. J. (2007). *Enabling occupation II: Advancing an occupational therapy vision of health, well-being and justice through occupation.* CAOT Publications ACE.

Townsend, E. A., Polatajko, H. J., & Canadian Association of Occupational Therapists. (2013). *Enabling occupation II: advancing an occupational therapy vision for health, well-being, and justice through occupation* (2nd ed.). Canadian Association of Occupational Therapists.

Townsend, E. A., & Wilcock, A. A. (2004). Occupational justice and client centred practice: A dialogue in progress. *Canadian Journal of Occupational Therapy, 71*(2), 75–87. https://doi.org/10.1177/000841740407100203

Trzepacz, D., Guerin, B., & Thomas, J. (2014). Indigenous Country as a context for mental and physical health: Yarning with Nukunu Community. *The Australian Community Psychologist, 26*(2), 38–53. https://groups.psychology.org.au/Assets/Files/Trzepacz-ACP-26-2-Dec-2014.pdf

Turpin, M., Garcia, J., & Iwama, M. K. (2024). *Using occupational therapy models in practice: A field guide* (2nd ed.). Elsevier.

Werner, C. M., Altman, I., & Oxley, D. (1985). Temporal aspects of home: A transactional perspective. In I. Altman & C. M. Werner (Eds.), *Home environments* (Vol. 8, pp. 1–32). Plenum.

World Health Organisation. (2001). *International Classification of Functioning, Disability and Health.* World Health Organization.

World Health Organization. (2025). *Social determinants of health.* https://www.who.int/health-topics/social-determinants-of-health#tab=tab_1

CHAPTER 28

The occupational therapy practice process

Stephen Isbel, Louise Gustafsson, and Alexandra Logan

Authors' positionality statement

This chapter has been written by three academics of white, Anglo-Australian heritage. We recognise that our cultural, historical, and social backgrounds have shaped how we understand and interpret the world. We are conscious of the social and institutional advantages associated with our racial and cultural identities and acknowledge that this may have introduced bias into our writing.

We are committed to ongoing critical reflection on our positionality and its impact on our work. Throughout this chapter, we have made an effort to include perspectives beyond our own, aligned with the chapter's Objectives. Our goal is to contribute to an inclusive and equitable academic dialogue by being transparent about our viewpoints and by actively seeking to understand and reflect diverse experiences.

Key terms

- Occupational therapy process
- Canadian Occupational Therapy Practice Process Framework
- Occupational Therapy Intervention Process Model
- MOHO-Therapeutic Reasoning Process

Objectives

Upon completion of this chapter, the reader will be able to:

- Articulate the importance of using an occupation-centred practice process
- Describe the main features of the Canadian Occupational Therapy Practice Process Framework, the Occupational Therapy Intervention Process Model, and the MOHO-Therapeutic Reasoning Process
- Understand how to apply three occupational therapy processes

DOI: 10.4324/9781003495666-31

28.1 Introduction

The occupational therapy process provides guidance that helps occupational therapists adopt an occupation-centred approach when working with individuals, groups, communities, or populations. It is not formulaic or linear but rather a flexible, theory-driven process that acknowledges that every individual, group, community, and population is unique as is the context in which the process takes place. This chapter will describe three different occupational therapy process models and demonstrate their application through a case study to show how they can be utilised in practice.

Occupational therapists use *occupation models* and *process models* to guide all aspects of their practice to assess, evaluate and apply occupational therapy interventions. The types and roles of occupation models are explored in Chapter 25. This chapter focuses on three different *process models* which guide occupational therapists in what to consider and how to apply occupation-focused interventions.

28.2 The Canadian Model of Occupational Participation: the model underpinning the COTIPP

The Canadian Occupational Therapy Inter-relational Practice Process (COTIPP) is the process model developed from the Canadian Model of Occupational Participation (CanMOP) (Egan & Restall, 2022a) which is newest version of the original Canadian Model of Occupational Performance (and Enabling) (Canadian Association of Occupational Therapists, 1997). The details of the CanMOP are explored in detail in Chapter 25.

The key aspects of the CanMOP that are relevant to the COTIPP are that it focuses on the occupations that give purpose and meaning to human activity, while acknowledging the importance of the context in which the occupations takes place, the influence on the past on current occupational performance and the importance of relationships in occupational performance. A diagrammatically representation of the CanMOP can be seen in Figure 28.1

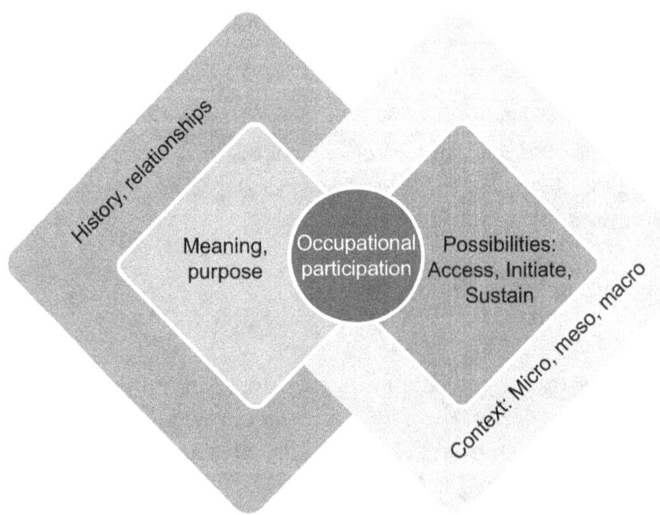

Figure 28.1 Canadian Model of Occupational Participation (CanMOP)

(Egan & Restall, 2022b, p. 7)

28.3 Process 1: The Canadian Occupational Therapy Practice Process Framework

At the core of the COTIPP lies the essential process underpinning occupational therapy practice: building and sustaining relationships. Surrounding this core, the framework includes three additional foundational processes that are used in practice: understanding context; reflecting and reasoning; and applying a justice, equity, and rights-based perspectives.

The framework also outlines six action domains that describe how therapists facilitate occupational participation: connecting; exploring occupational participation; seeking understanding and defining purpose; co-designing priorities, goals, outcomes, and plans; testing the plan, exploring changes, and refining it; and planning for transitions. These processes are fluid, and interact with each other meaning that occupational therapists are continuously building and sustain relationships, seek to understand the context in which occupations take place, reflect and reason, and apply justice, equity and rights-based perspectives. The underlying approach of the COTIPP is described along with the foundational processes and six action domains. Refer to Figure 28.2 when reading about these aspects of the COTIPP.

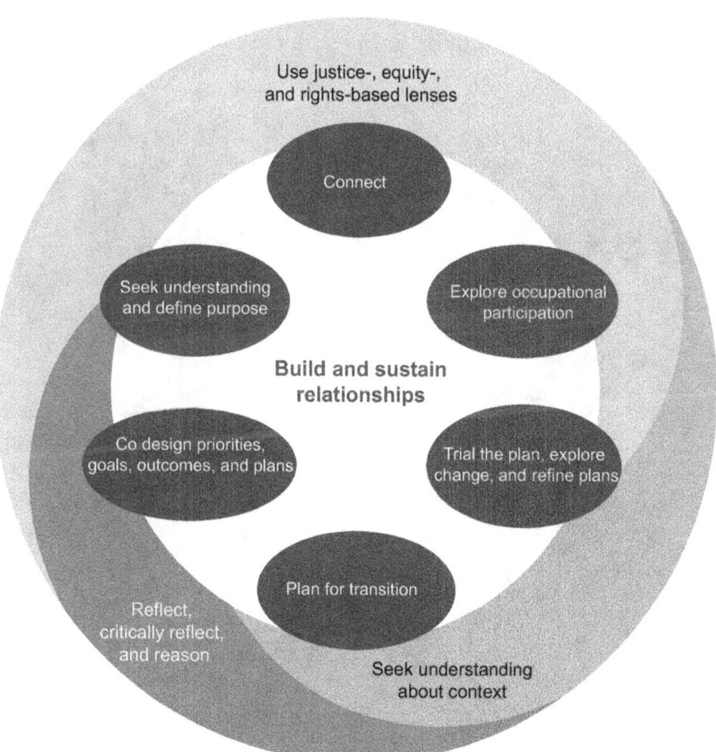

Figure 28.2 Canadian Occupational Therapy Practice Process Framework

(Restall et al., 2022, p. 122)

28.4 Essential underlying approach

At the core of the COTIPP is the process of occupational therapy practice building and sustaining relationships through collaborative relationship-focused occupational therapy. This is important, as 'the purpose of the COTIPP is to describe the collaborative, inter-relational, and rights-based practice of occupational therapy' (Restall et al., 2022 p. 121). Collaborative relationship-focused occupational therapy acknowledges the importance of client-centred occupational therapy while also highlighting the need to develop sustainable relationships by being aware of aspects such as self-determination, justice, equity and rights in any therapeutic relationship (see Chapter 25 for detail on these terms). As underpinned in the CanMOP, collaborative relationship-focused occupational therapy highlights the nuanced aspect of occupational therapy and the importance of integrating contextually relevant information into decision making. A diagrammatical representation of collaborative relationship-focused occupational therapy that is seen at the core of the COTIPP is presented in Figure 28.3

28.5 The three foundational processes of the COTIPP

There are three foundational processes in the COTIPP: seek to understand context; reflect, critically reflect, and reason; and use justice-, equity-, and rights-based lenses.

28.5.1 Seek to understand context

Context can be complex and includes factors like the natural and built environment, location, laws and legislation, societal and cultural norms, expectations, individual

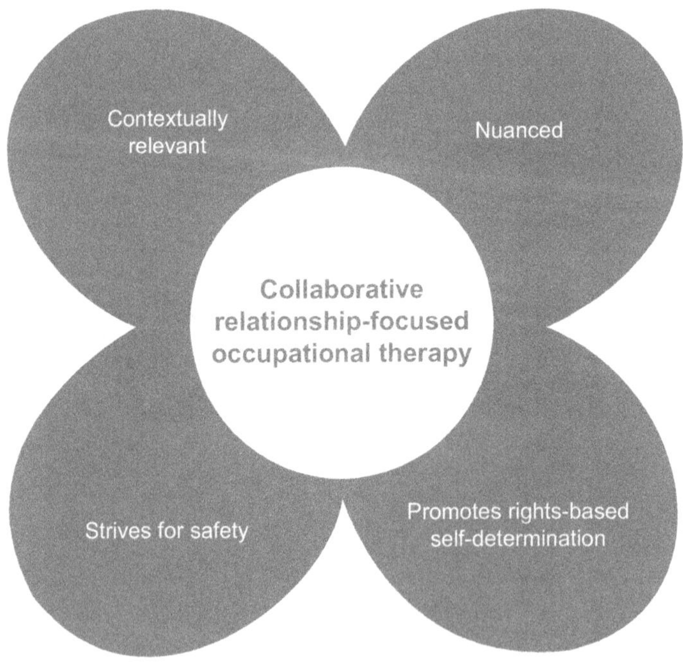

Figure 28.3 Collaborative relationship-focused occupational therapy

(Restall & Egan, 2022, p. 101)

beliefs and behaviours, and the ways in which power plays out with families and communities. The COTIPP views context in the broadest possible way recognising that different aspects of context influence each other. For example, the National Disability Insurance Scheme (policy context) has allowed many people with disability to access occupational therapy (practice context). Understanding both the therapist context and the practice context is important in occupational therapy practice and involves developing the skill and taking the time to critically reflect on practice.

28.5.2 The therapist context

The physical, social, political, and cultural contexts in which we work and live shape the way we view and treat others. The way we shape our own identities can be influenced by factors such as sexual orientation, religion, ethnicity, gender, and age. The ways we treat others are influenced by conscious and unconscious biases that take critical reflection to identify and address. This can include an acknowledgment that some people enjoy a privileged position over others in society and actively acknowledging this in any therapeutic relationship we engage in.

28.5.3 The practice context

Where occupational therapy takes place is important to the occupational therapy process. The history, rules and expectations of the place where occupational therapy takes place along with the values, social norms, expectations of the people who work in the practice setting and those who access the practice setting are important to consider. It is important for occupational therapists to consider their often-privileged position in the practice context and critically reflect on their own background, personal beliefs and assumptions in the occupational therapy process.

28.5.4 Reflect, critically reflect, and reason

Reflection requires a process of noticing what is occurring during occupational therapy (reflection during practice) and thinking about what to change or do differently in subsequent sessions. For example, an occupational therapist may be working with a child for the first time in a large multi-purpose therapy space and during the session the child is distracted by specific items in the space. During the session the therapist may remove the specific distractions (reflection during practice) and decides after the session that subsequent sessions will be held in a smaller, less distracting space (reflection on practice).

Critical reflection is a process that can identify and challenge deeper and systematic influences that occur in the occupational therapy process. For example, an occupational therapist may be working for an Aboriginal and Torres Strait Islander health service run out a of rural hospital. The therapist notices that many of the clients of the service miss important follow-up appointments following surgery. Critically reflecting on the potential reasons for this reveals that there are historical, cultural and systematic reasons clients of the service do not feel safe attending these appointments. Critically reflecting on these reasons is a starting point in trying to address the health inequality that exists when the clients of the service cannot safely access post-surgical treatment.

Practice reasoning is the process occupational therapists undertake when considering making, and refining decisions in practice (Greber et al., 2024). Reasoning in occupational therapy is influenced by many factors, including the context in which it takes place, the values and background of the therapist and client, therapist experience, and the resources available. Importantly reflection and critical reflection is important for effective practice reasoning

28.5.5 Use justice-, equity-, and rights-based lenses

Occupational therapists have a responsibility to promote a just society that upholds individuals' rights and ensures equitable access to occupational participation (Restall et al., 2022). One way they fulfil this responsibility is by applying a justice-, equity-, and rights-based perspective to their practice. This involves critically evaluating how their practice contexts and processes either support or hinder the justice, equity, and rights of the individuals and groups they serve and taking steps to reduce or eliminate barriers to participation in occupations (Restall et al., 2022).

By engaging in critical reflection and applying justice-, equity-, and rights-based perspectives, occupational therapists can evaluate their practice and take actions to enhance capabilities while addressing individual and systemic barriers to occupational participation. Promoting the rights of individuals, families, groups, communities, and populations to engage in occupations, and ensuring these rights through equitable opportunities for individuals and groups to choose the occupations and ways of being they value, are key steps toward advancing justice for all (Restall et al., 2022).

28.6 The six action domains of the COTIPP

The six action domains of the COTIPP are: i) connect; ii) seek, understand, and define purpose; iii) explore occupational participation; iv) co-design priorities goals outcomes and plan; v) trial the plan, explore change, and refine the plan' and vi) plan for transition.

28.6.1 Connect

This is the time when the occupational therapist first meets their client, which could be an individual, group, community, or population. This is the time to explore mutual expectations and develop rapport and the collaborative relationship required for an effective relationship (Restall et al., 2022).

28.6.2 Seek understand and define purpose

This action domain centres on collaboratively establishing the conditions under which the therapist and the individual or group will engage in their work together. The therapist and the individual or group jointly create an environment where information about experiences, desires, and priorities related to occupational participation can be openly shared. The therapist remains receptive to learning about occupations and occupational participation within the individual's or group's unique contexts, including identities, strengths, resources, challenges, history, and cultural significance (Restall et al., 2022).

28.6.3 Explore occupational participation

In this action domain, the therapist and the individual or group work together to create conditions for exploring the individual's or group's current concerns about occupational participation, their occupational aspirations, and perceived possibilities. Methods used in this domain may involve informal or formal co-assessment and co-evaluation aimed at highlighting occupational concerns and setting priorities for addressing them (Restall et al., 2022).

28.6.4 Co-design priorities, goals, outcomes, and plans

In this action domain, the therapist and the individual or group collaboratively establish the conditions for co-designing priorities, goals, outcomes, and plans by sharing perspectives on occupational concerns and potential solutions. The therapist aims to understand the meanings underlying the individual's or group's concerns and aspirations regarding occupational participation. The therapist actively listens to and values the individual's or group's knowledge, expertise, and experiences while also applying their own professional knowledge and expertise in occupational participation to co-design effective plans (Restall et al., 2022).

28.6.5 Trial the plan, explore change, and refine the plan

In this action domain, the therapist continues to develop and maintain collaborative relationships with the individual or group, testing the plan, assessing whether desired changes have been achieved, and adjusting as necessary. Both the therapist and the individual or group co-monitor and modify their relationship as therapy unfolds. For instance, the therapist may take a more directive role at the beginning and transition to a more supportive role as therapy progresses and the individual or group feels ready to take on greater responsibility (Restall et al., 2022).

28.6.6 Plan for transition

Planning for transition is characterised by the therapist listening to and seeking to understand the individual's or collective's perspective about transitioning from occupational therapy. The therapist summarises their perspective of what has been done together and the occupational participation outcomes achieved during therapy. The therapist seeks the perspective of the individual or collective on what has been done together and what has been achieved and this information is communicated with important associated people (Restall et al., 2022).

28.7 Process 2: Occupational Therapy Intervention Process Model

The Occupational Therapy Intervention Process Model (OTIPM) (Fisher & Marterella, 2019) outlines three phases in the occupational therapy practice process: i) evaluation and goal setting, ii) intervention, and iii) re-evaluation (see Figure 28.4).

28.8 Transactional Model of Occupation

The Transactional Model of Occupation (Fisher & Marterella, 2019) recognises that the person cannot be separated from their situational contexts (or elements) and that occupation and situational elements are interwoven to mutually shape and influence each other (Aldrich & Cutchin, 2013; Cutchin & Dickie, 2012). The occupation elements are composed of the observable aspects of the occupation (occupational performance) and the experience of doing the occupation (occupational experience), which result in participation (engagement in occupation). The transactional perspective asserts that people do not produce occupation, rather that occupations are a response to the situational elements.

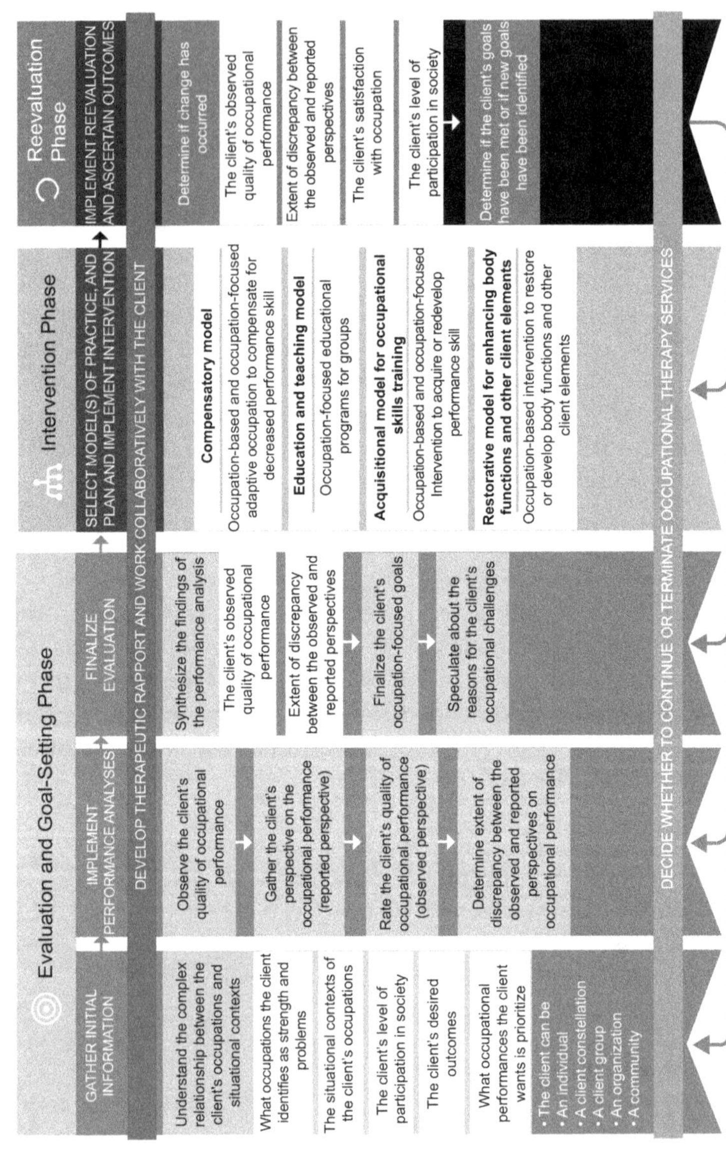

Figure 28.4 Occupational Therapy Intervention Process Model

(Fisher & Marterella, 2019)

The *geopolitical, sociocultural,* and *temporal* elements include geographic and economic influences; rules, regulations, and norms; and patterns, sequences, and rhythms. The *social* and *physical* elements (environments) include spaces, tangible objects, and people. The *task* and *client* elements describe what is expected during occupation (e.g., structure, tools, purpose, outcome) and influences that are internal to the client (e.g., age, gender, life stage; habits, routines, rituals, and roles; attitudes, beliefs, values; body functions) (see Figure 28.5) When applying the transactional model of occupation, the occupational therapist is reminded to not focus solely on the person but rather to explore how changes in situational elements can result in changes within occupation. The transaction model of occupation encourages the occupational therapist to consider the three elements of occupation throughout the OTIPM. That is, what is observed (occupational performance), the client's perspective (occupational experience), and what emerges when the individual values the experience and the doing (participation) (Fisher & Marterella, 2019).

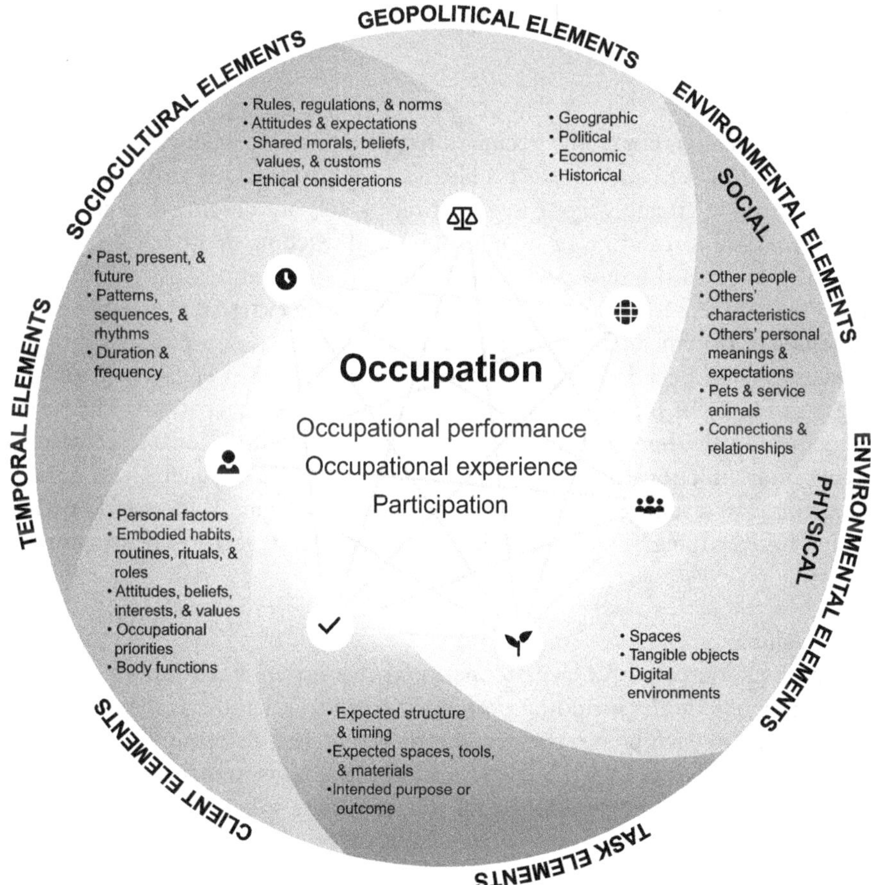

Figure 28.5 Transactional Model of Occupation

(Fisher & Marterella, 2019)

28.9 Evaluation and goal setting

Therapeutic rapport and a collaborative relationship are established in this phase and continue throughout the entire process. First, the occupational therapist *gathers the information* necessary to understand the interplay between the client's occupations and situational elements. There is an exploration of occupations considered strengths and problems by the client and the contexts of the occupations. The client's participation in society is explored, desired participation outcomes are identified, and occupations are prioritised for the performance analysis in the next step of the evaluation. *A performance (occupation) analysis* is conducted to observe the quality of performance in the chosen occupations. The performance is rated by the occupational therapist, and the client is asked to share their perspective of the occupational performance. Discrepancies between the therapist rating and client perspective are noted. In the final step, *finalise evaluation*, the observations of the occupational performance and discrepancies between the client and occupational therapist rating are considered. Next, the occupational therapist and client collaboratively discuss the performance analysis and develop occupation-focused goals. Finally, the occupational therapist and client consider possible reasons for the observed problems of occupational performance, leading to the intervention phase of the OTIPM.

28.10 Intervention

During the intervention phase, the occupational therapist and client collectively plan and implement approaches to address the problems of occupational performance and achieve the occupation-focused goals. Four intervention models are described: i) compensatory, ii) acquisitional, iii) restorative, or iv) education and teaching approaches. The compensatory model involves the introduction of adaptive equipment or assistive technology, alternative or compensatory strategies, and/or modifying external elements to influence occupational performance. The acquisitional model promotes occupational skill training and development of occupational performance through direct engagement in occupation (e.g., training that includes progressive grading of the occupation). The restorative model focuses on the remediation of impairments, and restoration or maintenance of underlying body functions or other client elements through engagement in occupation. The education and teaching model is applied to share occupation-focused knowledge or occupation-based strategies with individuals or groups using lectures or workshops.

28.11 Re-evaluate

Progress and the outcomes of the occupational therapy intervention are re-evaluated through various methods, including performance analyses and a review of the client's goals. At the end of each phase, the occupational therapist determines whether to continue or terminate services. In the re-evaluation phase, this may lead to the identification of new goals and re-entry into the most appropriate step in the OTIPM.

28.12 Process 3: Therapeutic Reasoning Process

The Therapeutic Reasoning Process (TRP) (Wolske et al., 2024) is an occupation focused, client-centred practice process that embeds the four concepts of the Model

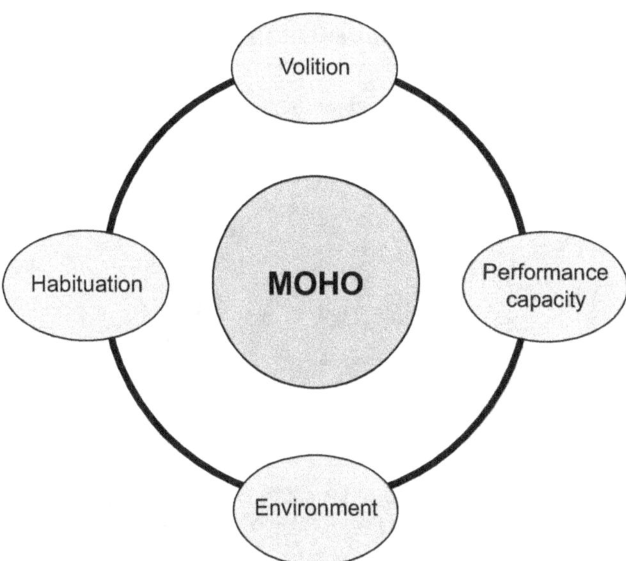

Figure 28.6 The Model of Human Occupation

(Taylor et al., 2024). Reproduced with permission

of Human Occupation (MOHO) (see Figure 28.6). The MOHO conceptual model is based on 'open systems' theory where the concepts of volition, habituation, performance capacity and the environment are seen as individual systems that have permeable boundaries (Taylor et al., 2023). Change in one concept can transfer and influence another concept. Understanding the reciprocal and dynamic nature of the MOHO concepts can support therapists in their reasoning, including decision making and problem solving, throughout the course of therapy.

Therapeutic reasoning is a progression from the earlier writings on clinical and professional reasoning (Mattingly, 1991; Mattingly & Fleming, 1994). The TRP places a greater emphasis on the dynamic and collaborative nature of working with clients addressing contemporary professional setting demands. See Figure 28.7, followed by a description of each step.

28.12.1 Step 1: Generate and ask questions to guide the reasoning process

Theory driven questions guide therapists to consider how volition, habituation and performance capacity are impacted by the external social and physical environment. This initial step is crucial in getting to know the person, their unique circumstances and the ways they 'do' their chosen occupations (occupational skills, performance, and participation). Information gathered on these concepts often raise broader questions relating to occupational identity (a sense of who one is and wishes to be as an occupational being), competence (how effective a person is in meeting their expectations for their occupational identity), and adaptation (the process of change that supports a person to meet occupational and environmental challenges and increase occupational competence, reaching their ideal occupational identity).

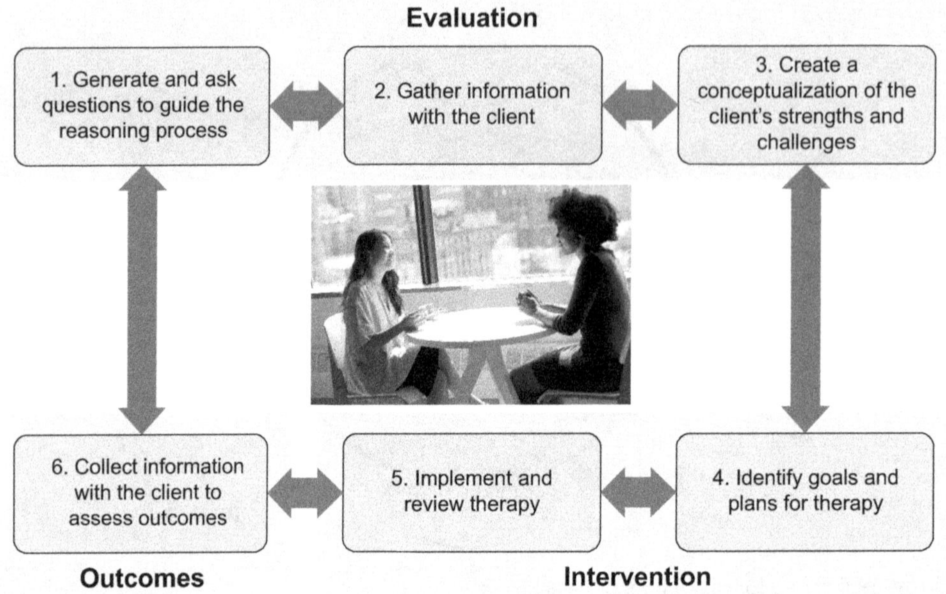

Figure 28.7 The Therapeutic Reasoning Process

(Kielhofner & Forsyth, 2008) Reproduced with permission

28.12.2 Step 2: Gather information with the client

The TRP is a form of procedural reasoning with the MOHO guiding the therapist's thinking at each step in the process. Therefore, the selection of structured and unstructured assessments can be used to answer the theory driven questions from step one. There are numerous standardised assessments that have been developed with the MOHO concepts as a foundation and are a logical method to collect information on these concepts. An example of a MOHO-based assessment tool is the Model of Human Occupation Screening Tool (MOHOST) (Parkinson et al., 2006). However, subscribing to the TRP does not mean therapists need to restrict their selection to only the MOHO assessments. Unstructured assessments such as informal observations and semi-structured interviews can also contribute valuable assessment information.

28.12.3 Step 3: Create a conceptualisation of the client's strengths and challenges

Conceptualisation draws the assessment data sources together to provide a uniquely occupational perspective to the client's life circumstance. The result of the conceptualisation is an occupational formulation. The purpose of the formulation is to highlight personal and environmental strengths. The formulation may also highlight functional limitations and environmental demands for consideration when setting goals and intervention planning. In this stage, therapists aim to collaborate with the client to create the occupational formulation, ensuring that the formulation reflects client priorities.

Collaboration underpins genuine and effective partnership needed to sustain positive therapy outcomes.

28.12.4 Step 4: Identify goals and plans for therapy

Despite humans being innately occupationally driven, many clients find framing goals for the future a challenge. This step in the TRP prompts the therapist to explore with the client what occupational changes the client may want from therapy. Understanding the subjective nature of change may support the therapist and client to solidify the desired goals and outcomes for therapy.

Occupational therapists may have a range of techniques and preferences (SMART goals or goal attainment scaling) for establishing and collaborating with clients to develop measurable goals. By following the TRP, therapists are prompted to consider the MOHO concepts that are reflected in the client's goal. This step supports therapists to remain aligned with the MOHO theory during the goal setting process to ensure goals and the subsequent intervention planning stay occupationally focused.

28.12.5 Step 5: Implement and review therapy

Humans are complex occupational beings. The TRP guides therapists' understanding of the uniqueness of people's occupational experience. The MOHO concepts form the basis for engaging a person in their meaningful occupations. This approach allows the therapist to consider interventions that work with a person's strengths and resources to enable occupational performance. Health and well-being outcomes are achieved when a client can participate in their meaningful occupations.

28.12.6 Step 6: Collect information with client to assess outcomes

This step can involve one or both of the following: Reflecting on goal attainment (Step 5) and/or re-administering of standardised assessments (Step 2). This step may not be the final step in the therapeutic process. In many instances, this might be considered an opportunity to evaluate therapy and move through other steps in the therapeutic process, such as developing new measurable goals to reflect a client's change in circumstances or health status. The client's subjective evaluation of the therapy is crucial in this step. Client satisfaction with the therapy process can contribute to valuable adaptations to later therapy and support the therapist to learn and develop as a therapist.

Up to this point in the chapter, an overview and application of three occupational therapy practice process models have been discussed. These process models are frequently used by Australian occupational therapists to guide their professional decision-making and actions. Understanding these models should follow a progression starting with an understanding of the occupational therapy model underpinning the process, then identifying the stages of the process model, then applying the model in a specific context (as demonstrated in Daisy's case), and finally analysing and evaluating the model's effectiveness. Table 28.1 uses Daisy's case study to illustrate how each process model can be applied with the same person and context. It also aligns the stages of each model to highlight their similarities and differences. Each model has taken Daisy's progression in slightly different directions to highlight specific parts of each process.

Table 28.1 Illustrating how each process model can be applied with the same person and context

Daisy is an 88-year-old woman who is a retired teacher, living independently by herself for 10 years since her husband passed away. While cleaning her windows at home, she slipped and fell, causing her to lose consciousness for about 5 minutes. She was admitted to hospital, where her concussion resolved well. She was discharged after 5 days to respite care in a local residential aged cared home with the plan of returning home after 3 weeks.

Daisy's daughter Miranda is worried that Daisy is not managing at home, given that her home is large, and she seems to be forgetting things a lot. Miranda says that while Daisy is independent in most everyday activities, she wonders if Daisy should move into a retirement village. Daisy is keen to get home and wants to remain there for as long as possible, but she does worry about falling again, as well as maintaining her garden that has 'gotten away' from her. Jaydon is the occupational therapist for Transitional Therapy and Care Program (TTCP), which is a service that supports older people to return home after a hospital stay. The following case study describes the journey and occupational therapy process that Daisy and Jaydon take during the respite care stay.

	COTIPP	OTIPM	MOHO–TRP
Assessment, goal setting, and planning	*Connect:* Jaydon first meets Daisy in respite care after a referral from hospital occupational therapist. Jaydon explains the role of occupational therapy and develops a rapport with Daisy by talking about the things she enjoys when at home. *Seek understanding and define purpose:* Jaydon attempts to build a relationship based on collaboration and co-creation by understanding Daisy's occupational history and current desires for occupational participation. Daisy and Jaydon agree that occupational therapy could be beneficial, and they agree to develop an occupation focused plan.	*Gather initial information* Jaydon explains occupational therapy and builds therapeutic rapport while seeking to understand Daisy as an occupational being. Jaydon explores the occupations that Daisy finds challenging and those that are not. This step concludes with Daisy identifying challenging occupations that are important to her.	*Generate and ask questions:* Prior to meeting Daisy, Jaydon reviews Daisy's referral information. He uses the MOHO concepts to organise the information and determine what further information is needed. The referral included information on motor and process skills, ability to complete dressing, and showering tasks and transfers. There was no information on Daisy's strengths, interests, values, home environment, cultural background, and routines. These information 'gaps' drive Jaydon to think about possible assessments he could administer to learn more about her occupational narrative. His experience informs him that Daisy will only provide this valuable information if she feels a level of trust and comfort in the therapeutic relationship.

(Continued)

Table 28.1 (Continued)

Explore occupational participation	*Implement performance analyses*	Jaydon contacts Daisy in the respite accommodation. He expresses empathy regarding her recent hospital admission. He picks up on her cheeky sense of humour and jokes with her about needing to send a search party after him if he doesn't make it through her overgrown garden. A time is made for a home visit when Daisy knows Miranda can attend.
Daisy explains that her main valued occupations are home-based craft activities and visiting her daughter each week for a meal. She is worried that some IADL occupations such as home maintenance and gardening are becoming very difficult, but she does not want to move.	Daisy has prioritised gardening and preparing breakfast. Jaydon observes Daisy i) preparing scrambled eggs and toast and ii) watering plants and removing dead leaves. Jaydon and Daisy discuss the occupational performance – Jaydon notes that performance was slow, and it was effortful for Daisy to prepare breakfast. There were times when Daisy appeared fatigued and at risk of tripping or falling. Daisy felt that, although slow, it was acceptable that there was extra effort because of her age. However, she realises that she may have been less active around home recently, and she is worried about falling again.	*Gather information:* Jaydon meets Daisy and Miranda at Daisy's home. After some brief introductions, Jaydon picks up on Daisy's Swan artwork near her front door. He asks if she is a fan of the Swans Australian League football team, and she responds that she has been a club member since she was in primary school.
Co-design priorities, goals outcomes, and plans		Jaydon explains his role on the TTCP and invites Daisy and Miranda to ask any questions.
Daisy clearly has a priority of returning home after respite care. She articulates that she is worried about falling at home and safely accessing her bathroom and back yard. She wants to continue to do her craft-based occupations and visit her daughter each week. Jaydon uses the use the Canadian Occupational Performance Measure (Law et al., 2014) with Daisy to articulate and quantify occupation-based goals.	*Finalise evaluation*	Jaydon decides that he will use an unstructured approach to gathering further information on Daisy's MOHO concepts. Daisy has an open communication style and appears to enjoy talking about her interests and routines. He also asks if Daisy can show him around the house and garden, which he explains is a good opportunity to observe her mobility and identify falls risks.
	Daisy and Jaydon discuss and finalise occupation-focused goals related to preparing breakfast and gardening.	

(Continued)

Table 28.1 (Continued)

Intervention	*Trial the plan, explore change, and refine the plan*	*Select model(s) or practice and plan*	In addition to this unstructured approach, the TTCP use an assessment protocol known as the Home Support Needs Assessment (HSNA). This screening tool provides data which Jaydon can use to generate a management plan and access funding for extra supports for Daisy. He runs through the assessment items with Daisy and Miranda to collect information on a range of daily living domains.
	As the goals Daisy has articulated relate to returning home to safely engage in personal care occupations and leisure occupations, the plan involves assessing her home for safety (Clemson, 1997), making changes to her home environment based upon the assessment, and testing if the changes have improved safety at home.	Daisy and Jaydon agree on a compensatory approach that includes the provision and education and training on the use of assistive equipment such as a kitchen trolley and stool and raised garden bed.	
	The home safety assessment identified several areas that needed addressing, and these were mainly minor home modifications to improve safety accessing the bathroom and front entrance. Daisy also was relieved when she was offered home maintenance services and gardening assistance as part of a Home Care Package (https://www.health.gov.au/our-work/hcp).	They also agree on an acquisitional approach which includes a graded training programme to build confidence with the assistive equipment while reducing effort during occupational performance.	*Create a conceptualisation of the client's strengths and challenges*
		Implement the plan/ intervention	During stages 1 and 2, Jaydon has been able to gather strands of subjective and objective information about Daisy's occupational narrative including her strengths and challenges surrounding returning home. Jaydon syntheses these strands to create a conceptualisation which provides an understanding of Daisy's occupational identity, competence and overall occupational adaptation after her fall. This provisional conceptualisation needs to be reviewed with Daisy and Miranda to ensure that Jaydon has understood correctly and provide opportunity to incorporate any information they feel is missing.
		Jaydon and Daisy trial and choose an appropriate kitchen trolley and stool that will support Daisy to engage in breakfast preparation on the ward and home. A home visit is conducted to ensure that the assistive equipment is appropriate for Daisy's home environment. The assessment of the home environment further identified the need for minor modifications in the bathroom and at the front entrance.	*Identify goals for therapy*

(Continued)

Table 28.1 (Continued)

		Daisy joins the ward-based breakfast group each day with the support of the therapy assistant to become confident and safe when using the kitchen stool and trolley and to gradually increase her ability to prepare breakfast with less effort. She also works alongside the therapy assistant to care for the raised garden beds in the nursing home garden. Daisy plans to purchase her own raised garden bed at home to enable her to stay engaged in an aspect of gardening.	Once Daisy is satisfied the conceptualisation is an accurate reflection of her situation, Jaydon works with her to establish some goals for the therapy. Daisy reiterates her desire to return home. Jaydon uses MOHO concepts to guide the Objectives that will underpin the steps to returning home. Jaydon considers personal causation* as one concept that would support the development of skills and behaviours to reach her goal of building competence in preventing falls.
Evaluation	*Trial the plan, explore change, and refine the plan; plan for transition* The minor home modifications were completed, and Daisy agreed that a graduated return home was a good idea. This involved spending some time at home during the day, then an overnight stay before leaving respite care. During these stays Daisy was able to safely access her home for her activities of daily living and her leisure occupations and safely access her front yard to be transported to her daughter's home for dinner.	*Re-evaluate* Daisy is observed performing the same two occupations, and her occupational performance is consistent with meeting the agreed-upon goals. Daisy describes her occupational experience as feeling safer and less fatigued, and she is less fearful of falling. The minor home modifications have been completed, and Daisy is discharged to her home with the newly acquired assistive equipment and her Home Care Package.	*Implement and review the therapy* Whilst in respite care, Jaydon asks Daisy to keep a record of the times of day when she feels most active and times when she feels her energy is low. This helps to identify a routine (habituation) that supports her to make the most of her day and reduce the risk of a fall when fatigued (performance capacity). Establishing a routine that supports successful completion of tasks aims to build self-efficacy (personal causation).

(Continued)

Table 28.1 (Continued)

After three weeks of respite, Daisy was satisfied that she would be safe at home and be able to do the occupations she wanted to do. Daisy was discharged from TTCP with the care transferring to her Home Care Package provider. She still was waiting on some gardening assistance and minor home maintenance tasks.	Jaydon also discusses Daisy's preference of alternative ways to complete some tasks that also reduces fatigue (personal causation). The HSNA-informed management plan has approved access to a Home Care Package for home modifications, including for grab rails in her bathroom and handrails for her garden so she can still get out and enjoy watering her plants (environment). Further gardening assistance was also included for larger tasks like pruning.

*Personal causation is a sense of capacity and self-efficacy.

28.13 Conclusion

Occupational therapy process models enable occupational therapists to work collaboratively with clients through the elements of assessment, intervention, and evaluation, although these are defined differently in different models. There are numerous processes available, and in this chapter, we have presented three examples: the Canadian Occupational Therapy Practice Framework, the Occupational Therapy Intervention Process Model, and the Model of Human Occupation Therapeutic Reasoning Process. A case study has been used to demonstrate how the interactions between the therapist and the client are guided by these processes with the aim to show that each one can be applied to the same client. The choice of practice process may depend on the therapist's preferred conceptual models, workplace requirements, client characteristics, and needs, among other factors. While our case study focused on an individual client, it is important to note that these practice processes can also be applied when working with groups, communities, and populations.

28.14 Summary

- The occupational therapy process is a way that occupational therapists can apply to support occupation-centred thinking and action when interacting with individuals, groups, communities, or populations.
- The Occupational Therapy Intervention Process Model (OTIPM) (Fisher & Marterella, 2019) outlines the steps required to implement occupation-centred reasoning throughout all phases of the occupational therapy process.
- The Canadian Occupational Therapy Inter-relational Practice Process (COTIPP) (Restall et al., 2022) aims to highlight the context specific, collaborative, and rights-based focus of occupational therapy.

- The Therapeutic Reasoning Process (Kielhofner & Forsyth, 2008) is an occupation focused, client-centred practice model that embeds the four elements of the Model of Human Occupation at each step of occupational therapy.

28.15 Review questions

- What are the three foundational processes and six action domains of the COTIPP?
- What are the three practice phases in the OTIPM?
- What are the seven steps of the MOHO-TRP?
- Name three similarities and three differences between the CPPF, OTIPM, and MOHO-TRP.

References

Aldrich, R. M., & Cutchin, M. P. (2013). Dewey's concepts of embodiment, growth, and occupation. Extended bases for a transactional perspective. In M. P. Cutchin & V. A. Dickie (Eds.), *Transactional perspective on occupation* (pp. 13–23). Springer.

Canadian Association of Occupational Therapists. (1997, 2002). *Enabling occupation: An occupational therapy perspective.* CAOT Publications ACE.

Clemson, L. (1997). *The Westmead Home Safety Assessment.* Coordinates Publications.

Cutchin, M. P., & Dickie, V. A. (2012). Transactionalism: Occupational science and the pragmatic attitude. In G. E. Whiteford & C. Hocking (Eds.), *Occupational science: Society, inclusion, participation* (pp. 23–37). Wiley-Blackwell.

Egan, M., & Restall, G. (2022a). The Canadian Model of Occupational Participation. In M. Egan & G. Restall (Eds.), *Promoting occupational participation: Collaborative relationship-focused occupational therapy* (pp. 74–95). CAOT Publications.

Egan, M., & Restall, G. (2022b). *Promoting occupational participation: Collaborative relationship-focused occupational therapy.* Canadian Association of Occupational Therapists.

Fisher, A. G., & Marterella, A. (2019). *Powerful practice. A model for authentic occupational therapy.* Center for Innovative OT Solutions Inc.

Greber, C., Isbel, S., Scanlan, J., & Garcia-Rojas, J. (2024). Practice reasoning in occupational therapy: Introducing the model of occupational therapy reasoning. In T. Brown, S. Isbel, L. Gustafsson, S. Gutman, D. Powers-Dirette, B. Collins, & T. Barlott (Eds.), *Human occupation: Contemporary concepts and lifespan perspectives* (pp. 113–139). Routledge.

Kielhofner, G., & Forsyth, K. (2008). Therapeutic reasoning: Planning, implementing, and evaluating the outcomes of therapy. In G. Kielhofner (Ed.), *A Model of Human Occupation: Theory and application* (4th ed., pp. 143–154). Wolters Kluwer.

Law, M., Baptiste, S., Carswell, A., McColl, M. A., Polatajko, H., Pollock, N., & Toomey, M. (2014). *Canadian Occupational Performance Measure* (5th ed.). CAOT Publications ACE.

Mattingly C. (1991). What is clinical reasoning? *American Journal of Occupational Therapy, 45*(11), 979–986. https://doi.org/10.5014/ajot.45.11.979

Mattingly, C., & Fleming, M. H. (1994). *Clinical reasoning: Forms of inquiry in a therapeutic practice.* F.A. Davis.

Parkinson, S., Forsyth, K., & Kielhofner, G. (2006). *Model of Human Occupation Screening Tool (MOHOST) v2.0.* Model of Human Occupation Clearinghouse, Department of Occupational Therapy, University of Illinois at Chicago. https://moho-irm.uic.edu/

Polatajko, H., Davis, J., Stewart, D., Cantin, N., Amoroso, B., Purdie, L., & Zimmerman, D. (2013). Specifying the domain of concern: Occupation as core. In E. Townsend & E. A. Polatajko (Eds.), *Enabling occupation II: Advancing an occupational therapy vision for health, well-being, & justice through occupation* (2nd ed., pp. 23–36). CAOT Publication ACE.

Restall, G., & Egan, M. (2022). Collaborative relationship focused occupational therapy. In M. Egan & G. Restall (Eds.), *Promoting occupational participation: Collaborative relationship-focused occupational therapy* (pp. 98–117). CAOT Publications.

Restall, G., Egan, M., Valavaara, K., Phenix, A., & Sack, C. (2022). Canadian Occupational Therapy Inter-Relational Practice Process Framework. In M. Egan & G. Restall (Eds.), *Promoting occupational participation: Collaborative relationship-focused occupational therapy* (pp. 121–150). CAOT Publications.

Taylor, R. R., Bowyer, P., & Fisher, G. (Eds.). (2023). *Kielhofner's Model of Human Occupation: Theory and application* (6th ed.). Lippincott Wolters Kluwer.

Wolske, J., Raber, C., Pépin, G., & Fisher, G. (2024). Therapeutic reasoning: Planning, implementing, and evaluating the outcomes of therapy. In R. R. Taylor, P. Bowyer, & G. Fisher (Eds.), *Kielhofner's Model of Human Occupation: Theory and application* (6th ed., pp. 161–187). Lippincott Williams & Wilkins.

CHAPTER 29

Occupational therapy assessment

*Ted Brown, Helen Bourke-Taylor, Susan Darzins,
and Melinda Cooper*

Authors' positionality statement

We are Western-educated occupational therapists with postgraduate qualifications working in leadership positions in Australia. We are white, cisgender, able-bodied, English-speaking Australian citizens. We acknowledge our white privilege, our Global North outlook, and the impacts of colonial hegemony on the Aboriginal and Torres Strait Islander peoples of Australia. We support decolonisation, racial equality, queer inclusivity, cultural sensitivity, social and occupational justice, and gender-affirmative and culturally safe and responsive health care and education.

Key terms
- Assessment
- Measurement
- Validity
- Reliability
- Psychometrics
- COSMIN
- Outcome measures
- Functional capacity assessment

Objectives
This chapter will allow the reader to:

- Provide an overview of the purpose and types of assessment in contemporary occupational therapy practice contexts
- Outline the domains that occupational therapists typically assess
- Describe the measurement/psychometric properties of assessments and the features of outcome measures

DOI: 10.4324/9781003495666-32

■ Describe aspects of the assessment of functional capacity
■ Apply principles of assessment in two practice contexts

29.1 Introduction

As part of professional practice, occupational therapists must be knowledgeable in their selection, administration, scoring, and interpretation of assessments for a broad range of clients. Assessment is one of the most fundamental, yet very complex, aspects of what occupational therapists do in their day-to-day practice. The purpose of assessment is to assist an occupational therapist to collaborate with clients to make reasoned and informed decisions about goal setting, therapy planning, intervention provision, and re-evaluation.

There are potentially harmful consequences for our clients if we select tests that are poorly structured, statistically inaccurate, culturally insensitive, or irrelevant for the person/population. Many standardised assessments are developed to assess skills, abilities, factors, and constructs that are deemed important by dominant culture, and occupational therapists need to be cognisant of this when working with diverse populations that may fall outside these cultural boundaries. Similarly, it is important to follow assessments' directions or training specifications to ensure that an assessment is administered and scored accurately. Incorrectly administered or scored assessments can have negative consequences for individuals or groups who participate in the occupational therapy assessment process.

This chapter will provide an introductory overview of the purpose, and types of assessments within an occupational therapy context. The skills and attributes typically assessed by occupational therapists will be described and the psychometric properties of standardised tests, scales and instruments will be outlined. Outcome measures used in occupational therapy practice will also be described. Finally, an overview of the assessment of functional capacity will be provided, and how assessment fits with the requirements of the National Disability Insurance Scheme, My Aged Care, Department of Veterans' Affairs scheme, private health insurance plans, or other compensable schemes where occupational therapists work.

29.2 Occupational therapy assessment

29.2.1 Types of assessment

Assessments may be categorised by purpose: descriptive, discriminative, predictive, and evaluative (Brown, 2012).

Descriptive assessments can establish an individual's baseline set of skills and occupational performance and participation needs as well as indicate if they fall within typically expected score ranges. Descriptive assessments provide a reference point or way of describing functional status to inform goal setting and intervention planning.

Discriminative assessments are norm-based scales that aim to distinguish between individuals or groups on some characteristic or underlying dimension. They determine whether a client is functioning in the specified range of typical development or performance and can classify individuals into groups of different abilities (e.g., above average, average, or below average) or discernible traits (e.g., introvert, extrovert, creativity, flexibility, assertiveness).

Predictive assessments attempt to predict future performance of a person's skills or abilities based on scores on a test administered at the present time. For example, high school grades of a student can predict their future academic success at university.

Evaluative assessments or outcome measures detect changes over at least two points in time. Evaluative assessments will provide both the occupational therapist and the client with an objective indication of meaningful progress during or following occupational therapy intervention.

29.2.2 How assessment information is gathered

In practice, occupational therapists use a mix of formal and informal assessments. Formal assessments have established protocols directing the method of administration, guidelines for standardised use, evidence of their validity and reliability, and standardised scores. Informal assessments (also known as dynamic or clinical observations) are less structured and formal in their administration. Often the assessor is less directive and observes the client completing tasks and daily occupations in naturalistic settings.

Assessments vary in how they elicit client perspectives and measure clients' occupational performance and occupational participation (Law et al., 2017). The perspective or performance of a client may be directly sought and measured (e.g., self-report), a person knowledgeable about the client's perspective or performance may be consulted (e.g., third party or proxy report), or the occupational therapist may score, rate or evaluate the client's perspective or performance. Some assessments use ratings of clients' performance by a trained professional while some assessments use client self-report.

29.2.3 Standardised assessments

Standardised assessments have a set of specific characteristics. They are designed to measure a defined construct, dimension, ability, or attribute that is subsequently operationalised into specific items (and related subscales) that are rated, answered, or performed by the clients being assessed. For example, self-concept is an overarching construct, and its sub-constructs (such as academic self-concept, social self-concept, athletic self-concept, and family self-concept) (Piers et al., 2018) are accessible through items considered to adequately represent the construct. Children's motor skills may be assessed through the completion of a series of standardised motor skill tasks (or items) rated by an experienced examiner using specific criteria. Examples of standardised motor skill assessments are the Bruininks-Oseretsky Test of Motor Proficiency – Third Edition (BOT-3) (Bruininks & Bruininks, 2024), and the Movement Assessment Battery for Children – Third Edition (Movement ABC-3) (Henderson & Barnett, 2023).

As stated, standardised tests have a manual or set of instructions describing use, application, and interpretation. The manual will typically contain details of how the test was developed, standardised, and validated. Test authors complete various psychometric studies that confirm or report on reliability, validity, responsiveness, interpretability, and utility features of the test. Authors of standardised tests typically gather a large dataset of scores, known as a normative sample. The normative sample often mirrors a population's traits (e.g., gender, age, ethnicity, socio-economic status, geographical distribution) based on census data. Test authors then use the standardisation sample to generate performance scores to compare test-takers against. Score examples include stanines, z-scores, T-scores, stanine scores, standard scores, percentile ranks, and age equivalents (Kubiszyn & Borich, 2015).

The final trait of a standardised test is its ongoing and iterative refinement and revision. A body of empirical literature is usually established about its measurement properties and its application in different contexts (e.g., with diverse client groups, applied in cross-cultural environments). This evidence is dynamic and continually supplemented by test-users and researchers; subsequently the test constantly evolves. The Model of Human Occupation Screening Tool (MOHOST) (Parkinson et al., 2006) is an assessment used by occupational therapists with a substantial body of empirical work published about its use, application and measurement properties.

29.2.4 What skills, attributes, and domains do occupational therapists assess?

Occupational therapists focus on and assess occupational performance, participation, and engagement. Occupational performance has been defined as the 'accomplishment of the selected occupation resulting from the dynamic transaction among the client, their context, and the occupation' (American Occupational Therapy Association [AOTA], 2020, p. 80). Occupational therapy assessment measures must be valid, reliable, responsive to change, clinically relevant, culturally appropriate, and occupation focused. Standardised assessments provide objective data that can help support and evidence the need for occupational therapy services and track progress (AOTA, 2020). Meaningful occupational therapy assessment should include consideration of aspects of the context and environment including cultural, personal, physical, social, temporal, attitudinal, economic, political, and virtual features. Table 29.1 offers examples of assessments commonly used by occupational therapists, mapped to the International Classification of Functioning, Disability and Health (ICF) (World Health Organization, 2001). The examples listed in Table 29.1 are not exhaustive.

29.2.5 Selecting psychometrically sound instruments and scales

Before selecting an assessment, occupational therapists need to be clear on the three crucial factors: 1) the *purpose* of the assessment; 2) the area(s) being assessed, such as the *person, environment,* or *occupation*; and 3) whether the measurement scale is psychometrically sound. The terminology about psychometric properties that occupational therapists adhere to aligns with the universal terminology and internationally recognised standards proposed by the COnsensus-based Standards for the selection of health Measurement INstruments (COSMIN) (Mokkink et al., 2023) (see https://www.cosmin.nl/). This taxonomy assists occupational therapists to make sound selection of outcome measures and to psychometrically evaluate assessments used in both clinical practice and in research.

The COSMIN taxonomy categorises measurement properties of health outcome measurement instruments into three domains: reliability, validity, and responsiveness. Table 29.2 provides an overview of the measurement properties, brief definitions (Mokkink et al., 2018), and examples of occupational therapy psychometric studies.

29.2.6 Assessing functional capacity

Occupational therapists assess an individual's functional capacity in many areas of practice, including driving assessments, work-related assessments, self-care assessments, or when providing services to clients through the National Disability Insurance Scheme (NDIS) and Veterans Affairs. The NDIS (2020) defines functional capacity as

Table 29.1 Standardised assessments often used by occupational therapists mapped to the International Classification of Functioning, Disability and Health

	Standardised assessment examples
Body Functions and Structures	■ Beery-Buktenica Developmental Test of Visual-Motor Integration 6th Edition (Beery VMI) ■ Bruininks-Oseretsky Test of Motor Proficiency, Third Edition (BOT-3) ■ Cognitive Assessment of Minnesota ■ Melbourne Assessment of Unilateral Upper Limb Function ■ Movement Assessment Battery for Children, Third Edition (Movement ABC-3) ■ Rivermead Behavioural Memory Test – Third Edition (RBMT-3)
Activities	■ Animated Movie Test (AMT) ■ Checklist of Leisure, Interests and Participation (CLIP) ■ Child-Initiated Pretend Play Assessment (ChIPPA) ■ Child Leisure Assessment Scale (CLASS) ■ Children's Assessment of Participation and Enjoyment/Preferences of Activities of Children (CAPE/PAC) ■ DriveSafe DriveAware ■ Pediatric Evaluation of Disability Inventory Computer Adaptive Test (PEDI-CAT) ■ Vineland Adaptive Behavior Scales, Third Edition (Vineland-3)
Participation	■ Activity Card Sort (ACS) ■ Home Support Needs Assessment (HSNA) ■ ICF-Measure of Participation and Activities Screener (IMPACT-S) ■ Impact on Participation and Autonomy (IPA) ■ Participation and Environmental Measure for Children and Youth (PEM-CY) ■ School Function Assessment (SFA) ■ Utrecht Scale for Evaluation of Rehabilitation-Participation (USER-Participation) ■ Y-PEM – Youth, Young-adult Participation and Environment Measure
Personal Factors	■ Usually assessed informally by asking questions in an interview format about a person's life and lifestyle, such as questions about gender identity, educational level, race, ethnicity, religion, age, fitness level, socioeconomic status, coping styles, literacy level, past and current life events, habits, and upbringing
Environmental Factors	■ Environmental Restriction Questionnaire (ERQ) ■ Home Falls and Accidents Screening Tool (HOME FAST) ■ Home Observation for Measurement of the Environment (HOME) ■ In Home Occupational Performance Evaluation (I-HOPE) ■ School Setting Interview (SSI) Version 3.0 ■ Westmead Home Safety Assessment (WeHSA) ■ Work Environment Impact Scale (WEIS) Version 2

'an individual's ability to be involved in life situations and to execute tasks or actions, with and without assistance (assistive devices and/or personal assistance)' (p. 11). Assessing functional capacity involves evaluating a person's abilities and skills to perform a range of daily occupations in home, work, and community environments.

Table 29.2 COSMIN properties, brief definitions (Mokkink et al., 2018) and examples of psychometric studies by Australian and New Zealand occupational therapists

Psychometric domain and definition	Measurement property	Definition of measurement property	Example of a published psychometric study by occupational therapists
Reliability: The degree to which the measurement is free from measurement error, and it contains the measurement properties internal consistency, reliability, and measurement error.	Internal consistency	Demonstrated strength of relationship between items within the scale/assessment.	Joyce, K., Bourke-Taylor, H.M., Wilkes-Gillan, S. (2017) Validity of the Assistance to Participate Scale with parents of typically developing Australian children aged 3–8 years. *Australian Occupational Therapy Journal, 64*(5), 381–390. https://doi.org/10.1111/1440-1630.12409 This study also investigates construct validity.
	Interrater reliability	Stability between raters for the same instrument.	Radia-George, C., Imms, C., & Taylor, N. F. (2014). Interrater reliability and clinical utility of the Personal Care Participation Assessment and Resource Tool (PC-PART) in an inpatient rehabilitation setting. *American Journal of Occupational Therapy, 68*(3), 334–343. https://doi.org/10.5014/ajot.2014.009878 This study also investigated clinical utility.
	Intrarater reliability	Stability on repeats of the instrument by the same rater (may be called test retest reliability).	Wu, O. K., Brown, T., Yu, M. L., Joshua, N., Wilson, C. J., & Campbell, H. C. (2023). Test–retest reliability and convergent validity of the Movement Assessment Battery for Children–third edition with Australian 3–6-year-olds and their parents. *Journal of Occupational Therapy, Schools, & Early Intervention*, 1–21. https://doi.org/10.1080/19411243.2023.2271480 This study also investigates construct validity.
	Measurement error	The extent to which changes in scores from the measurement scale are *not* due to changes in the true construct.	Muskett, R., Bourke-Taylor, H.M., Hewitt, A. (2017). Intrarater reliability of the Health Promoting Activities Scale. *American Journal of Occupational Therapy, 71*(4), 7104190010p1–7104190010p8. https://doi.org/10.5014/ajot.2017.021162 This study also investigates standard error of measurement and minimum detectable difference.

(Continued)

Table 29.2 (Continued)

Psychometric domain and definition	Measurement property	Definition of measurement property	Example of a published psychometric study by occupational therapists
Validity: The degree to which an outcome measure measures the construct it purports to measure and contains the measurement properties content validity (including face validity), construct validity (including structural validity, hypotheses testing, and cross-cultural validity\ measurement invariance), and criterion validity.	Content validity	Evidence that the measurement scale has relevant items, is comprehensive in the inclusion of items, and is easily comprehended by the person/people being assessed. Face validity means that experts agree that the items are representative of the construct being measured.	Hrdlicka, H. C., Meise, E., Corbett, J., Meyer, A., & Grevelding, P. (2024). Content validity testing of a novel cognitive screen, the Gaylord Occupational Therapy Cognitive (GOT–Cog), to improve inpatient occupational therapy treatment planning. *American Journal of Occupational Therapy, 78*(1), 7801345020. https://doi.org/10.5014/ajot.2024.050306
	Construct validity	The construct is stated and then measured to evaluate if the instrument measures what it purports to measure.	Darzins, S., Imms, C., Shields, N., Taylor, N.F. (2015). Responsiveness, construct and criterion validity of the Personal Care Participation Assessment and Resource Tool (PC-PART). *Health and Quality of Life Outcomes, 13*, 125. http://dx.doi.org/10.1186/s12955-015-0322-5 This study also investigates responsiveness and criterion validity.
	Structural validity	Whether all items are statistically grouped to belong to the same underlying construct.	Lyons, C., Brown, T. and Bourke-Taylor, H. (2018), The Classroom Environment Questionnaire (CEQ): Development and preliminary structural validity. *Australian Occupational Therapy Journal, 65*(5), 363–375. https://doi.org/10.1111/1440-1630.12474
	Cross-cultural validity	Whether an instrument from one population is relevant in a different population.	Sim, S.S., Bourke-Taylor, H.M., Yu, M-L., Fossey, E., Tirlea, L. (2022) Cross-Cultural Validation of the Chinese Version of the Health Promoting Activities Scale. *American Journal of Occupational Therapy, 76*(6), 7606205080. https://doi.org/10.5014/ajot.2022.049434

(Continued)

Table 29.2 (Continued)

Psychometric domain and definition	Measurement property	Definition of measurement property	Example of a published psychometric study by occupational therapists
	Criterion validity	Whether an instrument agrees with the gold standard for the same construct. Includes concurrent validity (do two measures agree?) and predictive validity (does the measure predict the outcome of interest?). Includes sensitivity and specificity.	Mackenzie, L. and Byles, J. (2018), Scoring the home falls and accidents screening tool for health professionals (HOME FAST-HP): Evidence from one epidemiological study. *Australian Occupational Therapy Journal*, 65(5), 346–353. https://doi.org/10.1111/1440-1630.12467 This study also investigates predictive validity, sensitivity, and specificity.
Responsiveness		The ability of an outcome measure to detect change over time in the construct to be measured. It refers to the validity of a change score.	Taylor, S., Elliott, C., McLean, B., Parsons, R., Falkmer, T., Carey, L. M., Blair, E., & Girdler, S. (2022). Construct validity, reliability, and responsiveness of the Wrist Position Sense Test for use in children with hemiplegic cerebral palsy. *Australian Occupational Therapy Journal*, 69(5), 637–646. https://doi.org/10.1111/1440-1630.12825 This study also investigates construct validity and reliability.

An Occupational Therapy Assessment of Functional Capacity (OTAFC) focuses on what a person's goals are for the future and then seeks to identify how they are managing general self-care and general day-to-day occupations and what challenges need to be addressed for them to make progress towards achieving those identified and agreed-upon goals. These are referred to as occupational performance issues and challenges (OPICs). An OTAFC will likely take more than one session, depending on the complexity of the person's situation, number of presenting OPICs, and number of funded hours included in their plan. Typically, an OTAFC will take six to eight hours of funding to complete. An OTAFC will include an occupational therapist speaking with a person about their occupational performance areas, including:

- Communication
- Cognition
- Psychosocial functioning
- Self-care

- Home management
- Community mobility
- Working
- Studying, learning, and education
- Leisure, recreation, and play pursuits
- Social participation and engagement
- Sleep and rest

An OTAFC may also involve a person completing a practical assessment using observation, interview and standardised assessments. If specific OPICs have been identified, then an occupational therapist may use informal and formal/standardised assessments to observe the person completing certain tasks, occupations, or daily functional activities to gather further information about the OPICs they are experiencing. This also assists the occupational therapist in making recommendations about the types of services, supports, therapy interventions, or equipment that they could suggest for enhancing the person's independence, safety, and functional skill development. A list of questions that occupational therapists can ask themselves when considering the most appropriate assessment to select to use as part of their professional practice is located in Table 29.3.

29.2.6.1 Vignette 29.1: NDIS paediatric scenario

Natalia, a 12-year-old girl with Down syndrome, had been a participant in the National Disability Insurance Scheme for several years and received occupational therapy services from Caitlin, an occupational therapist in private practice. In preparation for Natalia's transition to secondary school, Caitlin assessed Natalia for an up-to-date evaluation of her abilities to provide information to the new school and inform further intervention planning.

The family's initial goals for engaging with occupational therapy were to help improve Natalia's independence in school and home activities as well as increasing her ability to participate in community activities such as gymnastics and swimming lessons. After completing an updated occupational profile, Caitlin chose to administer

Table 29.3 Guide to selecting, learning and administering occupational therapy assessments: questions to consider

---

- What aspects of the person, occupation, or environment does the scale, instrument, or measure assess?
- What does the client want or need to change in their situation or living context to enhance occupational participation?
- What is the reliability and validity evidence of the scale, instrument, or measure?
- What type of training is required to administer the scale, instrument, or measure?
- How long does the scale, instrument, or measure take to complete?
- What is the cost of the scale, instrument, or measure to purchase?
- Is the scale, instrument, or measure appropriate for culturally diverse or vulnerable groups within society and for the person being assessed?
- What are the eligibility criteria for the funding scheme, and how does this align with assessment requirements and assessment selection?
- How many assessments has the client completed previously?

---

the PEDI-CAT, the PEM-CY, and the Movement ABC-3. The PEDI-CAT is an online caregiver questionnaire addressing the domains of daily activities, mobility, social/cognitive, and responsibility. It provided both norm-referenced scores, which Caitlin could use to evidence Natalia's need for ongoing assistance, and criterion-referenced scores that were useful for setting functional goals and tracking progress. The PEM-CY was also completed by a caregiver and asked about participation in the home, school, and community, along with environmental factors within each of these settings.

Caitlin used the test component of the Movement ABC-3 during the face-to-face assessment session to gather data about Natalia's fine and gross motor abilities from a body structure and function perspective. Natalia had previously been assessed with the Movement ABC-2, but this was several years prior. The PEDI-CAT and PEM-CY were completed separately by Natalia's parents. Upon completing and reviewing these assessments, Caitlin also decided to administer the Child and School forms of the Sensory Profile 2 (SP-2), as her findings suggested that sensory processing differences might also be affecting Natalia's participation.

Natalia achieved scores considerably below the average range for the Balance & Locomotion and Aiming & Catching domains of the Movement ABC-3, which correlated with her results on the PEDI-CAT Mobility domain, where Caitlin noted that functional tasks such as stepping in and out of the bath and bending down to pick up objects were areas of relative difficulty. Although Natalia also scored below average on the Manual Dexterity domain, this domain was an area of relative strength, and Caitlin made sure to note this in her report alongside a comment about Natalia's interest in cooking and art and craft activities. The PEM-CY highlighted that sensory factors in the environment were a likely barrier to Natalia's participation in community activities, and when analysing the results of the SP-2, Caitlin noticed that Natalia showed individual differences in the Sensitivity and Avoiding quadrants for both auditory and tactile input. Caitlin was able to use the combined results of these assessments to build a picture of Natalia's current participation, identify areas of strength and challenge, set goals for further intervention, and provide tangible strategies to help smooth the transition from primary to secondary school. She summarised these results into a report to be provided to school and the NDIS for future support planning.

29.2.6.2 *Vignette 29.2: My Aged Care scenario*

An occupational therapist, Anita, funded by the MyAgedCare Commonwealth Home Support Program, has been asked to provide occupational therapy services for Mrs Maria Kodanska, an 88-year-old woman living alone in her own suburban home. She has cataracts impacting her ability to see clearly and osteoarthritis in her left hip limiting her mobility, especially going up and down stairs. She recently tripped and fell over a carpet in her home and injured her left shoulder and wrist. She has also been forgetful. Last week she forgot a doctor's appointment and burnt a saucepan on the stovetop. She also becomes short of breath doing household tasks, and she can no longer walk to the local shops. Since her fall, Maria has become less confident about moving around in her home as well as outdoors.

Anita used a combination of informal conversation, valid standardised assessments, and informal observational assessment to gather clinically relevant information about (1) Maria's priorities for enhancing participation in her daily life occupations and routine, (2) additional supports needed to help Maria manage her personal and instrumental activities of daily living, (3) hazards in her home environment that could be eliminated to promote safer mobility in her home, (4) Maria's cognitive status and whether she may need to be further assessed for cognitive impairment, and (5) access into the home and for transfers in her bathroom and toilet.

1. Anita spent time getting to know Maria through informal conversation and observation of Maria making her a cup of tea while they spoke. She established that Maria's greatest concern and priority was to regain confidence moving around her home and outdoors and to remain living at home for as long as possible. She also observed that Maria moved cautiously and slowly and used walls and furniture to help steady her.

2. Anita then completed a standardised assessment with Maria, the Home Support Needs Assessment (HSNA) (Darzins & Darzins, 2018). The HSNA is conducted as a structured conversation covering the *self-care* and *domestic life* activities people need to manage to sustain life at home. Anita used this assessment to identify if Maria had unmet support needs and to estimate the risk to Maria's health associated with these unmet needs. She used the HSNA to identify priorities for action. They identified that Maria would benefit from mobility and assistive technology to help her remain independent. They also identified that Maria will need additional support for shopping, household cleaning, and garden maintenance. Anita established with Maria that further assessment of the home environment was needed to comprehensively identify falls risk hazards and to assess for minor home modifications.

3. Anita then completed the Home Falls and Accidents Screening Tool (Home FAST) (Mackenzie et al., 2000) with Maria, which examines a person's home environment to identify falls risks in their home environment. Several potential falls risks were identified including slippery floor surfaces in the kitchen and bathroom, several loose mats in the living room and bedroom, inadequate lighting in the kitchen and living rooms, clutter in most rooms in the house, no light switch accessible from Maria's bed, a shower over the bath in the bathroom, and a poorly secured grab rail along the stairs going to the first floor of the house.

4. Anita completed the Rowland Universal Dementia Assessment Scale (RUDAS) (Storey et al., 2004) with Maria. The RUDAS is a cognitive screening instrument for individuals presenting with suspected cognitive impairment in culturally and linguistically diverse populations. Anita noted that Maria experienced challenges in the registration, visuospatial orientation, visuoconstructional drawing, judgement, and memory recall cognitive domains, obtaining a total RUDAS score of 24/30.

Using the information gathered from these observational and standardised assessments, Anita was able to build a case for funding of minor home modifications to improve access and mobility, additional supports for shopping and cleaning, assistive technology, and garden maintenance. Anita also made a referral for physiotherapy to work with Maria on mobility and strengthening to enhance her mobility and confidence and recommended that Maria's cognitive skills be further investigated by her treating doctor.

29.2.7 Reporting assessment results

Interpreting and communicating results is an important step in the occupational therapy assessment process. In addition to providing useful information to clients and other stakeholders, reports are also used as evidence of the need for funding, services or accommodations. When writing an assessment report, the therapist should keep in mind the purpose of the report and the intended audience. Some funding bodies may require reports to be formatted in a specific way or include certain types of scores such as percentile ranks, while a parent is more likely to need a concise and practical summary of the assessment findings and a plan or suggestions for how to help their child. The tone of the report is also important. Taking a strengths-based approach to report writing is a way to convey assessment results in a manner that provides necessary scientific data about the client's needs and abilities but also acknowledges the possibilities we see within them (Dunn, 2017). For example, for a child who scores below the 2nd percentile on the PEDI-CAT Daily Activities domain: '(Child) is able to participate in personal activities of daily living such as dressing, toileting and eating when provided with physical and verbal support through each step of the task' as opposed to '(Child) requires maximal assistance for all self-care tasks'.

There are many artificial intelligence (AI) reporting tools available for occupational therapists and other professionals. Using AI to assist with administrative tasks such as report writing can be a valuable time and energy saver, but it is crucial to remember that AI is not infallible and should be used as an adjunct to the professional reasoning process rather than to replace therapists' own clinical reasoning. Care should be taken to protect any identifying information and sensitive client information by ensuring that the reporting tool has sufficient data privacy controls in place to maintain clients' confidentiality. Occupational therapists using AI for reporting should always critically appraise the outputs and use their training, knowledge and skills to interpret assessment results and make edits as necessary. The Australian Health Practitioner Regulation Agency (AHPRA) has developed a set of guidelines for the safe and appropriate use of AI in professional practice (see link: https://www.ahpra.gov.au/Resources/Artificial-Intelligence-in-healthcare.aspx).

29.3 Conclusion

Assessment is a vital part of the occupational therapy process. In professional practice with clients and families, occupational therapists use a wide range of tests and measures. Assessment is a key professional competency for occupational therapists, and it is important for therapists to stay informed about new assessments and revisions of existing ones. Occupational therapists need to use standardised assessments that provide clinically meaningful and valid information and to measure meaningful changes brought about from occupational therapy interventions, through repeated measurements. Use of standardised, valid assessments supports our professional reasoning, aids communication across the health team, can help us measure the benefits and impacts of our services, and can be useful for resource allocation.

29.4 Summary

- Assessments can be categorised as formal or informal; standardised or non-standardised; and self-report, performance-based, or proxy-report.

- Assessment assists with establishing a baseline of clients' occupational strengths, challenges, and interests; collaborative goal setting; and monitoring changes in clients' occupational performance.
- Occupational therapists typically assess clients' skills, interests, participation, and performance abilities in the areas of activities of daily living, self-management, play, leisure, work, education, social participation, and sleep.
- The COSMIN specifies that evidence of the following seven types of measurement properties should be reported about health-related instruments: internal consistency, reliability, measurement error, content validity, construct validity, criterion validity, and responsiveness.

29.5 Review and reflection questions

- What is the purpose of occupational therapists completing an assessment with a client?
- What is an outcome measure, and why do occupational therapists commonly use such assessments?
- What are four types of measurement properties highlighted in the COSMIN?
- What are four occupational performance areas that Occupational Therapy Assessment of Functional Capacity will often focus on?
- What are two examples of accommodations and adaptations of standardised assessment that can be made by occupational therapists when assessing clients?

References

American Occupational Therapy Association. (2020). Occupational Therapy Practice Framework: Domain and process, 4th edition. *American Journal of Occupational Therapy*, 74(Supp 2), 7412410010. https://doi.org/10.5014/ajot.2020.74S2001

Brown, T. (2012). Assessment, measurement, and evaluation/Why can't I do what everyone expects me to do? In S. J. Lane & A. C. Bundy (Eds.), *Kids can be kids: A childhood occupations approach* (pp. 320–348). F. A. Davis Co.

Bruininks, B. D., & Bruininks, R. H. (2024). *Bruininks-Oseretsky Test of Motor Proficiency – third edition examiner manual*. Pearson.

Darzins, S., & Darzins, P. (2018). *Home support needs assessment (HSNA)*. Darzins Consulting Pty Ltd.

Dunn, W. (2017). Strengths-based approaches: What if even the 'bad' things are good things? *British Journal of Occupational Therapy*, 80(7), 395–396. https://doi.org/10.1177/0308022617702660

Henderson, S. E., & Barnett, A. L. (2023). *Movement assessment battery for children, third edition test manual*. Pearson.

Kubiszyn, T., & Borich, G. (2015). *Educational testing and measurement* (11th ed.). Wiley & Sons Inc.

Law, M., Baum, C. M., & Dunn, W. (2017). *Measuring occupational performance: Supporting best practice in occupational therapy* (3rd ed.). Slack Incorporated.

Mackenzie, L., Byles, J., & Higginbotham, N. (2000). Designing the Home Falls and Accidents Screening Tool (HOME FAST): Selecting the items. *British Journal of Occupational Therapy*, 63(6), 260–269. https://doi.org/10.1177/030802260006300604

Mokkink, L. B., de Wet, H. C. W., Prinsen, C. A. C., Patrick, D. L., Alonso, J., Bouter, L. M., & Terwee, C. B. (2018). COSMIN risk of bias checklist for systematic reviews of patient-reported outcome measures. *Quality of Life Research*, 27(5), 1171–1179. https://doi.org/10.1007/s11136-017-1765-4

Mokkink, L. B., Terwee, C. B., & de Vet, H. C. W. (2023). COSMIN: Consensus-based standards for the selection of health status measurement instruments. In F. Maggino (Ed.), *Encyclopedia of quality of life and well-being research* (pp. 1215–1225). Springer. https://doi.org/10.1007/978-3-031-17299-1_595

NDIS. (2020). *Independent assessment selection of assessment tools*. Author. https://www.ndis.gov.au/about-us/history-ndis/archived-policy-proposals

Parkinson, S., Forsyth, K., & Kielhofner, G. (2006). *User's manual for the Model of Human Occupation Screening Tool (MOHOST) (version 2.0)*. The Model of Human Occupation Clearinghouse. https://moho-irm.uic.edu/default.aspx

Piers, E. V., Shemmassian, S. K., & Herzberg, D. S. (2018). *Piers-Harris 3: Self-concept scale*. Western Psychological Services.

Storey, J. E., Rowland, J. T., Basic, D., Conforti, D. A., & Dickson, H. G. (2004). The Rowland Universal Dementia Assessment Scale (RUDAS): A multicultural cognitive assessment scale. *International Psychogeriatrics, 16*(1), 13–31. https://doi.org/10.1017/s1041610204000043

World Health Organization. (2001). *International Classification of Functioning, Disability, and Health: ICF*. World Health Organization.

Core business

Occupation analysis, activity analysis, and task analysis

Lynette Mackenzie, Joanne Lewis, Judy Ranka, and Kylie Angelou

Authors' positionality statement

All authors are occupational therapy academics working within two academic programmes at the University of Sydney and Notre Dame University, Sydney. They all come from a western background from the United Kingdom, the United States, and Australia. Two are early career academics. All authors are involved in teaching at an undergraduate and master's entry level and conduct research in occupational therapy practice.

Key terms
- Occupation
- Activity
- Task
- Analysis
- Meaning
- Environment

Objectives
This chapter will allow the reader to:

- Define and differentiate between task analysis, activity analysis, and occupation analysis
- Identify how occupational therapists can use occupation analysis in their practice
- Identify factors to consider when conducting an occupation analysis
- Apply occupation analysis to different areas of practice

30.1 Introduction
When gathering information about an individual, the occupational therapist seeks to understand the daily life of that person. The therapist explores the perspective of the

DOI: 10.4324/9781003495666-33

individual about their most important or meaningful occupations. This essential phase of the occupational therapy practice process involves analysis of these important occupations. This analysis is called occupation analysis. There are three different levels of analysis: an occupation analysis, an activity analysis, and a task analysis. This chapter provides an overview of the three forms of analysis, along with illustrative practical examples, and to conclude the chapter, there are examples of occupation analyses.

30.2 Occupation, activity, and task analysis

Occupation is central to the practice of occupational therapy (Chard & Mesa, 2017), making occupation analysis an important aspect of practice. A review of occupational therapy literature indicates occupation and activity analysis are used in multiple ways. Occupation analysis is either considered synonymous with activity analysis (American Occupational Therapy Association [AOTA], 2020; Wilson & Landry, 2014) or each distinctly different from each other (O'Toole, 2011). While terms may be used interchangeably in practice and in some literature, this chapter considers them different. See the definitions in Table 30.1.

30.2.1 Occupation analysis

Examines engagement in an occupation that has meaning for a person while simultaneously considering the effect of and the dynamic relationship between personal factors and the specific contexts and environments of each unique individual (O'Toole, 2011). An occupation analysis is a comprehensive process designed to understand the values and meaning a person assigns to engagement in specific occupations within their own environments (Thomas, 2022). The person is central in this analysis with consideration of their body functions and structures, life experiences, habits, routines, values, and goals, along with the demands of the occupation within their unique environments and context for performance (O'Toole, 2011). Occupation analysis involves observing the person complete their occupations, ideally in the environments/contexts in which they occur.

30.2.2 Activity analysis

Identifies the overall demands of performing an activity within daily life. It is possible to conduct an activity analysis without reference to an individual. An activity analysis isolates and sequences the required actions; the typically used equipment while performing the activity; and the physical, cognitive, emotional, perceptual, sensory, and social

Table 30.1 Definitions of occupation analysis, activity analysis, and task analysis

Occupation analysis	'The process of exploring the transactional relationship between the characteristics of an occupation, the personal meanings attributed to the occupation by individuals, groups and communities, and the contribution of various factors to the performance of an occupation' (Mackenzie & O'Toole, 2011, p. 383).
Activity analysis	'The examination of the demands of an activity that stipulates the required skills and component tasks for successful completion of the activity' (Mackenzie & O'Toole, 2011, p. 378).
Task analysis	'The exploration of individual actions required by each of the components of an occupation' (Mackenzie & O'Toole, 2011, p. 385).

skills required to perform the activity (Perlman & Bergthorson, 2017; Reese Walter & Winston, 2025). An activity analysis does not typically relate to the specific skills of the individual or their unique environment or context and it does not relate to the meaning attributed to a particular activity or occupation. An activity analysis identifies potential areas of difficulty, ways of grading and adapting the activity, and the possible required supports to promote completion of the activity (Perlman & Bergthorson, 2017).

30.2.3 Task analysis

Is the examination of the set of actions required to achieve a specific step within an activity. It may involve a more detailed observation and analysis of the exact actions within specific contexts to complete the task. The purpose of a task analysis is to obtain a detailed understanding of the specific demands of the task and thus the required skills to undertake an activity. For example, a task analysis within the activity of cooking would analyse a specific step, such as peeling potatoes, by analysing grips required, grip strength, sensation in the hand, co-ordination of a vegetable peeler or knife, and standing tolerance if standing to conduct this task at the sink.

To illustrate the analysis of occupations, activities and tasks, two examples of analysing common activities of daily living follow: the first is making a cup of tea, and the second is bathing.

30.3 The example of making a cup of tea

The occupation of making a cup of tea is commonly used in practice. Figure 30.1 illustrates the three levels of occupation analysis, with the following section providing a more detailed description of each level of analysis for making a cup of tea.

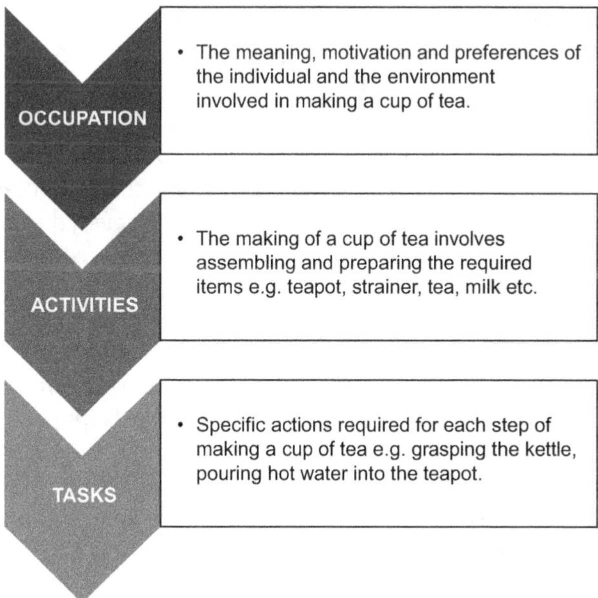

Figure 30.1 Levels of analysis involved in making a cup of tea

(Creek 1996; Fair & Barnitt 1999; Hannam 1997)

How someone makes tea depends on their culture, preferences, and environment. Occupation analysis helps therapists understand the personal meaning, habits, and routines behind the task, ideally observed in the person's own setting. Activity analysis focuses on the general skills, tools, and steps needed – like using a teabag versus a teapot. Tasks may include boiling water, selecting a cup, and pouring tea. Task analysis breaks down each step to identify specific actions and challenges. All three levels of analysis require attention to skills like vision, reach, strength, sensation, and cognition (O'Toole, 2011).

30.4 The example of bathing

Bathing varies by culture, values, and environment (McGraw & Drennan, 2009). The AOTA (2020) defines it as gathering supplies, washing, rinsing, drying, and transferring. Its meaning shifts across life stages – children may enjoy it, teens may resist or prolong it, and adults may use it to relax or energise. Frequency also differs. Occupation analysis must consider personal routines and beliefs. Environmental contexts (physical, temporal, cultural, social, institutional, and political) such as drought can change bathing methods (e.g., bucket baths). Occupational therapy focuses on the interaction between person, occupation, and environment (Polatajko et al., 2013; Whalley Hammell, 2013). Therapists use activity analysis to outline steps, tools, and skills, guiding assessment and intervention. Task analysis targets specific challenges, like reaching for shampoo, to inform therapy and adaptations.

30.5 Components involved in conducting a comprehensive occupation analysis

When conducting a comprehensive occupation analyses it is essential to consider three fundamental components: (1) the individual or personal factors, (2) the contexts (environments), and (3) the factors relating to the occupation. The complex dynamic relationship between these three components are recognised as key contributors to occupational performance by conceptual practice models such as the Person–Environment–Occupational Model (Law et al., 1996); the Person–Environment–Occupation–Performance Model (Baum & Christiansen, 2005), and the Occupational Performance Model Australia (Chapparo & Ranka, 2025). It is important to recognise that an occupational therapist may apply the components from within their chosen conceptual practice model when conducting an occupation analysis. This chapter applies the components of the model of occupation analysis developed by O'Toole (2011), as discussed in the following.

30.5.1 Individual components

Individual components are the intrinsic aspects of the individual typically related to the contextual components. This dynamic personal system consists of the expected roles of the individual, their personal values and beliefs, their spirit and their personality. Attributes and traits such as gender, age, weight, height, skills (physical, cognitive, communication, social, etc.), motivation, and emotional regulation are interwoven within the dynamic personal system. Individual components can act as a barrier or facilitator to performing the occupation. The individual components determine choices, expectations, capacities, and decisions when performing occupations (O'Toole, 2011, p. 11).

30.5.2 Contexts

The contexts of occupations (see Table 30.2) include the cultural context, spiritual context, political and institutional context, social context, physical context (natural, built, and

Table 30.2 Contexts considered in a comprehensive occupation analysis

Cultural	Provides the setting for and expectations of the occupation from within a cultural group, such as using your right hand to eat with your fingers or eating only leavened bread.
Spiritual	Provides the values and beliefs sustaining and motivating the individual, such as eating only after sunset during Ramadan or separation of those utensils for touching milk products from those used to touch meat products.
Political and institutional rules	Affects the availability and management of environments to allow performance of occupations within the environments, such as road rules and licensing to facilitate driving occupations.
Social	Includes the influence of family, friends, colleagues, pets, neighbours, and so on. They can be complex, sometimes producing unconscious expectations of occupational engagement, and may significantly affect occupational performance, such as being obliged to continue family sporting traditions not necessarily reflecting personal skills or preferences.
Physical	The built, natural, and temporal environments of the occupation. For some people there may be valued occupations, which are associated with specific locations or times of the day/times of the year, such as swimming only at the beach, jogging early in the morning, or eating Christmas pudding at Christmas time.
Sensory	Features within the environment that require use of sight, touch, hearing, smell, taste, and balance. Features include the intensity of sensory input as well as, for example, colour, pattern, texture, weight, sound, odour, flavour, moving parts, and surface stability.
Technological	A significant force affecting modern-day occupations; for example, demands of computer use for productive occupations require an individual to sit and focus on a computer screen for extended periods.
Socio-economic	The effect of the availability of resources and access to occupations; for example, not owning a car will necessitate accessing alternative forms of transport such as a public transport or walking.

temporal), technological contexts, and socio-economic contexts (O'Toole, 2011). Contexts interrelate and will have varying effects on the individual at a given time in their lifespan.

30.5.3 The occupation being analysed

Understanding an occupation is the starting point for its analysis. This involves examining what the person does, the context of their actions, and their values, routines, and environment. Occupational structure (O'Toole, 2011) refers to societal or governmental expectations that shape access to occupations – for example, age restrictions on driving. Family routines also influence engagement, such as bedtime rituals. Environmental factors, like weather, can affect times when tasks like gardening are performed.

30.6 How to conduct an occupation analysis

1. *Selecting the occupation to analyse*: Determining which occupation to analyse must be a collaborative process involving the person to determine priority concerns. As occupations fundamentally relate to individual meaning and motivation, it is essential that the decision to analyse an occupation be collaborative and person centred.

2. *Be careful not to assume anything about the occupation*: An occupational therapist must be aware of their own personal opinion or idea of what is important or meaningful in an occupation. This awareness ensures that the personal values and expectations of the therapist do not affect the occupation analysis being conducted for and with another person.

3. *Use a conceptual framework to guide occupation analysis:* For the occupation analysis examples in this chapter, the framework by O'Toole (2011, p. 11) is used.

4. *Occupation analysis needs to be consistent with person-centred goals*: It is essential that the occupation analysis undertaken be consistent with person-centred goals when developing occupational therapy interventions.

5. *Conduct an interview with the person (or significant others if appropriate) to determine priorities for occupation analysis*: This is an important step to identify the personal meaning for certain occupations held by the person and therefore the priority for analysis and any interventions following the analysis. An interview will also enable the therapist to understand how and where an occupation is usually performed and the typical use of equipment.

6. *Consult with any significant others*: It may be useful to consult any family members or other carers who may be able to provide an important perspective on the usual practices of the person and their capacity to undertake occupations.

7. *Observation of engagement in the occupation*: One way to gather information for an occupation analysis is to observe the person undertaking the occupation. This may involve paying attention to the tasks involved and recording how the person performs each of the observable components of the occupation. This process would ideally be conducted in the environment where the person typically performs the occupation but on occasions may need to be in a simulated environment, for example, in a hospital or community centre.

8. *Collect any assessment findings of relevance to the occupation*: Some assessment results will provide information about the capacity of the person to undertake some of the required actions of the occupation – for instance, range of motion, endurance capacity, memory, and so on.

30.7 Completed case studies of occupation analysis

The two case studies presented have been analysed according to the components of occupation analysis presented by O'Toole (2011, p. 11).

Case study 1: A completed occupation analysis with Harold

Harold, 73, was admitted after falling while walking his dog, resulting in a right (dominant) humerus fracture requiring surgical fixation. He's in significant pain and wears a lightweight cast. He also experiences shortness of breath with exertion and is unsteady on his feet. Harold lives alone in a two-storey house with the bathroom upstairs. He's a retired teacher, uses reading glasses, and values his appearance. Active in his community, he volunteers at the local library. His main goal is to shower independently. His bathroom has a shower over the bath with a curtain, and the toilet is in the same room (see Table 30.3).

Table 30.3 Occupation analysis of Harold showering

Component	*Aspects of analysis*
The occupation of showering	**Steps involved:** ■ Assembling items required for showering (towel, change of clothes, etc.) ■ Accessing the bathroom, the shower recess or the shower over the bath ■ Operating taps ■ Setting the water temperature ■ Undressing ■ Stepping into the shower area ■ Accessing toiletries ■ Lathering ■ Washing body ■ Washing hair ■ Rinsing ■ Turning taps off ■ Stepping out of shower area ■ Drying body ■ Dressing **Required skills:** ***Physical demands:*** such as standing or sitting balance. Harold must step over the edge of the bath to shower and has only one arm to assist with the transfer, especially if there are no rails to assist. Pain may limit his endurance. Observing Harold dressing will identify any difficulties he may have dressing or undressing. Hand function and strength. Harold has only one hand to use and has to use a plastic bag to encase his cast when showering. Harold may have difficulty accessing and holding shampoo or body wash, as well as managing the towel to dry himself with two hands. ***Sensory demands:*** Adequate vision and sensation; for example, Harold may have difficulty reading labels with small print without glasses on in the shower. Water temperature will affect showering. ***Cognitive demands:*** Such as motor planning, memory, and problem solving. Harold plans these activities to carry them out successfully. ***Psychosocial demands:*** Harold values his appearance and is actively involved in social activities, so showering is a priority for him. **Required values:** Harold prefers to shower first thing in the morning to invigorate himself for the day and to prepare for going out. **Occupational structures:** Harold lives alone so can take his time showering, although he will have to be much more aware of safety precautions. Harold can also organise his own system for storing towels and clothing during showering. **Circumstances:** ***Time and age:*** Harold did not want homecare assistance for showering, as his preference was having a shower early in the morning and such assistance could not be arranged at a particular time. ***Place:*** The shower over the bath for Harold is situated in the bathroom on the same level as his bedroom. ***Season:*** Harold wanted to be independent in showering so he could have additional showers if needed in hot weather. ***Equipment and safety:*** Harold had a shower hose and was willing to accept a bath board and purchase a non-slip bathmat to make his showering safer. Harold preferred not to use a sponge bath at a sink as an alternative.

(Continued)

Table 30.3 (Continued)

Component	Aspects of analysis
Individual factors relevant to showering	**Roles:** The role of self-maintainer and volunteer were important to Harold. **Meaning and values:** Harold values his appearance and has a history of formal relationships with others from his teaching role. He values showering for his appearance and presentation. **Spirituality:** Harold derives satisfaction and feelings of hope for the future by being able to keep himself presentable to his self-determined high standard. **Age, gender, and personal skills:** Harold has always valued and been able to shower independently throughout his life. **Motivation:** Harold was motivated to engage in showering, as self-presentation was important to maintain his roles. **Cognition:** Harold needed to be able to plan showering and needed to know and remember the sequence of steps and the required equipment when showering. **Sensory capacity:** Harold experiences pain in his injured arm which restricts movement. Harold is able to distinguish hot and cold water when showering. **Physical capacity:** Harold has the use of only one arm, experiences shortness of breath, and is unsteady on his feet. Thus, he will take longer to shower, will have to be careful to maintain safety, and will have to adapt his dressing techniques. **Emotional regulation:** It is important to consider the emotional response Harold has to his difficulties when showering, especially if experiencing pain during this occupation.
The contexts relevant to showering	**Cultural context:** Harold had cultural expectations about cleanliness, insisting on showering despite his physical status. He also valued his privacy, preferring not to have assistance with showering. **Spiritual context:** Harold has no spiritual beliefs affecting his showering. **Institutional context:** The following regulations require consideration when assisting Harold to shower, especially if he requires modifications to his showering environment. Regulations about temperature of hot water, water restrictions and usage, design of shower recesses and bathrooms (building codes and standards), costs of a water supply, and so on may affect showering or possible adaptations. **Social context:** Harold lives alone, so he needs to be fully independent in showering to safely undertake this at home. **Physical context:** Harold has a shower over his bath and thus requires a bath board or bath seat and training in how to safely transfer using the bath seat to shower. **Sensory context:** Harold's bathroom is well lit by artificial lighting, and there is a window which provides natural light and ventilation. He is experiencing pain, and water temperature may be something that exacerbates his pain. Labels on toiletries are in small print, but Harold has sufficient visual acuity to read them. **Technological context:** Currently Harold does not have any technical changes such as water-saving devices, methods of temperature control, or automated devices such as tap sensors in his bathroom. **Socio-economic contexts:** This will affect the resources available for Harold to undertake showering or pay for assistive equipment or bathroom modifications.

Case study 2: A completed occupation analysis with Petrina

Petrina, 49, was treated for breast cancer with surgery, radiation, and chemotherapy. She now has lymphoedema in her right arm, limiting shoulder and wrist movement, and peripheral neuropathy, causing foot tingling and hand sensitivity. Chemotherapy also led to cognitive issues – poor concentration, memory, and planning – along with ongoing fatigue. A former part-time childcare worker, she hasn't returned to work and is unsure how to manage her health while resuming job tasks.

An occupation analysis would usually be carried out through a workplace assessment at Petrina's place of employment (see Table 30.4).

Table 30.4 Occupational analysis of Petrina's work in childcare

Component	Aspects of analysis
The occupation of childcare work	Steps involved: • Preparing materials and equipment for children's education and recreational activities. • Managing children's behaviour and guiding their social development. • Conducting activities for children. • Entertaining children by reading and playing games. • Supervising and assisting children in recreational activities. • Supervising and assisting the daily routine of children (e.g. food preparation, dressing, eating, resting and sleeping). • Supervising and assisting with the hygiene of children (e.g. toileting, nappy changing and medications). Required skills: *Physical demands:* walking and standing (long periods); lifting and carrying up to 20 kg); sitting (small chairs or on floor); crawling; kneeling; squatting; forward bending to low levels; overheard reaching, ladder and stair climbing, pushing, pulling, manual dexterity gripping/grasping, fine motor skills. *Sensory demands:* adequate hearing and visual acuity to monitor child safety and changes in details, hot/cold discrimination, pressure discrimination with hands through touching and sensing with hands, body awareness and coordination, balance and stability. *Cognitive demands:* attention and concentration to ensure the safety and well-being of children; problem solving to quickly assess, address, and resolve conflicts or issues with children; planning and organising daily lessons and activities; following schedules and timelines; communicating effectively with children, parents, and colleagues, both verbally and in writing. *Psychosocial demands:* Working as part of a team, demonstrating empathy and patience, providing emotional and social support for children, regulating own emotions and stress levels, dealing with challenging behaviours or situations, having positive relationships with children, parents, and colleagues.

(Continued)

Table 30.4 (Continued)

Component	*Aspects of analysis*
	Required values: Petrina loves working with children and is committed to her work. **Occupational structures:** Petrina was employed 30 hours per week. Hours of childcare centres are likely to be 7.00am–7.00pm, and different shifts would be required. Patrina's return to work (duties, tasks, and hours) would need to be negotiated with her employer. **Circumstances:** *Time and age:* Paid employment is likely to be a necessary occupational role for Petrina, as she is 49 years old and still several years away from retirement. The more time she is absent from work, the less likely she will return to work. *Place:* The location of Petrina's employment and travel to and from the workplace would need to be considered and assessed through a workplace assessment. Petrina's ability to drive may need to be assessed due to her physical, sensory, and cognitive impairments. *Season:* Petrina may have certain restrictions for sun exposure and difficulty managing hot weather due to her medication and menopausal symptoms. *Equipment and safety:* A workplace assessment would provide exact details on the type of equipment Petrina would need to where adaptive technology could be used to support her employment. This may include equipment to support her upper limb weakness and sensory changes or technology to support her cognitive impairments to help minimise the impact work performance and ensure the safety of the children.
Individual factors	**Roles:** Being a worker is an important role for Petrina. **Meaning and values:** Petrina values her work and being employed. Her mother and father both worked and have instilled strong work ethics. She strives to role model strong work ethics to her children. **Spirituality:** Working with children and supporting families brings Petrina joy and a sense of purpose in her life. Her work is central to her personal identity. **Age, gender, and personal skills:** Petrina has been a childcare worker for 12 years, and she values the relationships she has with children and their families. She has been able to help families navigate difficult situations with their children and is able to support parents in their roles. She is 49 years old and plans to work in childcare until her retirement. **Motivation:** Petrina previously valued her work; however, the change in health status may now impact her capability and confidence and hence motivation to work. **Cognition:** Petrina has difficulty with sustained attention and concentration, working memory, planning and organising novel tasks, and problem solving in high-pressure situations. This may impact her ability to drive to and from work, provide the necessary supervision to ensure child safety, and plan activities for children in the required structure and timeframes required. **Sensory capacity:** Petrina experiences hypersensitivity and reduced temperature discrimination in her hands. This may impact her ability to perform feeding tasks with children. She also has numbness in both her feet regularly throughout the day, which worsens when standing for long periods of time. She may need to modify postures or tasks to reduce long periods of standing.

(Continued)

Table 30.4 (Continued)

Component	Aspects of analysis
	Physical capacity: Petrina experiences swelling and pain in her right upper limb, with reduced movement in the shoulder, elbow, and wrist. She experiences changes in body temperature and fatigue, requiring rest periods during the day. This may impact her ability to physical support children (e.g. lifting, carrying, supporting, patting, or feeding).
	Emotional regulation: Petrina has had difficulty regulating her emotions, often becoming teary and upset over previously minor issues. She believes this is due to the ongoing side effects she is experiencing after breast cancer treatment but also the psychological impact of what the future may hold. This may impact her ability to manage children with behavioural or emotional difficulties or deal with challenging staff circumstance at work in an effective and rational manner.
The contexts relevant to childcare work	**Cultural context:** Through a workplace assessment, the culture of the workplace will need to be explored in relation to management and colleagues supporting workplace rehabilitation for people with illness where modified duties and hours may be needed.
	Spiritual context: Petrina will need to adapt her approaches to parents with different spiritual beliefs that may affect caring for their children.
	Institutional context: Working with children in Australia requires specific government checks, as well as a level of fitness that may need to be assessed by a doctor to ensure the health and wellbeing of children, as a vulnerable population. There are certain regulations on the ration of staff to children and the level of qualifications needed when working with children. Modifications (including assistance technology) would need to first ensure the safety of children. Childcare programmes and activities must be delivered be in accordance with government policy learning outcomes.
	Social context: Childcare centres are a place to develop the social skills of children, and this is facilitated by childcare workers. Collaboration and communication with parents and guardians are essential to ensure the wellbeing of children. Effective teamwork amongst the team of childcare workers is essential for continuity of care for children.
	Physical context: A workplace assessment would need to determine the specific requirements of the workplace in terms of indoor and outdoor spaces, access, floor and ground surfaces, distances, heights and weights of equipment, seating options, and staff retreat areas.
	Sensory context: It could be anticipated that a childcare centre will generally have loud noises, strong odours, and bright light. Any items Petrina may be required to lift, handle, or carry will need to be investigated as the sensory impairments in her hands and feet may render her unsafe.
	Socio-economic contexts: Petrina is receiving sickness-based government benefits. She does not have a compensable injury and does not have income protection, so she is not receiving any other entitlements. This may also affect her ability to access an occupational therapist to do a workplace assessment.
	Technological context: Through the Employment Assistance Fund, Petrina may be able to access assistive technology to assist her with manual handling tasks and help with planning and organising daily tasks and routines to assist her memory and planning difficulties.

30.8 Conclusion

Occupation, activity, and task analysis are core skills for occupational therapists. They help identify the demands of occupations, individual capabilities, and environmental factors that support or hinder participation. This analysis guides the grading or adaptation of tasks and informs targeted interventions. It is central to clinical reasoning – assessing engagement, setting meaningful goals, and enabling desired outcomes. Occupation analysis is especially important when challenges affect performance, allowing for tailored support to enhance participation.

30.9 Summary

- Occupation analysis, activity analysis, and task analysis are related. A task analysis informs an activity analysis, which in turn informs the occupation analysis.
- Occupation analysis considers the dynamic relationship between the occupation, the person, and the contexts/environments.
- Individual values and skills, occupational structures, and particular circumstances affect the occupation.
- Aspects of the person including their designated roles; their motivation; values; and cognitive, communicative, emotional, physical (including sensory), and social skills inform an occupation analysis.
- Specific contexts including cultural, spiritual, political and institutional, social, physical (natural, built, temporal), technological, and socio-economic support occupation, which is an important component of an occupation analysis.

30.10 Review and reflection questions

- What is the relevance of an occupation analysis to occupational therapy practice?
- What is the difference between an occupation analysis, an activity analysis, and a task analysis?
- Choose two contexts and suggest how they might support or challenge occupational performance.
- List three aspects of the person to be incorporated into an occupation analysis. Suggest how they might be incorporated in practice.
- Choose an occupational structure and explain how it affects occupational choices.

References

American Occupational Therapy Association. (2020). Occupational Therapy Practice Framework: Domain and process, 4th edition. *American Journal of Occupational Therapy*, 74(Supp. 2), 7412410010p1–7412410010p87. https://doi.org/10.5014/ajot.2014.682006

Baum, C. M., & Christiansen, C. H. (2005). Person–environment–occupation–performance: An occupation-based framework for practice. In C. H. Christiansen, C. M. Baum, & J. Bass-Haugen (Eds.), *Occupation therapy: Performance, participation and well-being* (pp. 243–266). SLACK Inc.

Chapparo, C., & Ranka, J. (2025). The Occupational Performance Model (Australia): Constructs, structure, propositions, and utility for occupational therapy practice. In M. N. Ikiugu, S. D Taff, S. Kantartzis, & N. Pollard (Eds.), *Routledge companion to occupational therapy: Theories, concepts and models* (pp. 93–107). Routledge, Taylor & Francis Group. https://doi.org/10.4324/9781003526766-10

Chard, G., & Mesa, S. (2017). Analysis of occupational performance: Motor, process and social interaction skills. In M. Curtin, M. Egan, & J. Adams (Eds.), *Occupational therapy and physical dysfunction: Promoting occupation and participation* (7th ed, pp. 217–243). Elsevier.

Creek, J. (1996). Making a cup of tea as an honour's degree subject. *British Journal of Occupational Therapy, 59*(3), 128–130. https://doi.org/10.1177/030802269605900310

Fair, A., & Barnitt, R. (1999). Making a cup of tea as part of a culturally sensitive service. *British Journal of Occupational Therapy, 62*(5), 199–205. https://doi.org/10.1177/030802269906200504

Hannam, D. (1997). More than a cup of tea: Meaning construction in an everyday occupation. *Journal of Occupational Science: Australia, 4*(2), 69–73. https://doi.org/10.1080/14427591.1997.

Law, M., Cooper, B., Strong, S., Stewart, D., Rigby, P., & Letts, L. (1996). The person–environment–occupation model: A transactive approach to occupational performance. *Canadian Journal of Occupational Therapy, 63*(1), 9–23. https://doi.org/10.1177/000841749606300103

Mackenzie, L., & O'Toole, G. (2011). Glossary. In L. Mackenzie & G. O'Toole (Eds.), *Occupation analysis in practice* (p. 383). Wiley-Blackwell.

McGraw, C., & Drennan, V. (2009). Assisting older people with bathing. *Journal of Community Nursing, 12*, 15–16. http://search.proquest.com/docview/208560794/

O'Toole, G. (2011). What is occupation analysis? In L. Mackenzie & G. O'Toole (Eds.), *Occupation analysis in practice* (pp. 1–24). Wiley-Blackwell.

Perlman, C., & Bergthorson, M. (2017). Task, activity and occupational analysis. In M. Curtin, M. Egan, & J. Adams (Eds.), *Occupational therapy for people experiencing illness, injury or impairment* (7th ed., pp. 192–206). Elsevier.

Polatajko, H. J., Davis, J., Stewart, D., Cantin, N., Amoroso, B., Purdie, L., & Zimmerman, D. (2013). Specifying the domain of concern: Occupation as core. In E. A. Townsend & H. J. Polatajko (Eds.), *Enabling occupation II: Advancing an occupational therapy vision of health, well-being and justice through occupation* (2nd ed., pp. 13–36). CAOT Publications ACE.

Reese Walter, J., & Winston, K. (2025). Therapeutic occupations and modalities. In H. Pendleton (Ed.), *Pedretti's occupational therapy: Practice skills for physical dysfunction* (9th ed., pp. 731–750). Elsevier Inc.

Thomas, H. (2022). *Occupation-based activity analysis* (3rd ed.). SLACK Inc.

Whalley Hammell, K. R. (2013). Client-centred practice in occupational therapy: Critical reflections. *Scandinavian Journal of Occupational Therapy, 20*(3), 174–181. https://doi.org/10.3109/11038128.2012.752032

Wilson, S. A., & Landry, G. (2014). *Task analysis: An individual, group, and population approach* (3rd ed.). American Occupational Therapy Association.

Understanding human occupation

Ted Brown, Aislinn Lalor, Luke Robinson, Jess Archer, and Kim Weigle-Reese

Authors' positionality statement

We are all Caucasian, cisgender, English-speaking, university-educated occupational therapists who acknowledge our white privilege, Global North perspective, and inherent biases. We endorse the social justice principles of anti-sexism, anti-racism, anti-discrimination, and anti-oppression. We acknowledge First Nations Australians, who are the traditional owners and carers of the land on which we live, and their collective wisdom related to country. We respect the dynamic and constantly evolving range of daily occupations that all people, families, communities, and organisations engage in and the positive health and wellbeing benefits that occupational engagement brings.

Key terms
- Activities of daily living
- Caring occupations: self-care, personal care, and caring for others
- Co-occupations
- Occupational participation
- Occupational performance

Objectives
This chapter will allow the reader to:

- Define occupation, occupational performance, and occupational participation
- Provide an overview of the types of daily occupations people typically engage in
- Provide an overview of different ways of classifying human occupation
- Identify factors that may impact the occupations that a person chooses to engage in
- Identify and describe occupational performance issues and challenges

DOI: 10.4324/9781003495666-34

31.1 Introduction

This chapter unpacks the concept of human occupation, addressing the historical and theoretical classification of occupations, as well as the various contextual factors that influence occupational performance and occupational participation. Occupations are recognised as dynamic, evolving, and influenced by complex interactions between individual, cultural, social, environmental, and systemic contexts. Traditional approaches to classifying and labelling occupations often fail to account for diverse, nuanced, and culturally specific experiences, including the influence of socio-economic status; cultural beliefs; and access to resources, time, and technology. Moreover, less traditional or socially non-sanctioned occupations are frequently excluded from these classifications, highlighting the importance of adopting inclusive, trauma-informed, client-centred, and culturally sensitive approaches in occupational therapy practice. By considering subjective meanings of occupations and moving beyond prescribed classification systems, occupational therapists can better address the unique needs, goals, and lived experiences of clients, fostering more meaningful and inclusive therapeutic practices.

All humans engage in and perform occupations daily, and this is often referred to as occupational performance. Human occupations and occupational performance are essential for a person's health and well-being. A person can engage in various occupations, including self-care, work, volunteering, play, leisure, education, sleep, caring for others, and social participation. The types and range of occupations engaged in or performed changes and shifts from childhood to adulthood and older age. Occupational performance is also impacted by a variety of factors external and internal to each person. Occupational therapists aim to promote and maximise client, family, and community health, well-being, life satisfaction, dignity, and social connectedness through occupational performance and engagement. We recognise that human occupations are constantly changing and evolving.

This chapter will provide an overview of occupational performance, the types of occupations people engage in or perform, the factors and contexts that impact the occupations that humans engage in, the evolution of the conceptualisation of human occupation, and finally, the occupational performance issues and challenges that humans may experience. Finally, it is not possible to include or mention every type of occupation that humans may engage in since we are very complex beings, and so too are the vast array and plethora of the daily occupations we participate in.

31.2 An overview of human occupation

31.2.1 Defining key terms

Occupations are defined in several different ways. In the Occupational Therapy Practice Framework – 4th edition (OTPF-4), *human occupations* are defined as daily 'personalized activities that people do as individuals, in families, and with communities to occupy time and bring meaning and purpose to life' (American Occupational Therapy Association [AOTA], 2020, p. 7412410010p79). Human occupations have been categorised and defined in several different ways (see Table 31.1). *Occupational participation,* in the Canadian Model of Occupational Participation (CanMOP), refers to 'having access to, initiating, and sustaining valued occupations within meaningful relationships and contexts' (Egan & Restall, 2022, p. 76), whereas in the Model of Human Occupation (MOHO), it represents the engagement in work, play, and self-care activities that are related to a person's cultural environment and that are wanted and potentially needed for a person's health and well-being (Taylor et al., 2023). A related concept, *occupational performance* involves the completion of a daily occupation resulting from the dynamic interaction between a person, their environment, and the occupation itself (AOTA, 2020).

It is also salient to mention that some occupational therapy authors, including the authors of the CanMOP, have suggested that it is not necessary to label or classify types of human occupation for two main reasons (Egan & Restall, 2022). First, predefined categories of human occupation may cause other significant or relevant types of occupations to be disregarded or ignored, and second, an already established set of occupational categories may impose a biased view while also not taking into consideration the scope, importance, intricacies, and subtleties of those occupations for individuals, families, groups, organisations, or communities that occupational therapists may be engaging with (Egan & Restall, 2022).

We take on board the reasons mentioned by Egan and Restall (2022), but we will provide an overview and taxonomy of the primary types of occupations humans engage as a starting point only. We do not infer that it is prescriptive and all-inclusive. Instead, each individual, family, community, or organisation that an occupational therapist engages with should be viewed as having its own unique repertoire of occupations.

There are a variety of factors that can affect individual occupational performance. These may include age, gender identity, socio-economic status, religious beliefs, cultural beliefs, ethnicity, living environment (e.g., urban, rural, low- and lower-middle-income countries), family composition, political views, social connectedness, community participation, physical and mental health status, languages spoken, access to technology, geographical location, and education attainment, to name a few (AOTA, 2020; Taylor et al., 2023). Societal, institutional, and systemic factors can also impact a person's occupational performance. When one or more of these factors impact, or could impact, an individual's ability to successfully select, arrange, or complete daily occupations, they have encountered an occupational performance issue (OPI) or challenge (Townsend & Polatajko, 2013).

31.2.2 Considerations of factors and contexts impacting occupations

Recognising evolutionary shifts in occupations is essential for occupational therapy practice, as it enables therapists to focus on client-centred interventions that address the unique meanings everyone brings to their experiences in constantly changing environments. Occupational therapy theory emphasises the complex interplay between various factors and contexts that can impact and influence engagement and participation in human occupation. Understanding how these can enable or restrict engagement and participation is essential for enhancing occupational performance and promoting health and well-being. Such factors and contexts may include, but are not limited to:

- **Individual/Personal Factors:** These consider an individual's intrinsic characteristics, such as age, gender identity, physical and mental health status, intelligence, languages spoken, roles (parental, sibling, carer, worker, etc.), socio-economic status, religious/spiritual beliefs, culture, ethnicity/social identity, or social/political views.
- **Physical Environment:** The natural and hand-made physical context in which individuals engage and participate in occupations, including their home, workplace,

and community, can either facilitate or hinder occupational performance. Accessibility, safety, and the availability of resources (such as technology) are critical components of the physical environment that impact engagement.

- **Social Environment:** Social interactions, attitudes, and relationships can shape occupational performance. Support from family, friends, and community members can enhance motivation and participation, while social isolation may lead to decreased engagement in meaningful activities.
- **Cultural Factors:** Cultural beliefs and values inform individuals' perceptions of acceptable occupations and influence their choices throughout different life stages. Understanding cultural context is crucial for occupational therapists to provide culturally sensitive interventions that align with clients' values.
- **Temporal Context:** The timing of occupational engagement is significant, as life stages, transitions, and the rhythm of daily life can affect the types of occupations people choose and prioritise.
- **Occupation Characteristics:** The nature of the occupation (complexity, duration, and significance) also influences occupational performance. Ensuring occupations match an individual's skills and interests can enhance motivation and success and facilitate occupational performance.
- **Policy and Systemic Factors:** Broader societal policies, healthcare systems, and economic conditions can impact access to resources and opportunities for occupational engagement.
- **Interpersonal and Community Factors:** These can include composition of family or household members, community participation, living environment (e.g., urban, rural, remote; low- and middle-income countries), social capital/connectedness, access to technology, or climate.

When one or more of these factors or contexts impact, or can impact, an individual's ability to successfully 'choose, organize, and satisfactorily perform meaningful occupations', they have encountered an occupational performance issue or challenge (OPIC) (Townsend & Polatajko, 2013, p. 181). Considerations and examples of types of occupations, occupational performance issues or challenges for each of the occupations are illustrated in Table 31.1. It is important to note that a single occupation may fit into more than one type of occupation listed in Table 31.1. For example, the occupation of going for a walk with a friend may be an active, outdoor, social, life-giving, leisure occupation in and of itself. Table 31.1 also includes a column titled 'Proximity to others' which refers to whether occupations can be performed in individual, group (e.g., reciprocal, cooperative, collective), family, and/or community environments.

31.3 Evolution of the conceptualisation of human occupations

The way that occupational therapists categorise and conceptualise occupations has seen several paradigm shifts as the profession has grown and matured, moving beyond traditional models that separate occupations into categories of self-care, work, and play (Kielhofner, 2002) or self-care, productivity, and leisure (Townsend & Polatajko, 2013). Critics of these earlier categorisations describe them as unnecessarily limiting and potentially dismissive of occupations that cannot be as neatly classified (Egan &

Table 31.1 Examples of human occupation, the proximity to others when completed, and related occupational performance issues or challenges (OPICs)

Occupation	Definition	Examples	Proximity of others	OPICs
Activities of daily living	Routine activities intended to take care of one's body and maintain physical health and wellbeing, safety, and homecare (adapted from AOTA, 2020, p. 7412410010p30)	Bathing/showering, toileting/toilet hygiene, dressing, eating, feeding, meal preparation, functional mobility, personal hygiene and grooming, sexual activity, health management, financial management, shopping, laundry, housework	■ individual ■ reciprocal/ cooperative ■ collective/ groups/family	Difficulty with dressing due to arthritis and associated joint pain, making it difficult to use fasteners, buttons, and zippers
Play occupations	'Activities that are intrinsically motivated, internally controlled, and freely chosen and that may include suspension of reality . . . exploration, humour, risk-taking, contests, and celebrations' (AOTA, 2020, p. 7412410010p34)	Exploration play; practice play; pretend play; games with rules; constructive play; symbolic play; obtaining, using toys, equipment, and supplies	■ individual ■ parallel ■ reciprocal/ cooperative ■ collective/ groups/family ■ community	An individual may struggle to initiate or maintain play with peers because of poor balance skills, poor language skills, shyness, or social anxiety
Leisure and recreation occupations	■ Leisure is described as 'free time' away from work and required activities such as eating, sleeping, and educational pursuits ■ Recreation is a diversion, pastime, hobby, or interest that a person chooses to participate in that promotes enjoyment, pleasure, restoration, and relaxation	Going for a walk in a natural setting, completing a puzzle, reading a book, listening to music, planting a garden, playing soccer or basketball; it can also include self-selected occupations viewed as fun, relaxing, and pleasurable but also risky or unsanctioned: smoking, alcohol consumption, gambling, skydiving, mountain climbing, recreational drug use, and excessive screen-time use	■ individual ■ parallel ■ reciprocal/ cooperative ■ collective/ groups/family ■ community	An individual is unable to participate in formal sporting competition as a result of socio-economic status, gender identity, or accessibility of leisure environments
Education occupations	'Activities needed for learning participating in the education environment' (AOTA, 2020, p. 7412410010p33)	Academic, non-academic, extracurricular, technological, and vocational education activities; attending school; parents and caregivers passing on family histories and cultural traditions; intergenerational storytelling	■ individual ■ reciprocal/ cooperative ■ collective/ groups/family ■ community	A child has difficulty completing reading and writing tasks in a classroom environment due to dysgraphia, dyslexia, or dyspraxia

(Continued)

Table 31.1 (Continued)

Occupation	Definition	Examples	Proximity of others	OPICs
Productivity/ work occupations	Paid occupations related to developing, producing, delivering, or managing goods and services	Examples are largely dependent on the job type and context (e.g., a healthcare worker may engage in very different work occupations in comparison to a landscape gardener); however, most workers will engage in employment seeking, acquisition, performance, participation, and maintenance activities	■ individual ■ parallel ■ reciprocal/ cooperative ■ collective/ groups	A person has difficulty prioritising responsibilities or meeting deadlines due to traumatic brain injury leading to decreased efficiency, problem solving, and decision making
Volunteering occupations	Occupations where individuals are not paid or remunerated for their contributions (e.g., donate their time and skills), and they choose to engage in activities of their own volition	Helping at non-profit organisations, fundraising for a charity, looking after animals, visiting care homes, providing services at a homeless shelter or soup kitchen	■ individual ■ parallel ■ reciprocal/ cooperative ■ collective/ groups ■ community	A lack of knowledge, accessibility, opportunity, or training may make an individual feel unprepared or lack the skills for a specific volunteer role, leading to apprehension to participate
Sleep and rest occupations	'Activities related to obtaining restorative rest and sleep to support healthy, active engagement in other occupations' (AOTA, 2020, p. 7412410010p32)	■ Having a bath, meditating, reading, listening to music quietly ■ Napping, sleep preparation, sleep participation	■ individual ■ parallel ■ family	A person is unable to engage in quiet relaxation as a result of anxiety or to maintain a healthy sleep routine as a result of a stress disorder

Table 31.1 (Continued)

Occupation	Definition	Examples	Proximity of others	OPICs
Social participation occupations	Occupations that involve interacting, caring, communicating, cooperating, problem solving, compromising, accommodating, understanding, appreciating, and sharing with one or more other people either face to face or remotely using a device (e.g., Zoom video conferencing)	Working on a team on a group project, attending a family birthday party, playing on a basketball team, speaking to a friend on your phone, attending a community bingo game, attending a religious celebration with family and community members	■ parallel ■ reciprocal/ cooperative ■ collective/ groups/family ■ community	A person is unable to participate in community centre-based activities following the suspension of a driver's licence because of epileptic seizures
Planetary health and green-related occupations	Occupations related to promoting planetary health, reducing people's carbon footprint, decreasing polluting activities, and positively responding to climate change initiatives	Riding a bicycle, driving an electric car, planting trees, purchasing products that are made from recycled materials, recycling household waste, upcycling and creative reuse of waste or unwanted materials, growing your own food in a garden and recycling wastewater	■ individual ■ reciprocal/ cooperative ■ collective/ groups/family ■ community	Individuals working in fields related to planetary health may experience burnout or compassion fatigue due to a sense of being overwhelmed by the nature of environmental issues; this may lead to impacts with their motivation and productivity
Technology-related occupations	Occupations that require the use, application, and engagement with technology and related devices to complete tasks	Sending a text message on a mobile phone, writing an essay on a computer, online banking, using artificial intelligence to answer a question, watching a YouTube clip, using social media platforms, looking at Google Maps for directions when driving	■ individual ■ parallel ■ reciprocal/ cooperative ■ collective/ groups/family ■ community	A person is unable to engage in online banking due to cognitive issues with memory, problem solving, and decision making due to dementia

(Continued)

Table 31.1 (Continued)

Occupation	Definition	Examples	Proximity of others	OPICs
Caring occupations	Caring occupations can be either formal or informal and involve helping other people and/or animals to engage in purposeful and meaningful occupations. Caring occupations can also be for oneself	Self-care or personal care occupations such as grooming, bathing, meal preparation, feeding, toileting, and parenting; health management and maintenance occupations such as wound care, medication management, aid and equipment maintenance and operation; leisure and recreation occupations such as travel, exercise, play, socialising, and engaging in hobbies; or productive occupations such as interpreting, translating, or transcribing materials	■ individual ■ parallel ■ reciprocal/ cooperative ■ collective/ groups/family ■ community	A person has difficulty maintaining their carer role due to the unrelenting nature of providing ongoing care as a result of compassion fatigue or physical and emotional exhaustion
Lifestyle occupations that can impact one's health, well-being, and safety **Indoor and outdoor occupations**	Activities that may negatively impact one's health and wellbeing or the safety of others and the community. Connection to these activities may provide people with a sense of identity, risk, and reward and are often embedded in a social occupation ■ Indoor: occupations that are completed in internal, inside, or sheltered environ-ments ■ Outdoor: occupations that are completed in external, natural, or outside environments	Gang membership, addiction (smoking/ vaping, social media, drugs, alcohol), criminal, violence, extreme sports, destructive self-care (self-harm, disordered eating, driving faster than the speed limit), smoking, alcohol consumption, gambling, skydiving, mountain climbing, and recreational drug use ■ Indoor: sleeping in a tent, having a shower in an indoor bathroom, reading a book in a library, cooking pasta sauce on a stove in an indoor kitchen, working at a desk in an office building, driving a car or riding on a tram ■ Outdoor: hiking in forest parkland, swimming at an ocean beach, cutting the grass outside, picking berries in a garden, cooking food on a barbeque on a patio or balcony, rowing a boat on a river in the open air	■ individual ■ parallel ■ reciprocal/ cooperative ■ collective/ groups/family ■ community ■ individual ■ parallel ■ reciprocal/ cooperative ■ collective/ groups/family ■ community	A person having trouble being able to safely engage in recreational drug use (as a risk minimisation strategy) due to social, legal, and financial constraints Indoor: poor lighting and physical environment accessibility may hinder an individual's ability to engage in working from home Outdoor: adverse weather conditions may limit the safe participation in hiking, gardening, camping, or swimming

Table 31.1 (Continued)

Occupation	Definition	Examples	Proximity of others	OPICs
Sedentary, quiet, and passive occupations	■ Sedentary: occupations that do not require a person to exert large amounts of energy, are not too physically taxing, and do require large amounts of movement ■ Passive and quiet: occupations that do not require a person to be active, make decisions about what they do, or take responsibil-ity for their actions, or could be activities that involve very little mental or physical effort	■ Sedentary: spending screen time on a device, sitting watching a movie on TV, working at a computer at a desk, being a passenger on a bus or tram ■ Passive and quiet: lounging, sunbathing, napping, listening to music, watching TV, scrolling through pictures while on a screen device	■ individual ■ parallel ■ reciprocal/ cooperative ■ collective/ groups/family ■ community	Sedentary: neck and back pain may be a result of prolonged sitting that could limit further engagement in watching a movie on TV Passive and quiet: feelings of loneliness and anxiety because of limited social interaction while being at home alone
Active and engaged occupations	Occupations that require a person to be physically active and exert energy within their daily living environments; occupations that require physical exertion, coordinated movement of the body, gross and fine motor skills, and maintaining balance against gravity	Playing soccer; jogging; swimming; walking; cutting the grass; digging up a garden; juggling; dancing; yoga; typing at a computer keyboard; throwing, catching, and kicking a ball	■ individual ■ parallel ■ reciprocal/ cooperative ■ collective/ groups/family ■ community	A person being unable to participate in soccer, swimming, dancing, or riding a bicycle due to a knee injury resulting in a knee reconstruction and subsequent reduced mobility
Cognitive-oriented occupations	Occupations that require memory, attention, logic, reasoning, processing information, reflecting, critical thinking, making decisions, selective attention, and visual and auditory processing	Reading a report, writing an essay, completing mathematical calculations, recalling memories, making decisions about daily tasks, learning a new application on your device, and solving problems	■ individual ■ parallel ■ reciprocal/ cooperative ■ collective/ groups/family ■ community	An individual cannot complete a written assessment task at university due to difficulty maintaining attention or understanding the marking criteria

(Continued)

Table 31.1 (Continued)

Occupation	Definition	Examples	Proximity of others	OPICs
Life-giving, sustaining, and creative occupations	Occupations that provide meaning, insights, joy, happiness, calmness, inner strength, refreshment, reflection, recollection, and healing; occupations that involve creative expression, imagination, originality, purpose, knowledge, motivation, lateral thinking, and desire	Yoga, meditating, reading a book, keeping a diary, praying, creating artworks, writing a story or a poem, painting a picture, arranging flowers, making a collage out of pictures, knitting a sweater, weaving a rug, designing a garment, decorating a room in a house, planning a party, designing a menu for a meal, building a piece of furniture out of wood	■ individual ■ parallel ■ reciprocal/ cooperative ■ collective/ groups/family ■ community	An individual having limited engagement in creative artworks due to financial constraints to source and supply resources for the creative activities
Ritual-related occupations	'Symbolic actions with spiritual, cultural, or social meaning contributing to the client's identity and reinforcing values and beliefs. Rituals have a strong affective component and consist of a collection of events' (AOTA, 2020, p. 7412410010p41)	'Some rituals (e.g., those associated with certain holidays) are associated with different seasons or times of the year . . . whereas others are associated with times of the day or days of the week (e.g., daily prayers, weekly family dinners)' (AOTA, 2020, p. 7412410010p13). Rituals and ceremonies are also a feature of Aboriginal and Torres Strait Islanders and Māori cultures	■ individual ■ reciprocal/ cooperative ■ collective/ groups/family ■ community	Being unable to participate in family traditions during birthdays and anniversaries that are meant to provide comfort or connection because of grief linked to the passing of a family member
Cultural occupations	Activities and practices that individuals engage in that enable them to reflect and connect with their cultural identity, traditions, and heritage and provide a sense of belonging, meaning, and connection	Storytelling, traditional dance or music practices, traditional dress or cultural attire, festivals or celebrations, culturally significant food or meal gathering/ preparation, connection to Country	■ individual ■ parallel ■ reciprocal/ cooperative ■ collective/ groups/family ■ community	A group may feel disconnected from their cultural heritage due to relocation or assimilation, making it challenging for them to engage in cultural practices

Table 31.1 (Continued)

Occupation	Definition	Examples	Proximity of others	OPICs
Religious/ spiritual occupations	Occupations that refer to activities and practices that individuals engage in to fulfil their spiritual or religious needs	Meditation, prayer, rituals, or other services that foster a sense of connection, meaning, or purpose	■ individual ■ parallel ■ reciprocal/ cooperative ■ collective/ groups/family ■ community	A group has limited access to religious texts, materials, or spaces for worship due to financial constraints, or inability to drive may restrict engagement in meaningful personal or communal practices

OPICs: Occupational performance issues or challenges

Restall, 2022). These categories are thought to predispose occupational therapists to biased notions of occupations that tend to favour privileged, urban, individualist, classist, ableist, and culturally specific perspectives (Kantartzis & Molineux, 2011), while perspectives about First Nations people remain largely unexplored (Gibson et al., 2020). Westernised categories are insufficient to capture diverse experiences of the relationships between occupation and human health, development, and wellbeing (Mahoney & Kiraly-Alvarez, 2019). Categorisation of occupation is important to explore however considering that the way categories are defined and aligned is dependent on the subjective and nuanced meaning that the individual and/or community place on the occupation.

By adding a temporal aspect to the classification of occupations, Harvey and Pentland (2010) propose that occupations can be categorised according to the allocation of time spent on necessary, contracted, committed, and free-time occupations. While this categorisation arguably retains some of the traditional categories discussed earlier, in linking time and occupation, there are also increased opportunities for defining the meaning and value that people attach to occupations. For instance, an individual might undertake paid work as a house cleaner (a contracted occupation), but this same individual may also undertake unpaid household cleaning as part of maintaining their own living environment (a committed occupation). The use of time links the occupation of household cleaning yet changes the way the occupation is categorised by the individual by altering the meaning, purpose, values, and priorities that can be attached to engaging in the occupation (Johnson & Dickie, 2019). Indigenous communities take this idea further by connecting past, present, and future temporality across generations with cultural occupations and co-occupations such as yarning, knowledge translation, and participating in ceremonial business (Gibson et al., 2020; Ryan et al., 2020).

With the continuous growth of global connectivity, traditional barriers to occupational engagement such as geographic distance, time zones, language, and cultural boundaries are gradually receding (Pemberton & Cox, 2015). This shift brings about new challenges at the intersection of time and occupations, increasingly blurring the lines between necessary, contracted, committed, and free-time occupations. Occupations that once were considered restorative and health promoting could contribute to health reduction if occupational balance is not maintained. Nowadays, people often find themselves multitasking and engaging in multiple occupations simultaneously and at an accelerated rate which impacts their sense of occupational presence and engagement (Pemberton & Cox, 2015). The ability to be contactable 24/7, multitask across different occupations, and readily access information and services using the internet and technology have all influenced occupational possibilities. They have also changed how different generations perceive the meaning and value of the occupations they engage in, as their sense of occupational presence and synchronicity with time has changed (Pemberton & Cox, 2015).

As social and political attitudes have progressed in Australia and Aotearoa New Zealand, the occupational therapy profession has transitioned to become more trauma informed and focus on a harm-minimisation approach to health and wellbeing (MacRae, 2024). This change has also led to a decrease in the bias and stigma associated with non–health-promoting and less socially acceptable occupations. These activities are sometimes referred to as dark occupations, alternative occupations, or unsanctioned occupations in the literature. Traditionally they've been considered deviant from more socially accepted occupations that are presumed to be positive, beneficial, and to promote health and well-being, yet these occupations still fulfil a need or offer value to the individuals engaging in them (Twinley, 2023). For instance, joining a gang might involve participation in illegal activities and violence, yet it also may provide connection, security, and belonging. This demonstrates how an occupation may provide a sense of meaningful connection and social engagement for the individual while other aspects of the occupation are potentially detrimental to their health. Acknowledgment of the subjective experiences and meaning associated with occupations and the categories used to define them can help occupational therapists to move beyond their own bias, assumptions, and misunderstandings to better support the wants and needs of the individual or group (Twinley, 2023).

31.4 Conclusion

This chapter explores the multifaceted nature of human occupation, emphasising its dynamic and evolving characteristics influenced by individual, cultural, social, environmental, and systemic contexts. The critique of the traditional classification systems highlights some of their limitations in capturing the diverse and nuanced experiences of occupations and acknowledges the need for advocating for more inclusive, trauma-informed, and culturally sensitive approaches in occupational therapy. By moving beyond rigid classification systems, occupational therapists can foster more meaningful and inclusive therapeutic practices while also highlighting the significance of considering less traditional or socially non-sanctioned occupations, which are often overlooked.

In summary, this chapter underscores the importance of understanding the subjective meanings of occupations to better address the unique needs and goals of clients and calls for a holistic view of daily occupations, recognising their complexity and the various factors that influence them. It encourages occupational therapists to adopt flexible, client-centred approaches that respect the diverse experiences and meanings individuals attach to their occupations, ultimately promoting health, well-being, and social connectedness.

31.5 Summary

- Human occupation is essential for a person's health and wellbeing
- Human occupations are dynamic and influenced by a variety of internal and external factors
- There is debate in the field about the need to formally categorise types of occupations, but it can be helpful in some contexts
- Individuals presenting with occupational performance issues or challenges (OPICs) may require assistance from an occupational therapist

31.6 Review and reflection questions

- What are the key factors that can impact individual occupational performance?
- Why do some occupational therapy authors argue against the need to classify types of human occupation?

- What is the significance of understanding the subjective meanings of occupation in occupational therapy?
- Reflect on a time when you engaged in an occupation that was not traditionally classified or socially sanctioned. How did this occupation impact your wellbeing and sense of identity?

References

American Occupational Therapy Association. (2020). Occupational Therapy Practice Framework: Domain and process-fourth edition. *American Journal of Occupational Therapy*, 74(Supp 2), 7412410010p1–7412410010p87. https://doi.org/10.5014/ajot.2020.74S2001

Egan, M., & Restall, G. (2022). The Canadian model of occupational participation. In M. Egan & G. Restall (Eds.), *Promoting occupational participation: Collaborative relationship-focused occupational therapy* (pp. 77–95). Canadian Association of Occupational Therapists.

Erlandsson, L. K. E., & Eklund, M. (2001). Describing patterns of daily occupations – a methodological study comparing data from four different methods. *Scandinavian Journal of Occupational Therapy*, 8(1), 31–39. https://doi.org/10.1080/11038120120035

Gibson, C., Dudgeon, P., & Crockett, J. (2020). Listen, look & learn: Exploring cultural obligations of Elders and older Aboriginal people. *Journal of Occupational Science*, 27(2), 193–203. https://doi.org/10.1080/14427591.2020.1732228

Harvey, A., & Pentland, W. (2010). What do people do? In C. H. Christiansen & E. A. Townsend (Eds.), *Introduction to occupation: The art and science of living* (2nd ed., pp. 101–133). Pearson.

Johnson, K. R., & Dickie, V. (2019). What is occupation? In B. A. Boyt Schell & G. Gillen (Eds.), *Willard & Spackman's occupational therapy* (13th ed., pp. 2–10). Wolters Kluwer.

Kantartzis, S., & Molineux, M. (2011). The influence of Western society's construction of a healthy daily life on the conceptualisation of occupation. *Journal of Occupational Science*, 18(1), 62–80. https://doi.org/10.1080/14427591.2011.566917

Kielhofner, G. (2002). *A Model of Human Occupation: Theory and application* (3rd ed.). Williams & Wilkins.

MacRae, A. (2024). Philosophical worldviews of mental health. In A. MacRae (Ed.), *Cara and MacRae's psychosocial occupational therapy: An evolving practice* (4th ed., pp. 3–17). Routledge.

Mahoney, W. J., & Kiraly-Alvarez, A. F. (2019). Challenging the status quo: Infusing non-Western ideas into occupational therapy education and practice. *The Open Journal of Occupational Therapy*, 7(3), 1–10. https://doi.org/10.15453/2168-6408.1592

Pemberton, S., & Cox, D. L. (2015). Synchronisation: Coordinating time and occupation. *Journal of Occupational Science*, 22(3), 291–303. https://www.doi.org/10.1080/4427591.2014.990496

Ryan, A., Gilroy, J., & Gibson, C. (2020). #Changethedate: Advocacy as an on-line and decolonising occupation. *Journal of Occupational Science*, 27(3), 405–416. https://doi.org10.1080/14427591.2020.1759448

Taylor, R. R., Bowyer, P., & Fisher, G. (2023). *Kielhofner's Model of Human Occupation: Theory and application*. Wolters Kluwer.

Townsend, E., & Polatajko, H. (2013). *Enabling occupation II: Advancing occupational therapy vision for health, well-being and justice through occupation* (2nd ed.). CAOT Publications ACE.

Twinley, R. (2023). *Illuminating the dark side of occupation: International perspectives from occupational therapy and occupational science*. Routledge.

CHAPTER 32

Developing and participating in occupations across the life course

Kylie Wales, Simon Leadley, Kate Garam, Claire Lynch, Loretta Sheppard, and Aislinn Lalor

Authors' positionality statement

All authors acknowledge the traditional owners of the land on which they wrote this chapter: Awabakal, Boon Wurrung and Bunurong Country, Wurundjeri, and Wadawurrung Country. The authors are from predominantly middle-class families/whānau and acknowledge their white privilege. The authors come from across western, global north countries Aotearoa New Zealand, Australia, and Ireland as well as currently living in Australia with various ancestries, including English, Irish, and Scottish. All authors identify as cisgender and are either married or in a heterosexual relationship. The team comprises various ages, including Baby Boomers, GenX, and Millennials. Each author is an occupational therapist with varied experience as a practitioner, researcher, and educator. All authors bring diverse knowledge and experiences, including support of family and friends with chronic and/or life-shortening illnesses; advocating for the rights of people with illnesses, disability, and mental health challenges to participate in their chosen life roles; and contributing to an environment where all can thrive. We acknowledge the role of carers in supporting well-being across the lifespan and life course. The team all value and seek to understand the lived/living experience(s) of individuals and communities, recognising the contribution to knowledge generation, education, and translation of evidence. More broadly, the authors see the importance of diverse perspectives in strengthening communities, including western/non-western, Indigenous, disability, and inter/multigenerational. All are strong allies of occupational justice and human rights and value the contribution that this brings to practice.

Key terms
- Occupation
- Occupational participation
- Life course
- Life course theory
- Occupational patterns

DOI: 10.4324/9781003495666-35

Objectives

Upon completion of this chapter, the reader will be able to:

- Describe the lifespan/life course theory from an occupational perspective
- Describe participation in occupation across the life course and key points of transition
- Discuss the unique contexts of individual, family, and community influence on occupational patterns
- Recognise how the occupational therapy role is situated in the context of the individual, families, and their communities

32.1 Introduction

Participation in occupations commences in early infancy and continues throughout life, providing a basis for lifelong development, health, and wellbeing. Occupational development can be understood as the range of occupations that one engages in, which are based on the individual's choice as well as their contextual factors including interpersonal, cultural, and societal influences (Womack & Bagatell, 2024). These influences result in the formation of occupational patterns (Womack & Bagatell, 2024). Positive factors that may influence occupational development include but are not limited to 1) interpersonal encounters during participation in valued occupations; 2) opportunities to participate in important cultural occupations; and 3) having adequate resources, such as finances, to support participation (Womack & Bagatell, 2024). Conversely, occupational development can be impacted by a range of factors including: 1) significant events, such as illness, injury, disability, experience of trauma/family breakup, poverty, and loss of financial security; 2) unfair/discriminatory institutional factors or governmental policies, colonialism, capitalism; 3) conflict; and 4) natural disasters and climate change events (Womack & Bagatell, 2024). Such interruptions not only alter the way we engage in occupations but also the time and the priority placed on them.

Predictable, balanced, and health-promoting occupational patterns and opportunities for full participation in a range of occupations are vital for an individual's ongoing occupational development (Hocking & Sutton, 2024; Womack & Bagatell, 2024). Given the multitude of occupations across the life course, this chapter provides a snapshot of common everyday occupations at different time points. The vignettes illustrate the diversity of occupations and demonstrate how a person's or whānau/family or mob's participation in occupations may change, therefore influencing their life course and occupational patterns. These vignettes are written using a *strengths*-based approach aimed at seeing multiple 'aspects of people within their authentic lives; all behaviours and characteristics are neutral or positive features' (Dunn, 2017). Readers are invited to consider traits that may traditionally be viewed as negative or a deficit to consider how these may be seen as strengths. Additionally, recovery and trauma-informed approaches, inclusive of occupational, biopsychosocial, and ecological views of human development, should be considered. Occupational needs continuously change over the life course of a person, family/whānau/mob, or community, and occupational therapists are uniquely placed to understand the impact of this continual change.

32.2 An occupational perspective of life course theory

Traditional western developmental theory has positioned development and growth to occur in a linear or pyramidal progression that encompasses universal and predictable changes. As a more contemporary approach, life course theory (LCT) adopts a holistic perspective of traditional western developmental theory, recognising the dynamic transactions that occur between a person's genetic makeup (nature) and their environment (nurture). LCT acknowledges traditional developmental theories (e.g., stages of development or psychosocial theories) but also adopts a multicultural and non-linear perspective that accounts for historical and contextual factors and views humans and occupational development as embedded in the environment, not separated from it (Womack & Bagatell, 2024).

LCT asserts that life transitions are pivotal points in development (e.g., starting school or work) and recognises a person's agency (i.e., ability to make choices) and the interdependent nature of our social lives (e.g., family, friends). LCT acknowledges that the time and place in which a person is born serves as a pathway for development and that development is affected by common life changes (e.g., moving house), unexpected events, and factors at an individual, societal, cultural, and historical level (e.g., disability, socioeconomic status, an economic recession, effects of colonialism). From an occupational perspective, transactional processes that occur between the person and the environment shape occupational development, patterns of occupation, occupational choices, and future potential to participate in occupations (Womack & Bagatell, 2024).

Occupational therapists draw on a broad range of occupational therapy frameworks and models when delivering interventions (Womack & Bagatell, 2024). However, the focus of the occupational therapist is on *participation* in meaningful everyday activities, a focus emphasised in the Canadian Model of Occupational Performance (CanMOP) (Egan & Restall, 2022). The CanMOP highlights the collaborative relationship needed between all stakeholders, including the occupational therapist, the individual, family, and/or communities (Egan & Restall, 2022). As such, readers may notice language used throughout this chapter aligns closely with the CanMOP.

To help explain an occupational approach to LCT, the following section will present a range of vignettes that provide a snapshot of common life events or transitions/changes and unexpected events and how these influences may impact participation in occupations. The reason for discontinuing an occupation, continuing an occupation, or starting a new one is not just about individual preferences but the influence of the contexts in which we live.

32.2.1 Infant (up to a year old)

In early infancy the family supports the child to develop and explore their world. Early occupations of infancy include eating and sleeping. Play, socialising, and participating in their family's daily routine can enhance a child's growth and cognitive and physical development and prepare them for roles and occupations of childhood (Whitney, 2024).

Lilli

At six months old, Lilli spends much of her day exploring her environment through movement and touch, sleeping, feeding, and socialising with those around her. Lilli has started to sit up by herself, grasp and place small objects, and play with cause-and-effect toys. She is beginning to remember things and is very keen to practice social interactions by making sounds, laughing, and interacting with familiar people. Her three-year-old brother often sits with her on the floor playing peek-a-boo, which makes her giggle and reach for him to communicate 'more'. Every day there are new things that come her way, sometimes overwhelming her and other times exciting and stimulating her. During family mealtimes, she is showing interest in food by smelling and exploring the textures through touch and taste but still relies on the comfort and closeness of breastfeeding to soothe and calm her. Sometimes she feels so tired but can't close her eyes; there is so much to see and listen to! And all she really needs are her parents to rock and comfort her and help her busy body and mind to rest and feel at peace.

32.2.2 Childhood (1–12 years)

Childhood is when interests are explored and children develop their social skills and have continued opportunities to develop physical and cognitive abilities. A family continues to support a child's growth; however, the child starts entering the broader community environment (Whitney, 2024).

Mira

Four-year-old Mira loves socialising and being active, particularly with music. Mira's dad picks her up from kindergarten on Tuesdays and together they groove to music in the car on their way to pick up her brother, Aki, from dance classes. Each week Mira stands outside the class watching Aki and his peers twirl and leap to the music; she longs to join them. Dad says to her, 'That looks fun, hey?' Mira replies, 'Can I dance like that too, Dad? I want to.' He replies, 'Ummm, I am not sure, perhaps we can find a way.'

Later that night, Dad talks with Mum about the glee in Mira's face; however, the uncertainty due to her diagnosis of cerebral palsy means that she may fall, not be able to follow the steps, and be laughed at. Mum says maybe a dance school won't let her join, and they need some help to find a way.

Dad, Mum, and Mira meet with her occupational therapist the next week and discuss the goal of joining a dance class. The occupational therapist agrees, 'Yes, let's find a way to help you dance, Mira. You have great rhythm.' The family and occupational therapist make an appointment to meet with the dance school to discuss the next steps.

32.2.3 Adolescent to adulthood (13–17 years)

During adolescence there is often an exploration of relationships and roles outside of the family unit as well as the development of more independent occupations such as engaging in paid employment (Bourke-Taylor et al., 2024).

Jas

Jas is 16 years old. Adjusting to a changing body and wrestling with their identity, they are caught between longing for the secure feelings of childhood and urging onwards towards adulthood. Keen to explore their sexuality whilst grappling with the fear of judgement and the excitement of self-discovery, their days appear idle at times. Gone are the satisfaction and meaning once found in childhood games, yet the tasks of adulthood seem just that – tasks.

There is a strangeness and disconnection that comes with simultaneous fear and excitement and paralysis and energy. So much time is spent 'lazing around'. Yet holding still while churning inside feels like a full-time job. The rhythm of participating in school, sports, friends, homework, and household chores, which has carried them along without too much thought, seems elusive now. And lately, a heaviness has crept into everything, making it hard to get up in the morning, hard to communicate with others, and hard to understand (or care about) what others are thinking or doing and bringing moodiness and unhappiness.

32.2.4 Adulthood, young adult (17–59 years)

Adulthood is often a time for multiple life transitions, including those associated with relationships, career, starting a family, and living out of home (Bourke-Taylor et al., 2024).

Kai

Kai is a 36-year-old tane/man, who identifies with his Māori and Scottish whakapapa/ancestry. He has two tamariki/young children with his ex-wife Stacey – his daughter Hunu (7 years old) and his son Hemi (5 years old). They share custody of the tamariki since their divorce three years ago. Kai says, 'I loved my childhood, growing up in a kāinga, or home filled with aroha/love, with my whānau, family, in a rural community in Aotearoa New Zealand.' Kai then moved to a large city to complete his apprenticeship as a builder. After qualifying, Kai worked as a builder for 12 years before starting his own building business.

Kai works long hours running his small business and has minimal time for leisure pursuits such as rugby, hunting or fishing. He says, 'I would like to spend more time with my tamariki and my new partner Aroha, but the long hours in my job, my business, and my other whānau commitments are causing me lots of stress.' Kai is also experiencing chronic back pain and reports, 'I'm worried about how my back pain might impact my ability to work as a builder and I'm feeling depressed.' Kai is also supporting his father (75 years old), who lives alone in a small, rural coastal town and who recently had a stroke. Kai says, 'I am not sure how much longer my father can live on his own, and if or how I can reduce my hours of work to support him, and still pay the bills like the mortgage, cope with my back pain, and have time with my tamariki and partner.' The combination of his paid work, financial and health-related concerns, and his whānau commitments are leaving Kai feeling worried and stressed.

32.2.5 Adulthood, older adult (60–84 years)

Older adulthood is a phase where potential decline in abilities, like hearing and vision, as well as cognitive functions such as memory and processing speed, can occur. Concurrently, older adults often display their wisdom and creativity and may continue in working roles, including volunteering or caring for others.

Mary

Mary, aged 68, recently had an unexpected transition into retirement following redundancy. Unlike her husband Tom, aged 71, who planned his retirement and is currently volunteering at the local Refugee Support Centre, Mary feels lost without her career in retail management, which once provided her with purpose, leadership, and daily structure. Watching Tom thrive while she feels empty and unproductive creates a strain on their relationship; his well-meaning attempts to involve her in his pursuits often lead to frustration and resentment. This sense of isolation affects her relationships with her children and grandchildren, who sense her depression but are unsure how to help. Many of her friendships are fading as well. Although Mary knows she has much to offer, the sudden loss of her professional identity has left her yearning for meaningful engagement and a renewed sense of purpose. Where does she start to reconnect with her loved ones? Can she find a way to contribute to her community?

32.2.6 Older, older adult (85+ years)

Older, older adulthood can be a time where individuals may experience increased impairments, complications of chronic conditions like dementia or cardiovascular disease, and have a higher likelihood of needing some form of supported living. Supported living may be increased supports to remain living in their own home or transitioning into a residential aged care home, where there is a greater reliance on staff for assistance with tasks of daily living.

Matt

Matt, aged 85, lives with his partner Chris in regional Victoria. Matt's wife died 15 years ago following a cancer diagnosis and Matt cared for her for a couple of years. After the passing of his wife, Matt reconnected with Chris whom he had known in his youth. Initially, Matt's adult children were surprised by the relationship but came to appreciate their bond. In recent years, Matt's health has declined; he has experienced multiple falls at home and daily tasks like bathing, dressing, and cooking have become increasingly difficult. Chris, though physically well, is experiencing some cognitive decline and requires some support, which Matt feels responsible to provide. Navigating funding options has been overwhelming. The idea of moving into town to supportive living may be an option, but leaving behind their much-loved home and community is daunting. Can they afford to move, and what support might they need? These concerns worry them both; however, despite these challenges, their bond remains strong.

All the vignettes illustrate the importance of understanding the multifaceted needs of each stage of life, including physical, cognitive, emotional, and social health. Occupational therapists have a key role across the life course in enhancing the quality of life through tailored interventions that enhance participation in occupations and support the needs of the individual and the communities in which they live.

32.3 The role of occupational therapists in promoting and supporting occupational participation

Focusing on occupations that provide purpose and meaning to individuals or community groups, occupational therapists can support individuals and communities to engage in their chosen occupations. This can occur by taking a rights-based and equity approach; considering the context; and using strategies such as adapting occupations, modifying the environment, and collaborating or advocating for the individual with a lived experience to achieve their goals (Gillen, 2024). Using an evidence-based approach, the occupational therapist draws on their clinical expertise, information from the practice context, research evidence, and the individual's goals/values in planning for intervention (Hoffman et al., 2023).

The occupational therapist must thoroughly understand the person's life, exploring the occupations they currently engage in and what occupations they have previously participated in and aspire to undertake. Standardised tools should be used to ensure valid and reliable assessments of current function (descriptive assessments), to predict future abilities (predictive assessments), or to understand the performance in reference to a criterion (performance-based assessments) (Laver-Fawcett & Cox, 2021). Combining occupational therapists' observations that are structured using occupational models like the Kawa model (Iwama & Matsubara, 2024) with standardised assessments provides contextual information that can be used to enrich and triangulate assessment findings and plan for intervention (Laver-Fawcett & Cox, 2021).

The occupational therapist works collaboratively with the person/s to identify those occupations that bring meaning and purpose to their life, co-designing the goals and interventions to achieve desired outcomes (de las Heras de Pablo & Muñoz, 2024; Egan & Restall, 2022). Working with different population groups may require targeted approaches. For example, knowledge of what features and occupations are typical during a person's life course and how these can be influenced by physical or mental health concerns are important for an occupational therapist to know when supporting a person who is using an occupational therapy service.

In the case of Lilli (see vignette), to support mastery of skills and development through maximising opportunities in daily routines, the occupational therapist works in partnership with Lilli and her family to co-design interventions. This approach enhances and builds Lilli and her family's skills while encouraging engagement in everyday life, such as playing with differently textured toys, advice on how to play with the toys, and how to offer and engage with food at mealtimes. Through play activities, Lilli can develop fine and gross motor strength; self-care; and cognitive, emotional, and social communication skills. Play provides children with the opportunity to develop proficiency, enabling them to have choices and control over their world (Cronin, 2021). The occupational therapist provides early intervention through family-centred practice

(FCP) and works closely with the family to support participation in occupations such as bathing, eating, and play (Frolek Clark & Kingsley, 2020).

A child's environment influences their options and access to participate in occupations. By considering the child and their environmental context (Frolek Clark & Kingsley, 2020) and using FCP principles, the occupational therapist can increase participation in occupations for the child and their community. For Mira, dance is a focal occupation. Collaborative practice (Occupational Therapy Australia, 2016), advocating, engaging, and building a relationship with the dance school and family will enable Mira to engage in this meaningful occupation while creating an environment to support her motor, cognitive, and social skills. The occupational therapist can continue to partner and consult with the dance school, Mira, and her family to adapt and grade the classes to be inclusive and support sustainable participation. The opportunity to develop dance classes inclusive of all ability levels can support Mira's interests and abilities across the life course and create opportunities for others in her community.

Occupational therapists should focus on participation in meaningful occupations alongside a person/family-centred recovery and trauma-informed approach when working alongside people with mental health concerns. This provides an opportunity for the individual to address their needs in a safe, effective, and age-appropriate way. Occupational therapy interventions, alongside interdisciplinary approaches, should support the individual's development, health and wellbeing (Swarbrick, 2024). These can include reducing barriers to participation, using occupations as a medium for its benefits, connecting socially and developing supportive relationships, or fostering occupational skill development (Swarbrick, 2024). In the case of Jas, the occupational therapist could explore with Jas the journey they are on and their hopes, spirituality, volition, and occupational identity, alongside developing occupational patterns (e.g., habits, routines) that support their wellbeing (Cahill et al., 2020). Similarly, the occupational therapist's focus for Kai and his mental health may be his occupational goals and strategies that help him cope with and overcome his stress and challenges. The transitions across the life course may create challenges in identifying meaningful occupations. The occupational therapist can support Mary in identifying occupations that are meaningful to her and what roles she wishes to fulfil in her retirement (Eagers et al., 2019; Eagers et al., 2020).

When working with individuals who have experienced a sudden, unexpected change in function, such as Kai's father, who had a stroke, the therapist may adopt different strategies to achieve participation in meaningful but also necessary occupations for everyday life, such as self-care tasks. Compensatory strategies incorporate task adaptation or modification, whereas restorative strategies focus on enhancing functional ability, such as improving upper limb function after stroke (Stroke Foundation, 2023). Changes in function may be more gradual, such as those experienced by Matt. The occupational therapist may support Matt's continued participation in self-care activities through environmental modifications (Stark et al., 2017) or engagement in fall prevention programmes, such as Stepping On (Clemson et al., 2004). In addition, the therapist may also work to support Matt and Chris in their reciprocal caregiving roles (Micklewright & Farquhar, 2023). Support to the caregiver may also be provided during palliative care, where the occupational therapist is focused on enhancing participation in meaningful occupations for both the individual and caregiver (American Occupational Therapy Association, 2020).

Occupational therapists advocate for individuals, families, communities, and populations, particularly where there are historical and contextual inequities that are impeding their occupational rights and their participation in occupations, which might limit their development and potential for future participation (Egan & Restall, 2022; Lysack et al., 2024). In Matt's case, the occupational therapist may advocate (American Occupational Therapy Association, 2020; Egan & Restall, 2022) and support him and his partner to understand the health system and how to achieve his participation goals in this context.

In all instances, the occupational therapist engages in critical reflection alongside the individual and their families to inform reasoning and decision-making as well as evaluating outcomes (Chisholm & Schell, 2024). Through this reflection, the therapist can provide person/family/group-centred services that support occupational patterns and maximise participation in occupations across the life course.

32.4 Conclusion

This chapter explored how occupational patterns change across the life course and used vignettes to highlight how individuals' experiences of occupations are influenced by their unique context. The focus of the occupational therapist is to enhance participation in meaningful and necessary occupations for the individual through collaboration and by continually evaluating the intervention's effectiveness in partnership with the person and their families.

32.5 Summary

- Occupations contribute to an individual's occupational development, occupational patterns (habits, routines, roles, rituals), and identity at all ages.
- The type of occupations and their meanings continually evolve across the life course.
- The context in which an occupation is or will be performed must be considered so that inequitable opportunities for participation in occupations are identified and addressed.

32.6 Review and reflection questions

- Describe three ways in which occupations may evolve or change across the life course.
- How do a person's unique characteristics influence the development of occupational patterns?
- How have your occupational patterns changed over your life? Think about key transition points in your life, such as starting school, entering tertiary study, or entering the un/paid workforce.
- Reflect on the current occupations in which you engage. Select three and consider the meaning and value that you ascribe to each and what this has meant for your occupational development.

References

American Occupational Therapy Association. (2020). Occupational Therapy Practice Framework: Domain and process – fourth edition. *American Journal of Occupational Therapy*, 74(Supp 2), 7412410010p1–7412410010p87. https://doi.org/10.5014/ajot.2020.74S2001

American Occupational Therapy Association. (2023). End-of-life care and the role of occupational therapy. *American Journal of Occupational Therapy, 77*(Supp 3), 7713410210. https://doi.org/10.5014/ajot.2023.77S3002

Baker, N. A., Tickle-Degnen, L., & Marfeo, E. E. (2024). Evidence-based practice: Integrating evidence to inform practice. In G. Gillen & C. Brown (Eds.), *Willard & Spackman's occupational therapy* (14th ed., pp. 438–453). Wolters Kluwer.

Bourke-Taylor, H., Sin Sim, S., & Rassafiani, M. (2024). An occupational therapy perspective on families, occupation, health, and disability. In G. Gillen & C. Brown (Eds.), *Willard & Spackman's occupational therapy* (14th ed., pp. 180–198). Wolters Kluwer.

Brown, T., Isbel, S., Gustafsson, L., Gutman, S., Dirette, D. P., Collins, B., & Barlott, T. (2025). Introduction to human occupation: Contemporary concepts and lifespan perspectives. In T. Brown, S. Isbel, L. Gustafsson, S. A. Gutman, D. Powers Dirette, B. Collins, & T. Barlott (Eds.), *Human occupation: Contemporary concepts and lifespan perspectives.* (pp. 3–28). Routledge.

Cahill, S. M., Egan, B. E., & Seber, J. (2020). Activity and occupation based interventions to support mental health, positive behavior, and social participation for children and youth: A systematic review. *American Journal of Occupational Therapy, 74*(2), 7402180020p1–7402180020p28. https://doi.org/10.5014/ajot.2020.038687

Chisholm, D., & Schell, B. A. B. (2024). Overview of the occupational therapy process and outcomes. In G. Gillen & C. Brown (Eds.), *Willard & Spackman's occupational therapy* (14th ed., pp. 282–298). Wolters Kluwer.

Clemson, L., Cumming, R. G., Kendig, H., Swann, M., Heard, R., & Taylor, K. (2004). The effectiveness of a community-based program for reducing the incidence of falls in the elderly: A randomized trial. *Journal of the American Geriatrics Society, 52*(9), 1487–1494. https://doi.org/10.1111/j.1532-5415.2004.52411.x

Cronin, A. (2021). Development in the preschool years. In A. Cronin & M. Mandich (Eds.), *Human development and performance throughout the life span* (2nd ed., pp. 248–271). Cengage.

de las Heras de Pablo, C. G., & Muñoz, J. P. (2024). Therapeutic relationships and person-centered collaboration: Applying the intentional relationship model. In G. Gillen & C. Brown (Eds.), *Willard & Spackman's occupational therapy* (14th ed., pp. 468–481). Wolters Kluwer.

Dunn, W. (2017). Strengths-based approaches: What if even the 'bad' things are good things? *British Journal of Occupational Therapy, 80*(7), 395–396. https://doi.org/10.1177/0308022617702660

Eagers, J., Franklin, R. C., Broome, K., & Yau, M. K. (2019). The experiences of work: Retirees' perspectives and the relationship to the role of occupational therapy in the work-to-retirement transition process. *Work, 64*(2), 341–354. https://doi.org/10.3233/WOR-192996

Eagers, J., Franklin, R. C., Broome, K., Yau, M. K., & Barnett, F. (2020). Current occupational therapy scope of practice in the work-to-retirement transition process: An Australian study. *Scandinavian Journal of Occupational Therapy, 29*(6), 495–510. https://doi.org/10.1080/11038128.2020.1841286

Egan, M., & Restall, G. (2022). Collaborative relationship-focused occupational therapy. In M. Egan & G. Restall (Eds.), *Promoting occupational participation: Collaborative relationship-focused occupational therapy. 10th Canadian occupational therapy guidelines* (pp. 97–117). Canadian Association of Occupational Therapists.

Frolek Clark, G., & Kingsley, K. L. (2020). Occupational therapy practice guidelines for early childhood: Birth–5 years. *American Journal of Occupational Therapy, 74*(3), 1–42. https://doi.org/10.5014/ajot.2020.743001

Gillen, G. (2024). Occupational therapy interventions for individuals. In G. Gillen & C. Brown (Eds.), *Willard & Spackman's occupational therapy* (14th ed., pp. 343–365). Wolters Kluwer.

Hocking, C., & Sutton, D. (2024). Contribution of occupation to health and well-being. In G. Gillen & C. Brown (Eds.), *Willard & Spackman's occupational therapy* (14th ed., pp. 111–122). Wolters Kluwer.

Hoffman, T., Bennett, S., & Del Mar, C. (2023). Introduction to evidence-based practice. In T. Hoffman, S. Bennett, & C. Del Mar (Eds.), *Evidence-based practice across the health professions* (4th ed., pp. 1–13). Elsevier.

Iwama, M. K., & Matsubara, A. (2024). The Kawa (river) model. In G. Gillen & C. Brown (Eds.), *Willard & Spackman's occupational therapy* (14th ed., pp. 599–616). Wolters Kluwer.

Laver-Fawcett, A. J., & Cox, D. L. (2021). *Principles of assessment and outcome measurement for allied health professionals: Practice, research and development* (2nd ed.). Wiley-Blackwell.

Lysack, C. L., Adamo, D. E., & Galvaan, R. (2024). Social, economic, and political factors that influence occupational performance. In G. Gillen & C. Brown (Eds.), *Willard & Spackman's occupational therapy* (14th ed., pp. 224–242). Wolters Kluwer.

Micklewright, K., & Farquhar, M. (2023). Occupational therapy interventions for adult informal carers and implications for intervention design, delivery and evaluation: A systematic review. *British Journal of Occupational Therapy*, 86(2), 90–100. https://doi.org/10.1177/03080226221107924

Occupational Therapy Australia. (2016). *Occupational therapy guide to good practice: Working with children.* https://connect.otaus.com.au/resources/details/078858ae-b81b-4ada-8566-233dc86245ed

Stark, S., Keglovits, M., Arbesman, M., & Lieberman, D. (2017). Effect of home modification interventions on the participation of community-dwelling adults with health conditions: A systematic review. *American Journal of Occupational Therapy*, 71(2), 1–11. https://doi.org/10.5014/ajot.2017.018887

Stroke Foundation. (2023). *Clinical guidelines for stroke management.* https://informme.org.au/guidelines/living-clinical-guidelines-for-stroke-management.

Swarbrick, M. (2024). Providing wellness-oriented occupational therapy services for persons with mental health challenges. In G. Gillen & C. Brown (Eds.), *Willard & Spackman's occupational therapy* (14th ed., pp. 1106–1118). Wolters Kluwer.

Whitney, R. V. (2024). Human occupations of infants, toddlers, and preschoolers. In T. Brown, S. Isbel, L. Gustafsson, S. Gutman, D. Powers Dirette, B. Collins, & T. Barlott (Eds.), *Human occupation* (1st ed., pp. 453–472). Routledge. https://doi.org/10.4324/9781003504610-29

Womack, J. L., & Bagatell, N. (2024). Transformations of occupations: A life course perspective. In G. Gillen & C. Brown (Eds.), *Willard & Spackman's occupational therapy* (14th ed., pp. 100–110). Wolters Kluwer.

CHAPTER 33

Emerging areas of occupational therapy practice

Marina Ciccarelli, Bronwyn Paynter, Helen Jeffery, Leigh Tesch, Carole James, Jessica Francis, and Karen Below

The authors acknowledge Kauwanu Ivan-Tiwu Copley, OAM, as cultural broker for Aboriginal and Zenadth Kes Peoples' knowledge.

Authors' positionality statement

The seven authors of this chapter are female, university-educated, occupational therapists with collective experiences across diverse practice areas in Australia and New Zealand. Six authors acknowledge their perspectives are shaped by white, western, English-language privilege, and one author by Māori ways in harmony with the land. All are committed to improving the health, well-being, and inclusion of the diverse communities which they serve. This is evidenced by their occupational therapy practice that is underpinned by respect for all people and their natural environments and through innovative application of ancient, grassroots, and emergent technologies and media.

Key terms
- Innovation
- Design thinking
- Person-occupation-environment
- Re-imagining practice
- Artificial intelligence
- Local and global health and wellbeing

Objectives
This chapter will allow the reader to:

- Describe contemporary examples of occupational therapy practice that emerged to meet community needs or fill a service gap

DOI: 10.4324/9781003495666-36

- Explain design thinking and how it aligns with an occupational therapy professional practice process framework when innovating occupational therapy practice
- Describe innovative approaches in occupational therapy services from the perspectives of occupational therapists in Australia and Aotearoa New Zealand
- Discuss the roles of evidence-based, collaborative, sustainable, and ethical decision making in the development, implementation, and evaluation of innovative occupational therapy practice

33.1 Introduction

Multiple factors influence the health and wellbeing of individuals, families, communities, and nations. During the 2020s, the world experienced many 'once-in-a-generation' phenomena that presented significantly affected humanity and the environment, as well as the dawn of access to artificial intelligence (AI) by the wider community. Recent examples include international political conflicts and wars affecting global economies and supply chains of food commodities and other resources; post-COVID-19 chronic skills shortages particularly in health and the housing construction industries; natural disasters associated with climate change leading to food insecurity and forced displacement of people; a developing realisation of potential benefits and threats of accessible AI on daily life; and exponential growth in worldwide rates of chronic health conditions, especially mental illness.

Throughout these challenges and opportunities, the theoretical underpinning of occupational therapy – that humans are occupational beings and that engagement in occupations is important to promote health and well-being – remains relevant and important. From 'going back to the future' and re-connecting with traditional occupational therapy practice reimagined for today's society to futuristic applications of AI, this chapter describes emergent occupational therapy practice through the lens of an innovation framework and discusses why and how, in this era of significant global change, occupational therapy practice must evolve to remain relevant and responsive to community needs.

33.2 Innovating by design

Innovation is the process of turning a creative idea into a viable solution to address an identified need. Innovation starts when it becomes apparent that a change is needed. The innovation can be a product, service, business model, or strategy that is novel and useful. Occupational therapists can be innovators at all stages of their professional life including being a student on placement, starting in a graduate role, and as an experienced practitioner managing a service. So, how do you begin an innovation? Having an iterative co-design process with the consumer (client or patient) can help determine the best possible solution to meet the need(s). Stanford Design Thinking Process (see Figure 33.1 and Table 33.1) is a five-stage iterative process that provides a roadmap for innovation (Hasso Plattner Institute of Design at Stanford, n.d.).

Several factors can foster or hinder innovation including funding to support development, implementation, and evaluation; technologies required; stakeholders, including consumers (person factors); policies and legislative requirements (environment factors); and accountability for efficacy, safety, and ethics. Innovation does not have to

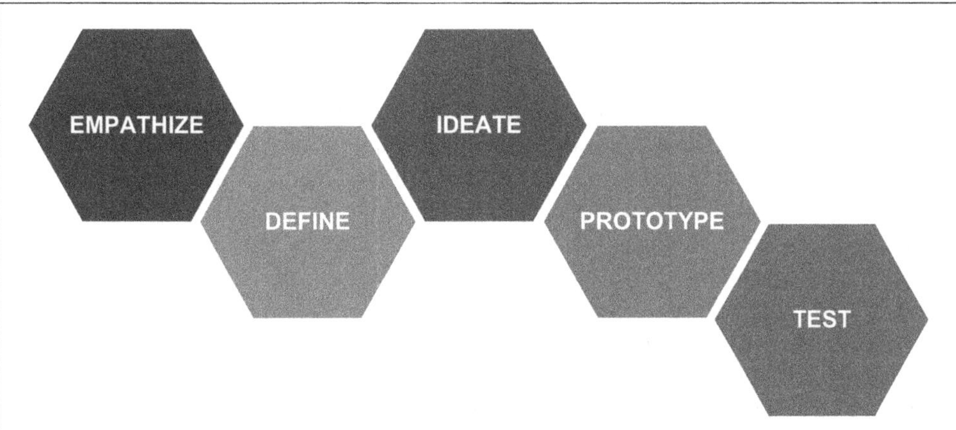

1. Understand experiences of the consumer(s) to whom you provide service and/or the organisation in which you work (Empathise).
2. Identify needs of your consumer(s) and/or organisation (Define).
3. Consider all the possible ways to address the identified need – this is best done using a co-design process (Ideate).
4. Develop a low fidelity version of a solution – again, best done through co-design (Prototype).
5. Trial the solution with your consumer(s) and/or organisation (Test). Get feedback and refine as required until the solution meets the identified need.

Figure 33.1 The Stanford Design Thinking Process

(Hasso Plattner Institute of Design at Stanford, n.d.)

Table 33.1 Alignment of the Stanford Design Thinking Process with the CPPF

Stanford Design Thinking	*Canadian Practice Process Framework*
	Enter/initiate (make contact);
	Set the stage (confirm how you will work with the consumer)
Empathise and define the problem	Assess/evaluate the consumer's occupational performance
Ideate and prototype	Agree on Objectives and plan with the consumer
Test, feedback, and refine	Implement plan
	Monitor/modify (iterative process of feedback and refinement)
Evaluation of the innovation	Evaluate outcomes

be a brand-new concept and can be occupational therapists working in an improved way or repurposing a previous solution to address a different need, or with a different consumer group, or at a different time in history. Four examples are provided here that illustrate occupational therapy practice that has or will emerge through innovative thinking to address identified needs.

33.2.1 Example 1. Back to the roots – nature-based occupational therapy

Multiple social, economic, and lifestyle factors contribute to the development of chronic health conditions, which affect all body systems and place increasing demands on health services. Globally, chronic conditions account for three-quarters of premature deaths and affect participation in occupations. Occupational therapy practice is influenced by understanding the dynamic, interdependent relationships between people, their natural and built environments, and occupational engagement (see Figure 33.2). Humans' diverse relationships with nature are influenced by culture, opportunity, and experiences of and with nature over generations. These include knowing humans are a part of and inextricably linked to nature; perceiving nature as a resource to benefit people or an asset to own; and a backdrop for participation in occupations. Research evidence supports humans' physiological links with nature and aligns with Indigenous practices that encompass connection, respect, and responsibility towards nature. The Māori whakataukī – *ko au ko te taiao, ko te taiao ko au* (I am the environment, the environment is me) and Aboriginal and Torres Strait Islander lore include land as a place for healing and to draw strength from. Nature encompasses everything around, above, and below us including oceans, skies, and stars, and informs cultural practices of Aotearoa and Australia.

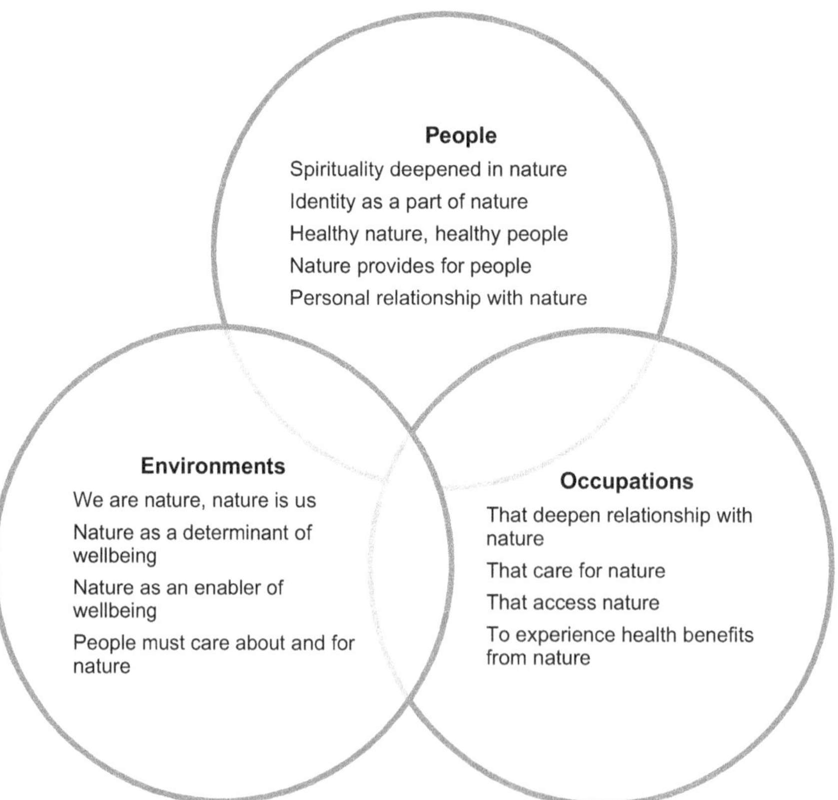

Figure 33.2 The interrelationships among people, the natural environment, and occupations

The shift towards industrialised and urbanised lifestyles has diminished humans' access to nature, affecting the health of nature and people. The Māori Peoples of Aotearoa and Australian Aboriginal and Torres Strait Islander Peoples have embodied ancestral wisdom and practices supporting their symbiotic relationship with nature. Despite Western colonisation, these knowledges and practices are not lost. This ancestral wisdom, augmented by Western science, supports nature as a determinant/enabler of wellbeing. Incorporating this into occupational therapy is innovative and a return to practice that is fundamental to humanity.

Everything humans need to thrive is within nature. Nature influences all body systems including circadian rhythms and co-regulation of the nervous system. Deep knowledge of the influence of nature's rhythms on humans is evidenced in the maramataka (Māori lunar calendar) and Australian Indigenous calendars. Health and wellbeing are enhanced through attunement to nature's rhythms, such as sleep cycles attuned to light and dark, and eating cycles in harmony with seasons. Equally important are nature's influences on the nervous system. For example, birdsong and trickling water are calming, viewing nature enhances healing, touching animals reduces blood pressure, eating natural whole foods is nutritional, and aromas directed to the limbic system trigger emotions (Willis, 2024). Integrating nature into occupational therapy practice in public health, health promotion, and goal-directed therapy profoundly benefits people and the planet.

Humans' thriving is dependent on a symbiotic relationship – as nature cares for us, so we must care for nature. Environmental problems such as depletion, extinction, pollution, and climate change are caused by people and affect people. The concept of eco-social occupational therapy (Simó Algado & Townsend, 2015) includes the everyday doing of ecology and provides a pathway for occupational therapy to respond to the imperative that humans must incorporate ecology into our sense of self and act to rectify damage to nature.

Occupational therapists can facilitate engagement with nature to support prevention and/or self-management of chronic health conditions:

- *Build spirituality* through deeper connections to the earth and the universe via facilitated experiences of awe and being a part of something bigger than self, for example, astronomy, meditation and contemplation in nature, mindfulness in and of nature, watching natural history documentaries, and following Indigenous seasonal calendars.
- *Build ecological identity* through occupations that deepen awareness of self as inseparable from ecological homes and relationships, for example, environmental education, awareness of physiological relationships with nature, gardening, or photography across seasons.
- *Build an ethic of care for nature* via occupations that care for nature, promote enjoyment in nature, and build understanding of nature as family, for example, individual and community gardens, reforestation projects, and conservation volunteering.
- *Build awareness of nature* and positive impact on wellbeing by noticing nature, for example, birdwatching, nature photography, star gazing, cloud watching, and noticing sensory experiences in nature (see Figure 33.3).

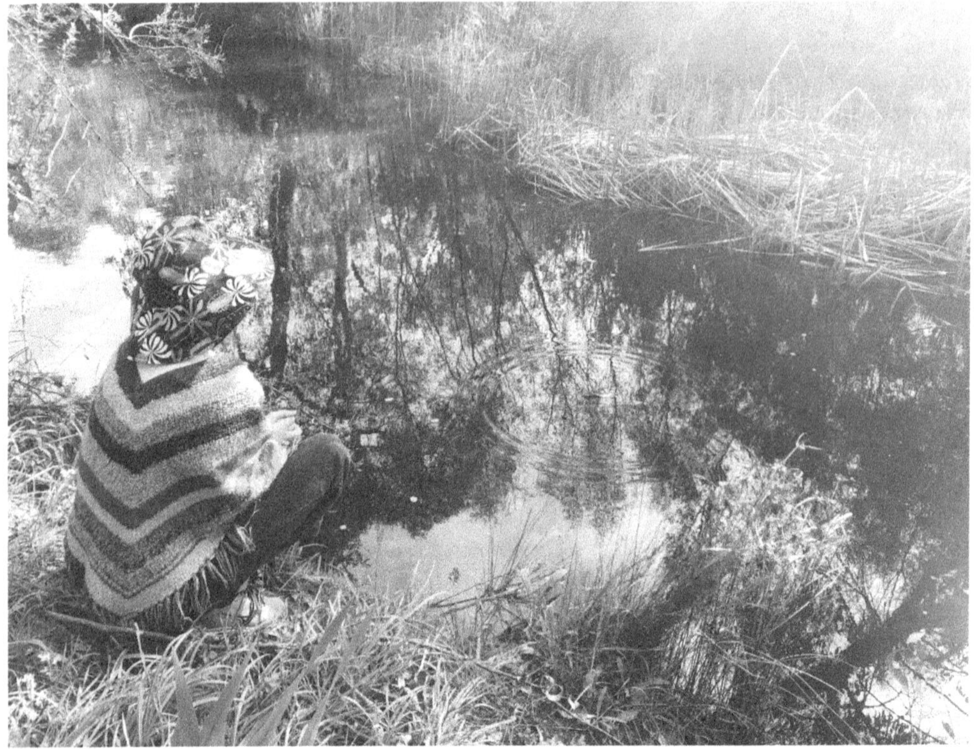

Figure 33.3 An occupational therapist facilitates awareness of nature at a wellbeing festival

(Image credit: Wellness Wander, 2023)

- *Build gratitude for nature* through occupations that fulfil human needs, for example, hunting, fishing, and foraging or growing food.
- *Build awareness of humans' physiological relationship with nature*, for example, breathing in phytoncides reduces cortisol (stress hormone), soil bacteria improve mood, and being in nature improves attention, focus, empathy, and social connection.
- *Build resilience to harmful effects* of urban environments and overuse of technology through routinely accessing the restorative power of nature.
- *Build routines that maintain health* through accessing everyday nature, for example, bringing nature inside (indoor plants, pets, art), and building eco-identity.

Some may consider this an innovative approach to occupational therapy, but it is simply a return to acknowledging that humans are indigenous to earth and supports practices that work for people and for nature.

33.2.2 Example 2. For arts' sake

People may experience significant stress and vulnerability when accessing health and wellbeing services. A person's ability to engage in meaningful occupation is influenced by their agency within their environment; however, many healthcare environments including acute care hospitals can be noisy and hectic, with an organisational focus on efficiencies in service delivery. The consumer's experience and personhood can be overlooked, which can affect their healthcare outcomes. There is a need and opportunity to innovate to support person-centred occupational therapy services within under-resourced and demanding healthcare environments.

For millennia, the arts have been used to express and share stories to make sense of the human experience. There is growing evidence that including the arts in healthcare environments is associated with reducing pain, anxiety, and stress among inpatients; providing health consumers the opportunity for self-expression and a collective voice; and promoting health messages and social connectedness (Fancourt & Finn, 2019). The benefits of arts-based occupation are not new to occupational therapy, but the challenge is how these opportunities can be re-imagined into 21st-century healthcare.

One example is the establishment of Inscape Tas, an arts and health organisation that engages professional artists to work with patients, their families, and staff. This evolved from a nurse and an occupational therapist recognising the need for consumers to have agency and voice in healthcare. Using funds from a bequest, they followed an iterative design thinking process, empathising and exploring with consumers, while influenced by relational arts and community development processes. Artistry enriches the experiences of people with complex medical situations, low mood and/or cognitive challenges, or those in long stay admissions (see Figure 33.4). Inscape Tas artists receive professional development and mentoring, and listen, empathise, and respond with nuanced adaptations of art media and activities (Ford et al., 2018).

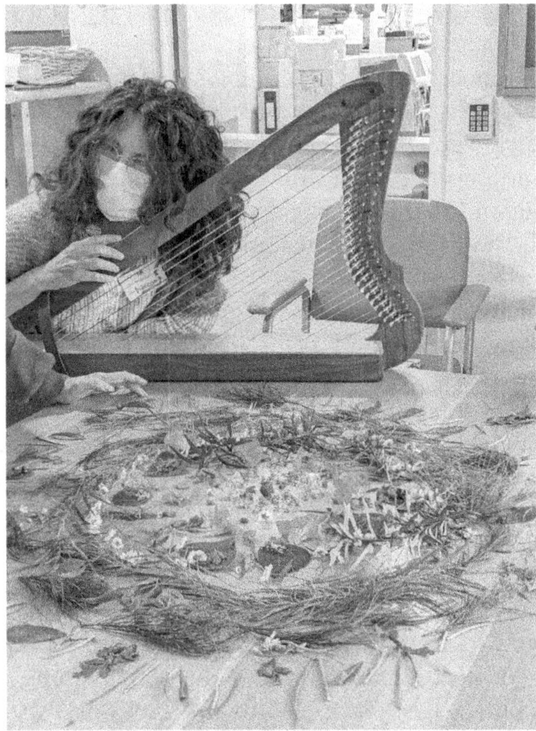

Figure 33.4 An Inscape Tas musician engages with a patient who is creating a floral mandala

Person-centredness is essential to this innovation and two case studies illustrate this approach. 'Molly' was admitted to an acute hospital after a fall and presents with delirium and short-term memory loss. Molly relaxes as she listens to live music played by an Inscape musician. Careful listening to her story reveals Molly was a ballroom dancer and previously ran her own business. An artist paints her a 'life-scape' artwork, illustrating important moments of Molly's life. Staff and visitors admire the artwork displayed at Molly's bedside and ask her about its significance. Molly remembers and engages socially – her personhood is acknowledged beyond that of being an inpatient on a busy ward.

'Greg' is struggling with behaviours and psychological symptoms of dementia during his hospital admission. An artist encourages Greg to engage in a nature-based art activity, placing petals and leaves in a mandala, and he becomes immersed in the sensory and physical nature of the activity. Greg smells the fragrance of an herb and tells stories of family dinners, and despite his current difficulties, in this moment he is present to being capable and occupationally functional. A poet records Greg's story, and together the words and images are captured into a booklet that Greg folds and keeps in his pocket.

For Molly and Greg, these were opportunities to engage in fundamentals of occupational therapy – 'doing, being, becoming, and belonging' (Wilcock, 1996). They were able to 'do' meaningful occupation, despite their presenting deficits and restrictions. 'Doing' arts is both active and passive (e.g. listening to music or appreciating artwork). Arts engagement supports them to 'be' in the present and to 'belong' with others around them. In 'becoming', there is opportunity for Molly and Greg to re-story their experiences of illness, to reflect, and to make sense and meaning of the disruption in their life journeys.

This foundational understanding of occupational therapy can be an enabler for innovation. Our skills in listening, problem solving, and adaptation can help explore situations, ideas, and potential solutions. By working with clients, and respectfully partnering within and beyond the healthcare environment, opportunities emerge for new ways of working and re-discovering and transforming practices. Ongoing reflection, feedback, evaluation, and documentation is critical for developing robust and responsive initiatives like Inscape Tas.

Experiencing someone's story through artwork, film, or spoken word can strengthen empathy and understanding of them. Clients' lived experiences combined with research evidence are key drivers for innovation in practice. Occupational therapists identify needs, explore potential solutions, and develop and evaluate emerging practices that respond to our clients and environments. Leaning into our understanding of occupation, the qualities of the arts, and our clients' stories can resource us to think broadly about possibilities. Nurturing our creativity will enrich innovative practice.

33.2.3 Example 3. Healthy @ Work

Work is an important occupation for many. Occupational therapists' have a long history in work-related practice beginning with rehabilitation of World War 1 soldiers: progressing to occupational rehabilitation and expanding to promoting health and wellbeing through engagement in good work environments (Andersen & Reed, 2017). Good work extends beyond managing health and safety; promotes wellbeing, workers' personal development, self-determination, a sense of meaning, and fulfilment. It is a key determinant of health and wellbeing of employees, families, and society (AFOEM, 2022).

Workplaces can influence the physical, mental, economic, and social wellness of workers, and offer the infrastructure and opportunity to embed policies and practices to improve workers' wellness (WHO, 2010). Keeping workers well at work is financially sound practice (Foster, 2016). Despite workplace health-promotion initiatives to improve employees' health and work-related outcomes such as improved employee engagement, creativity, innovation, enhanced productivity, and organisational profits (Mental Health Commission of Canada, 2013), worker health is often not core business for many organisations.

Occupational therapists are well placed to work collaboratively with organisations to identify workers' health issues and creatively co-design evidence-based interventions for implementation and subsequent evaluation. Occupational therapists consider the worker (person), their work activities (occupations), and the social and physical environments at the workplace. They bring interdisciplinary stakeholders together to navigate industry-specific health problems. Using co-design processes and end-user engagement in intervention development creates trust and assists in the implementation and sustainability of health outcomes into practice (Wolfenden et al., 2016). Developing and maintaining relationships with diverse stakeholders, (e.g. union officials, human resources representatives, engineers, safety and health professionals) creates a genuine understanding of feasibility and acceptability when designing and implementing an intervention and evaluating its effectiveness. Awareness of the economic state and any industrial relations concerns of a particular industry is essential because these factors can assist or hamper worker engagement. Early engagement and ongoing consultation with worksite employee representatives and management is necessary for feedback on health and wellbeing interventions, progress, and outcomes.

Mental illness is a global health concern and is the focus in this example of how occupational therapy researchers worked with the mining industry to understand the health challenges and collaboratively developed frameworks to promote worker health and wellbeing. An interdisciplinary team including occupational therapists, collaborated with stakeholders from a regional mining industry, local health services, and researchers from the University of Newcastle's Institute for Energy and Resources (University of Newcastle, 2024) to create a roadmap to address emerging health issues. The roadmap recognised mental health as a major health concern to be addressed. The Blueprint for Mental Health and Wellbeing was developed (Minerals Council of Australia, 2022) in collaboration with the Minerals Council of Australia (industry association). This national blueprint is a framework to promote worker wellbeing and reduce risks and impacts of mental illness in the mining industry. It identifies key directions and recommends evidence-based strategies to guide companies' responses to their workers' mental health issues.

Assessing the prevalence and effects of mental health issues in the mining sector involved regular engagement with site-level management, supervisors, and employee representatives to collect accurate information used in the co-design of workplace mental health interventions. The Working Well Mental Health Program was established and involved expansion of Mates in Mining, a peer-support mental health and suicide prevention programme. Program evaluation provided evidence to support implementation of the Blueprint for Mental Health and Wellbeing to help the mining industry prioritise this critical health issue.

Using a similar co-design process, the Blueprint for the Management of Overweight and Obesity in the New South Wales (NSW) mining industry was created and RESHAPE, a framework for a sustainable workplace approach to healthy weight for NSW mining, was developed. RESHAPE was embedded into existing organisational policies and procedures to evaluate workplace problems and collect measurable outcomes targeted to workplace wellness initiatives. By using knowledge of the interactions among the environment (workplace), occupations (good work), and the person (worker), occupational therapists have united stakeholders in the work wellness space, acknowledging our holistic approach to health and occupation.

33.2.4 Example 4. Artificial intelligence–supported occupational therapy practice

Artificial intelligence is increasingly accessible to mainstream society and is transforming how occupational therapists practice in Australia and New Zealand. Occupational therapists face evolving professional practice challenges including workforce shortages and associated productivity demands; rising service delivery costs; more accountability to reduce human error and improve consumer outcomes; and rising expectations of consumers for access to personalised and accessible occupational therapy services. Innovation using AI should incorporate design thinking through iterative problem solving and a user-centred approach, to ensure that AI tools address genuine needs by first understanding the challenges faced by clinicians and consumers, then co-creating effective solutions. Creative use of AI that prioritises users' needs over novelty can drive innovative solutions to support occupational therapists in service delivery, administration, and business management, and enhance efficiencies, safety, and improve consumer outcomes.

Integrating AI innovations into occupational therapy practice requires careful consideration of several factors. Policies that support the ethical use of AI, robust data privacy frameworks, and infrastructure investments are critical enablers. Organisational cultures that embrace innovation and provide time and training opportunities for staff will facilitate AI adoption. Conversely, barriers such as limited access to technology, resistance to change, and ethical concerns about data use must be addressed. The Australian Health Practitioner Regulation Agency emphasises the importance of maintaining high standards of care when integrating AI into practice while recognising its potential to improve health outcomes and create more person-centred health delivery (Australian Health Practitioner Regulation Agency, 2024).

Ethics is paramount to the application of AI into occupational therapy practice, and processes must be established that view AI as a complement to, not replacement for person-centred care, and that maintain consumers' informed consent and data privacy. Education on the ethical implications and responsible use of AI should be integrated into occupational therapy education curricula to prepare future practitioners. While AI may be a useful tool in practice, it does not replace the clinical judgment and decision-making of the occupational therapist. Occupational therapists deciding to use AI should keep privacy, data management, and ethical considerations in mind and ensure they are following the applicable practice and legislative standards (College of Occupational Therapists of Ontario, 2024).

Generative AI can produce multimodal outputs that can automate and streamline occupational therapists' administrative tasks. For example, ambient listening AI 'listens' to a health professional's session with a consumer, filters important information, and automatically transcribes a clinical note. Preliminary research on this AI use demonstrates its benefits for improving documentation quality, reducing documentation time, and increasing clinician presence with consumers (Balloch et al., 2024). Occupational therapists can use AI-powered software to analyse consumer information to guide treatment plans, monitor progress through its integration into therapy-based apps and wearable technologies, and simplify documentation using practice management software. When combined with other emergent technologies, like augmented and virtual reality technology, AI signals powerful advancements in the delivery and experience of occupational therapy services. Agentic AI, designed to perform complex, multi-step tasks (Built In, 2024), is imminent and will enable greater advancements in practice.

The practical applications of AI represent a potential radical shift in occupational therapy practice. As AI rapidly evolves, the affordances and challenges this technology presents will likely have changed by the time this book is published. The changing pace of AI and its application to innovative occupational therapy practice necessitates ongoing professional development and adaptability. Predictions suggest AI could replace clinical decision making within our lifetimes (Hatherley et al., 2024), signalling the need for systemic changes in healthcare delivery models. Occupational therapists are adaptable professionals and should embrace the innovation opportunities and leverage AI to enhance consumer outcomes.

33.3 Conclusion

This chapter presented innovation as a feature of occupational therapy practice that emerges to meet the identified needs of individuals, families, organisations, and communities. Occupational therapists at all stages of their professional journeys can be responsive to the changing needs of society through innovative practice. Design thinking can guide occupational therapists to develop practice innovations using a stepwise process that aligns well to occupational therapy practice process frameworks, and is driven by interactions among the person, their occupations, and their environments.

33.4 Summary

- Occupational therapists in Australia and New Zealand are responding to the changing and diverse occupational needs of people in contemporary society.
- Occupational therapists demonstrate innovation in the application of design thinking approaches to create co-design partnerships; modify environments; and empower individuals, groups, and communities to achieve health and wellbeing through active participation in meaningful occupations.
- Innovative emergent occupational therapy practice should consider collaborative and/or co-designed, sustainable, and ethical decision making in the development, implementation, and evaluation of programmes and services.

33.5 Review and reflection questions

- Select one of the examples of re-imagined occupational therapy practice initiatives described in this chapter. Identify the unique need and explain how the innovation described enhances health and wellbeing through participation in meaningful occupation for the target population.

- Consider the bicultural and multicultural natures of contemporary Australian and New Zealand societies. How might the innovative practice initiatives/programmes described in this chapter be relevant across different socio-demographic groups in the community? What adaptations to the initiatives may be required to increase inclusion?

- What aspect(s) of occupational performance do the innovations aim to impact? For example, are there modifications to the environment(s) or how the environment(s) are selected, adaptations to the how occupations are performed, or changes to the person's capacities or relationship with the occupation or environment?

References

Andersen, L. T., & Reed, K. L. (2017). *The history of occupational therapy: The first century* (1st ed.). Routledge.

Australasian Faculty of Occupational and Environmental Medicine [AFOEM]. (2022). *Australasian consensus statement on the health benefits of work* [Online]. https://www.acrrm.org.au/docs/default-source/all-files/aust-consensus-statment_health-benefits-work_and-background.pdf?sfvrsn=6a4f87eb_2

Australian Health Practitioner Regulation Agency. (2024). *Meeting your professional obligations when using artificial intelligence in healthcare* [Online]. https://www.ahpra.gov.au/Resources/Artificial-Intelligence-in-healthcare.aspx

Balloch, J., Sridharan, S., Oldham, G., Wray, J., Gough, P., Robinson, R., Sebire, N. J., Khalil, S., Asgari, E., Tan, C., Taylor, A., & Pimenta, D. (2024). Use of an ambient artificial intelligence tool to improve quality of clinical documentation. *Future Healthcare Journal*, *11*(3), 100157–100157. https://doi.org/10.1016/j.fhj.2024.100157

Built In. (2024). *What are AI agents?* [Online]. https://builtin.com/articles/ai-agents

College of Occupational Therapists of Ontario. (2024). *What should occupational therapists consider if using artificial intelligence (AI) in practice?* https://www.coto.org/resources/what-should-occupational-therapists-consider-if-using-artificial-intelligence-ai-in-practice/

Fancourt, D., & Finn, S. (2019). *What is the evidence on the role of the arts in improving health and well-being? A scoping review*. World Health Organization. https://iris.who.int/handle/10665/329834

Ford, K., Tesch, L., Dawborn, J., & Courtney-Pratt, H. (2018). Art, music, story: The evaluation of a person-centred arts in health programme in an acute care older persons' unit. *International Journal of Older People Nursing, 13*(2), e12186. https://doi.org/10.1111/opn.12186

Foster, N. (2016). *Workplace health and safety law in Australia* (2nd ed.). LexisNexis Butterworths.

Hasso Plattner Institute of Design at Stanford. (n.d.). *An introduction to design thinking: Process guide*. https://web.stanford.edu/~mshanks/MichaelShanks/files/509554.pdf

Hatherley, J., Kinderlerer, A., Bjerring, J. C., Munch, L. A., & Threlfall, L. (2024). The FHJ debate: Will artificial intelligence replace clinical decision making within our lifetimes? *Future Healthcare Journal, 11*(3), 100178. https://doi.org/10.1016/j.fhj.2024.100178

Mental Health Commission of Canada. (2013). *Psychological health and safety in the workplace – Prevention, promotion, and guidance to staged implementation*. Quebec, Canada. https://

mindscount.org/resources/psychological-health-and-safety-in-the-workplace-prevention-promotion-and-guidance-to-staged-implementation/

Minerals Council of Australia. (2022). *Blueprint for mental health and wellbeing.* https://minerals.org.au/wpcontent/uploads/2022/12/MCA_Mental_Health_Blueprint.pdf

Simó Algado, S., & Townsend, E. A. (2015). Eco-social occupational therapy. *British Journal of Occupational Therapy, 78*(3), 182–186. https://doi.org/10.1177/0308022614561

Townsend, E., & Polatajko, H. (2007). *Enabling occupation II: Advancing an occupational therapy vision for health, well-being, & justice through occupation.* CAOT Publications.

University of Newcastle. (2024). *Newcastle's Institute for Energy and Resources.* https://www.newcastle.edu.au/research/centre/nier

Wilcock, A. A. (1996). *The relationship between occupation and health. Implications for occupational therapy and public health.* University of Adelaide.

Willis, K. (2024). *Good nature: The new science of how nature improves our health.* Bloomsbury Publishing.

Wolfenden, L., Williams, C. M., Wiggers, J., Nathan, N., & Yoong, S. L. (2016). Improving the translation of health promotion interventions using effectiveness-implementation hybrid designs in program evaluations. *Health Promotion Journal of Australia, 27*(3), 204–207. https://doi.org/10.1071/HE16056

World Health Organization [WHO]. (2010). *Healthy workplaces: A model for action.* https://www.who.int/publications/i/item/9789241599313

CHAPTER 34

Occupational therapy process and assistive technology

Libby Callaway, Natasha Layton, Emma Gee, Erin Georgiou, and Sandy Rutherford

Authors' positionality statement

We are all female Caucasian, English-speaking, university-educated occupational therapists, descendant of immigrants from the United Kingdom and Europe. Four people in our authorship group are Australian citizens, and one is an Aotearoa New Zealand citizen who identifies as tauiwi Pākehā and tangata tiriti. We bring personal or professional experiences of assistive technology through clinical work, research, and/or having our own lived or family experiences of the use of assistive technology due to disability, health, or age-related conditions. We acknowledge the systems and structures that afford us unearned privilege. We are committed to improving our understanding and practice around decolonising research, guided by Indigenist and decolonising perspectives, epistemic justice, and people with lived experiences different than our own.

Key terms
- Assistive technology
- Assistive products
- Service provision
- Personnel
- Person-centred practice
- Participation outcomes

Objectives
This chapter will enable the reader to:

- Identify contemporary definitions of assistive technology (AT) and international classification of and terminology for assistive products
- Understand the AT ecosystem that occupational therapists work in across the lifespan
- Learn about existing models of practice and evidence to inform occupational therapy process in the field of AT

DOI: 10.4324/9781003495666-37

■ Gain insight to global, local and lifespan experiences of AT interventions for both people who use assistive technology and occupational therapists

34.1 Introduction

Assistive technology (AT) is an umbrella term for assistive products and their related systems and services. *Assistive products* enable a person to optimise functioning and reduce disability (International Standards Organization [ISO], 2023, p. 7) and are most effective when provided with *assistive services*, that is, skilled assessment; product selection; fitting, training, and use; and maintenance and review (Layton et al., 2022; World Health Organization [WHO] & UNICEF, 2022). Assistive products are always used within the context of an environment and can be considered within a 'technology chain' with environmental interventions or home modifications. For example, some fixtures and fittings such as handrails are classified as assistive products (see Class 18 in Table 34.1).

AT can help maintain or improve a person's functioning across the domains of cognition, communication, hearing, mobility, self-care, and vision. Timely and effective AT provision can also enable health, well-being, inclusion, and participation (WHO & UNICEF, 2022). The provision of AT-enabled interventions should be person centred and often may involve a team of professionals, including occupational therapists (Layton et al., 2022). This is because AT is a key intervention used by occupational therapists to maintain or enhance occupational performance and participation (Akyurek et al., 2017; American Occupational Therapy Association [AOTA], 2016). While occupational therapists may share similar competencies with other professionals in AT provision, the grounding of an occupational therapist's professional reasoning and theoretical foundation in occupation is a unique point of difference (Sarsak et al., 2023).

34.2 People-centred AT practice

In 2022, the first Global Report on Assistive Technology provided clear direction on work to improve access to AT globally (WHO & UNICEF, 2022). The WHO 5P People-Centred AT Model, detailed in the Global Report, illustrates an AT ecosystem focused upon the goals and needs of the person using AT. The WHO 5P model (see Figure 34.1) places the person using AT at the centre of intersecting relationships between assistive products, the personnel who advise on and provide these products (including occupational therapists), provision systems, and overarching policies that guide the funding of assistive products and services (WHO & UNICEF, 2022).

Introducing Emma

I was working as a qualified occupational therapist when I survived a stroke in 2005, at the age of 23. My world suddenly changed from me being an independent adult to needing support for all activities every day. As a stroke survivor, it has been a 19-year rehabilitation journey including the use of assistive technology, home modifications, or other environmental interventions at every step in the process. To read more about my experience, go to www.emma-gee.com.

In following sections in this chapter, I describe the assistive products I use across many product classes (see Table 34.1). I also discuss the occupational therapy process used by therapists collaborating with me to get good AT outcomes linked to my goals and needs.

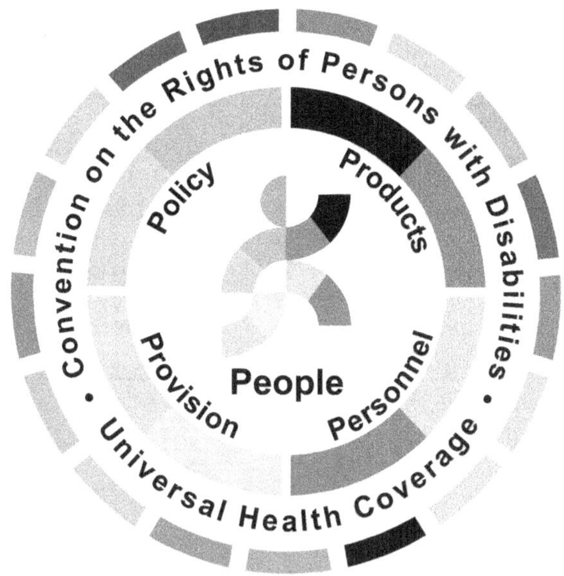

Figure 34.1 The WHO 5P people-centred AT model

Table 34.1 Assistive products and environmental interventions Emma uses

Product class (ISO, 2023)	*Examples of assistive product used*
Class 4 – Assistive products for measuring, stimulating, or training physiological and psychological functions	■ Back support for pain management ■ Pill cutter ■ Focused task lighting
Class 9 – Assistive products for self-care activities and participation in self-care	■ Height-adjustable shower chair ■ Custom-made eye patch for eye protection
Class 12 – Assistive products for activities and participation relating to personal mobility and transportation	■ Four wheeled walking frame with seat and basket ■ Three wheeled motorised scooter
Class 15 – Assistive products for domestic activities and participation in domestic life	■ Sensor rubbish bin ■ Cup holder for walking frame ■ Clothes drying rack ■ Air fryer ■ Retractable garden house
Class 18 – Furnishings, fixtures, and other assistive products for supporting activities in indoor and outdoor human-made environments	■ Grab rails in shower recess ■ Rubber threshold ramp at backdoor
Class 22 – Assistive products for communication and information management	■ Eyeglasses ■ eBook reader ■ Software for writing editing, organising, and storing text and multimedia materials
Class 24 – Assistive products for controlling, carrying, moving, and handling objects and devices	■ Long handled pick-up stick ■ Container openers ■ Motorised door and blind openers

(Continued)

Table 34.1 (Continued)

Product class (ISO, 2023)	Examples of assistive product used
Class 27 – Assistive products for controlling, adapting, or measuring elements of physical environments	■ Smart lighting ■ Non-slip strips in shower recess ■ Humidifier for vision
Class 28 – Assistive products for work activities and participation in employment	■ Ergonomic desk chair ■ Vision Australia keyboard ■ Task-focused lighting for work ■ Footrest
Class 30 – Assistive products for recreation and leisure	■ Recumbent bicycle

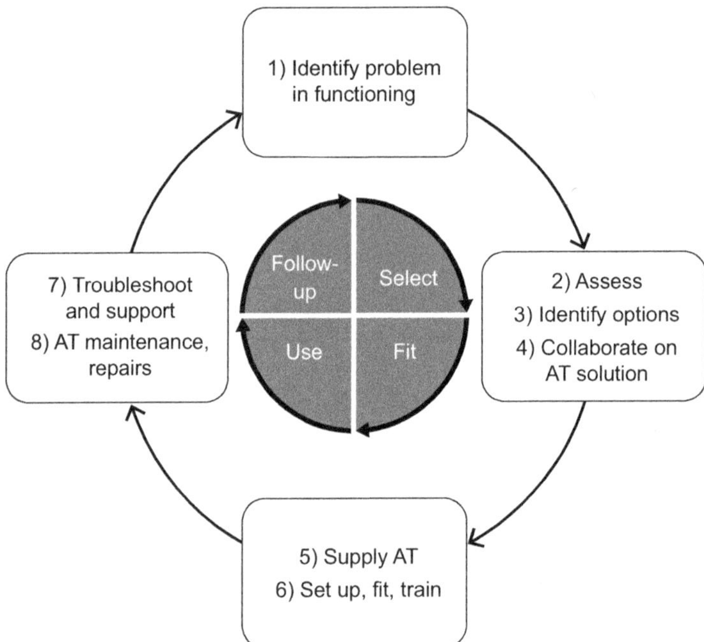

Figure 34.2 AT service provision steps

(Layton et al., 2022; WHO & UNICEF, 2022)

34.3 AT practice steps

The WHO and UNICEF (2022) have summarised AT service provision into four core steps. These are: (1) selecting, (2) fitting, (3) using, and (4) following up AT. These four steps are shown in Figure 34.2, linked to eight more detailed steps compiled in a recent literature review: (1) identifying a problem in functioning; (2) assessing goals and needs; (3) identifying options to try; (4) collaboratively determining the AT solution; (5) supplying assistive product/s or other environmental interventions like home modifications; (6) set up, fitting, and training and the use phase of AT, including (7) troubleshooting and supporting use; and (8) product maintenance and repairs for safe working life and evaluation of effects of the assistive product/s on functioning (Layton et al., 2022).

34.4 Occupational therapy process and AT

Occupational therapists understand occupational participation to be an outcome of the transaction between a person, their environment or context, and the occupations or activities they need or want to do (Akyurek et al., 2017; Law et al., 1996). The profession's holistic perspective, along with a broad scope of practice across assistive product categories, means that occupational therapists are important members of the AT ecosystem (AOTA, 2016; Layton et al., 2022). Within the AT personnel workforce, occupational therapists have a significant scope of practice across all AT practice steps. This includes advice on the selection of *assistive products* to meet a person's occupational performance goals and needs; provision of *assistive services* advising on product choice, setup, and fitting; training on their use for both the person who needs the AT as well as significant others who may assist the person to use the product (like family members or paid support workers); and *measurement of AT outcomes* achieved (Steel & Layton, 2016).

Chapter 29 describes *occupational therapy assessment* in more detail; however, specific to interventions that include AT, occupational therapists may use varied methods including published assessment tools, functional observation, and customised approaches. These approaches closely consider, analyse, and document body functions and structures; activities and participation; and personal and environmental factors that may be a barrier or enabler to functioning (WHO, 2018). Importantly, task, activity, and occupation analysis are all central to both occupational therapy assessment and intervention planning in the field of AT (see Chapter 30). The effectiveness of AT as an *occupational therapy intervention* depends upon the relationship between the assistive product, the context of its use, and the goals of the person using the AT (Akyurek et al., 2017; Federici & Scherer, 2017). Linked to assessment, *measuring AT outcomes* is also an important part of occupational therapy practice and can help to avoid product under-use or abandonment.

34.5 Occupational therapy scope of practice across assistive product classes

Occupational therapists may help people consider assistive products across all eleven ISO9999 product classes (ISO, 2023). Although occupational therapists frequently recommend low-risk or low-cost AT in everyday practice to enable occupational performance (e.g., long-handled bathing or dressing assistive products for self-care; pencil grips or other writing aids for education or work tasks), other assistive products require more in-depth levels of training, supervision, and mentoring and/or the development of advanced scope of occupational therapy practice (e.g., robotics; alternate computer access systems like voice or eye gaze controls; powered mobility products; smart home technology systems) (AOTA, 2016).

> ## Occupational therapy process and AT – Emma's experience
>
> I have worked with occupational therapists throughout every stage of my stroke rehabilitation, from my initial hospitalisation through to living in my own home now. Occupational therapists have worked with me to assess my goals and needs and recommend certain assistive technology interventions based on this assessment process. When trying new AT, design elements like product weight, colour, and other aesthetics are important to consider. Testing the products in the environments where I am going to use them (rather than only in a showroom) is also important. Occupational therapists also write reports to justify National Disability Insurance Scheme (NDIS) funding for mid- or high-cost assistive products, as well as any services I need. They have had an important role in setting up and educating both myself and other people – like my support workers – on how to use the AT, particularly more complex or high-risk AT. Collaborative problem solving of any unexpected issues that arise, and plans for routine maintenance, have also been important so I can get the AT outcomes I need.

34.6 Occupational therapy theory and AT

New technologies enter the marketplace every day, and it is not possible for an occupational therapist to maintain in-depth knowledge across all assistive products available. Occupational therapy practice models and frameworks therefore play an important role in guiding effective AT practice, enabling occupational therapists to evaluate assistive products whilst considering the interaction of the person, the environment, and their desired occupations (see Chapter 28). In addition to discipline-specific models of practice, the International Classification for Functioning, Disability and Health (ICF) provides a useful framework to guide occupational therapy practice, classifying assistive products and technology as environmental factors that may pose barriers or be enablers to activities and participation (Steel & Layton, 2016; WHO, 2018). For further application of the ICF within occupational therapy practice in the field of AT within Australia's NDIS, see Vignette 1 in Chapter 3.

34.7 Occupational therapy practice and AT with communities

AT, home modifications, and other environmental interventions are essential facilitators of independent living and participation for the one in five Australians and one in four Aotearoa New Zealanders living with disability (AIHW, 2024; Whaikaha Ministry of Disabled People, 2024). Occupational therapists work across the lifespan, providing assistive products and services for children, adults, and older people that support individuals to be included and participate in occupations they want or need to do (Sarsak et al., 2023). AT is provided by occupational therapists for people with a range of health-, age-, or disability-related AT needs and with various conditions that the person may be born with or acquire which impact functioning (Layton et al., 2022; WHO, 2018).

As part of culturally safe occupational therapy practice, it is also important to consider different perspectives on the use of AT. Occupational therapy associations internationally are revising accreditation and competency standards to be culturally responsive and are engaging in critical reflection of what it takes to move from individualistic to relational allyship (Whalley Hammell et al., 2022) and how to enact decolonisation in occupational therapy courses (Rudman et al., 2021). Specific to First Nations communities in Australia and Aotearoa New Zealand, there is only a small body of literature to guide culturally safe and respectful AT practice for occupational therapists and other AT advisors. Of the evidence that does exist, there is a focus on decolonising Western approaches with Māori and Aboriginal and Torres Strait Islander people and their families (Whānau or mob) (Boland et al., 2020; iLA, 2024). More research led by and with these communities is necessary to guide AT practice, and genuine engagement by occupational therapists is required, as exemplified through this community listening approach to uncovering First Nations perspectives on AT (iLA, 2025).

34.8 Occupational therapy ethics in practice using AT

Ethical occupational therapy practice in the field of AT is guided and regulated by occupational therapy professional associations and regulatory bodies in Australia and Aotearoa New Zealand, and the individual practitioner's capability or scope of practice (see also Chapter 7) occupational therapy professional registration requirements and ethical codes identify that practicing clinicians must act with integrity, honesty, and transparency and disclose any real, perceived, or potential conflicts of interest when making recommendations regarding, or providing, assistive products and/or services. There are a range of ways actual, potential, or perceived conflict of interest can occur for occupational therapists working in the field of AT. These could include completing assessments that recommend supports and equipment that financially benefit the occupational therapist, prescribing supports and referring to an organisation that gives them incentives or gifts, or having a conflicted relationship when prescribing complex AT from specific providers (National Disability Insurance Scheme, 2024). These conflicts must be closely considered and mitigated against within ethical occupational therapy AT practice (AOTA, 2016).

34.9 AI, AT, and occupational therapy

Occupational therapists must also consider ethical practice in relation to the growing field of artificial intelligence–enabled AT (Kaelin et al., 2024). AI-enabled AT exist and are growing across almost all assistive product classes. Occupational therapists are now using AI in practice across assessment and within interventions, as well as for report writing and other administrative tasks and education (Canadian Occupational Therapy Association, 2023). Guidance to manage the risks and the benefits of AI-enabled AT in occupational therapy practice focuses on maintaining or enhancing a person's occupational performance and participation, considering occupational justice and respect for diversity, and transparency regarding use and respect for the privacy of data (AOTA, 2016; Kaelin et al., 2024). Because AI is emerging technology which offers potential to bring with it both challenges and opportunities, as well as risks and rewards (Smith et al., 2023), both Australian and New Zealand governing bodies have invested in frameworks and guidance on the use of AI in health and disability care which occupational therapy practice can be informed by (Office of the Prime Minister's Chief Science Advisor, 2023; Silvera et al., 2022).

34.10 Evidence-based occupational therapy practice in the field of AT

Because AT is considered in relation to each person's goals and needs, as well as the contexts in which they use assistive products or environmental interventions, it is proposed that the focus of evidence-based occupational therapy practice is not on the technology itself but the use of assistive products and services as part of a dynamic system of occupational therapy-related interventions (AOTA, 2016). This is because the highly individualised provision and training on the use of AT, as well as the environments in which AT is used, makes the traditional evidence from an evidence-based practice paradigm (i.e., evidence drawn from well-designed clinical trials and subsequent meta-analyses) difficult to obtain. Moreover, AT continues to rapidly advance, often forging ahead of published evidence available to guide practice. It is therefore also important to consider non-empirical evidence that can inform practice (Hoffman et al., 2023).

Adding to this challenge, a recent review of international clinical practice guidelines in the area of complex and progressive conditions for adults demonstrated the significant evidence gap that exists in relation to AT, with only 7% of guidelines identified mentioning AT as an intervention and a range of different terminology used to describe assistive products (Callaway et al., 2025). Some guidance in relation to particular populations is available in the form of evidence reviews by funders of AT, such as the review by Australia's National Disability Insurance Agency on AT interventions to support children (National Disability Insurance Agency, 2023). There are reviews on specific assistive product classes led by occupational therapists (see, for example, Charlton et al., 2025 and Karlsson et al., 2018). Given the challenges noted, however, occupational therapists must stay informed of current and emerging technological advances and consider the best evidence available combined with occupational therapy models to guide practice, whilst continuing to hone their skills in functional performance, task and activity, and environmental analysis and adaptations to enhance performance outcomes (AOTA, 2016).

34.11 Vignette 1

Sarah is a 20-month-old child with cerebral palsy. She lives at home with her parents, who have dedicated themselves to supporting individualised developmental opportunities for Sarah since she came home from the hospital. Sarah is a bright and sociable child who likes to be involved in play with her parents and other children.

Sarah's early motor assessments with an occupational therapist found that, at 20 months of age, Sarah is able to sit with support and pull herself along the floor but cannot crawl, pull herself to stand, or take any steps.

Sarah's parents highly value the goal of Sarah being able to move around independently. Sarah's mother is now planning to return to work, and the family are beginning to consider what Sarah's experience of childcare may be. Her parents are worried about how Sarah will be included in this environment and if she will be able to move around and play with other children. They have begun to discuss with Sarah's occupational therapist how to best facilitate her participation goals at childcare, and the therapist reassured the family that participation goals involving assistive products for mobility can assist alongside goals for motor skill development (Livingstone & Field, 2014). Working collaboratively with the family, the occupational therapist demonstrated, took step-by-step photos of, and wrote up an activity-based programme they could complete with Sarah at home to assist motor skill development. The occupational therapist also worked through the WHO four-step process (WHO & UNICEF, 2022) to identify possible options for assistive technology that might facilitate Sarah's safe access and participation in the childcare environment with other children.

34.11.1 Selecting AT

Sarah's barriers to participation in the childcare environment were identified to be linked to her motor changes impacting mobility. Therefore, assistive products for mobility were considered the best option to facilitate Sarah to keep up with her peers for social and play engagement and inclusion (Bray et al., 2020). Based on Sarah's current function as well as her capacity for continued development, both an introductory attendant and self-propelled (Scooot Mobility Rider – https://askned.com.au/children/scooter-boards-and-trolleys/leckey-firefly-scooot/) and more advanced powered mobility device (Wizzybug – https://askned.com.au/children/childrens-wheelchairs/childrens-powered-wheelchairs/wizzybug-powered-wheelchair/) were selected and trialled with Sarah and her parents in the home and childcare environments. It was important that the options trialled could be accessed through hire or loan schemes (rather than purchase) so that suitability of the products could be regularly reviewed and exchanged in response to Sarah's continuing development and growth (Botelho, 2021).

34.11.2 Fitting AT to the user's goals and needs

Sarah was able to begin practising use of the Scooot independently once the control was demonstrated to her and her parents by the occupational therapist. The occupational therapist was aware the Scooot would be useful for moving around indoors, but it would not suitable for accessing the outdoors area and playground at childcare (due to the tanbark surfacing). The Wizzybug was suitable for outdoors access and play, but Sarah needed more time to learn the skills to safely and independently use the Wizzybug when others were present in her environment. The Wizzybug controller was set up on Sarah's right side so she could reach it using her dominant hand.

34.11.3 Using AT

A written training plan for practise was put in place by the occupational therapist to ensure opportunities for Sarah to practise and build confidence in using both the Scooot at home in her familiar environment before commencing Scooot use at childcare. Through a total of three occupational therapy sessions, structured opportunities were offered for Sarah and her parents to practice with the powered mobility option with graded skill introduction. Following these sessions, further parent education and a plan for regularly practice by Sarah with her parents was put in place at home. The occupational therapist arranged to attend the childcare initially with Sarah to support both her and childcare staff to familiarise with use and charging of the Scooot and safely navigating the environment with full supervision. A collaborative plan for graded introduction of use of the Scooot with small modifications to the environment and play spaces was also made. This included removing any unnecessary furnishings that could impede independent environmental exploration and clearing passageways for Sarah to move alongside her friends for side-by-side and interactive play.

34.11.4 Following up AT use

To ensure successful progress, the occupational therapist followed up with Sarah and her family to review and update the activity-based home programme as her skills developed. These reviews also allowed for monitoring of Sarah's readiness to transition to graded use of the Wizzybug into the childcare environment. As part of follow up, the occupational therapist facilitated discussion with Sarah and her parents about expanding Sarah's participation opportunities as her safe use of mobility assistive products progressed. This ensured that her continued capacity for learning and early childhood development was promoted both within and outside of the home.

34.12 Occupational therapy and AT outcomes

The WHO identifies 'follow up' as an important step in the AT process. This should include measuring outcomes achieved via the provision of assistive products and services. Measuring outcomes is important to evaluate how AT has worked for the person, any additional customisation or training/education on use that may be needed, and whether the person's goals and needs have been met. Occupational therapists need to consider the ways outcomes can be assessed, and following are some examples of published measures that may be used across different domains:

- The ICF checklist (version 2.1a clinician form) provides a detailed set of *bodily functions and structures* to be considered, as well as *impairments* that may be experienced (https://www.who.int/publications/m/item/icf-checklist).
- Outcome measures relating to AT interventions for *activities* or *occupational performance* may include the Australian Therapy Outcomes Measures (https://austoms.com/) or Canadian Occupational Performance Measure (https://www.thecopm.ca/).
- Measures relating to the *assistive products and/or services* may include, for example, the Quebec User Evaluation of Satisfaction with Assistive Technology (QuEST 2.0) (Demers, Weiss-Lambrou & Ska, 2002) or the Psychosocial Impact of Assistive Devices Scale (www.piads.at).
- *Context* is also important to consider, and examples of measures that occupational therapists may utilise in collaboration with an AT user include the Residential Environment Impact Scale (version 4.0 short or long form) (for details, go to https://moho-irm.uic.edu/productDetails.aspx?iid=5) or section 3 of the ICF Checklist (version 2.1a clinician form), focused on environmental barriers and enablers (WHO, 2003).

34.13 Vignette 2

Marion is a divorced 61-year-old woman diagnosed with motor neurone disease (MND) two years ago. She lives at home alone in a single level three-bedroom house. Marion previously worked as a high school teacher but had to retire early due to significant fatigue and the progression of MND symptoms. She has three adult children. Her two daughters live in Auckland, and she speaks on the phone with them most days. Marion's son lives in America, and Marion video calls him each Sunday. Marion has a large network of friends and colleagues who she is in regular contact with and check in on her often. She has a large package of care which enables her to live at home.

Marion requires a hoist for all transfers in and out of her wheelchair and on and off her bed and shower commode. She is assisted to shower using a shower/commode chair and dress on her hospital bed. Marion visits her hairdresser once a week to have her hair washed and styled. She is dependent on others for all cooking, cleaning, and household tasks.

Marion was provided with a multifunction power chair following her first wheelchair and seating assessment with an occupational therapist and physiotherapist. However, she is now having difficulty using a standard joystick to move the wheelchair. Marion has very limited hand function, and her muscles fatigue very quickly. She frequently has to rest her hand and sometimes gets stuck in the hallway of her home or on her way to her hairdresser located at the local shops. Marion is no longer able to hold her phone or use the touch screen on it. She uses the tilt and recline functions on her power chair to redistribute pressure and reduce the likelihood of a pressure injury. She also has a pressure-relieving cushion to reduce the risk of skin breakdown. Her home has been modified following involvement of a community occupational therapist, who arranged for a ramp at her front door and a stepless wet area shower to be installed.

Marion wishes to remain at home for as long as she can. She describes feelings of fear of something happening to her in between visits from her carers, as she cannot summon help using her mobile phone. She can only be in contact with friends and family when someone else is in the house to assist her. Marion is also no longer able to operate her television. She is keen to explore the use of an alternative joystick and her mobile phone connected via Bluetooth to her wheelchair to enable her to operate her phone and television via her wheelchair joystick.

34.13.1 Selecting AT

As Marion's condition is progressive, it is important to think about how current AT provisions could be modified in the future so she can continue use (National Institute for Health and Care Excellence, 2016). This information is carefully and sensitively shared with Marion by the occupational therapist. Funding is also dependent on meeting eligibility criteria, and every item which has a cost must be well justified to the funder. Marion is eligible because she is a New Zealand citizen, she has a physical disability which will persist longer than 6 months, and her disability impacts her ability to compete everyday tasks around her home. Bluetooth is a function that is already present in her current wheelchair, and she already has a smart phone which works well with the make of wheelchair she uses. Provision of these additional features means Marion will be able to remain in her home, move around in it, and communicate effectively to summon help if needed. It is also possible to use these features via a head array in the future if Marion can no longer operate the joystick on her wheelchair as the symptoms of MND progress. An alternative joystick can be positioned at the elbow, foot, or other location if needed. It was important to check that the mount for the mobile phone and the joystick were able to be fitted to Marion's wheelchair as they come from different suppliers.

Marion's goals were explored and recorded using the Wheelchair Outcome Measure (Mortenson et al., 2007), which is based on the ICF, to record baseline and outcome

Table 34.2 Marion's baseline and outcome rating on the Wheelchair Outcome Measure

Participation goals in and around home	Importance	Satisfaction (baseline, before AT intervention)	Satisfaction (outcome, post-AT intervention)
To use the joystick on my wheelchair to access my phone to talk with and video call friends and family.	10/10	1/10	10/10
To feel more confident in my ability to summon help when needed.	10/10	1/10	8/10
To access my smart TV to watch movies on Netflix using the joystick on my wheelchair.	8/10	2/10	10/10
To be able to drive my wheelchair around the house without needing a rest or getting stranded in the hallway.	10/10	4/10	8/10
Participation goals outside of home or in my community	Importance	Satisfaction (baseline, before AT intervention)	Satisfaction (outcome, post-AT intervention)
To use my wheelchair to go to my hairdresser at the local shops.	7/10	2/10	8/10

measurement of wheelchair provision on participation as well as body structures and functions (see Table 34.2).

34.13.2 Fitting AT to the user's goals and needs

A personal alarm (pendant and wrist alarm) was explored, but Marion was unable to activate the alarm button due to weakness in her upper limbs. A larger grooved mushroom joystick handle was trialled on her power wheelchair, and Marion was able to drive her wheelchair with less effort and fatigue and control the joystick with ease. The community occupational therapist observed that Marion was able to operate her phone via this joystick on her wheelchair after the Bluetooth connection was set up and demonstration was provided to her. This setup and use was video recorded and the video sent to Marion to show her carers to enable them to assist her with any troubleshooting if needed.

34.13.3 Using AT

With training from the occupational therapist, therapy assistants from the wheelchair and seating service were able to visit Marion twice to practice using her new technology. They also went with her to her hairdresser to check if she was able to manage to drive this distance with the new joystick.

34.13.4 Following up AT use

Marion was encouraged to contact the occupational therapist if she experienced any difficulties using the modifications to her wheelchair. After Marion had been using the new setup for four weeks, the therapist phoned her to revisit her responses on the

Wheelchair Outcome Measure (see Table 34.2). MND symptoms progress rapidly, and so Marion was put on the review list as a Priority One client to be seen again in six months rather than the usual two years.

34.14 Conclusion

Assistive technology is fundamental to enablement and inclusion and a core intervention within the scope of occupational therapy practice. Provision of assistive products and services can be improved by collaboration with people who use AT in their own lives whilst also striving for and reflecting on the congruence between occupational therapy theory, process, and outcomes (Steel & Layton, 2016). The 5P people-centred AT model, working definitions, and practice steps from the World Health Organization offer useful considerations for occupational therapists when collaborating with AT users to address their assistive product and service goals and needs.

34.15 Summary

- Assistive technology (AT) includes both products and services, and occupational therapists are key personnel in the AT ecosystem.
- Person-centred practice by occupational therapists holds central the goals and needs of the person using AT, the occupational performance they want or need to achieve, and the context of their occupational performance.
- AT interventions are often used by occupational therapists concurrently with rehabilitative or habilitative approaches and for people of all ages and abilities.
- The grounding of an occupational therapist's professional reasoning and theoretical foundation in occupation is important, with a primary goal of AT being to maintain or enhance functioning linked to meaningful occupational participation.
- Occupational therapists provide AT assessments, advice on both assistive products and services, and interventions that include AT as a core area of practice.
- Whilst evidence-based practice is strongly encouraged, the rapid growth in technology (including in AI-enabled AT) means that research gaps exist and occupational therapists will need to draw on evidenced theoretical models and frameworks to guide practice.
- Measuring AT outcomes is important in occupational therapy practice and may focus on the person using AT and changes in functioning achieved; their occupational performance within activities undertaken, evaluation of effectiveness of assistive products and/or services, and/or measurement of the person's context of use.

34.16 Review and reflection questions

- The World Health Organization describes assistive technology as an umbrella term — what two core concepts fit under the umbrella of assistive technology?
- What five components (beginning with P) are described in the 5P people-centred AT model?
- List the eight AT service provision steps.
- Which AT service provision steps may an occupational therapist have a role in?

- What are some of the ways occupational therapists can stay informed of current and emerging technological advances and consider the best evidence to guide practice?
- Can you think of an example of risks that may be posed in the use of AI-enabled AT and how occupational therapists may play a role in reducing or mitigating that risk?

References

Akyurek, G., Kars, S., Celik, Z., Koc, C., & Cesim, Ö. B. (2017). Assistive technology in occupational therapy. *InTech.* https://doi.org/10.5772/intechopen.68471

American Occupational Therapy Association (2016). Assistive technology and occupational performance. *American Journal of Occupational Therapy, 70*(Supp 2), 7012410030p1–7012410030p9. https://doi.org/10.5014/ajot.2016.706S02

Australian Institute of Health and Welfare (AIHW). (2024). *People with disability in Australia.* Author. https://www.aihw.gov.au/reports/disability/people-with-disability-in-australia/contents/summary

Boland, P., Jones, B., Stanley, J., Graham, F., Perry, M., & Levack, W. (2020). Using a Māori model of health to analyse the use of equipment by New Zealand Māori post-stroke. *New Zealand Journal of Occupational Therapy, 67*(2), 19–26.

Botelho, F. H. F. (2021). Childhood and assistive technology: Growing with opportunity, developing with technology. *Assistive Technology, 33*(Supp 1), 87–93. https://doi.org/10.1080/10400435.2021.1971330

Bray, N., Kolehmainen, N., McAnuff, J., Tanner, L., Tuersley, L., Beyer, F., Grayston, A., Wilson, D., Edwards, R. T., Noyes, J., & Craig, D. (2020). Powered mobility interventions for very young children with mobility limitations to aid participation and positive development: The EMPoWER evidence synthesis. *Health Technology Assessment, 24*(50), 1–194. https://doi.org/10.3310/hta24500

Callaway, L., Bragge, P., Ego, C., Delafosse, V., Lennox, A., Hill, K., & Layton, N. (2025). A review of international clinical guidelines that inform the use of assistive technology to support adults living with progressive or complex conditions. *Disability and Rehabilitation: Assistive Technology.* https://doi.org/10.1080/17483107.2025.2449993

Canadian Occupational Therapy Association. (2023). *Occupational therapy, artificial intelligence and technology.* Author. Retrieved November 17, 2024, from https://caot.ca/document/8063/OT%20&%20AI_Final%20Copy_EN.pdf

Charlton, K., Murray, C., Layton, N., Ong, E., Farrar, L., Serocki, T., & Attrill, S. (2025). Manual wheelchair training approaches and intended training outcomes for adults who are new to wheelchair use: A scoping review. *Australian Occupational Therapy Journal, 72*(1), e12992. https://doi.org/10.1111/1440-1630.12992

Demers, L., Weiss-Lambrou, R., & Ska, B. (2002). Development of the Quebec User Evaluation of Satisfaction with Assistive Technology (QUEST). *Technology and Disability, 14*(3), 101–105. https://doi.org/10.3233/TAD-2002-14304

Federici, S., & Scherer, M. (Eds.). (2017). *Assistive technology assessment handbook.* CRC Press.

Hoffman, T., Bennett, S., & Del Mar, C. (2023). *Evidence-based practice across the health professions* (4th ed.). Elsevier.

iLA. (2024). *LiveUp better practice guide for culturally safe information about assistive products.* Author. https://www.ilaustralia.org.au/rethink-ageing/resources-research

iLA. (2025). *First Nations perspectives on assistive technology (AT) and home modifications (HM) service provision: A community listening report.* https://www.ilaustralia.org.au/docs/default-source/research-and-projects/first-nations---community-listening-report.pdf?sfvrsn=48dcac8c_1

International Standards Organization. (2023). *Australian/New Zealand Standard™ assistive products – Classification and terminology (AS/NZS ISO 9999:2023)*. Author.

Kaelin, V. C., Nilsson, I., & Lindgren, H. (2024). Occupational therapy in the space of artificial intelligence: Ethical considerations and human-centered efforts. *Scandinavian Journal of Occupational Therapy*, 31(1), 2421355. https://doi.org/10.1080/11038128.2024.2421355

Karlsson, P., Allsop, A., Dee-Price, B. J., & Wallen, M. (2018). Eye-gaze control technology for children, adolescents and adults with cerebral palsy with significant physical disability: Findings from a systematic review. *Developmental Neurorehabilitation*, 21(8), 497–505. https://doi.org/10.1080/17518423.2017.1362057

Law, M., Cooper, B., Strong, S., Stewart, D., Rigby, P., & Letts, L. (1996). The Person-Environment-Occupation Model: A transactive approach to occupational performance. *Canadian Journal of Occupational Therapy*, 63(1), 9–23. https://doi.org/10.1177/000841749606300103

Layton, N., O'Connor, J., Fitzpatrick, A., & Carey, S. (2022). Towards co-design in delivering assistive technology interventions: Reconsidering roles for consumers, allied health practitioners, and the support workforce. *International Journal of Environmental Research and Public Health*, 19(21), 14408. https://doi.org/10.3390/ijerph192114408

Livingstone, R., & Field, D. (2014). Systematic review of power mobility outcomes for infants, children and adolescents with mobility limitations. *Clinical Rehabilitation*, 28(10), 954–64. https://doi.org/10.1177/0269215514531262

Mortenson, W. B., Miller, W. C., & Miller-Pogar, J. (2007). Measuring wheelchair intervention outcomes: Development of the wheelchair outcome measure. *Disability and Rehabilitation: Assistive Technology*, 2(5), 275–285. https://doi.org/10.1080/17483100701475863

National Disability Insurance Agency. (2023). *Assistive technology interventions to support children: An evidence snapshot*. Author. https://dataresearch.ndis.gov.au/research-and-evaluation/market-stewardship-and-employment/assistive-technology-interventions-support-children

National Disability Insurance Scheme. (2024). *Conflicts of interest in the NDIS provider market*. Author. https://www.ndis.gov.au/providers/provider-compliance/conflicts-interest-ndis-provider-market

National Institute for Health and Care Excellence. (2016). *Motor neurone disease: Assessment and management*. Author. https://www.nice.org.uk/guidance/ng42/resources/motor-neurone-disease-assessment-and-management-pdf-1837449470149

Office of the Prime Minister's Chief Science Advisor. (2023). *Capturing the benefits of AI in healthcare for Aotearoa New Zealand – Full report*. Author. https://doi.org/10.17608/k6.OPMCSA.24814101

Rudman, M. T., Flavell, H., Harris, C., & Wright, M. (2021). How prepared is Australian occupational therapy to decolonise its practice? *Australian Occupational Therapy Journal*, 68(4), 287–297. https://doi.org/10.1111/1440-1630.12725

Sarsak, H. I., Kamadu, A., Pearlman, J., Goldberg, M., Kandavel, K., & Augustine, N. (2023). A perspective on occupational therapy and assistive technology: Research, contributions, challenges and global initiatives. *WFOT Bulletin*, 79(2), 1–9. https://doi.org/10.1080/14473828.2023.2196794

Silvera, D., Packer, K., Higgins, L., Walker, J., Niven, P., Li J., Byrnes, J., Khanna, S., Liu, D., & Freyne, J. (2022). *Framework for artificial intelligence enabled assistive technology as supports under the National Disability Insurance Scheme: Final report*. Commonwealth Scientific and Industrial Research Organisation. https://dataresearch.ndis.gov.au/research-and-evaluation/market-stewardship-and-employment/markets-and-innovations-research

Smith, E. M., Graham, D., Morgan, C., & MacLachlan, M. (2023). Artificial intelligence and assistive technology: Risks, rewards, challenges, and opportunities. *Assistive Technology*, 35(5), 375–377. https://doi.org/10.1080/10400435.2023.2259247

Steel, E. J., & Layton, N. (2016). Assistive technology in Australia: Integrating theory and evidence into action. *Australian Occupational Therapy Journal*, 63(6), 381–390. https://doi.org/10.1111/1440-1630.12293

Whaikaha Ministry of Disabled People. (2024). *Appendix: Disabled people population and life outcome statistics*. Author. https://www.whaikaha.govt.nz/about-us/corporate-publications/annual-reports/annual-report-2024/appendix

Whalley Hammell, K., Laliberte Rudman, D., Zafran, H., Schmidt, J., Bunting, K., Bulk, L., Grenier, M., Desormeaux-Loreau, M., Lee, M., Jarus, T., & Ben Mortenson, W. (2022). Unbecoming change agents. *Canadian Journal of Occupational Therapy, 89*(2), 96–102. https://doi.org/10.1177/00084174221089708

World Health Organization. (2003). *ICF checklist, version 2.1a: Clinician form*. World Health Organization.

World Health Organization. (2018). *International Classification of Functioning, Disability and Health (ICF)*. Author. https://www.who.int/standards/classifications/international-classification-of-functioning-disability-and-health

World Health Organization [WHO] & the United Nations Children's Fund [UNICEF]. (2022). *Global report on assistive technology*. Authors. https://www.who.int/publications/i/item/9789240049451

CHAPTER 35

Sustainability and occupational therapy

Tenelle J. Hodson, Tracey Parnell, and Keri McMullan

Authors' positionality statement

The authors recognise the impact that their world view and experiences have had on the writing of this chapter. All authors have brought their lived experiences, knowledge, and values to the chapter, including a mix of rural, regional, and metropolitan upbringings and knowledge of feminist theory, critical disability studies, eco-health principles, and decolonisation. Two authors have not completed any formal study in relation to sustainability, with their own interests and research growing their insight into this area. One author was formerly a biodiversity ranger. All authors share a deep appreciation for sustainability and how it facilitates the achievement of occupational participation, justice, health, and wellbeing. All authors are non-Indigenous to their countries of residence. Tenelle J. Hodson and Tracey Parnell are both non-Indigenous, white Australians and pay respect to the Traditional Custodians of the lands on which they live and work. Keri McMullan is Pākehā (New Zealand European) and Tangata Tiriti (acknowledging their responsibility of active citizenship by virtue of te Tiriti o Waitangi). Keri pays respect to the people of Ngai Tahu, Kāti Māmoe and Waitaha, who are the custodians of their birthplace: Ōtākou, Te Wai Pounamu. All authors recognise that issues of sustainability disproportionately impact the Traditional Custodians of the countries they live in and that the Traditional Custodians hold knowledge of practices which are vital to facilitate sustainability. The missing voices of Aboriginal, Torres Strait Islander, and Māori Peoples is a recognised limitation of this chapter, as these insights are invaluable. Finally, the authors understand that their cisgender or cishetero-passing, middle-class, tertiary educated, able-bodied position in society has afforded them privilege in how they experience the world and their understanding of it.

Key words
- Environmental sustainability
- Social sustainability

DOI: 10.4324/9781003495666-38

- Economic sustainability
- Occupational justice

Objectives
This chapter will allow the readers to:

- Understand three key aspects of sustainability: environmental, social, and economic
- Develop an understanding of how sustainability relates to occupational therapy practice
- Develop an appreciation for the role occupational therapists can play in sustainability
- Identify how occupational therapists can approach practice in a more sustainable manner and why this is important

35.1 Introduction

Sustainability can be defined as 'meeting the needs of the present without compromising the ability of future generations to meet their own needs' (World Commission on Environment and Development, 1987). For occupational therapists, sustainability plays a pivotal role in ensuring future generations have the conditions available to them to enable occupational participation. Drolet et al. (2020) suggest that occupational therapists should promote sustainable occupations that consider intergenerational occupational justice or 'mokopuna decisions': planning for future generations' wellbeing. The United Nations (UN; n.d.) posits that there are three relevant areas for consideration in terms of sustainability: environmental, social, and economic. Optimal sustainability initiatives target all three components simultaneously although there are situations where initiatives may preference one element over others.

The main body of this chapter starts with a general overview of sustainability before discussing three aspects of sustainability and how occupational therapy can contribute to each of these. Environmental sustainability is discussed first to reflect the urgent need for climate action to ensure that the global context can support occupational participation. Following this, social sustainability is discussed to reflect that at the heart of occupational therapy is a focus on justice and equity to enable people to live meaningful and fulfilling lives through participation in the occupations they need and want to do. Finally, the need for occupational therapists to consider and contribute to economic sustainability will be discussed to demonstrate how the profession can show its unique value in sustaining economies.

35.2 Sustainability – Mātiro whakamua | Look beyond the horizon, beyond the obvious

To achieve sustainability, there is a need to uphold all three elements of sustainability. For instance, for environmentally sustainable actions to be normalised, they must be socially and economically acceptable and equitable. Occupational therapists are well placed to address sustainability by promoting occupational participation that considers environmental, social, and economic issues associated with daily occupations (Hudson & Aoyama, 2008). The World Federation of Occupational Therapy (WFOT) 2012 position statement on sustainability and sustainable practices recognised the interconnected relationship between occupational participation, health, wellbeing, and environmental sustainability. Over time the focus on sustainability has shifted to include issues of social and economic sustainability. Sustainable reasoning requires looking beyond the obvious in daily practice, which can be difficult when addressing what may appear to be the most pressing and obvious needs of individuals and collectives. To facilitate sustainable reasoning, professional reasoning must evolve from focusing on specific situations to considering downstream environmental, social, and financial costs (Hess & Rihtman, 2023).

Advocacy is an important component of the role of occupational therapy in sustainability initiatives and involves speaking publicly about issues of interest and justice to promote the rights of individuals and collectives (Gonclaves et al., 2025). For example, occupational therapists may be involved in advocating for policies that support environmental sustainability and occupational justice through promoting green spaces in urban areas, or they may work with marginalised communities who are disproportionately affected by climate change disasters to support recovery efforts. By advocating with and for individuals and collectives to promote sustainability, occupational therapists make valuable contributions to environments, policies, and practices that support health and wellbeing.

35.2.1 Environmental sustainability & occupational therapy – Ka ora te whenua, ka ora te tangata | When the land is well, the people are well (Tiwaiwaka). The interconnection of all living beings

The biggest threat to environmental sustainability is climate change, resulting from exploitative, unsustainable practices often undertaken to enable participation in daily occupations. Climate change has been described as 'the biggest global health threat of the 21st century' and has the potential to impact how people engage in daily occupations now and in the future (Costello et al., 2009, p. 1693). Given both the impact that occupations have on the environment, as well as the impact extreme weather events are having on occupational participation, occupational therapists can have a key role to play in preventing, addressing and responding to environmental sustainability challenges. Before continuing with an exploration of environmental sustainability, the authors would like to recognise the incredible work that Indigenous leadership is doing in this space, despite not being the peoples who have driven climate change, that is, the Global North.

An occupational justice perspective posits that enabling occupations harmful to the environment, and thus to future generations' health and opportunities, is unethical. In addition to considering future generations, climate change is already negatively impacting marginalised communities, requiring an intersectional perspective. For example, Indigenous peoples, people with disabilities, older adults, younger children, and rural and remote people are all more likely to be adversely impacted by the effects of climate change and climate change related disasters (Intergovernmental Panel on Climate Change, 2022). Both the Occupational Therapy Board of Australia (OTBA) and the Occupational Therapy Board of New Zealand | Te Poari Whakaora Ngangahau o Aotearoa (OTBNZ) outline competency standards that stipulate the requirement for occupational therapists to uphold occupational justice and consider intersectionality. For instance, within the OTBA's Competency Standards (2018) reference is made to *addressing issues of occupational justice in practice* and *managing the influences of values and culture.* The OTBNZ requires occupational therapists to be responsive to te Tiriti o Waitangi (the country's founding document), which guarantees active protection over whenua | land and other taonga | treasures.

While recognising that individual action is only a component of climate action, occupational therapists' unique focus on occupational participation allows a focus on everyday actions that are either environmentally sustainable or not, and to promote or transition away from such actions (Dieterle, 2020; Hess & Rihtman, 2023). Working alongside other people's values, and in the practicalities of daily living, occupational therapists can support sustainable change. The profession's skillset includes supporting people through occupational transitions, adapting to new ways of meaningful participation, modifying equipment, and facilitating habit change. These transferable skills can help people to adopt new ways (or return to old ways) of environmentally sustainable doing.

Occupational therapists can also offer a role in adaptation as climate change will require significant occupational transitions. For example, land displacement, ecological changes impacting food systems, and changes to disease patterns will all impact where and how people live (Costello et al., 2009). Occupational therapists can assist individuals and collectives to adapt to such changes. As with all transitional spaces, unknown occupational adaptations will reveal themselves over the course of time (Smith et al., 2020).

35.2.2 Social sustainability & occupational therapy. He waka eke noa | We are all in this together

Social sustainability is focused on the creation of systems and structures that support social justice and equity, uphold human rights, and build a society where all individuals have opportunities to participate regardless of their background or circumstances (Eizenberg & Jabareen, 2017). Addressing systemic issues such as poverty, inequality, and discrimination, the outcomes of social sustainability efforts include equitable access to basic needs like healthy food, and provision of services such as education, healthcare, and employment opportunities. Social sustainability is closely aligned with an occupational justice perspective (Wilcock & Townsend, 2000) and a rights-based approach to occupational therapy practice (Crawford, 2017), with an aim that current and future societies provide opportunities for occupational participation for all. Occupational therapy has a significant role in promoting social sustainability through approaches grounded in occupation that promote inclusion and connection, enhance quality of life, support health and wellbeing, advocate for accessibility, empower marginalised groups, foster community development, and facilitate meaningful participation in occupations.

In considering social sustainability it is important to note that each individual or collective has different needs, and these needs are linked to contemporary and contextual societal and social issues (Assefa & Frostell, 2007; Ly & Cope, 2023), for instance the ongoing effects of colonialism and systems of oppression. Additionally, social sustainability is likely to hold different meanings and potential for different people, requiring culturally responsive practice. Vallance et al. (2011) suggest that sustaining current social systems and structures for some people may be an overwhelmingly negative experience. For example, remote communities lacking necessary infrastructure and services to support health, education and capacity building are unlikely to want to maintain the status quo. They are more likely to want to advocate for change to such systems to improve opportunities for community members, and then to sustain the positive changes. For such change to occur, there is a need to uphold and respect Tino Rangatiratanga – the need for marginalised communities to self-determine especially in response to the ongoing impacts of historic and current abuses and disenfranchisement. Working towards such changes is not an easy, but important, with Ly and Cope (2023, p. 15) discussing the 'complexity and heterogeneity of current social life' and the simultaneous need to develop approaches to social sustainability that are responsive to the immediate context and issues.

Social sustainability efforts involve addressing historical and systemic barriers that prevent individuals and collectives from fully participating in society and creating systems that provide equitable opportunities for meaningful participation both now and into the future. Collaborative development of community strategies supports individuals and collectives to respond to current social issues and empowers them to take an active role in shaping their environment and future. The publication *Doing Our Best: Individual and Community Responses to Challenging Times* (Whiteford et al., 2022) contains numerous examples of Australian communities collaborating to connect, provide support, and build capacity during times of adversity such as the global pandemic and the 2019/2020 Australian Black Summer bushfires. Galvaan and Peters (2013) provide a framework to guide occupation-based community development that supports practice focused on addressing social inequalities and promoting occupational justice. Practices that promote equitable occupational participation and inclusion of marginalised communities are essential for achieving social sustainability.

As an example, when considering town planning and development of shared built environments an occupational perspective could make an important contribution to enhance the value of project outcomes subsequently promoting social sustainability. Involvement of occupational therapy at policy development and planning stages of community projects can promote a focus on social sustainability through highlighting how such projects can link spaces and services, connect people, facilitate occupational participation, enable accessibility, and promote health and wellbeing. Parnell and Wilding (2010) demonstrated how deliberate design incorporating universal design principles (Centre for Excellence in Universal Design, n.d.), and ongoing maintenance of town pathway loops connect community members to health care centres, shopping precincts, schools, aged care services, childcare centres, green spaces, and sporting and social facilities. Such intentional design promotes occupational participation and has the potential to support social sustainability.

35.2.3 Economic sustainability & occupational therapy. Nā tō rourou, nā taku rourou ka
ora ai te iwi | With your food basket and my food basket the people will thrive

Economic sustainability accentuates that there is a need to achieve a balance between the economic needs of today's society and those of the future. The Australian and New Zealand governments have identified key challenges for the economic sustainability of each country, which reflect current economic ideals of growth and wealth. While this section will address these challenges and the role occupational therapists can play in economic sustainability as it is currently perceived, it is also argued that a shift in economic principles is required to ensure sustainability, with this argument being presented at the end of this section.

The Australian and New Zealand governments have outlined key risks to the economic success of each country (Department of the Prime Minister and Cabinet, 2024). These risks include reduced household consumption, reduced global growth, an ageing population, rising demand for care and support services, climate change and net zero transformation, technological and digital transformation, continued geopolitical risks and fragmentation, seismic and volcanic events, cyber incidents, and disease outbreaks (Department of the Prime Minister and Cabinet, 2024; Reserve Bank of New Zealand |Te Pūtea Matua, 2024). Occupational therapists can play a key role in helping to address many of these areas, including the ageing population, rising demand for care and support services, and climate change. For instance, in relation to climate change, the Australian government is creating an authority to manage the transition of workers in emissions-intensive industries to access new employment or improve their employment prospects (Department of the Prime Minister and Cabinet, 2024; Organisation for Economic Co-operation and Development, 2023). Occupational therapists could facilitate the occupational transition for these workers, into new roles aligned with their existing skills. Occupational therapists are experts in assisting people to live with autonomy and good health in the community and therefore well placed to play a role in addressing economic threats introduced from the ageing population and increasing demand for care and support services. Consequently, occupational therapists may play a pivotal role in guiding public policy in these areas.

Narrowing the focus to economic sustainability of health systems, more specific challenges exist. Funding of health systems is fragmented in Australia, with contributions from federal, state, and private funding (Angeles et al., 2023). This approach creates budget silos, leading to gaps in services and reduced efficiencies. There is a focus on paying for reactive services rather than prevention, with 1.8% of spending focused on the latter. Out-of-pocket expenses can prevent people from engaging in preventative measures such as allied health services until their health reaches a crisis point–an approach evident in both country's health systems. Consequently, preventative measures that could ensure that health issues are managed in primary health services at a reduced cost, are replaced with an increase in hospital presentations, often with more deleterious results for the person and the economy (Angeles et al., 2023; Gorman & Horn, 2022; Jeffreys et al., 2024). Exacerbating this, people who tend to have the highest out of pocket costs are also likely to have higher health needs, including those living outside capital cities, couples with children, people with chronic health conditions, and Indigenous peoples (Jeffreys et al., 2024). In addition to out-of-pocket expenses, people living outside urban hubs have greater difficulty accessing allied health services due to a lack of professionals in these areas, increasing care costs. Providing services closer to home is advantageous for people's health and wellbeing, the economy, and for reducing emissions to meet environmental targets. While these are only a few examples of current inefficiencies in how funds are spent in health systems, they provide an indication of potential opportunities for efficiencies.

There are clear opportunities for occupational therapists and occupational therapy as a profession to contribute to economic sustainability. For instance, occupational therapy as a profession may help to address the shortages of occupational therapists in rural and regional areas, to ensure chronic conditions are managed in a primary care setting (Gorman & Horn, 2022). Occupational therapists can assist with helping people to age in place, reducing risks of falls and injuries within the home and the number of hospital presentations (Gorman & Horn, 2022). However, as a profession, occupational therapy is inadequately demonstrating its ability to contribute to economic efficiencies, with a need for further health economic evaluations to be undertaken (Green & Lambert, 2017).

There are, however, limitations to current assumptions around economic growth results and its relationship with better health and wellbeing. Such assumptions do not take into consideration social and environmental impacts and tend to only benefit a small portion of society. The need and want for purchasing more does not necessarily lead to increased health and happiness. Baum (2015) posits that areas that require a change include preoccupation with economic growth, the indicators used for economic and social development, international economic systems and multinational corporations, fair taxation, and fair terms of global trade. Jones (2019) argues for addressing the colonial roots of the current global economic system which drives climate change and measures of inequity. Such changes extend far beyond the profession of occupational therapy, requiring commitment at national and international levels, however the profession can play a role in advocating for change.

35.3 Illustrative scenario

You are a government-employed occupational therapist working in a rural community in Australia. Your caseload includes individuals from birth to end of life. You have identified reoccurring issues with access to assistive technology (AT). Trials and repairs are difficult to coordinate as many equipment providers cannot visit your town or do not offer extended trials. This situation has resulted in some individuals ceasing to use AT following supply as it has been unsuitable or they have adapted while waiting the long periods of time without appropriate AT. You are concerned about the risks this poses to individuals, the impact of discarded AT on the environment, and the costs associated with replacing unsuitable AT. Furthermore, there are multiple accessibility barriers for people with mobility issues and visual impairments who are only able to access certain parts of the town due to poorly designed pathways, curbs, and storefronts. You apply a sustainability lens to address these issues at a micro, meso, and macro level.

35.3.1 Micro level

You make small but impactful changes to your practice, spending more time to explore an individual's environment and their goals related to AT. You utilise the equipment pool (meso-level) to explore individuals' likes and dislikes related to equipment, streamlining your equipment trials. You contact equipment providers and discuss your exploration of different options with individuals and the reasoning for requested trials of equipment. You find that this approach increases the likelihood of providers agreeing to visit the town, which is further enhanced by coordinating multiple trials on one day. Additionally, you seek mentorship from a senior occupational therapist working in a nearby regional centre who has demonstrated success with funding approvals, enhancing the success and outcomes of the equipment applications for the people you work with.

35.3.2 Meso Level

You discuss with your manager the possibility of introducing an equipment pool where unused AT can be donated and used for trial, temporarily used, or redistributed to others who may benefit. Your manager is supportive; however, they have concerns around the safety of this equipment. You discuss this issue with the health service's equipment and maintenance team who are responsible for maintaining equipment used within the health service. They state that for the equipment pool to be feasible, they would need to hire an additional staff member one day per week. You discuss this with the health service manager, who then completes a cost evaluation and approves the equipment pool including appropriate staffing.

35.3.3 Macro level

At a macro level you advocate for more accessible infrastructure in the town. You write to council and request a meeting to discuss the current experiences of AT users in the town. Drawing on feedback from your individuals, you outline how improved access presents multiple benefits for AT users and the broader community. You also discuss the economic benefits that such changes can have, including reducing need for support services, increasing the ability of AT users to pursue productive occupations, and reducing the likelihood of complaints made against council for injuries due to poorly designed and maintained pathways. You also advocate for a council access advisory group to advise the council on ongoing barriers to community participation. Through these activities, you challenge ableist and ageist cultural perspectives at the macro level.

35.4 Conclusion

In this chapter, readers have been introduced to the concept of sustainability. Three aspects of sustainability (environmental, social, and economic) have been explored with a particular focus on their relationship with occupational therapy practice. Sustainability refers to the practice of addressing current needs without compromising the ability to meet the needs of future generations. In the context of health and wellbeing, sustainability is focused on a balanced approach that integrates environmental health, social equity, and economic viability. Such an approach ensures that the health and wellbeing of individuals and collectives are supported over the long term. The occupational therapy profession has much to contribute to sustainability efforts, and indeed there is a requirement from professional bodies that occupational therapists meaningfully engage in sustainability work. Through a focus on sustainable approaches to practice that include encouraging participation in occupations that consider the environmental, social, and economic impacts, occupational therapists are well placed and should aim to promote occupational justice for current and future generations.

35.5 Summary

- Sustainability can be defined as 'meeting the needs of the present without compromising the ability of future generations to meet their own needs' (World Commission on Environment and Development, 1987).
- Sustainability can be best achieved when its three core areas (environmental, social, economic) are addressed in an integrated and balanced manner.

- Occupational therapists can contribute to achieving sustainability by promoting environmentally sustainable practices, ensuring social equity, and considering economic factors in their interventions.
- An awareness of intersectionality and occupational justice is pivotal to sustainability efforts within occupational therapy, ensuring equitable occupational participation for individuals and collectives now and in the future.
- Occupational therapists have the skills to collaborate with other professionals and communities to develop sustainable practices, community recovery strategies, and policies that enhance long-term health, well-being, and inclusion.

35.6 Review questions

- Describe in your own words what sustainability means.
- What role do occupational therapists play in promoting environmental sustainability?
- What role do occupational therapists play in promoting social sustainability?
- What role do occupational therapists play in promoting economic sustainability?

35.7 Reflection questions

- What is one element of your practice that you can change to make it more sustainable?
- Is there one aspect of sustainability that you are more drawn to? Why is this?

References

Angeles, M. R., Crosland, P., & Hensher, M. (2023). Challenges for Medicare and universal health care in Australia since 2000. *The Medical Journal of Australia, 218*(7), 322–329. https://doi.org/10.5964/mja2.51844

Assefa, G., & Frostell, B. (2007). Social sustainability and social acceptance in technology assessment: A case study of energy technologies. *Technology in Society, 29*(1), 63–78. https://doi.org/10.1016/j.techsoc.2006.10.007

Baum, F. (2015). Healthy economic policies. In F. Baum (Ed.), *The new public health* (4th ed., pp. 419–446). Oxford University Press.

Centre for Excellence in Universal Design. (n.d.). *The 7 principles.* https://universaldesign.ie/about-universal-design/the-7-principles

Costello, A., Abbas, M., Allen, A., Ball, S., Bell, S., Bellamy, R., Friel, S., Groce, N., Johnson, A., Kett, M., Lee, M., Levy, C., Maslin, M., McCoy, D., McGuire, B., Montgomery, H., Napier, D., Pagel, C., Patel, J., de Oliveira, J. A., . . . Patterson, C. (2009). Managing the health effects of climate change: Lancet and University College London Institute for Global Health Commission. *Lancet (London, England), 373*(9676), 1693–1733. https://doi.org/10.1016/S0140-6736(09)60935-1

Crawford, E. (2017). Continuing the dialogue: A rights-approach in occupational therapy. *Australian Occupational Therapy Journal, 64*(6), 505–509. https://doi.org/10.1111/1440-1630.12416

Department of the Prime Minister and Cabinet. (2024). *Corporate plan 2024–2025.* Commonwealth of Australia. https://www.pmc.gov.au/sites/default/files/resource/download/corporate-plan-2024-25.pdf

Dieterle, C. (2020). The case for environmentally-informed occupational therapy: Clinical and educational applications to promote personal wellness, public health and environmental sustainability. *World Federation of Occupational Therapists Bulletin, 76*(1), 32–39. https://doi.org/10.1080/14473828.2020.1717055

Drolet, M. J., Désormeaux-Moreau, M., Soubeyran, M., & Thiébaut, S. (2020). Intergenerational occupational justice: Ethically reflecting on climate crisis. *Journal of Occupational Science*, 27(3), 417–431. https://doi.org/10.1080/14427591.2020.1776148

Eizenberg, E., & Jabareen, Y. (2017). Social sustainability: A new conceptual framework. *Sustainability*, 9(1), 68. https://doi.org/10.3390/su9010068

Galvaan, R., & Peters, L. (2013). *Occupation-based community development framework.* https://vula.uct.ac.za/access/content/group/9c29ba04-b1ee-49b9-8c85-9a468b556ce2/OBCDF/index.html

Gonclaves, M. V., Roquete, D. E., De Almeida, G., & Bardi, G. (2025). Advocacy. In M. Curtin, M. Egan, Y. Prior, T. Parnell, R. Galvaan, K. Sauve-Schenk, & D. Cezar Da Cruz (Eds.), *Occupational therapy for people experiencing illness, injury or impairment: Promoting occupational participation* (pp. 270–284). Elsevier.

Gorman, D., & Horn, M. (2022). Challenges to health system sustainability. *Internal Medicine Journal*, 52(8), 1293–1458. https://doi.org/10.1111/imj.15873

Green, S., & Lambert, R. (2017). A systematic review of health economic evaluations in occupational therapy. *British Journal of Occupational Therapy*, 80(1), 5–19. https://doi.org/10.1177/0308022616650898

Hess, K. Y., & Rihtman, T. (2023). Moving from theory to practice in occupational therapy education for planetary health: A theoretical view. *Australian Occupational Therapy Journal*, 70(4), 460–470. https://doi.org/10.1111/1440-1630.12868

Hudson, M. J., & Aoyama, M. (2008). Occupational therapy and the current ecological crisis. *British Journal of Occupational Therapy*, 71, 545–548. https://doi.org/10.1177/030802260807101210

Intergovernmental Panel on Climate Change. (2022). Summary for policymakers. In H.-O. Pörtner, D. C. Roberts, M. Tignor, E. S. Poloczanska, K. Mintenbeck, A. Alegría, M. Craig, S. Langsdorf, S. Löschke, V. Möller, A. Okem, & B. Rama (Eds.), *Climate change 2022: Impacts, adaptation and vulnerability* (pp. 3–33). https://doi.org/10.1017/9781009325844.001

Jeffreys, M., Ellison-Loschmann, L., Irurzun-Lopez, M., Cumming, J., & McKenzie, F. (2024). Financial barriers to primary health care in Aoetearoa New Zealand. *Family Practice*, 41(6), 995–1001. https://doi.org/10.1093/fampra/cmad096

Jones, R. (2019). Climate change and Indigenous health promotion. *Global Health Promotion*, 26(3_suppl), 73–81. https://doi.org/10.1177/17579759198297

Ly, A. M., & Cope, M. R. (2023). New conceptual model of social sustainability: Review from past concepts and ideas. *International Journal of Environmental Research and Public Health*, 20(7), 5350. https://doi.org/10.3390/ijerph20075350

Occupational Therapy Board of Australia. (2018, February 20). *Australian occupational therapy competency standards 2018.* https://www.occupationaltherapyboard.gov.au/Codes-Guidelines/Competencies.aspx

Occupational Therapy Board of New Zealand. (2022, January). *Competencies for registration and continuing practice for occupational therapists.* https://www.otboard.org.nz/document/5886/7569%20OTBNZ%20%E2%80%93%20Competencies%20for%20practice%20FINAL%20G.pdf

Organisation for Economic Co-operation and Development. (2023). *OECD economic surveys Australia.* https://doi.org/10.1787/1794a7c9-en

Parnell, T., & Wilding, C. (2010). Where can an occupation-focused philosophy take occupational therapy? *Australian Occupational Therapy Journal*, 57(5), 345–348. https://doi.org/10.1111/j.1440-1630.2010.00860.x

Reserve Bank of New Zealand | Te Pūtea Matua. (2024). *Financial stability report.* www.rbnz.govt.nz/financial-stability/financial-stability-report

Smith, D. L., Fleming, K., Brown, L., Allen, A., Baker, J., & Gallagher, M. (2020). Occupational therapy and environmental sustainability: A scoping review. *Annals of International Occupational Therapy*, 3(3), 136–143. https://doi.org/10.3928/24761222-20200116-02

United Nations. (n.d.). *The 17 goals.* https://sdgs.un.org/goals

Vallance, S., Perkins, H. C., & Dixon, J. E. (2011). What is social sustainability? A clarification of concepts. *Geoforum, 42*(3), 342–348. https://doi.org/10.1016/j.geoforum.2011.01.002

Whiteford, G., Wicks, A., de Jong, D. C., Copland, L., Kearney, J., McSweeney, S. C., Millsteed, J., Moss, E., Murphy, L., Perez, M., Searle, K., Thomsen, K., Wiseman, L., & Pitts, D. (2022). *Doing our best: Individual and community responses to challenging times.* Occupational Therapy Australia. https://otaus.com.au/media-and-advocacy/doing-our-best

Wilcock, A. A., & Townsend, E. (2000). Occupational terminology interactive dialogue. *Journal of Occupational Science, 7*(2), 84–86. https://doi.org/10.1080/14427591.2000.9686470

World Commission on Environment and Development. (1987). *Report of the World Commission on Environment and Development: Our common future.* www.un-documents.net/our-common-future.pdf

World Federation of Occupational Therapy. (2012). *Position statement: Environmental sustainability, sustainable practice within occupational therapy.* http://www.wfot.org/resources/environmental-sustainability-sustainable-practice-within-occupational-therapy

The role of occupational therapy in primary health care in Australia and Aotearoa New Zealand

Emma George, Annette Peart, Ben Sellar, James Sunderland, and Sarah Redfearn

Authors' positionality statement

The Australian authors, Emma George, Annette Peart, and Ben Sellar, are non-Indigenous occupational therapists who acknowledge the traditional custodians of the land on which they live, play, work, and learn. In all their roles and practices, they value principles of equity and justice and the importance of meaningful occupation for health and wellbeing. For the first time, this chapter welcomes co-authorship with colleagues from Aotearoa New Zealand, James Sunderland and Sarah Redfern. They practice in line with Te Tiriti o Waitangi and recognise this as the founding, and living, document that guides New Zealand/Aotearoa. James identifies as Māori with whakapapa to Ngāti Maniapoto.

Key terms
- Primary health care
- Equity
- Empowerment
- Social justice
- Social determinants of health
- Community

Objectives
This chapter will allow the reader to:

- Recognise primary health care as a model and a field of practice for occupational therapy
- Describe the principles of primary health care, including the context of decolonisation
- Differentiate between upstream, midstream, and downstream approaches in primary health care
- Identify primary health care example from Aotearoa New Zealand and Australia

DOI: 10.4324/9781003495666-39

36.1 Introduction

Primary health care is both a model and a field of practice. Principles of primary health care strongly reflect principles of client-centred practice and participation in meaningful occupation. Occupational therapists can apply primary health care principles in all settings and when working with people, families, communities, and populations. Occupational therapists in primary health care focus on promoting health and preventing illness through meaningful occupation and addressing environmental factors. This chapter introduces the 'upstream, midstream, downstream' model as a tool for planning and practice. Examples of primary health highlight roles, opportunities, and actions in the primary health care context.

36.2 Primary health care

Primary health care is a model and a field of practice. It emerged as a model of community-based health service delivery following the World Health Organization's (WHO) Declaration of Alma-Ata (WHO, 1978) where health was recognised as a human right and an important worldwide goal. Over time primary health care has grown through numerous World Health Organization initiatives. The principles of primary health care (equity, empowerment and social justice) influence advocacy for universal health coverage, progress towards the United Nation's Sustainable Development Goals, strengthening health systems, and building global health partnerships.

Primary health care was designed and has always strived to be more than primary care and yet there remains confusion and debate about the context and definition. Primary care refers to the first point of call when people seek help for health concerns. Primary care services within this structure should be basic, accessible, affordable, and essential (Baum, 2016). Primary health care is more than primary care and should be integrated and coordinated to address the social determinants of health (Baum, 2016). These are the circumstances in which people are born, grow, live, work, and age (World Health Organization, 2025). The social determinants of health are shaped by the way that society is structured, reinforced by political choices and leadership. Primary health care offers a holistic approach that considers the context of social determinants of health for people, families, communities, and populations.

Primary health care as a field of practice promotes individual and community participation in prevention, curative, and rehabilitative services. This includes but is not limited to education, nutrition, access to clean water and sanitation, maternal and child health, family planning, immunisation, disease control, treatment, and the provision of essential drugs. A primary health care approach emphasises the need for an international commitment to health, more responsible use of the world's resources, and peace.

The principles of primary health care are aligned with occupational therapy's commitment to person-centred practice and participation in meaningful occupation (Galheigo, 2005; Tse et al., 2003). Occupational therapists work with people, individually or in groups or communities, and promote participation in ways that focus on personal, occupational, and environmental enablers and barriers to health (Occupational Therapy Board, 2018). For example, a review by Donnelly et al. (2023) identified occupational therapy with older populations included managing chronic conditions, participating in community services, health promotion, and falls prevention. Across multiple primary health care settings, occupational therapists in Australia and Aotearoa/New Zealand work as clinicians, educators, supervisors, administrators, managers, project officers, consultants, coordinators, programme directors, researchers, advocates, support staff, and more.

36.3 Aotearoa New Zealand context

Aotearoa New Zealand is a bicultural nation, encompassing both Māori and Pākehā (all non-Māori individuals). This unique cultural landscape necessitates that all health-related decisions consider the principles established in Te Tiriti o Waitangi (Treaty of Waitangi), which serves as a foundational document guiding the relationship between Māori and the Crown. For example, in 2018, the He Ara Oranga report, commissioned to address the inadequacies within the mental health and addictions services in New Zealand, highlighted several critical areas for improvement, one of which emphasised the need to enhance access and choice in primary care settings (New Zealand Government, 2018). The report recommended the establishment of the Integrated Primary Mental Health and Addiction programme, aimed to align health services more closely with the obligations outlined in Te Tiriti o Waitangi, specifically focusing on equity in accessing mental health services for all New Zealanders, particularly Māori.

In Aotearoa New Zealand, primary health organisations (PHOs) are community-based, not-for profit entities that coordinate and deliver primary health care to enrolled populations. They are responsible for ensuring primary care services meet the needs of people in community. This is an example of the overlap between primary care and primary health care.

36.4 Australian context

Primary health care in Australia is provided by Aboriginal Community Controlled Health Organisations, publicly funded community health services, not-for-profit organisations, and private operators. These services are funded through Australia's universal health insurance scheme, Medicare, ensuring that some services are low- or no-cost, state- or territory-funded (predominantly community health services). Primary health networks are federally funded, regionally based primary health care planning organisations that commission organisations to deliver services and population health programmes (Windle et al., 2023). Aboriginal Community Controlled Health Organisations of which there are 147 around Australia, are locally governed and were originally designed to address the inability of mainstream primary health care services to engage with Aboriginal communities. As such, primary health care services delivered by ACCHOs address social determinants of health and health inequities, as well as providing advocacy, community empowerment, and capacity building (Pearson et al., 2020).

36.5 Key principles of primary health care

Equity, empowerment, and social justice are the three principles of primary health care (Taylor et al., 2020). Together these principles create a foundation for addressing health and the social determinants that impact people and populations. Occupational therapists working in primary health care require critical reflexivity to ensure their practice aligns with key principles. This is especially important when addressing systemic barriers and health inequities.

36.5.1 Equity

Equity is about fairness. Equity is an ethical concept that can be defined as the absence of disparities in health and is connected to advantage and disadvantage (Braveman & Gruskin, 2003). If equity is about fairness, then equality can be described as sameness. Health equity focuses on the fair distribution of resources so people who need the most support have access to it. Achieving equality in service provision but providing the same services to all people does not necessarily translate to equity, because some people need more services or different services. For example, in Figure 36.1, if all four people were provided with equal services (the same size bike), participation would remain unequal. However, when an adapted bike is provided for the person who uses a wheelchair and suitably sized bikes are provided for other people, resources are equitable, and all people can participate.

36.5.2 Empowerment

Empowerment is a process that seeks to redress inequalities in health and promote participation to bring about personal, social, and political change (Keleher & MacDougall, 2021; Laverack, 2006). Empowerment is often confused with the provision of education, skills, and resources, but this ignores the power relationships that determine

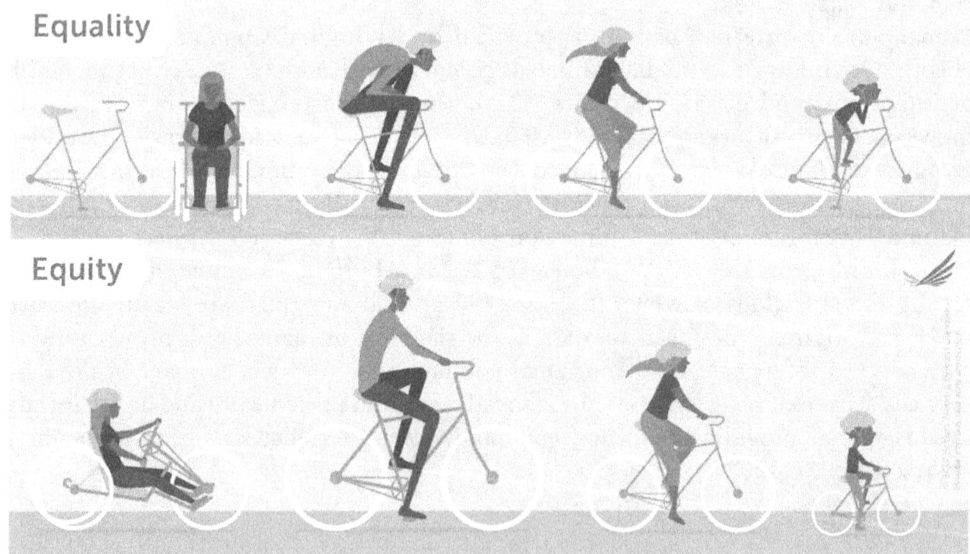

Figure 36.1 A commitment to health equity demonstrates a commitment to fair and just policies and service provision for people and communities who need it the most

(rwjf.org/en/library/infographics/visualizing-health-equity.html). Reproduced with permission

what is provided and whether that provision has meaningful impact. Empowerment requires partnership with people, families, and communities on issues of importance to that community and determined by the community. A commitment to empowerment involves supporting people to participate and goes beyond tokenistic consultation or collaboration towards decision making and community ownership (George et al., 2024; Taylor et al., 2020). Working in health involves power relationships between different stakeholders, especially between health professionals, regarded as the experts, and the clients or communities with whom they work. Health professionals must challenge notions of power and privilege and provide opportunities for self-determination and control over decision-making processes and enable access to resources to address disparities in social determinants of health (Keleher & MacDougall, 2021).

Decolonisation goes further than empowerment as it seeks to reimagine and rearticulate power by questioning and resisting colonial knowledges and systems that threaten Indigenous ways of being (Gibson, 2020; Sium et al., 2012). Empowerment can often mean providing knowledge to people who haven't had access to it, while decolonising practices acknowledge that the knowledge provided, and assumption that it is needed, may be doing the harm. Indigenous occupational therapists from Australia, Aotearoa New Zealand, and further abroad have provided important direction, learning, and leadership on decolonising occupational therapy (Emery-Whittington & Te Maro, 2018; Gibson, 2020; Gibson et al., 2015; Ramugondo, 2015). Key features of decolonisation include prioritising Indigenous voice and self-determination, building genuine relationships, sharing power, and working together to break down systemic barriers (Gibson, 2020). These actions demonstrate a commitment to decolonisation that goes beyond simply understanding that Indigenous peoples have been disadvantaged or colonial settlers advantaged by colonisation to the need to actively redress inequities (Emery-Whittington & Te Maro, 2018). Importantly, decolonisation may feel uncomfortable and threatening to non-Indigenous people, as it requires them to question and disrupt their own knowledge and power.

36.5.3 Social and occupational justice
Social justice is an ethical concept based on human rights, fairness, and equity in society (Keleher & MacDougall, 2021). Specifically, it relates to the fair and equitable distribution of opportunities for social, political and economic participation. This emphasis on participation is strongly aligned with occupational therapy, which has increasingly focussed on global connection, social injustice, and closing the gap in health status caused by avoidable health disparities (Bailliard et al., 2020; Hammell, 2017). Occupational justice is a discipline specific concept aligned with social justice, and, while too broad to define easily (Serrata Malfitano et al., 2016), it is becoming central to contemporary practice frameworks (Bailliard et al., 2020) and focuses on the rights of all people to participate in diverse, meaningful, balanced occupations that maximise their potential (Hocking, 2017).

36.6 Upstream, midstream, downstream model
Examples of primary health care can be seen through the 'upstream, midstream, downstream' model, part of a broader conceptual framework to identify relationships between social determinants and health (WHO, 2025). In this model, the main components

are grouped into upstream (macro), midstream (intermediate), or downstream (micro) factors with an associated approach to primary health care. For example, upstream factors include education, employment, income, and housing determinants. Upstream approaches are focused on keeping people healthy in the first place and often focus on public policy and the environment (Orleans, 2000). Midstream factors include psychosocial processes and health behaviours. Midstream approaches address behaviour to prevent illness or limit risk factors. Midstream approaches focus on perceived individual choices but target communities and groups.

Downstream factors primarily involve the functioning of various body systems. Downstream approaches treat illness and provide rehabilitation for individual people, representing a selective primary health care approach. The World Federation of Occupational Therapists (2024) position statement on Occupational Therapy and Primary Care outlines roles for professional practice that are upstream by design, that is, prevent health-damaging behaviours and illness (e.g. social inclusion policy); midstream, that is, enhance and maintain health for people with chronic health problems (e.g. assistive technology and lifestyle programmes); and downstream, that is, promote quality of life in palliative care (e.g. carer support and pain or fatigue management).

36.6.1 Example 1: Access and choice service

The Access and Choice programme in Aotearoa New Zealand represents a significant evolution in making mental health, wellbeing, and addiction services across Aotearoa New Zealand more accessible and equitable. Access and Choice aims to address disparities in mental health care, particularly for Māori, Pacific peoples, youth, and rural communities, by tailoring services to meet their unique needs, regardless of age. Launched in 2019, the Access and Choice programme is designed to provide timely, free, and easily accessible mental health, wellbeing, and addiction services through integrating behavioural health support into primary care settings, reducing the barriers often associated with specialist services.

In this programme, the placement of health improvement practitioners (HIPs), health coaches, and support workers in primary care provides a downstream approach, ensuring that help is available at the point of need. HIP roles are modelled on behavioural health consultant roles in the United States and a body of research supporting improved primary care outcomes for people and families/Whanau (Bryan et al., 2009; Ogbeide et al., 2018; Robinson & Reiter, 2016; Torrence et al., 2014). The HIP role is trans-disciplinary: any registered health professional with a 'talking therapy' component to their qualification can train as a HIP, making for a diverse, multiskilled workforce. Occupational therapists are particularly suited to the role with their skills utilising occupation as an intervention. The model is grounded in acceptance and commitment therapy principles and flexible enough to accommodate other evidence-based approaches such as motivational interviewing and cognitive behavioural therapy.

The Access and Choice programme is highly accessible: HIPs are available free of charge for same day 30-minute consultations at the clinic. The model features immediate, in-person 'warm handovers' from team members to the HIP rather than referrals. There is a strong educational component to the work of HIPs as they teach the team and patients a 'skills before pills' approach to health care. The hope is that attention to the mind–body connection becomes a normal part of primary health care.

HIPs use downstream approaches by working collaboratively with people to plan behavioural strategies that help clients align to their values and aspirations. The HIPs contribute to upstream projects, for example, involvement in community garden projects and championing national health campaigns for smoking cessation. The role also involves being familiar with the data for their clinic population so they can offer midstream interventions, health pathways, prevention strategies, and sessions aiming to increase wellbeing for the whole population.

The Access and Choice programme seeks to create a more responsive and inclusive health system by fostering collaboration between healthcare providers and communities. This initiative represents a significant step towards improving mental health outcomes, normalising behavioural health care, and reducing the stigma associated with seeking help in Aotearoa New Zealand.

36.6.2 Example 2: Lean On Me

The Lean On Me project was run in Clare, a regional town in South Australia, to support vulnerable families to find safe, secure, and affordable housing. Housing is a crucial determinant of health for families and communities and a major problem in Clare as more families moved into the region to escape family violence and the cost of living closer to the city. Many families with limited income, personal transport, and social and family supports were living in a regional town with minimal public infrastructure in the form of public transport, public housing, or government services. Guided by the principles of social justice and health as a human right, the need to support families to make this transition and maintain participation in education, work, and social activity was identified by local community members.

In 2019 the Lean On Me project was established as a partnership between local community members, stakeholders, and organisations and two University of South Australia final year occupational therapy students to develop sustainable community-controlled supports for vulnerable communities to transition to housing in the region. Over several months the students worked closely with the Community Development Coordinator from the Clare Valley Children's Centre and members of the Lions Club along with 100 community members and stakeholders from local schools, non-government organisations, and volunteer groups to collaboratively analyse the community needs and resources and then decide on a response.

Relationships, partnership, and collaboration were crucial to the project and allowed for collective decision making to occur. The community decided to establish a Furniture Shed where second-hand furniture could be donated and then sold at affordable prices to those who could pay or provided free to people who couldn't. The Furniture Shed would serve as a means through which to equitably distribute basic material resources for daily life and occupational participation. Importantly, as a local, community-controlled resource, the Furniture Shed was not reliant upon government grants and thus less vulnerable to external factors such as policy or government changes, representing greater self-determination about how the shed runs, who it supports, and how the resources it generates are redistributed through the community.

The Furniture Shed has continued to operate and grow over the last five years, servicing the needs of the local community through the provision of affordable furniture.

Community members have donated over 3500 items, and the income generated has supported over $45,000 in local projects. This project is exemplary because it:

1. Promoted self-determination by involving community members in the decision-making process and ensuring the outcome is controlled by the community.
2. Promotes equity, social, and occupational justice by redistributing material and financial resources amongst the community.
3. Fosters sustainability by drawing employing community strengths and resources without reliance on external funding.

Local community projects such as Lean On Me demonstrate how the principles of primary health care need not involve large-scale systems but can be applied in local communities with minimal resources to achieve meaningful outcomes.

36.7 Conclusion

There are many opportunities for occupational therapy in primary health care and for occupational therapists to demonstrate principles of equity, empowerment, and social justice in occupational therapy service provision. Primary health care that is comprehensive is holistic and focuses on social determinants of health. The challenge for occupational therapy is to effectively integrate primary health care into core occupational therapy practice and continue to take a leadership role to promote health and well-being for people, families, communities, and populations.

36.8 Summary
- Primary health care is both a model and a field of practice.
- Primary health care addresses the social determinants of health.
- Principles of primary health care are equity, empowerment, and social justice.
- Client-centred practice and participation in meaningful occupation reflect principles of primary health care.
- Occupational therapists who work in primary health care demonstrate commitment to equity, empowerment, and social justice.

36.9 Review and reflection questions
- What are the key features of comprehensive primary health care?
- How does a commitment to person-centred practice demonstrate a commitment to equity?
- How does decolonisation extend and enhance the principle of empowerment?
- Describe the different ways that occupational therapists work in upstream, midstream, and downstream areas of practice.

References

Bailliard, A. L., Dallman, A. R., Carroll, A., Lee, B. D., & Szendrey, S. (2020). Doing occupational justice: A central dimension of everyday occupational therapy practice. *Canadian Journal of Occupational Therapy, 87*(2), 144–152. https://doi.org/10.1177/0008417419898930

Baum, F. (2016). *The new public health* (4th ed.). Oxford University Press.

Braveman, P., & Gruskin, S. (2003). Defining equity in health. *Journal of Epidemiology and Community Health, 57*(4), 254–258. https://doi.org/10.1136/jech.57.4.254

Bryan, C. J., Morrow, C., & Appolonio, K. K. (2009). Impact of behavioral health consultant interventions on patient symptoms and functioning in an integrated family medicine clinic. *Journal of Clinical Psychology, 65*(3), 281–293. https://doi.org/10.1002/jclp.20539

Donnelly, C., Leclair, L., Hand, C., Wener, P., & Letts, L. (2023). Occupational therapy services in primary care: A scoping review. *Primary Health Care Research & Development, 24*, e7. https://doi.org/10.1017/S1463423622000123

Emery-Whittington, I., & Te Maro, B. (2018). Decolonising occupation: Causing social change to help our ancestors rest and our descendants thrive. *New Zealand Journal of Occupational Therapy, 65*(1), 12–19.

Galheigo, S. M. (2005). Occupational therapy and the social field. Clarifying concepts and ideas. In F. Kronenberg, S. S. Algado, & N. Pollard (Eds.), *Occupational therapy without borders: Learning from the spirit of survivors* (pp. 87–98). Elsevier.

George, E., Ritchie, T., Ryan, A., Fisher, M., Baum, F., & Mackean, T. (2024). "Listen with your ears and eyes and heart and your minds and your soul": Implications for decolonising consultation and occupational therapy from case studies on "Closing the Gap" policy implementation. *Australian Occupational Therapy Journal.* https://doi.org/10.1111/1440-1630.12960

Gibson, C. (2020). When the river runs dry: Leadership, decolonisation and healing in occupational therapy. *New Zealand Journal of Occupational Therapy, 67*(1), 11–20.

Gibson, C., Butler, C., Henaway, C., Dudgeon, P., & Curtin, M. (2015). Indigenous peoples and human rights: Some considerations for the occupational therapy profession in Australia. *Australian Occupational Therapy Journal, 62*(3), 214–218. https://doi.org/10.1111/1440-1630.12185

Hammell, K. W. (2017). Critical reflections on occupational justice: Toward a rights-based approach to occupational opportunities. *Canadian Journal of Occupational Therapy, 84*(1), 47–57. https://doi.org/10.1177/0008417416654501

Hocking, C. (2017). Occupational justice as social justice: The moral claim for inclusion. *Journal of Occupational Science, 24*(1), 29–42. https://doi.org/10.1080/14427591.2017.1294016

Keleher, H., & MacDougall, C. (2021). *Understanding health* (5th ed.). Oxford University Press.

Laverack, G. (2006). Improving health outcomes through community empowerment: A review of the literature. *Journal of Health, Population and Nutrition, 24*(1), 113–120. http://www.jstor.org/stable/23499274

New Zealand Government. (2018). *He Ara Oranga: Report of the government inquiry into mental health and addiction.* https://mentalhealth.inquiry.govt.nz/inquiry-report/he-ara-oranga

Occupational Therapy Board. (2018). *Australian occupational therapy competency standards 2018.* https://www.occupationaltherapyboard.gov.au/Codes-Guidelines/Competencies.aspx

Ogbeide, S. A., Landoll, R. R., Nielsen, M. K., & Kanzler, K. E. (2018). To go or not go: Patient preference in seeking specialty mental health versus behavioral consultation within the primary care behavioral health consultation model. *Families, Systems, & Health, 36*(4), 513–517. https://doi.org/10.1037/fsh0000374

Orleans, T. C. (2000). Promoting the maintenance of health behavior change: Recommendations for the next generation of research and practice. *Health Psychology, 19*(1), 76–83. https://doi.org/10.1037/0278-6133.19.suppl1.76

Pearson, O., Schwartzkopff, K., Dawson, A., Hagger, C., Karagi, A., Davy, C., Brown, A., Braunack-Mayer, A., & Leadership Group guiding the Centre for Research Excellence in Aboriginal Chronic Disease Knowledge Translation and Exchange (CREATE) (2020). Aboriginal community controlled health organisations address health equity through action on the social determinants of health of Aboriginal and Torres Strait Islander peoples in Australia. *BMC Public Health, 20*(1), 1859. https://doi.org/10.1186/s12889-020-09943-4

Ramugondo, E. L. (2015). Occupational consciousness. *Journal of Occupational Science, 22*(4), 488–501. https://doi.org/10.1080/14427591.2015.1042516

Robinson, P. J., & Reiter, J. T. (2016). *Behavioral consultation and primary care: A guide to integrating services* (2nd ed.). Springer.

Serrata Malfitano, A. P., Gomes da Mota de Souza, R., & Esquerdo Lopes, R. (2016). Occupational justice and its related concepts: An historical and thematic scoping review. *OTJR: Occupation, Participation and Health, 36*(4), 167–178. https://doi.org/10.1177/1539449216669133

Sium, A., Desai, C., & Ritskes, E. (2012). Towards the "tangible unknown": Decolonization and the Indigenous future. *Decolonization: Indigeneity, Education and Society, 1*(1), I–XIII. https://jps.library.utoronto.ca/index.php/des/article/view/18638/15564

Taylor, J., O'Hara, L., Talbot, L., & Verrinder, G. (2020). *Promoting health: The primary health care approach* (7th ed.). Elsevier.

Torrence, N. D., Mueller, A. E., Ilem, A. A., Renn, B. N., DeSantis, B., & Segal, D. L. (2014). Medical provider attitudes about behavioral health consultants in integrated primary care: A preliminary study. *Families, Systems, & Health, 32*(4), 426–435. https://doi.org/10.1037/fsh0000078

Tse, S., Penman, M., & Simms, F. (2003). Literature review: Occupational therapy and primary health care. *New Zealand Journal of Occupational Therapy, 50*(2), 17–23.

Windle, A., Javanparast, S., Freeman, T., et al. (2023). Evaluating local primary health care actions to address health inequities: Analysis of Australia's Primary Health Networks. *International Journal for Equity in Health, 22*, 243. https://doi.org/10.1186/s12939-023-02053-8

World Federation of Occupational Therapists. (2024). *Occupational therapy and primary care.* https://wfot.org/resources/occupational-therapy-and-primary-care

World Health Organization. (1978). *Declaration of Alma-Ata.* https://cdn.who.int/media/docs/default-source/documents/almaata-declaration-en.pdf?sfvrsn=7b3c2167_2

World Health Organization. (2025). *World report on social determinants of health equity, 2025.* https://www.who.int/teams/social-determinants-of-health/equity-and-health/world-report-on-social-determinants-of-health-equity

Occupational therapy in population health and health promotion in Australia and Aotearoa New Zealand

Kate Gledhill, Simon Leadley, and Kim Weigle-Reese

Authors' positionality statement

All authors acknowledge the traditional owners of the land on which they wrote this chapter: Awabakal, Boon Wurrung and Bunurong, Wurundjeri, and Wadawurrung Country. The authors are from predominantly middle-class families/whānau and acknowledge their white privilege. The authors come from across western, global north countries Aotearoa New Zealand, Australia, and America, all currently living in Australia with various ancestries, including English, Irish, German, and Scottish. All authors identify as Gen X, cisgender, and heterosexual. Each author is an occupational therapist with varied experiences as practitioners, researchers, and educators. All authors bring diverse knowledge and experiences, including support of family and friends with chronic and/or life-shortening illnesses and advocating for the rights of people with illnesses, disabilities, and mental health challenges to participate in their chosen life roles, creating an environment where all can thrive.

Key terms
- Population health
- Health promotion
- Determinants of health
- Culture
- Health literacy
- Cultural safety
- Equity

Objectives
This chapter will allow the reader to:

- Define population health, illness prevention, and health promotion
- Distinguish between illness prevention and health promotion

DOI: 10.4324/9781003495666-40

- Describe how occupational therapists can work in the areas of population health, illness prevention, and health promotion

37.1 Introduction

A core aim of occupational therapy practice is to create and facilitate opportunities for people to participate in meaningful occupations to promote health and well-being (World Federation of Occupational Therapists [WFOT], 2012). In contemporary practice, the 'client' is not limited to the individual but can include family, carers, communities, collectives, organisations, or populations and, in Indigenous communities, Mob and Iwi (Occupational Therapy Board of Australia [OTBA], 2018).

In Australia and Aotearoa New Zealand (NZ), people are developing ongoing health conditions earlier in life, and the population is ageing (Australian Institute of Health and Welfare [AIHW], 2024a; New Zealand Ministry of Health [MOH], 2023). To address this and ensure the health system is sustainable, occupational therapists require a population health perspective that incorporates health promotion. This perspective involves changing the focus of occupational therapy from individuals to populations and implementing strategies at local, regional, and national levels to enable people to increase control over (and improve) their health. Occupational therapists bring a unique perspective to population health through their focus on humans as occupational beings who influence their health through what they do within their environment (Wilcock & Hocking, 2015).

37.2 What is health?

'Health' is a familiar term often used in everyday communication. In healthcare, different models describe or define health. In Western health systems, the biomedical model is often used to understand health. According to the biomedical model, health is an individual's responsibility and refers to an objective biological state characterised by the absence of illness (Germov, 2019). In contrast, the social model defines health as a social construct influenced by factors such as living and working conditions, and political and social environments. Health is seen as a societal responsibility (Germov, 2019), especially true for Indigenous peoples such as Māori and Aboriginal and Torres Strait Islander peoples, for whom health means a holistic and inclusive concept that incorporates Mob and Iwi, cultural values, and a strong connection to land and environment (Redvers et al., 2022). More information about this can be found in Chapters 15–17 of this book.

In 1946, the World Health Organization (WHO) defined health as 'a state of complete physical, mental and social well-being and not merely the absence of disease or infirmity' (WHO, 1946, para. 1). The WHO reviewed this definition in the Ottawa Charter for Health Promotion (WHO, 1986), positioning health as 'a resource for everyday life, not the objective of living. Health is a positive concept emphasizing social and personal resources, as well as physical capacities' (para. 3). In 1997, WHO committed to develop an international strategy for health, affirming health as 'a basic human right essential for social and economic development' (WHO, 1997, para. 3). The Jakarta Declaration provided an international direction and goal 'to increase health expectancy and to narrow the gap in health expectancy between countries and groups' (WHO, 1997, para. 3) into the 21st century. These historical documents continue to shape our understanding of health and underpin efforts to improve health at a population level.

37.3 What is population health?

Population health refers to 'an aggregate of people who may or may not know each other but share at least one characteristic such as age, race, ethnicity, gender, health habit or condition, geographical location, cultural identity, socioeconomic status, or education' (Muriithi, 2024, p. 366) and has two key aims.

The first aim is to understand patterns of health and disease at community, state, and national levels. In Australia and Aotearoa New Zealand, health conditions such as cancer, cardiovascular disease, arthritis, musculoskeletal conditions, mental ill health, substance use disorders, and injuries have major impacts on people's lives and contribute significantly to the burden of disease. Burden of disease refers to the loss of health and well-being due to premature mortality, morbidity, and disability (AIHW, 2024b; MOH, 2023).

The second aim of population health is to identify and address health inequalities to improve population health and well-being. Health inequalities are observable and measurable differences in health status between population groups (Hosseinpoor et al., 2023). The distribution of health and disease in a population follows a social gradient, where people in the lowest socioeconomic groups are more likely to live with health conditions and die prematurely than those in the highest socioeconomic groups (AIHW, 2016). Population groups such as Māori, Aboriginal and Torres Strait Islander people, and Pacific Peoples; those in rural and remote areas; culturally and linguistically diverse populations; people with disabilities; members of LGBTQIAP2S communities; veterans; and prisoners experience disparities in health status compared to the general population (AIHW, 2024b; MOH, 2023). To address health inequalities, population health needs to consider the distribution and accessibility of health services and focus on health equity.

37.4 What influences population health?

What people do each day, or their occupations, are amongst the determinants that contribute to health and wellbeing outcomes. Determinants that positively influence health are called protective factors, and those that negatively influence health are called risk factors (AIHW, 2024a). Protective factors such as regular physical activity, restorative sleep, or meaningful social activities help prevent illness and maintain health and wellbeing. Conversely, risk factors, such as engagement in risky occupations like the use of alcohol and drugs, increase the likelihood of physical or mental health problems. In the long term, this can result in chronic conditions that further limit people's participation in occupations and perpetuate ill health or disability (AIHW, 2024a; Hocking & Sutton, 2024). Modifiable risk factors are within a person's ability to change for example physical activity, social participation and connection.

However, people's capacity to make choices about their daily activities is influenced by population-level determinants beyond their control. Social determinants of health –

the conditions in which people are born, grow, live, work, and age – and the association with people's health and health inequities are well supported by evidence (Lysack et al., 2024). Additionally, other determinants of health, such as economic, political, cultural, and environmental determinants, have also been recognised (AIHW, 2024b). Indigenous worldviews include a more holistic, nature-based, and interconnected view about determinants that relate both to people's and, more broadly, the planet's health (Redvers et al., 2022). Different conceptual models explain the influence of social determinants on people's health and wellbeing and how health inequities occur.

A recent concept developed by Canadian Indigenous communities uses the metaphor of a tree (see Figure 37.1). In this model, proximal determinants include factors such as participation in occupations, housing, social inclusion; intermediate determinants

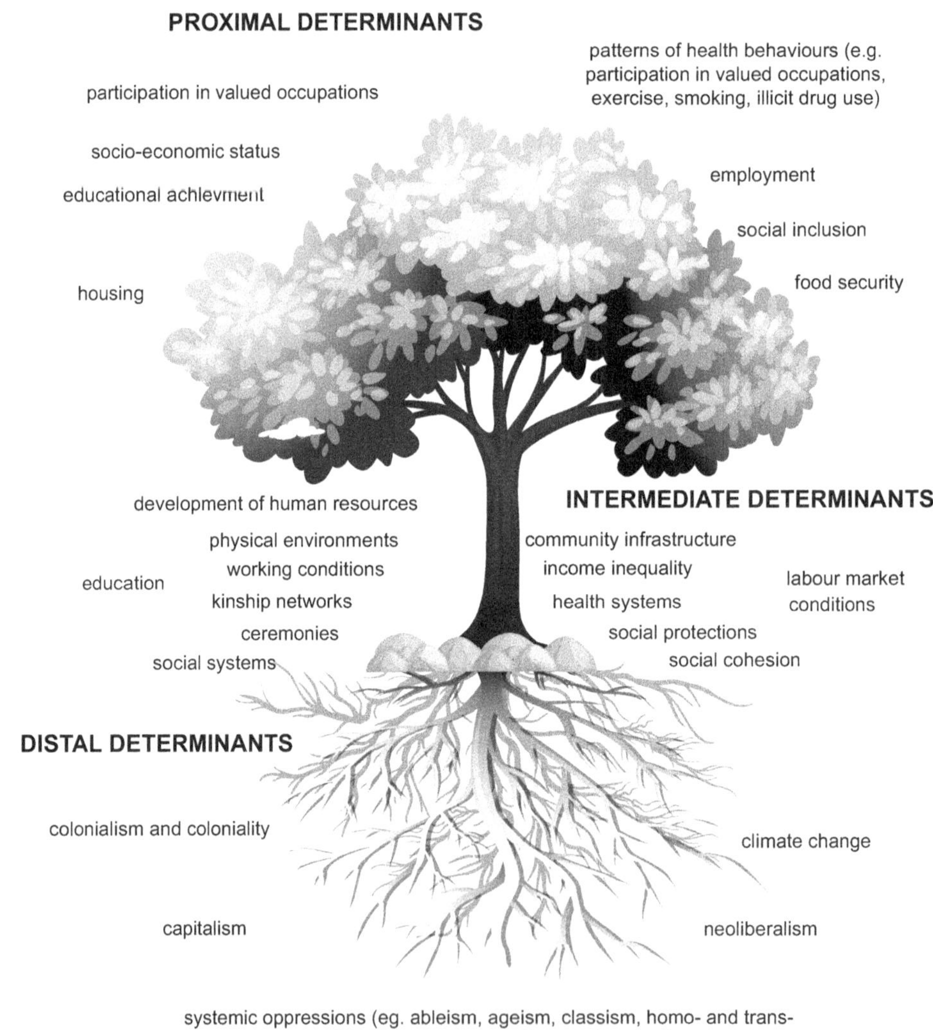

Figure 37.1 Multi-layered determinants of health, well-being and occupation

(Trentham et al., 2022)

include factors such as social networks and cohesion, employment conditions, and the physical environment; and distal determinants include the impacts of colonialism, neoliberal policies, and the effects of climate change (Egan & Restall, 2022). This model, developed from an occupational lens, originates from an Indigenous worldview, inclusive of connections with the environment, the harmful legacy of colonialism, and widespread negative economic ideologies like capitalism.

37.4.1 Culture

Having an awareness of our behaviour and how it impacts culturally diverse groups is crucial in reducing health inequalities within populations. Culture refers to ideas, meanings, beliefs, knowledge, values, and ways of being shared by a particular group but also includes concepts such as language, arts/expression, and customs and traditions (Beagan, 2015). Culture may encompass ethnicity; gender; sexual orientation; religion; ability; physical appearance; socioeconomic status; and connection to family, community, and country, which intersect to shape unique individuals and communities. Important cultural associations for First Nations peoples in Australia include the concept of 'mob' or a grouping of peoples based on shared place or Country. In Aotearoa New Zealand, for Indigenous Māori peoples, this includes 'hapū', or a collection of whānau/families in a region with shared whakapapa/ancestry, and 'Iwi', a larger tribe consisting of several hapū.

Culture is both individual and collective, making it complex, multilayered, and evolving (Agner, 2020). Culture influences how individuals view and seek healthcare and also influences health practitioners' perspectives. Developing cultural humility, a lifelong learning process, is integrated into university curriculum and is emerging as an important factor in reducing the power differential in healthcare interactions (American Occupational Therapy Association [AOTA], 2020). This involves self-reflection, understanding implicit bias (feelings, thoughts, stereotypes, subconscious perceptions) and explicit bias (conscious beliefs about a group) and considering systemic issues when working with diversity (Agner, 2020; AOTA, 2020; MOH, 2023). Cultural safety, a term introduced in the 1990s by Māori nurses in Aotearoa NZ, seeks awareness of differences, decolonisation, power inequity, reflective practice, and empowering clients to determine if they feel safe within the healthcare encounter (Curtis et al., 2019).

37.4.2 Health literacy

Health literacy can be defined through both a personal and an organisational lens. Personal health literacy explores the individual's ability to locate, understand, and utilise information and services to make informed health-related decisions and actions (Yinusa-Nyahkoon & Berger, 2024). An organisation's responsibility is to be equitable in enabling individuals in this process. Improving health literacy is a key strategy in population health to empower people to improve their health and prevent illness and disability. Health literacy is influenced by individual factors such as age, gender, race, education, language, sensory abilities (e.g., eyesight and hearing), geographical location, socio-economic status, and cultural background. Environmental components of health literacy, such as infrastructure, policies, processes, systemic oppression, working conditions, social systems, and power inequity and relationships, also impact patient referral pathways, coordination of care, and hospital layouts (Yinusa-Nyahkoon & Berger, 2024). Health care professionals need to identify how, what, where, and when to communicate information for comprehension and to check for understanding (Yinusa-Nyahkoon & Berger, 2024). Occupational therapists have a role in developing individual and organisational health literacy by creating accessible, equitable, and inclusive policies, programmes, and resources.

These determinants of health can be addressed together to achieve better health outcomes for populations. The case study gives an example of an intervention that focused on culture and health literacy simultaneously.

37.5 Case study: Occupational therapy in action – addressing population determinants

An occupational therapist in an outpatient oncology unit runs activity-based 'stress management' and 'understanding cancer and recovery' education groups. They noticed that patients from culturally and linguistically diverse (CALD) backgrounds were under-represented and observed that those who attended rarely applied the information and skills taught. The occupational therapist explored factors contributing to the lower attendance rates of CALD patients.

They found differences in oncology consultations between Australian-born and overseas-born patients and investigated social determinants contributing this. Using data from the Australian Bureau of Statistics, they established a higher proportion of people who spoke a language other than English at home in the local area. Literature revealed cultural differences in healthcare interactions, with doctors spending less time discussing cancer with immigrants, especially those with interpreters (Theodosopoulos et al., 2024). The therapist hypothesised lower health literacy among CALD patients might be a factor.

To ensure equitable access, the therapist raised cultural awareness among the oncology team through education packages and co-designed flyers with CALD patients using pictures and minimal text. They also included video clips in session content and employed the 'teach-back' technique to reinforce key information. 'Teach-back' refers to patients' demonstration of their understanding of the information provided (Yen & Leasure, 2019). These measures improved the cultural competency of the team and the health literacy of the patients.

37.6 Promoting health

The Ottawa Charter (WHO, 1986) defined health promotion as 'a process of enabling people to increase control over, and to improve, their health' (para. 1). The view that health is a resource for life (WHO, 1986) is consistent with occupational therapy's stance that health provides the physical, mental and social capacities that enable people to do what they want, need or are expected to do.

Health promotion originated in health education but now goes beyond a focus on individual behaviour and lifestyles to address a wide range of social and environmental determinants. The Ottawa Charter (WHO, 1986) identified five health promotion action areas: i) build healthy public policy, ii) create supportive environments, iii) strengthen community actions, iv) develop personal skills, and v) reorient health services. Developing personal skills and creating supportive environments are central to occupational therapy practice, while the remaining action areas encourage occupational therapists to work with communities to develop policies to create sustained change within health services and other settings. Health promotion initiatives that use combinations of the five actions are more effective than single-track approaches (WHO, 1997).

37.7 Preventing illness and disability

Health protection approaches focus on protecting the population from communicable diseases, such as sexually transmissible infections or coronavirus outbreaks, while prevention approaches focus on chronic health conditions and injuries, such as diabetes or repetitive strain industry. From a prevention perspective, the optimal outcome of intervention is the absence of illness or disability, which represents good health. Three levels of prevention are identified: i) primary, ii) secondary, and iii) tertiary (AOTA, 2020).

Primary prevention initiatives are aimed at healthy populations, prior to the development of risk factors, designed to prevent any progression to a physical or mental health condition. Secondary prevention initiatives target populations who are 'at-risk', because they have been exposed to risk factors or are showing early signs or symptoms of a health condition. The aim of secondary prevention is to address risk factors and early symptoms to stop or slow the progression of symptoms or disability and, ideally, return individuals to optimal health. Finally, tertiary prevention targets populations who have been diagnosed with an ongoing health condition or disability and refers to interventions to prevent the progression and complications of health conditions and their reoccurrence. The case study provides an example of how primary, secondary, and tertiary prevention initiatives can be applied.

37.8 Case study: occupational therapy in action – illness and disability prevention

A pair of occupational therapy students were assigned to a project to support the development of children's school readiness skills in a kindergarten. The kindergarten was in a suburb where many children were from low-income, single-parent families. The early childhood educator recognised early life experiences and education as health determinants and wanted to prevent further disadvantage. After consulting with educators, parents, children, teachers, and local primary schools and reviewing the literature, the students proposed three interventions.

The first primary intervention involved educating educators and parents on children's emotional and behavioural development and using play to enhance early life experiences and prevent problems. The second intervention, based on secondary prevention, involved early childhood educators identifying children who experienced trauma or showed signs of developmental delay for further assessment and intervention. The third intervention, based on tertiary prevention, involved occupational therapists working with children diagnosed with behavioural disorders. The therapist also provided consultations to educators and parents to extend intervention across home and educational environments and share perspectives on referral processes with students. During the project, the students also created a resource of information booklets and play activities and developed referral pathways with the local community health service. An evaluation found the referral process was simple and clear to educators and parents, and the education sessions improved parents' understanding of school readiness and increased educators' confidence in identifying behavioural and emotional issues.

37.9 Occupational therapy's role in fostering health and well-being of individuals, communities, and populations

Occupational therapy contributes a person-centred and occupational focus to address health inequalities and improve population health and well-being. Population health approaches are often incorporated into occupational therapists' clinical roles, for instance when conducting quality improvement projects, while others may be employed in a health promotion, illness prevention, or population/public health roles in a variety of health care, education, workplace, and community settings (Muriithi, 2024). Adopting a population health approach, where the most beneficial impact occurs from micro/meso/macro-systematic interventions (Muriithi, 2024; Lynch et al., 2023), challenges occupational therapy to adopt a wider lens to address the broader determinants of health and well-being including equitable participation in occupations.

Occupational therapy conceptual models of practice, such as the Model of Human Occupation (MOHO), Person-Environment-Occupation model (PEO), Do Live Well, and others, are inclusive of environmental factors that influence individual, families, and community health (Muriithi, 2024). As these frameworks indicate, population health approaches may incorporate occupation as a means to improve health and well-being or as an end in itself to support participation and advance occupational justice (Muriithi, 2024). In a population health context, evaluation of process, impact, and outcomes establishes how an intervention is implemented; whether the intervention met its Objectives; and its long-term effects on participation, health, and well-being (Muriithi, 2024; Toto & Ching, 2024). Examples of evaluating occupationally focused population health programmes include the community and population health practice (CPHP) paradigm by Scaffa and Reitz (2020, as cited in Muriithi, 2024). Additionally, the population health programme evaluation guidelines by the AOTA includes ten outcome measures such as assessing occupational participation and performance, occupational justice, and wellbeing (Muriithi, 2024).

37.10 Conclusion

In this chapter, population health, illness prevention, and health promotion were discussed in relation to contemporary occupational therapy practice. Population health, illness prevention, and health promotion are related concepts integrated in the daily practice of occupational therapy. Occupational therapy and population health share many similarities including:

- A commitment to professional, ethical, and evidence-informed practice;
- An ecological approach that considers people and what they do within their environment;
- Working towards equity and social justice.

Occupational therapy contributes a unique occupation focus and a person-centred perspective to population health. The ability to work with communities and populations, as well as individuals and groups, is now specified in the contemporary education of occupational therapists and recognised as a required competency for all occupational therapists (OTBA, 2018). Occupational therapy models of practice and emerging frameworks provide a solid foundation for addressing determinants of health and supporting the participation, health, and well-being of communities and populations.

37.11 Summary

- Occupational therapists are increasingly providing services to groups, communities, and populations.
- Population health aims to understand patterns of health and disease and identify and address health inequalities.
- There are similarities between occupational therapy and population health approaches in that both focus on the relationships between what people do in their environments and their health and well-being.
- Population health interventions must go beyond individual behaviours and lifestyles to address broader determinants of health, such as culture and health literacy.
- Occupational therapists contribute a person-centred and occupational perspective to population health.

37.12 Review questions

- What is a population, and why is it important for occupational therapists to take a population health perspective?
- What are the key differences between the biomedical model and social model of health?
- What are the two aims of population health?
- You are working as an occupational health and safety advisor at a large organisation and have been asked to develop a programme for employees to prevent occupational overuse injuries. What type of prevention approach would you use and why?
- Think of a health promotion initiative (e.g. SunSmart, This Girl Can, Movember). Based on the Ottawa Charter (WHO, 1986), which health promotion actions are used? What occupations do these initiatives involve?

References

Agner, J. (2020). Moving from cultural competence to cultural humility in occupational therapy: A paradigm shift. *American Journal of Occupational Therapy*, 74(4), 7404347010p1–7404347010p7. https://doi.org/10.5014/ajot.2020.038067

American Occupational Therapy Association. (2020). Educator's guide for addressing cultural awareness, humility, and dexterity in occupational therapy curricula. *American Journal of Occupational Therapy*, 74(Supp 3), 7413420003p1–7413420003p19. https://doi.org/10.5014/ajot.2020.74S3005

Australian Institute of Health and Welfare. (2016). *Australia's health 2016: Health across socioeconomic groups* (Cat. no. AUS 199). AIHW.

Australian Institute of Health and Welfare [AIHW]. (2024a). *Australia's health: Topic summaries*. AIHW. https://www.aihw.gov.au/reports-data/australias-health/summaries

Australian Institute of Health and Welfare [AIHW]. (2024b). *Australian burden of disease study 2024*. AIHW. https://www.aihw.gov.au/reports/burden-of-disease/australian-burden-of-disease-study-2024

Bailliard, A. (2024). Occupational justice. In G. Gillen & C. Brown (Eds.), *Willard & Spackman's occupational therapy* (14th ed., pp. 139–160). Wolters Kluwer.

Beagan, B. L. (2015). A critique of cultural competence: Assumptions, limitations, and alternatives. In C. L. Frisby & W. T. O'Donohue (Eds.), *Cultural competence in applied psychology: An evaluation of current status and future directions* (pp. 123–138). Springer.

Curtis, E., Jones, R., Tipene-Leach, D., Walker, C., Loring, B., Paine, S.-J., & Reid, P. (2019). Why cultural safety rather than cultural competency is required to achieve health equity: A literature review and recommended definition. *International Journal for Equity in Health*, *18*(1), 174–181. https://doi.org/10.1186/s12939-019-1082-3

Egan, M., & Restall, G. (2022). Collaborative relationship-focused occupational therapy. In M. Egan & G. Restall (Eds.), *Promoting occupational participation: Collaborative relationship-focused occupational therapy* (pp. 97–117). Canadian Association of Occupational Therapists.

Germov, J. (Ed.). (2019). *Second opinion: An introduction to health sociology* (6th ed.). Oxford University Press.

Hamilton, K. A., Letts, L. J., Larivière, N., & Moll, S. E. (2023). Revisiting the Do-Live-Well health promotion framework: A citation content analysis. *Canadian Journal of Occupational Therapy*, *90*(3), 297–302. https://doi.org/10.1177/00084174221149268

Hocking, C., & Sutton, D. (2024). Contribution of occupation to health and well-being. In G. Gillen & C. Brown (Eds.), *Willard & Spackman's occupational therapy* (14th ed., pp. 111–122). Wolters Kluwer.

Hosseinpoor, A. R., Bergen, N., Kirkby, K., & Schlotheuber, A. (2023). Strengthening and expanding health inequality monitoring for the advancement of health equity: A review of WHO resources and contributions. *International Journal for Equity in Health*, *22*(49). https://doi.org/10.1186/s12939-022-01811-4

Hyett, N., Kenny, A., & Dickson-Swift, V. (2019). Re-imagining occupational therapy clients as communities: Presenting the community-centred practice framework. *Scandinavian Journal of Occupational Therapy*, *26*(4), 246–260. https://doi.org/10.1080/11038128.2017.1423374

Lynch, H., Moore, A., O'Connor, D., & Boyle, B. (2023). Evidence for implementing tiered approaches in school-based occupational therapy in elementary schools: A scoping review. *American Journal of Occupational Therapy*, *77*(1), 1–11. https://doi.org/10.5014/ajot.2023.050027

Lysack, C. L., Adamo, D. E., & Galvaan, R. (2024). Social, economic, and political factors that influence occupational performance. In G. Gillen & C. Brown (Eds.), *Willard & Spackman's occupational therapy* (14th ed., pp. 224–242). Wolters Kluwer.

Minister of Health. (2023). *New Zealand health strategy*. Ministry of Health. https://www.health.govt.nz/publications/new-zealand-health-strategy#mig

Muriithi, B. A. K. (2024). Occupational therapy evaluation and intervention for communities and populations. In G. Gillen & C. Brown (Eds.), *Willard & Spackman's occupational therapy* (14th ed., pp. 366–377). Wolters Kluwer.

Occupational Therapy Board of Australia. (2018). *Australian occupational therapy competency standards 2018*. https://www.occupationaltherapyboard.gov.au/Codes-Guidelines/Competencies.aspx

Redvers, N., Celidwen, Y., Schultz, C., Horn, O., Githaiga, C., Vera, M., Perdrisat, M., Mad Plume, L., Kobei, D., Kain, M. C., Poelina, A., Rojas, J. N., & Blondin, B. (2022). The determinants of planetary health: An Indigenous consensus perspective. *Lancet Planet Health*, *6*(2), e156–e163. https://doi.org/10.1016/S2542-5196(21)00354-5

Theodosopoulos, L., Fradelos, E. C., Panagiotou, A., Dreliozi, A., & Tzavella, F. (2024). Delivering culturally competent care to migrants by healthcare personnel: A crucial aspect of delivering culturally sensitive care. *Social Sciences*, *13*(10), 530. https://doi.org/10.3390/socsci13100530

Toto, S. K., & Ching, K. (2024). Occupational therapy practice through the lens of primary health care. In G. Gillen & C. Brown (Eds.), *Willard & Spackman's occupational therapy* (pp. 1175–1196). Wolters Kluwer.

Trentham, B. (2022). Occupational (therapy's) possibilities: A queer reflection on the tangled threads of oppression and our collective liberation. *Canadian Journal of Occupational Therapy*, *89*(4), 346–363. https://doi.org/10.1177/00084174221129700

Wakefield, M. K., Williams, D. R., Le Menestrel, S., & Flaubert, J. L. (2021). Social determinants of health and health equity. In M. K. Wakefield, D. R. Williams, S. Le Menestrel, & J. L. Flaubert (Eds.), *The future of nursing 2020–2030: Charting a path to achieve health equity* (pp. 31–58). The National Academies Press. https://doi.org/10.17226/25982

Wilcock, A. A., & Hocking, C. (2015). *An occupational perspective of health.* SLACK Inc.

World Federation of Occupational Therapists. (2012). *Definitions of occupational therapy from member organisations.* http://www.wfot.org/ResourceCentre.aspx

World Health Organization. (1946, June 19–22). *Preamble to the constitution of the World Health Organization.* Paper presented at the International Health Conference, New York.

World Health Organization. (1986, November 21). *The Ottawa Charter for Health Promotion.* Paper presented at the First International Conference on Health Promotion, Ottawa.

World Health Organization. (1997, July 21–25). *Jakarta declaration on leading health promotion into the 21st Century.* Paper presented at the Fourth International Conference on Health Promotion, Jakarta. http://www.who.int/healthpromotion/conferences/previous/jakarta/declaration/en/

Yen, P. H., & Leasure, A. R. (2019). Use and effectiveness of the teach-back method in patient education and health outcomes. *Federal Practitioner: For the Health Care Professionals of the VA, DoD, and PHS*, *36*(6), 284–289. https://cbrhl.org.au/wp-content/uploads/2020/11/Use-and-Effectiveness-of-the-Teach-Back-method.pdf

Yinusa-Nyahkoon, L., & Berger, S. (2024). Best practices for health education. In G. Gillen & C. Brown (Eds.), *Willard and Spackman's occupational therapy* (14th ed., pp. 378–390). Wolters Kluwer.

CHAPTER 38

Occupational therapy practice in regional, rural, and remote Australia

Monica Moran, Carol McKinstry, and Michael Curtin

Authors' positionality statement

As authors of this chapter, we acknowledge that we are Western-educated occupational therapists who have lived and worked in rural areas for most of our working lives. Our occupational therapy perspectives have been shaped by our professional experiences both in Australia and internationally and by our commitment to social and occupational justice, culturally safe and responsive practice, and equitable access to health services for all people. We recognise that the social determinants of health have an important impact on health inequalities. We acknowledge that we have much to learn from Indigenous and other non-Western approaches to social and emotional wellbeing.

Key terms
- Rural practice
- Occupational therapy
- Workforce
- Rural service delivery

Objectives
This chapter will allow the reader to:

- Describe differing lived experiences of people in rural Australia
- Describe and apply the Modified Monash Model
- Recognise rural contexts of health care service
- Grasp the diversity of, and identify successful strategies for, rural occupational therapy practice
- Understand options for rural student placements

DOI: 10.4324/9781003495666-41

38.1 Introduction

Australia is a large country (7,672,024 km²) with a relatively small population of approximately 27 million people (Australian Bureau of Statistics, 2024). Approximately 25% of Australians live in regional, rural, and remote areas (Australian Institute of Health and Welfare, 2024a). Consistent with the National Rural Health Alliance (NRHA) (2025), this chapter refers to the phrase 'regional, rural and remote locations' collectively as 'rural'. Rural is an umbrella term that encompasses non-metropolitan geographical, political, economic, cultural, and spiritual contexts across Australia.

38.2 Life in rural areas

It is recognised that people living in rural parts of Australia 'make a profound contribution to the economic and social fabric of the nation' (National Rural Health Commissioner, 2019, p. 5) and that people living in these communities can experience higher levels of social participation and inclusion than people living in metropolitan settings (McIntosh et al., 2019; Wilkins et al., 2022). The NRHA (2025, p. 3) states that people living in rural areas have many positive experiences, including that they are more likely to engage in volunteering and less likely to report loneliness, have high satisfaction with relationships and future security, have low levels of financial stress related to housing, and have a sense of community connectedness.

However, the Australian Institute of Health and Welfare (AIHW) (2024a) suggests that people living in rural areas 'can face unique challenges due to their geographic location and often have poorer health outcomes than people living in metropolitan areas' (p. 94). Some of these unique challenges include poor internet access and mobile phone reception, low rates of completion of secondary school and reduced participation in higher education, low incomes on average, and high levels of unemployment (NRHA, 2025, p. 3). Poorer health outcomes increase the more remote the population is with higher rates of health risk factors (e.g. smoking, alcohol consumption, physical inactivity, and being overweight), burden of disease (as measured by the health impact of disease on a population in a given year in terms of dying and living with disease and injury – disability-adjusted life years [DALYs]), potentially avoidable death (i.e. deaths among people under 75 years considered preventable due to individual or primary health/hospital care), and hospitalisations (AIHW, 2024b). Life expectancy is generally lower the more remote the area where a person lives (NRHA, 2025).

Poorer health outcomes have been associated with several factors, including 'challenges of geographic spread, low population density, limited infrastructure, as well as the higher costs of delivering rural . . . health care' (AIHW, 2024b, p. 265). In part the reduced access to health care is due to a significant decline in the number of health care professionals, or hours of health professionals' service, as remoteness increases (Battye et al., 2019; Grant et al., 2022; Hayes et al., 2023; Johnsson et al., 2019). The inequitable distribution of health professionals in rural Australia negatively impacts health, wellbeing, and economic participation (National Rural Health Commissioner, 2019). In addition, many people living in these areas must travel to towns and cities that are regional hubs, as well as to major cities, to access specialised health services.

38.3 Modified Monash Model location classification system

To determine the relationship between locations with health outcomes, health workforce and resource needs, and influence the development and implementation of federal, state and territory government policies and priorities, a system to classify and distinguish different locations, the Modified Monash Model (MMM), was developed (Department of Health, 2024; Services for Australian Rural and Remote Allied Health, 2015). The MMM is a location classification system used to identify the disparities in access to health services across Australia (Department of Health, 2024). This model has been used, for example, to determine financial incentives, such as subsidised housing and other allowances, to attract and retain health professionals to offer services in MMM regions 4–7 (AIHW, 2024b).

There are seven location categories in the MMM (Department of Health, 2024). These are listed in Table 38.1. The location of the MMM categories on a map of Australia is illustrated in Figure 38.1.

38.4 Occupational therapy workforce distribution

There were 34,143 registered occupational therapists in Australia on 30 March 2025 (Occupational Therapy Board of Australia, 2025), indicating continued growth, with

Table 38.1 Modified Monash Model categories (based on Australian Government Department of Health and Aged Care, n.d.). Population numbers recorded in the brief description for each category are based on 2023 data provided by National Rural Health Alliance (2025)

MMM category	Brief description
Modified Monash 1 (MM1)	Metropolitan area: major cities, accounting for approximately 70% of Australia's population. Population: 19,195,844
Modified Monash 2 (MM2)	Regional centres: areas within 20km road distance of a town with a population greater than 50,000. Population: 2,443,271
Modified Monash 3 (MM3)	Large rural towns: areas within 15km road distance, of a town with a population between 15,000 and 50,000. Population: 1,670,624
Modified Monash 4 (MM4)	Medium rural towns: areas within 10km road distance, of a town with a population between 5,000 and 15,000. Population: 1,010,381
Modified Monash 5 (MM5)	Small rural towns: other regional areas. Population: 1,825,015
Modified Monash 6 (MM6)	Remote communities: remote mainland areas and remote islands less than 5 kms offshore. Population: 294,605
Modified Monash 7 (MM7)	Very remote communities: Very remote areas and island communities more than 5km offshore or less than 5km offshore with a population less than 1000 and no bridges to the mainland. Population: 209,138

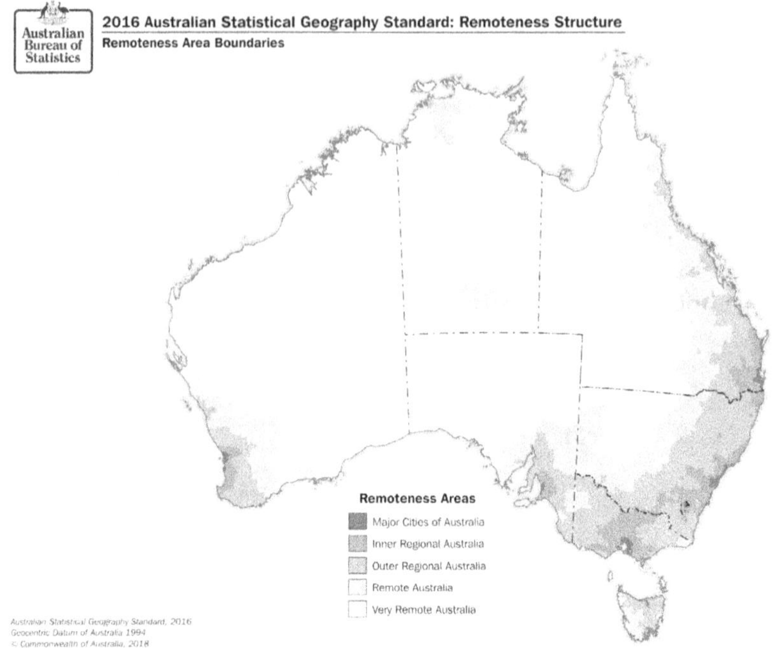

Figure 38.1 Map of the Modified Monash Model regions

(Department of Health, 2024)

Table 38.2 Occupational therapist practice locations in 2022

Level of remoteness	Number of registered and employed occupational therapists
Major cities	19,369
Inner regional	3,769
Outer regional	1,438
Remote	180
Very remote	64

a 7.7% increase between June 2023 and June 2024. The demand for occupational therapy services as part of a rural health workforce is anticipated to continue growing as the populations in rural areas become older and rates of chronic diseases increase (AIHW, 2024a). An overview of the number of occupational therapists working in different locations in Australia is provided in Table 38.2.

Due to ongoing legislative and policy changes, such as the National Disability Insurance Scheme, practice areas occupational therapists are working in have changed and continue to evolve. In 2022 there had been an increase in the number of occupational therapists working in the practice areas of paediatrics, disability, and mental health (Table 38.3). More occupational therapists are working in the community, particularly in the private sector, rather than in institutional settings such as hospitals

Table 38.3 Australian occupational therapists' practice areas (Australian Government Deparmtnet of Health and Aged Care, 2024)

Practice area	2021	2022
Paediatrics	5744	6469
Disability	4025	4516
Aged care	3613	3551
Rehabilitation	3444	3474
Mental health	2759	2955
Other	1565	2089
Occupational health	1525	1203
Neurological	745	808
Hand therapy	743	773
Palliative care	188	230
Driving assessment	90	109

(Occupational Therapy Australia [OTA], 2023). Occupational therapists are also increasingly working in consumer-directed care services (OTA, 2023) where consumers have control over their funded packages and determine who will provide their services, although choice of services may be limited in rural settings where there are fewer occupational therapists available. Costs associated with rural and remote private practice can be higher due to increased travel costs and lower economies of scale, which may not be necessarily factored into funding structures (OTA, 2023).

38.5 Building the occupational therapy rural workforce

Recruiting occupational therapists to rural positions will not address the disparities in rural health outcomes unless there are sound strategies to support therapists to stay and build their professional expertise. A study by Wakerman et al. (2019) reported that in 53 Northern Territory remote clinics, allied health turnover was as high as 80%, with half of these staff leaving within 12 months. This revolving door of employment means that service provision is disjointed, and the costs associated with recurring recruitment eats into rural health budgets that could be better spent on direct service delivery.

Kumar et al. (2020) and Dymmott et al. (2022) suggest that complex factors contribute to recruiting and retaining staff, including prior exposure to rural experiences, being included in the workplace and the community, feeling supported, and being exposed to a diverse caseload which provides opportunities to have a positive impact. The relationship between these factors and retention is mediated by personal and professional satisfaction (Dymmott et al., 2022). Cosgrave et al.'s (2018) study of rurally based allied health professionals and nurses working in community mental health reinforced the importance of both personal and professional expectations being met for these professionals to remain in rural positions.

Continuing or long-term contract positions provide opportunities for therapists to 'find their feet' within the workplace and within the community. Wakerman et al. (2019) recommend the provision of flexible working arrangements to allow health personnel to manage the demands of rural living, upskill and build their expertise, and move between areas of specialisation.

Working in rural locations requires a different skill set than working in a metropolitan area, due to caseload diversity and the prevalence of clients with complex, chronic conditions such as diabetes, arthritis, and mental illness (AIHW, 2018; Dymmott et al., 2022; Kumar et al., 2020), as well as higher frequencies of injury (NRHA, 2025). The broad-based, unique, and specialised practice skills required to meet the needs of rural populations means that occupational therapists require diverse continuing professional development (CPD), focusing on both the variety and complexity of clinical presentations, as well as administrative competencies. Pang et al. (2024) found that CPD was essential for rural allied health professionals because it contributed to providing career fulfilment, as well as workforce retention. However, accessing CPD can be a significant ongoing challenge. Relevant training often involves travel and accommodation away from the workplace and therapists need to strongly advocate for their CPD needs to be met. As digital connectivity improves in rural locations opportunities are increasing for rural therapists to undertake CPD, supervision and mentoring via online platforms. Membership of professional associations enables rural therapists to develop their professional networks, take on leadership roles and access evidence-based online CPD.

Participating in the community via informal interactions, sports, leisure, and cultural events are strategies to prevent social isolation and establish local networks (Dymmott et al., 2022; Kumar et al., 2020). Strategies for connection can contribute positively to self-management and self-care by increasing personal and professional support networks.

Allied health professionals who work in rural locations are encouraged to build strong, trusting relationships and genuine partnerships with First Nations communities and peoples (Tamwoy et al., 2022). This will include valuing and learning from First Nations worldviews and knowledges, and being open to 'changes in personal capacity, organisational mindset, and policy for the system to engage authentically with Aboriginal and Torres Strait Islander Peoples' (Tamwoy et al., 2022, p. 820). By learning to work in a culturally safe way, being self-reflective, and taking time to engage with community members, allied health professionals and students will learn to appreciate the strengths of the First Nations peoples in the communities in which they work and as well as contributing to their own personal growth (Green et al., 2025).

A rapid review conducted by Battye et al. (2019) on behalf of Services for Australian Rural and Remote Allied Health (SARRAH) found that there was emerging evidence of the positive impact of the 'rural pipeline' on the factors that influenced recruitment and retention of allied health professionals in rural areas of Australia (Table 38.4). The 'rural pipeline' refers to 'recruiting students from rural backgrounds, delivering regional training, exposure during training to rural curriculum and placement, and then building opportunities for regional postgraduate training' (Battye et al., 2019, p. 4).

38.6 Undertaking placements in rural areas

Ensuring that new graduates have knowledge of and a positive attitude towards rural work opportunities is essential. This may be best achieved by students completing a successful rural placement (Green et al., 2025). University programmes are identifying the importance of preparing graduates for rural practice. This involves designing a curriculum that embeds appropriate skills for rural practice and provides students with access to quality rural placements. An increasing number of Australian universities have established occupational therapy courses in regional areas while other courses require students to undertake at least one placement in a rural area.

Table 38.4 Summary of factors that influence recruitment and retention of allied health professionals in rural areas across the profession lifespan (Source: Battye et al., 2019, p. 5)

Elements	University	Early career	Establishing career	Mature Career
Attraction and selection	■ Describe the role and service environment ■ Market and promote rural practice and lifestyle professional and personal benefits			Re-entry programmes and support
Training pipeline	Quality student placements	Rural clinical and non-clinical skills and capability development	Advanced CPD	
Mentoring, supervision and support	Co-design support strategies with allied health stakeholders			
Accreditation and recognition	Nationally accredited postgraduate education programmes for rural and remote practice and transferrable qualifications			
Underpinning components				
Incentives	■ Financial incentives tailored to career and life stages ■ Non-financial incentives – e.g. partner/spouse employment, community connection			
Supportive work environment	For example, adequate staffing and leave relief, effective workplace, sustainable service delivery model			
System capability	Enable allied health professionals to work to their full scope of practice			
Recognition of allied health contribution	Building the evidence for: ■ Allied health intervention in rural ■ Workforce strategies ■ Cost effective service models			

Rural placements provide students with exposure to environments that demand innovation and creative clinical reasoning, often with fewer resources and more distributed service delivery models. Conversely students are exposed to the benefits of rural practice, with smaller close-knit multidisciplinary teams, supportive communities, and opportunities to extend their learning. Many students who complete placements in their final years of university return to take up professional roles in rural locations. Luka's practice story (Box 38.1) illustrates the benefits for students of study close to their rural home. To increase the number of allied health students (including occupational therapy students) experiencing regional, rural, and remote placements, the Commonwealth government has over the past 20 years developed and funded 19 Departments of Rural Health (DRH) attached to universities. The impact of DRH programmes is evaluated annually to evidence their positive impact on rural health workforce growth. The following quote from a Rural Health Service employer articulate how valuable student placement programmes are in increasing exposure to rural practice opportunities and building the rural allied health workforce:

I currently have four staff members in my team who completed a DRH rural placement in the region. Completing a placement gives students an understanding of our rural context and they make social connections here, so their willingness to apply for roles in our region is increased.

WA rural director of Community Health Service 2020

Box 38.1
Luka: A long and winding road to becoming an occupational therapist

Luka grew up in a rural town with a population of 6,000 people about 2 hours' drive from the nearest city and university. He always wanted to work in a health field and completed his high school work experience at the local public hospital where he saw a range of allied health professionals at work. He was very interested in the occupational therapist's role when he observed her work on home modifications for a local man who had sustained a serious injury. However, he worried that he did not have the academic or life skills to cope with university in the city.

In his final year of high school, he applied for a university bridging programme offered at the local Regional University Study Hub (RUSH) in his town. The RUSH provided a place for Luka to study and complete a one-year preparation programme that helped him improve his academic reading and writing skills as well as time management and workload prioritisation.

Over the course of the year Luka realised that he would not have a competitive score to achieve direct access into a university occupational therapy programme at the end of the bridging programme; however, he found out that he could apply to study a Bachelor of Health Sciences (BHSc) programme that would allow him to study some of the first-year subjects of occupational therapy and that if he maintained a good grade point average, he would be able to apply to transfer to the occupational therapy programme after one year. The fact that he could study the BHSc first-year programme remotely at the RUSH in his hometown was a strong incentive, and Luka continued his quest to become an occupational therapist.

He passed all the requirements of the first-year BHSc and was able to apply for direct entry to the occupational therapy programme. Finally, after two years, Luka was ready to start his occupational therapy journey. However, the programme was not offered remotely, and he realised that he would need to be on campus for tutorials, labs, and practical sessions. The cost of living away from home was prohibitive, and Luka had existing commitments at home where he was also a carer for his mother who had a chronic illness. He negotiated with his occupational therapy lecturers that he would drive to university three days per week for essential face-to-face learning and attend other learning activities remotely. This placed a significant time and financial burden on him but allowed him to continue to live at home, and he was relieved that he was able to meet his family obligations.

As Luka moved into third year of his programme the prospect of attending full-time placements weighed heavily on him. The university negotiated two consecutive placements with supervising therapists based in his local town, the first at a private paediatric service and the second at the local hospital where he had first been exposed to occupational therapy. Luka enjoyed the learning experiences he was exposed to during these placements.

Going into his final year of study Luka knew that he would face further challenges to complete his final long placement. Again, working closely with the university placement coordinator, he accepted a role emerging interprofessional placement at a small school in a remote community setting alongside two social work students and one speech pathology student. The placement was facilitated by a DRH and included the provision of a long-arm clinical supervisor, comfortable accommodation, and a vehicle for the students. Having access to no-cost accommodation was a game changer for Luka. He also received a scholarship from a local not-for-profit organisation that helped him with the day-to-day costs of being away from home as well as funding to help with care for his mother.

Luka revelled in the role emerging placement. His previous study experiences had prepared him to be autonomous and goal directed. He valued the on-site Aboriginal introduction and orientation that involved a visit to sites of significance to the local Aboriginal community and a Clinical Yarning training session. Luka knew how important it was to practice in a culturally sensitive way, and Clinical Yarning provided him with a new skill set.

At the end of his long placement Luka was proud of the work he and his student colleagues had accomplished, and he knew they developed a strong foundation programme to hand on to the next interprofessional student team. Luka was surprised at how much he enjoyed staying in the DRH accommodation, and he made some lifelong friends with students from other universities and other professions.

At the end of his degree, he reflected that his rural student journey to become an occupational therapist was long and demanding, but he learned to be solution focused and resourceful as he pursued his career goal. He developed and used skills of organisation, self-management, and negotiation to navigate the challenges of university study whilst living rurally and managing carer responsibilities. Tapping into rural support services such as the RUSH and DRH and local scholarship opportunities, as well as leaning into university support networks, allowed him to enter his chosen career. Going forward Luka planned to advocate for rural students to have greater access to rural and remote occupational therapy study via RUSH so that more students could enter the profession. He is now employed as a valued team member in the local hospital in his hometown where he first learned about occupational therapy.

38.7 Conclusion

Practice in rural areas offers many opportunities, rewards, and challenges for occupational therapists. Understanding the geographical, social, and cultural contexts for practice is essential for occupational therapists to successfully participate in the rural health workforce. Implementing a variety of strategies that assist in managing these unique challenges is critical for personal and professional development and sustainability.

38.8 Summary

- Rural is an umbrella term that encompasses non-metropolitan geographical, political, economic, cultural, and spiritual contexts across Australia.
- Life expectancy is generally lower the more remote a person lives.
- The inequitable distribution of health professionals in rural Australia negatively impacts health, wellbeing and economic participation.
- Modified Monash Model (MMM) is a system of seven categories used by governments to classify and distinguish different locations.
- Working in rural locations requires a different skill set than working in a metropolitan area, due to caseload diversity and the prevalence of clients with complex, chronic conditions as well as higher frequencies of injuries.
- University programmes are identifying the importance of preparing graduates for rural practice, including developing rural practice education placements.
- Working in a rural or remote region can provide many exciting opportunities for occupational therapists.

38.9 Review questions

- Describe the influence of level of remoteness on occupational therapy workforce distribution.
- How can new graduates working in rural locations sustain their professional development needs?
- Explain the benefits and challenges associated with providing occupational therapy services in rural settings.
- Having read the practice stories, how would you seek out more information about working rurally?

References

Australian Bureau of Statistics. (2021 July–2026 June). *Remoteness structure*. ABS. https://www.abs.gov.au/statistics/standards/australian-statistical-geography-standard-asgs-edition-3/jul2021-jun2026/remoteness-structure

Australian Bureau of Statistics. (2024, March). *National, state and territory population*. ABS. https://www.abs.gov.au/statistics/people/population/national-state-and-territory-population/mar-2024

Australian Government Department of Health. (2015). *Telehealth*. http://www.health.gov.au/internet/main/publishing.nsf/content/e-health-telehealth

Australian Government Department of Health and Aged Care. (n.d.). *Modified Monash Model*. https://www.health.gov.au/topics/rural-health-workforce/classifications/mmm

Australian Government Department of Health and Aged Care. (2024). *About allied health care*. https://www.health.gov.au/topics/allied-health/about

Australian Institute of Health and Welfare. (2018). *Rural, regional and remote health: Indicators of health system performance.* https://www.aihw.gov.au/reports/rural-health/rural-regional-and-remote-health-indicators-of-health-system-performance/contents/table-of-contents

Australian Institute of Health and Welfare. (2024a). *Australia's health 2024: in brief, catalogue number AUS 249, AIHW, Australian Government.* https://www.aihw.gov.au/getmedia/6b19e493-0ebe-420f-a9a3-e48b26aace9f/aihw-aus-249-ib.pdf?v=202407151547339&inline=true

Australian Institute of Health and Welfare. (2024b). *Rural and remote health, AIHW, Australian Government.* https://www.aihw.gov.au/reports/rural-remote-australians/rural-and-remote-health

Australian Rural Health Education Network. https://arhen.org.au/for-health-students/about-udrhs/

Barrett, S., Howlett, O., Lal, N., & McKinstry, C. (2024). Telehealth-delivered allied health interventions: A rapid umbrella review of systematic reviews. *Telemedicine Journal and E-Health: The Official Journal of the American Telemedicine Association, 30*(6), e1649–e1666. https://doi.org/10.1089/tmj.2023.0546

Battye, K., Roufeil, L., Edwards, M., Hardaker, L., Janssen, T., & Wilkins, R. (2019). *Strategies for increasing allied health recruitment and retention in rural Australia: A rapid review.* https://www.nintione.com.au/?p=39942.

Baxter, J., Gray, M., & Hayes, A. (2011). *Families in regional, rural and remote Australia.* Australian Institute of Family Studies. https://aifs.gov.au/sites/default/files/publication-documents/fs201103.pdf

Cosgrave, C., Maple, M., & Hussain, R. (2018). An explanation of turnover intention among early-career nursing and allied health professionals working in rural and remote Australia – findings from a grounded theory study. *Rural and Remote Health, 18*(3), 4511. https://doi.org/10.22605/RRH4511

Department of Health. (2024). *Modified Monash Model.* https://www.health.gov.au/health-workforce/health-workforce-classifications/modified-monash-model

Dymmott, A., George, S., Campbell, N., & Brebner, C. (2022). Experiences of working as early career allied health professionals and doctors in rural and remote environments: A qualitative systematic review. *BMC Health Services Research, 22*(1), 951. https://doi.org/10.1186/s12913-022-08261-2

Grant, C., Jones, A., & Land, H. (2022). What are the perspectives of speech pathologists, occupational therapists and physiotherapists on using telehealth videoconferencing for service delivery to children with developmental delays? A systematic review of the literature. *Australian Journal of Rural Health, 30*(3), 321–336. https://doi.org/10.1111/ajr.12843

Green, E., Rasiah, R. L., Quilliam, C., Moore, L., Ridd, M., Ferns, J., Sheepway, L., Seaton, C., Taylor, C., & Fitzgerald, K. (2025). What do Australian university staff perceive are the features of high-quality rural health student placements? A sequential explanatory study. *BMJ Open, 15*(6), e098381. https://doi.org/10.1136/bmjopen-2024-098381

Hayes, K., Dos Santos, V., Costigan, M., & Morante, D. (2023). Extension, austerity, and emergence: Themes identified from a global scoping review of non-urban occupational therapy services. *Australian Occupational Therapy Journal, 70*(1), 142–156. https://doi.org/10. 1111/1440-1630.12844

Humphreys, J., Wakerman, J., Pashen, D., & Buykx, P. (2009) *Retention strategies and incentives for health workers in rural and remote areas: What works?* Australian Primary Health Care Research Institute.

Johnsson, G., Kerslake, R., & Crook, S. (2019). Delivering allied health services to regional and remote participants on the autism spectrum via video-conferencing technology: Lessons learned. *Rural and Remote Health, 19*(3), 5358. https://doi.org/10.22605/RRH5358

Kagi, E., Rasiah, R., & Moran, M. (2023). Experiences of primary health care nurses advancing their careers in a remote Western Australian location. *The Australian Journal of Rural Health, 31*(1), 41–51. https://doi.org/10.1111/ajr.12904

Kumar, S., Tian, E. J., May, E. Crouch, R., & McCulloch, M. (2020). 'You get exposed to a wider range of things and it can be challenging but very exciting at the same time': Enablers of and barriers to transition to rural practice by allied health professionals in Australia. *BMC Health Services Research*, 20, 105. https://doi.org/10.1186/s12913-020-4954-8

McIntosh, K., Kenny, A., Masood, M., & Dickson-Swift, V. (2019). Social inclusion as a tool to improve rural health. *Australian Journal of Primary Health*, 25(2), 137–145. https://doi.org/10.1071/PY17185

McKinstry, C., Quilliam, C., Crawford, N., Thompson, J., & Sizer, S. M. (2024). Location and access to health courses for rural students: An Australian audit. *BMC Medical Education*, 24(1), 806. https://doi.org/10.1186/s12909-024-05787-3

National Rural Health Alliance. (2025). *Rural health in Australia snapshot 2025*. https://www.ruralhealth.org.au/wp-content/uploads/2025/02/NRHA-Rural-Health-in-Australia-Snapshot-2025.pdf

National Rural Health Commissioner. (2019). *Rural allied health quality, access and distribution*. https://ahpa.com.au/wp-content/uploads/2019/08/190816-Rural-Remote-Discussion-Paper-response-FINAL.pdf

Occupational Therapy Australia. (2020). *Telehealth guidelines*. https://otaus.com.au/publicassets/553c6eae-ad6c-ea11-9404-005056be13b5/OTA%20Telehealth%20Guidelines%202020.pdf

Occupational Therapy Australia. (2022). *2022–23 pre-budget submission to Australian Government Treasury*. https://treasury.gov.au/sites/default/files/2022-3/258735_occupational_therapy_australia.pdf

Occupational Therapy Australia. (2023). *Workforce development project summary report*. https://otaus.com.au/files/images/WorkforceDevProject/Workforce_Development_Project_2023_Summary.pdf

Occupational Therapy Board of Australia. (2025) *Registrant data*. https://www.occupationaltherapyboard.gov.au/About/Statistics.aspx

Pang, M., Sayner, A., & McKenzie, K. (2024). Continuing professional development training needs of allied health professionals in regional and rural Victoria. *The Australian Journal of Rural Health*, 32(4), 763–773. https://doi.org/10.1111/ajr.13141

Regional University Study Hubs Program. https://www.education.gov.au/regional-university-study-hubs

Services for Australian Rural and Remote Allied Health (SARRAH). (2015). *Defining remote and rural context*. http://www.sarrah.org.au

Tamwoy, N., Rosas, S., Davis, S., Farthing, A., Houghton, C., Johnston, H., Maloney, C., Samulkiewicz, N., Seaton, J., Tuxworth, G., & Bat, M. (2022). Co-design with Aboriginal and Torres Strait Islander communities: A journey. *Australian Journal of Rural Health*, 30, 816–822. https://doi.org/10.1111/ajr.12918

Wakerman, J., Humphreys, J., Russell, D., Guthridge, S., Bourke, L., Dunbar, T., Zhao, Y., Ramjan, M., Murakami-Gold, L., & Jones, M. P. (2019). Remote health workforce turnover and retention: What are the policy and practice priorities? *Human Resources for Health*, 17(1), 99. https://doi.org/10.1186/s12960-019-0432-y

Wilkins, R., Vera-Toscano, E., Botha, F., Wooden, M., & Trinh, T. (2022). *The household, income and labour dynamics in Australia survey: Selected findings from waves 1 to 20*. Melbourne Institute of Applied Economic and Social Research. https://melbourneinstitute.unimelb.edu.au/__data/assets/pdf_file/0011/4382057/HILDA_Statistical_Report_2022.pdf

World Federation of Occupational Therapists. (2014). Position statement on telehealth. *International Journal of Telerehabilitation*, 6(1), 37–39. https://doi.org/10.5195/ijt.2014.6153

Case management in occupational therapy practice in Australia and Aotearoa New Zealand

Sue Lukersmith and Suzanne Patterson

Authors' positionality statement

Sue Lukersmith has worked in various roles across sectors in Australia and internationally, where she recognised case management as a critical component of person-centred integrated health and social care. As a therapist, researcher and academic, she has developed an international reputation as an expert on person-centred care coordination/case management.

Suzanne Patterson (she/her) is of Ngāi Tahu/Ngāti Mamoe descent. She has clinical experience across the mental health and addiction sector, specialising in supporting whaiora and whānau in child and adolescent services. A former case manager in Aotearoa and the United Kingdom, she now teaches on a nationwide programme equipping novice clinicians' skills and knowledge for entering the mental health workforce, including those undertaking case management roles.

Key terms
- Case management
- Occupational therapy
- Person-centred perspective

Objectives
This chapter will allow the reader to:

- Identify and discuss the key principles of case management practice
- Describe the work of case management and common actions performed by case managers
- Describe best practice in different models of case management
- Understand the difference and be able to differentiate between occupational therapy and case management practices

DOI: 10.4324/9781003495666-42

39.1 Background

Case management is a targeted, community-based, and proactive approach to care involving tasks related to assessment, care planning, reviewing options and services needed, and care coordination to integrate services around the needs of people with long-term conditions (adapted from World Health Organization [WHO], 2015). Case management is a multidimensional and collaborative process and emerged in the 1960's in response to the de-institutionalisation of people with long term mental health conditions (Mas-Exposito et al., 2013). Care coordination services were needed to support the person's return to living in a community setting. In the decades since, multiple factors have influenced the need for and increased the presence of case management services within health and social care systems. Some of these are:

- Increased complexity of health systems, cost of health and social care services, and fragmentation of services, as well as access to those services (Kelly et al., 2019). Consequently, the need for care coordination and integrated care has grown in most countries (WHO, 2015).
- The change in the perception of health and disability from an impairment/disease focus towards a holistic conceptualisation of health and functioning espoused in the biopsychosocial model (WHO, 2001). There is demand by clients and value-based health practitioners to adopt an empowerment and person-centred care approach beyond medical care (Lukersmith, Huckel et al., 2016; WHO, 2016)
- Recognition of the social determinants on health (e.g. low education, socio-economic status). Case management and navigation towards appropriate services contributes to reducing health inequities (WHO, 2011).

Since its inception, case management has evolved and is now used in many different settings, with clients of different ages and health conditions.

39.2 Key principles of case management

Principles articulate the foundation for case management behaviour and a chain of reasoning for their actions. Four fundamental principles underpin and guide case management practice, irrespective of the approach, model, or the contexts and systems in which case management occurs. The principles are:

Principle 1. Holistic perspective

- Recognise and consider all aspects of a person (physical, emotional, social, spiritual) and their unique environmental contexts (home, communities, culture, services) are inter-connected and influence their health, wellbeing, and participation (WHO, 2001).
- Maintain a biopsychosocial perspective of health, rather than focusing solely on illness pathology and symptom reduction (WHO, 2001).
- Ensure service delivery is culturally responsive and considers social determinants of health (WHO, 2011).

Principle 2. Person-centred approach

- View the client as the 'expert' in their own lives, who can take responsibility for their health, share knowledge, be informed and involved in all decision-making regarding their care and support services (WHO, 2016).

■ Understand, respect and value the client's right to determine their own goals, and co-create their plan for the appropriate services, supports, and case management they need to achieve their goals (Healthcare Improvement Scotland, 2015; International College of Person-centered Medicine, 2013; Lukersmith, Huckel et al., 2016).

Principle 3. Strengths-based approach

■ Identify and direct all actions towards building on the client's unique strengths, talents, experience, skills, supports, and resources.

■ Facilitate goal attainment, participation and ensure practices and clinical decisions align with client's motivations, values, and beliefs (Rapp, 2006; World Health Organization – European Regional Office [WHO-Euro], 2013).

Principle 4. Collaborative and proactive support

■ Collaborate with the client, their support networks, relevant inter-sector health, social, and education providers and organisations. Understanding these networks and systems and their interactions facilitates improved integrated client care and thereby recovery outcomes (Reeves et al., 2017; WHO, 2016).

■ Proactively plan, coordinate, and monitor the delivery of supports to the client.

39.3 The work of case managers

Case management is a key pillar of integrated care (WHO, 2015) and is defined as a complex intervention in that there are multiple interdependent and dependent actions involved (Craig et al., 2008). Case managers perform various actions, typically described as coordination or administrative actions, which change depending on the client and their needs, health condition, context, and service setting. Practice experience and research evidence tells us that in most case management roles, a range of different actions are performed (Kelly et al., 2019; Lukersmith et al., 2023). Case managers and their actions have been described as the 'relational glue', whereby the client is connected with the right health and social services to meet their needs (Stretton et al., 2022), and client progress is monitored.

There are numerous models, approaches, and roles in the case management sector referred to in the literature (Lukersmith, Millington et al., 2016). The title case management is not person-centred, and typically other titles are preferred. Some of the terms for case manager include care managers; local area coordinators; case manager; clinical/therapy or rehabilitation; medical, strengths-based; nursing; assertive community treatment; intensive; care coordination; care navigator; navigation; generalist, broker, traditional or standard; discharge planner; peer assisted; advocacy; and managerial. Indigenous terms may be used for culturally responsive models (Stretton et al., 2022).

This variation in what a case manager does, with whom, and when, makes understanding, tracking, training, or managing case managers across the different models difficult. Measuring and evaluating the impact of case management is challenging (Köpke & McCleery, 2015; Leonard et al., 2025). The Case Management Taxonomy (CMTaxonomy) was developed to map the different case management actions, definitions and critically analyse the relationships between actions. The CMTaxonomy provides a common language for case management practice, quality analysis, evaluation,

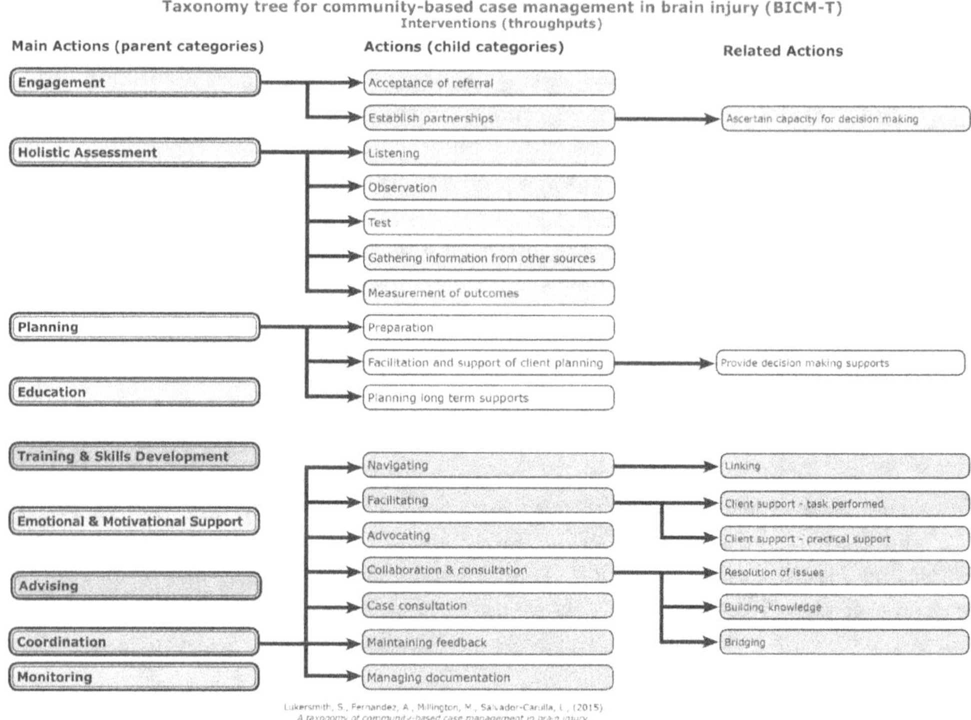

Figure 39.1 CMTaxonomy intervention 'tree' with the main actions, actions and related actions (reproduced with permission) (Lukersmith et al., 2015)

research, policy, service and resource planning (Lukersmith et al., 2015). Since its development, the CMTaxonomy has been used in both research and practice for people with a range of different health conditions and contexts. Figure 39.1 provides the CMTaxonomy Intervention 'tree' with the case manager's main actions, actions, and related actions. The case manager can map and record their actions to the CMTaxonomy, which also allows practitioners to consistently describe what they do in their reports, to their clients, other professionals, managers, funders, and policy makers.

All actions are defined in the CMTaxonomy glossary (Lukersmith et al., 2015). The CMTaxonomy also provides a service 'tree' which defines case management in terms of whether the service is mobile/non-mobile (community or office based), and the intensity of the case manager service provided to each client (Lukersmith et al., 2024). All the CMTaxonomy actions may not be used in each model. However, there are common actions across case management models. Each has benefits, disadvantages, variations, and adaptations to the setting, funding, and service structures in which they operate. Refer to Table 39.1 for examples of three different case management models used in Australia and Aotearoa New Zealand.

A generalist case manager is typically employed to provide practical guidance through a system and is often not mobile (e.g. through an insurance agency for a client injured at work, a discharge planner at hospital). Whereas a community-based case manager is typically employed by health or social service organisations (public,

Table 39.1 Examples of different case management models, approaches, theoretical description, best practice actions and period of involvement

Name/s of model and examples of titles (and period of involvement with the client)	*Theoretical description*	*Common best practice CM Taxonomy actions* performed, and definition*
Generalist, Broker, Medical case manager, Discharge Planner *Involvement is limited*	Impartial organisational or service, focuses approach on connecting the client to needed services and providers	■ Engagement: establish, develop, and maintain a relationship with the client ■ Assessment: through listening and gathering information from other sources (e.g. reports from therapists, doctors, teachers, vocational professionals) ■ Coordination: case consultation, maintaining feedback, managing documentation ■ Monitoring: continuous acquisition of information to evaluate the person's situation to determine their progress and anticipate problems ■ Related actions: actions that are less frequently performed to facilitate coordination (practical support and performing tasks e.g. making a medical appointment)
Community based case manager (Community CM), Care navigator, Care coordinator *Involvement can be brief or over months/years*	Tailored to the individual, person-centred and strengths-based focus to proactively enhance the person's recovery and progress towards participation in life roles and maintaining well being	■ Engagement: see generalist above ■ Assessment: see generalist above ■ Holistic assessment: assessment conducted by the case management through observation of functioning, testing and measurement of outcomes ■ Person-centred planning: supporting the person to develop their individualised plan including setting goals and identify support needs as well, as therapy and rehabilitation related goals ■ Advising: recommending a course to be followed, encourage change in function, environment, and attitude or behaviours to meet health needs and goals, and reduce risk ■ Coordination (see generalist above) ■ Proactive coordination: including navigation, facilitation, advocacy for services, and extensive collaboration ■ Education: Providing structured information to the person, and/or their family, other stakeholders in a manner conducive to improve knowledge about the person's condition, treatment, functioning, or strategies ■ Training and skill development: teaching, enhancing, or developing skills through context-specific practice to stakeholders (e.g. family member) ■ Emotional (and motivational support): providing the person (and others as appropriate) with comfort, empathy, or motivational support ■ Monitoring: (see generalist above) ■ Related actions: (see generalist above)

(Continued)

Table 39.1 (Continued)

Name/s of model and examples of titles (and period of involvement with the client)	*Theoretical description*	*Common best practice CMTaxonomy actions* performed, and definition*
Rehabilitation Case manager, Specialist case manager, Clinical case manager *Involvement can be brief or over months/years*	Involves a hybrid model where the health practitioner (e.g. occupational therapist) provides both clinical interventions to further enhance participation in life roles, and case management actions	■ Occupational therapy treatment relevant to the person's health condition and context (e.g. driving assessment, home modification design, hand therapy, graded return to work/training programme) ■ All or any of the actions described in community-based case manager approach

*Identified in research (Lukersmith et al., 2021; Stretton et al., 2022)

private, or non-governmental organisations [NGOs]) to provide holistic support to people with more complex health conditions (e.g. traumatic brain injury, spinal cord injury, severe mental illness, early childhood disability). The key to identifying the difference between a community-based case management and a hybrid rehabilitation case manager model is the addition of therapy-based treatments. In this model the case management service is mobile and there is contact with the client at home or community settings. Typically, services that provide a hybrid rehabilitation case manager model link the most appropriate professional (e.g. occupational therapist, physiotherapist, speech pathologist, social worker) to meet the client's needs for therapeutic treatment, but these therapeutic interventions should be recorded as separate to the case management actions.

39.4 Occupational therapists as case managers

Case management practice is not unique to occupational therapists. However, occupational therapists are considered well placed to assume case management roles. The profession's holistic, person-centred practice perspective, focus on functioning, promotion of client independence in activities, participation in life roles, and meaningful engagement with their community, parallel key principles of case management practice (Gentry et al., 2018; Kannenberg & Neville, 2018; Krupa & Clark, 1995; Robinson et al., 2016).

Moreover, occupational therapists have knowledge of illness pathology, human behaviour, occupational performance, and assessment expertise in functioning, task analysis, activity grading, and environmental adaptation (Krupa & Clark, 1995). They are skilled in assessment, evaluation, and using evidence-based interventions to facilitate client participation in the life domains of a client's choice (Boop et al., 2020; World Federation of Occupational Therapists, 2019). This lens ensures the provision of therapeutic pathways and continuums of care that are supportive and responsive to the client's fluctuating functioning and changing circumstances.

As a result of these skills and knowledge, occupational therapists are frequently employed in a dual role (hybrid model refer to Table 39.1), that of an occupational therapist and case manager. The dual role is present in numerous contexts in Australia and Aotearoa New Zealand. However, for reasons of policy, practice, quality appraisal, and evidence of effectiveness of both occupational therapy and case management practice, there is an unequivocal need to distinguish between the occupational therapy treatment and case management actions in practice. Therapeutic, evidence-based, occupational therapy interventions performed are different from the coordination, navigation, general monitoring, and support actions of case management (as defined in the CMTaxonomy).

39.5 The case management context

In Australia and Aotearoa New Zealand, case managers are employed in public and private health services, and NGOs; across settings of general practice to long term care and support; across the age spectrum; with a broad range of health conditions, although the case manager title varies.

39.5.1 Australia

Some examples of different sectors and titles are: *primary care* – 'care navigator/social prescriber' for people with chronic health conditions; *acute care hospital* – 'discharge planner'; *state community based rehabilitation* – 'rehabilitation case manager/case worker'; *state based insurance organisations* for people seriously injured at work or in a motor vehicle crash – 'case manager/service coordinator/service delivery coordinator, support advisor'; *National Disability Insurance Scheme* (NDIS) – 'local area coordinator/navigator/support coordinator/intermediary'. Case management is also used in other service systems such as education, legal services, domestic violence and correctional services. There are case managers employed in specialist positions for Aboriginal and Torres Strait Islander people and specialist Aboriginal and Torres Strait Islander organisations who provide case management services.

39.5.2 Aotearoa New Zealand

In Aotearoa New Zealand, case managers are predominantly employed within public health and insurance settings. This encompasses the national personal injury insurance scheme (Accident Compensation Corporation [ACC]), national health care services (i.e. Te Whatu Ora Health New Zealand, previously District Health Boards), and NGOs providing community-based support services in settings such as intellectual and physical disability, vocational rehabilitation, mental health and addiction, culturally based care (e.g. Māori and Pasifika organisations). There are also specialist case managers employed within health and social services due to holding relevant cultural knowledge, competence, and understanding of tikanga and culturally based care.

Vignette 39.1: Sally

The Person: Sally, 42-year-old New Zealand European, woman, sustained a mild traumatic brain injury; lived with her husband and two sons in a semi-rural community in Aotearoa New Zealand; employed fulltime as a workflow manager in a nationwide construction company.

The Context: Sally's symptoms included headaches, needing to rest more than usual, reduced concentration, difficulty completing her workload and activities of daily living, and fatigue after long periods at the computer. Following medical attention for her injury, a claim was submitted and accepted by the national personal injury scheme (i.e. ACC) and a care coordinator allocated.

Sally's Goals: Maintain her current employment and resume her role and responsibilities as a parent.

Generalist Case Management role:

1. Care coordinator contacted Sally to *establish a collaborative partnership* and conduct an *assessment through listening* to determine Sally's rehabilitation support needs.
2. After *clarifying* Sally's treatment goals, the care coordinator *advised* what services could be funded through ACC and *developed* an initial support plan.
3. Care coordinator *submitted the plan* to ACC and, when approved, *referred* Sally to:

    ■ Neuropsychologist to assess cognitive functioning (related to fatigue and concentration) and provide treatment.

    ■ Vocational rehabilitation provider for a workplace assessment and to provide liaison support with Sally's employer; facilitated a supported return to work programme.

    ■ Needs assessment team for a home and ADL assessment and provision of supported home help during Sally's rehabilitation.

4. Care coordinator *consulted* with service providers and *monitored* treatment provision and Sally's ongoing need for services.

Vignette 39.2: Ariki

The Person: Ariki, 19-year-old Māori man, referred for assessment by Community Mental Health Team (CMHT) due to low mood, and alcohol- and drug-induced psychosis symptoms; lived in shared accommodation and struggled to manage his finances and fulfil the expectations of his flatmates.

The Context: A keyworker from the CMHT *engaged* with Ariki to complete a *holistic assessment* and determined his *required supports* and *therapeutic goals. Through listening and establishing a relationship* with Ariki, the keyworker learned he grew up in foster care, had no connection to his Māori culture or whānau, and had experienced intermittent periods of homelessness. He had limited experience undertaking domestic living tasks or household management skills, left school at 14 years old, and had no previous work experience or qualifications. Ariki was physically assaulted during a period of homelessness and experienced distressing nightmares and flashbacks about the incident, contributing to his low mood and substance use.

Ariki's Goals: Support to manage his mood and distressing flashbacks; to remain in his current living situation; to gain full time employment.

Hybrid/Rehabilitation Case Manager role: Ariki and keyworker *collaboratively developed an individualised care plan* that included:

1. Keyworker *coordinated* physical and psychiatric consultations and facilitated regular appointments.
2. *Referred* to ACC funded psychology to address trauma symptoms.
3. *Referred* to community Kaupapa Māori service for support with his alcohol and drug use, to assist Ariki to learn domestic living and household management skills, and to assist with enrolment and attendance in training to facilitate employment.
4. Keyworker *advised* engaging with Kaupapa Māori cultural group to attend Maurakau sessions (Māori martial arts), learning karakia, waiata, and Māori tikanga to strengthen his cultural identity as a Māori man/tāne.
5. Keyworker *coordinated and facilitated* regular three-monthly *case conferences* to *assess and monitor* his progress.

Acknowledgement: Georgia Brown (NZROT)

Vignette 39.3: Michelle

The Person: Michelle, 48-year-old white woman; lived with her partner and two children in Sydney, Australia; sustained paraplegia (T6) following a motor vehicle crash. Prior to the injury, she worked four days per week as a teacher.

The Context: Michelle had no motor function and complete sensory loss from T6, resulting in total paralysis of trunk and lower extremities, moderate trunk stability, full control of her upper limbs, some compromise to her respiratory capacity and endurance, and autonomic dysfunction (loss of control of body temperature). She was referred to the Community Rehabilitation Case Manager (RCM)/occupational therapist) for treatment and case management three months prior to her discharge from the specialist spinal cord injury inpatient rehabilitation unit. Michelle had been provided with a wheelchair with power-assist for long distances. She had retrained and was mostly independent in self-care but needed stand-by assistance when she returned home for a further six months. She continued to require setup support and monitoring for toileting.

Michelle's Goals: Return home; resume roles as mother, partner, and teacher.

Hybrid case management role:

1. RCM engaged in *person-centred planning* with Michelle to identify her therapy and rehabilitation goals.
2. RCM *conducted and provided* occupational therapy assessments and interventions.
3. *Proactively collaborated and coordinated* with providers regarding specialist interventions to assist Michelle's return to work on a graduated programme and determined any environmental modifications needed.

4. *Connected* Michelle to incontinence product suppliers.
5. *Monitored* the family situation whether assessment was required for ongoing psychological support for Michelle, her partner, and children; liaised with the children's school as required.
6. RCM *evaluated and documented progress* and *overall rehabilitation costs, submitted the plan* to the government third party insurer (icareNSW).
7. RCM continued to *monitor* the services, supports, and ongoing progress of Michelle and her family.

39.6 Summary

- Case management is community-based, collaborative and relational – a key part of integrated care – involving assessment, planning, coordination, monitoring, and reviewing. There are numerous models, approaches, roles, and titles for case managers.
- Case managers should adopt a holistic perspective, person-centred, and strength-based approaches and be culturally responsive, collaborative, and proactive in their support of the client.
- Case managers work to connect the client with the right health and social services and supports, adapting actions in response to client needs, health condition, context, and the service setting.
- A common language (taxonomy) is essential to track case management activities for training, evaluation, and quality improvement. It is important to distinguish these actions from therapeutic occupational therapy interventions.

39.7 Review and reflection questions

- What are the four key principles underpinning case management models of service provision?
- In your state/province, where and by whom are case managers employed? Identify key tasks three of those case managers may be required to undertake.
- What are the similarities and differences between a broker and a community-based case management model?
- What are some of the skills and knowledge that occupational therapists might need to become successful case managers?
- What might be some common challenges for occupational therapists occupying case management roles?
- Why is it important to understand and differentiate between different models/approaches of case management?

References

Boop, C., Cahill, S. M., Davis, C., Dorsey, J., Gibbs, V., Herr, B., Kearney, K., Metzger, L., Miller, J., & Owens, A. (2020). Occupational Therapy Practice Framework: Domain and process fourth edition. *American Journal of Occupational Therapy*, 74(Supp 2), 1–85. https://doi.org/10.5014/ajot.2020.74S2001

Craig, P., Dieppe, P., Macintyre, S., Michie, S., Mazareth, I., & Petticrew, M. (2008). Developing and evaluating complex interventions: The new Medical Research Countil guidance. *BMJ*, 337. https://doi.org/10.1136/bmj.a1655

Gentry, K., Snyder, K., Barstow, B., & Hamson-Utley, J. (2018). The biopsychosocial model: Application to occupational therapy practice. *The Open Journal of Occupational Therapy*, 6(4), Article 12. https://doi.org/10.15453/2168-6408.1412

Healthcare Improvement Scotland. (2015). *Person-centred tools and approaches.* https://www.youtube.com/watch?v=T-SkAb52f58&list=PLzuTYNEZWHB7fT7_mgUKFRV_ZCbKpJsqs

International College of Person-centered Medicine. (2013). *2013 Geneva declaration on person-centred health research.* https://www.personcenteredmedicine.org/doc/2013_Geneva_Declaration_on_Person_Centered_Health_Research.pdf

Kannenberg, K., & Neville, M. (2018). Occupational therapy's role in case management. *American Journal of Occupational Therapy*, 72(2), 1–12. https://doi.org/10.5014/ajot.2018.72S206

Kelly, K. J., Doucet, S., & Luke, A. (2019). Exploring the roles, functions, and background of patient navigators and case managers: A scoping review. *International Journal of Nursing Studies*, 98, 27–47. https://doi.org/10.1016/j.ijnurstu.2019.05.016

Köpke, S., & McCleery, J. (2015). Systematic reviews of case management: Too complex to manage? *Cochrane Database of Systematic Reviews*, 1(1), Article ED000096. https://doi.org/10.1002/14651858.ED000096

Krupa, T., & Clark, C. C. (1995). Occupational therapists as case managers: Responding to current approaches to community mental health service delivery. *Canadian Journal of Occupational Therapy*, 62(1), 16–22. https://doi.org/10.1177/000841749506200104

Leonard, R., Linden, M. A., & Holloway, M. (2025). Case management for acquired brain injury: A systematic review of the evidence base. *Brain Injury*, 39(5), 337–358. https://doi.org/10.1080/02699052.2024.2438785

Lukersmith, S., Chung, Y., Du, W., Gibert, K., Salvador-Carulla, L., & Sarkissian, A. (2021). Mapping case management: A realist evaluation of characteristics and patterns. *International Journal of Integrated Care*, 20(3), Article 128. https://doi.org/10.5334/ijic.s4128

Lukersmith, S., Fernandez, A., Millington, M., & Salvador-Carulla, L. (2015). The Brain Injury Case Management Taxonomy (BICM-T): A classification of community-based case management interventions for a common language. *Disability and Health Journal*, 9(2), 272–280. https://doi.org/10.1016/j.dhjo.2015.09.006

Lukersmith, S., Huckel Schneider, C., Salvador-Carulla, L., Sturmberg, J., Wilson, A., & Gillespie, J. (2016). *What is the state of the art in person-centred care? An expert commentary. A report for an Australian Government policy agency.* University of Sydney.

Lukersmith, S., Millington, M., & Salvador-Carulla, L. (2016). What is case management? A scoping and mapping review. *International Journal of Integrated Care*, 16(4), 2. https://doi.org/10.5334/ijic.2477

Lukersmith, S., Salvador-Carulla, L., Chung, Y., Du, W., Sarkissian, A., & Millington, M. (2023). A realist evaluation of case management models for people with complex health conditions using novel methods and tools – What works, for whom, and under what circumstances? *International Journal of Environmental Research and Public Health*, 20(5), Article 4362. https://doi.org/10.3390/ijerph20054362

Lukersmith, S., Salvador-Carulla, L., & Millington, M. (2024). *The Case Management Taxonomy (CMTaxonomy).* University of Canberra. https://www.canberra.edu.au/research/centres/hri/research-projects/the-case-management-taxonomy

Mas-Exposito, L., Amador-Campos, J. A., Gomez-Benito, J., & Lalucat-Jo, L. (2013). Depicting current case management models. *Journal of Social Work*, 14(2), 133–146. https://doi.org/10.1177/1468017313477296

Rapp, C. (2006). *The strengths model: Case management with people with psychiatric disabilities.* Oxford University Press.

Reeves, S., Pelone, F., Harrison, R., Goldman, J., & Zwarenstein, M. (2017). Interprofessional collaboration to improve professional practice and healthcare outcomes. *Cochrane Database of Systematic Reviews*, 6(6), Article CD000072. https://doi.org/10.1002/14651858.CD000072.pub3

Robinson, M., Fisher, T. F., & Broussard, K. (2016). Role of occupational therapy in case management and care coordination for clients with complex conditions. *American Journal of Occupational Therapy, 70*(2), 7002090010p1-6. https://doi.org/10.5014/ajot.2016.702001

Stretton, C., Chan, W.-Y., & Wepa, D. (2022). Demystifying case management in Aotearoa New Zealand: A scoping and mapping review. *International Journal of Environmental Research and Public Health, 20*(1), 784. https://doi.org/10.3390/ijerph20010784

World Federation of Occupational Therapists. (2019). *Position statement: Occupational therapy and mental health.* WFOT. https://wfot.org/resources/occupational-therapy-and-mental-health

World Health Organization. (2001). *International classification of functioning, disability and health.* WHO. https://apps.who.int/iris/handle/10665/42407

World Health Organization. (2011). *Rio political declaration on social determinants of health.* WHO. https://www.who.int/publications/m/item/rio-political-declaration-on-social-determinants-of-health

World Health Organization. (2015). *WHO global strategy on integrated people-centred health services 2016–2026.* WHO. https://iris.who.int/handle/10665/155002

World Health Organization. (2016). *Framework on integrated, people-centred health services: Report by the Secretariat to 69th World Health Assembly (provisional agenda item 16.1).* WHO. https://apps.who.int/gb/ebwha/pdf_files/wha69/a69_39-en.pdf

World Health Organization – European Regional Office. (2013). *Roadmap: Strengthening people-centred health systems in the WHO European Region. A Framework for action towards coordinated/integrated health services delivery (CIHSD).* WHO-Euro.

CHAPTER 40

Leadership, advocacy and promotion in the occupational therapy profession

Dave Parsons, Angela Berndt, Michelle Bissett, and Angus Buchanan

Authors' positionality statement

As a team of four occupational therapists, comprising two males and two females, we bring a diverse range of experiences and perspectives to our work. We all hold PhDs and possess additional education and experience in leading and managing teams in academic and industry contexts. Our professional journeys have been shaped by our roles as educators, researchers, and practitioners, allowing us to understand the multifaceted nature of occupational therapy and its impact on individuals and communities. By integrating our varied experiences and insights, we aim to contribute meaningfully to the discourse on leadership and advocacy within occupational therapy. Our goal is to empower readers by increasing their knowledge in leadership, advocacy, and promotion viewed through an occupational therapy lens. Moreover, we strive to ensure that occupational therapy remains a dynamic and responsive discipline that meets the needs of those we serve.

Key terms
- Leadership
- Advocacy
- Promotion
- Change

Objectives
Upon completion of this chapter, the reader will be able to:

- Define the terms leadership, advocacy, and promotion and discuss these terms through an occupational therapy lens
- Understand the relevance of leadership in the practice of occupational therapists
- Recognise the synergies between the skills and competencies required for high-quality occupational therapy practice and those needed for effective leadership and advocacy

DOI: 10.4324/9781003495666-43

40.1 Introduction

This chapter provides a brief overview of the concepts of leadership, advocacy, and promotion through an occupational therapy lens, with a focus on the relevance of these concepts in the context of occupational therapy practice. Each of the terms will be defined, and their importance within the occupational therapy profession will be explained. It explores how occupational therapists, regardless of their role or setting, can influence change, support others, and raise the profile of the profession. Leadership is discussed as both formal and informal, with a focus on authenticity, emotional intelligence, and lifelong learning. Advocacy is presented as a core responsibility, highlighting the importance of working alongside individuals and communities to promote inclusion, equity and justice. The chapter also considers how occupational therapists can actively promote their work and the profession to a range of audiences. Each section provides examples to further illustrate how these concepts are embedded within occupational therapy practice. The importance of these concepts for both individual therapists and the profession, as a collective, is addressed.

40.2 Leadership

Leadership has been described as the process of an individual influencing a group or team to achieve a united goal (Northouse, 2015; Reed et al., 2019). Leadership skills are vital for occupational therapists as they give individuals the ability to positively influence change for themselves and their careers, their clients, and more broadly the profession and society.

Rodger (2011) interviewed emerging occupational therapy leaders and identified that leaders reported the following key characteristics: inspiring others, listening, facilitating change, having a vision, and strategic thinking. Rodger (2012) considered that everyone has the capacity to demonstrate leadership abilities and challenged all occupational therapists to see themselves as leaders. This may be within work teams, in occupational therapy departments, non-governmental organisations, voluntary boards, or within the wider profession.

All occupational therapists are required to be leaders whose primary focus is on the growth and well-being of people and communities. This is known as servant leadership, and leaders who practice this approach show characteristics such as listening, empathy, awareness (including self), persuasion, conceptualisation, foresight, stewardship, commitment to the growth of people, and building community (Canavesi & Minelli, 2022). Many of these characteristics reflect professional practice skills and expectations of occupational therapy practice.

Many people only view leadership as a formal role, but occupational therapists practice leadership every day, working closely with clients and their communities to bring about change. Simplistically, this can be described as 'Big L' leadership and 'Little l' leadership. 'Big L' leadership is evident in people who have defined roles and positions that inherently give them leadership responsibilities (Kotter, 2008). Examples include heads of departments, programme directors within universities, and coordinators of services such as rehabilitation units or community mental health facilities.

Little 'l' leadership can be described as the traits and behaviours that individuals exhibit where others perceive them to be 'good' leaders (Kotter, 2008). People who demonstrate this type of leadership, for example, have the courage to speak up when they see a conflict in their values, exhibit high emotional intelligence to resolve conflict, advocate for their patients or clients within a multidisciplinary team or suggest that their team consider a journal discussion group. There are many opportunities in occupational therapy practice to proactively see a need, take some action, and lead people to make a change.

Regardless of whether you hold a formal leadership role or practice 'Little l' leadership traits, authenticity is essential. Authentic leadership is an approach where leaders are genuine and act in a manner that is true to themselves. Authentic leaders understand their strengths, weaknesses, values, and beliefs; are aware of their biases, focus on the organisation's goals and mission, demonstrate empathy, have excellent communication, and look to the future (Duarte et al., 2021). 'Little l' leadership can be demonstrated as a student or new graduate – occupational therapists do not need formal titles to be leaders.

Good leaders are lifelong reflective learners, and lifelong learning is a key characteristic of effective leaders as they build their personal and professional capabilities (Vito, 2020). Lifelong learners can focus on improving themselves, are adaptable and resilient, and understand that their talents and abilities can be developed through effort and persistence. They are open to feedback, acquire new knowledge and skills that broaden their perspectives, and have proficiency in communication, empathy, and leadership values (Alla, 2024).

40.3 Change-makers

Occupational therapists have the potential to be change-makers in the systems and communities in which they work. Occupational therapists' unique understanding of the person, environment, and occupation (PEO) and the dynamic interactions (and transactions) between these domains provides a strong foundation on which occupational therapists can evoke and drive positive change. Change is inherently challenging; however, the positive impact that change can have – if done well and for the right reasons – makes it worthwhile.

Change often fails. It fails for various reasons, such as poor leadership, interpersonal conflict, insufficient environmental scanning and assessment, and/or poor execution of strategy (McGuier et al., 2024). To mitigate these risks, change leaders must employ emotional intelligence, set clear and achievable goals, foster strong communication and collaboration among stakeholders, and continuously evaluate and adapt their strategies to monitor their effectiveness in achieving the desired outcome (Errida & Lotfi, 2021). These skills are often well developed and come naturally for occupational therapists given their alignment with the necessary competencies essential to practice as occupational therapists in Australia and Aotearoa New Zealand, making occupational therapists ideal change makers.

Opportunities for change are often found in practice contexts under reform, such as the disability, mental health, and aged care sectors. However, change occurs in all practice contexts where occupational therapists work. Importantly, either as change leaders or stakeholders in change processes, occupational therapists can leverage their skills and entrepreneurial spirit to further the profession and improve outcomes for their patients, clients, and customers. Examples of where there is current scope for positive change and potential development include government policy, health system re-design, adoption of artificial intelligence, assistive technology, educational institutions, virtual and augmented reality technologies, big data, and telehealth delivery.

Another way occupational therapists can drive positive change is through entrepreneurship. While entrepreneurship is often viewed through the lens of commercial business development, there is a growing focus on the value of social entrepreneurship. Social entrepreneurship is an approach to developing, funding, and implementing solutions to social, cultural, or environmental issues with a strong focus on outcomes and less on financial profits (Reed et al., 2019; Zahra et al., 2009). Social entrepreneurship in modern society offers an altruistic, accountable, and inclusive form of entrepreneurship, derived from a social mission, that focuses on the benefits that society may gain, often working in areas such as poverty alleviation, health care, and community development (Pinto et al., 2024; Tan et al., 2005). Examples include exploring community-based employment enterprises for people with disabilities combined with addressing other pressing social needs, such as food insecurity or social isolation or supporting the development of micro-funding cooperatives to support refugee women developing their own small businesses.

While occupational therapy education programmes may touch on leadership and change management, further post-qualification experience and training will enable occupational therapists to gain the high-level and nuanced skills required to engage successfully in this area. Ideally, occupational therapists should undertake a self-assessment to determine their skill set and identify whether these are skills they need to develop through training and experience, seeking professional advice, or engagement in partnerships.

40.4 Advocacy

Historically, advocacy has been associated with human and civil rights movements and reflected an approach of standing up for people who are subjected to discrimination or marginalisation. Health professionals frequently undertake advocacy for, and in collaboration with, disadvantaged or vulnerable individuals or groups. Advocacy refers to the act or process of supporting a cause, idea or proposal (McKinnon et al., 2024).

Occupational therapists view advocacy as a part of their routine professional work (King & Curtin, 2014; McKinnon et al., 2024). Occupational therapy professional bodies such as the Occupational Therapy Board of New Zealand (2022) articulate that advocacy is a fundamental expectation of the therapist's role. Advocacy activities span the individual, group and population levels and are embedded as a core aspect of occupational therapy practice within theoretical practice frameworks, including the Occupational Therapy Practice Framework 4th edition (Boop et al., 2020) and others. The way occupational therapists enact advocacy requires careful consideration, especially when working with people from Indigenous and First Nations contexts, to respect reciprocity and knowledge sharing. In practice, this role enactment typically translates to ensuring that people's inclusion and participation in chosen and meaningful occupations is fair, equitable and just.

Advocacy can take different forms; is purposeful; is inherently a political act; must address power relationships, power redistribution, and the potential for unintended disempowerment; and thus requires reflective practice and other skills to be effective (Hunter & Pride, 2021; Taylor et al., 2021). Increasing attention to inclusion, co-design, and collaboration through community development and coalition building is occurring in occupational therapy practice. Kirsh (2015) suggest advocating with individuals and groups *on* specific issues, rather than *for*, leads to activation at an organisational level for changes to practices and action at a community level for changes in legislation and public awareness of professional issues (van Oort et al., 2023).

Advocacy and lobbying work together. Lobbying is the process and activities that occur to create a change in policy or services (Taylor et al., 2021). Taylor et al. (2021) use the example of the issue of youth safety and participation in occupations reliant on public transport. Advocacy may include working with young people to raise awareness of the risks of assault and other harms due to the lack of safe late-night transport, whereas lobbying might involve targeting the bus service administration or the city council to effect immediate change to accessibility.

The previous example describes a direct advocacy approach taken by occupational therapists, but advocacy can also be indirect. In these scenarios, therapists act on behalf of a community or client group or may foster or build skills in other people to enable them to advocate directly for themselves. In this way, advocacy reflects occupational therapy's practices and values. For example, King and Curtin (2014) interviewed therapists who worked with rehabilitation clients post-brain injuries. The therapists described the need to advocate for clients to receive funding from government organisations that would support their engagement in activities of daily living. In addition, these therapists also used their professional skills to educate and enable their clients to become self-advocates for their own needs. In contemporary occupational therapy practice, occupational therapists are expected to work with clients to enable them to become self-advocates (VanPuymbrouck et al., 2024).

Last, it is important to consider *professional advocacy*, where an individual or group works to strengthen a profession, identify problems at institutional levels, support systems change, contribute to legislative change and policy, and influence population-based decisions (McKinnon et al., 2024). Professional associations, such as Occupational Therapy Australia and Occupational Therapy New Zealand Whakaora Ngangahau Aotearoa, can collaborate, undertake projects, write submissions, use social media to raise awareness, and lobby to influence governments about health care provision and policies that affect people's engagement with occupations. In doing so, these organisations advocate for services that meet the needs of the client groups (Rogers & Hartstein, 2018). As members of their professional association, students are encouraged to engage and learn about professional advocacy as a foundational part of building their professional identity (McKinnon et al., 2024). Examples of this advocacy work include the implementation of the Australian National Disability Insurance Scheme (NDIS), services for veterans, submissions to Royal Commissions, and other government inquiries (see the Occupational Therapy Australia and Occupational Therapy New Zealand Whakaora Ngangahau Aotearoa website for other examples).

40.5 Promotion

Promotion, as defined by the *Oxford English Dictionary* (2015), refers to an activity that supports or encourages a cause or venture or endorses a particular view. Within the context of occupational therapy, promotion can be understood as the strategic advancement and political positioning of the profession. The promotion of occupational therapy, and the work of occupational therapists, is essential for raising awareness, fostering professional growth, and enhancing public and stakeholder understanding. Health professionals must actively promote their services to a range of audiences, including clients, other health care professionals, and the general public (Amiri & Ali, 2023). By doing so, they can influence the perception of the services they can offer, and enhance an understanding of their contribution towards health care provision (Yeo et al., 2025). Professional promotion is typically enacted through individual or collective approaches. Individually, occupational therapists should routinely describe and keenly promote their work in their practice with clients (Jacobs, 2012). This can be done in practice, for example, by therapists providing clear communication about the focus of occupational therapy in neurological rehabilitation or by discussing evidence for a planned falls-prevention programme.

Additionally, occupational therapists need to promote their work to other health professionals, policymakers, funders, and stakeholders (Jacobs, 2024). For example, therapists could promote the potential contribution occupational therapy could have in a new interprofessional clinic being established in a hospital or a new multicultural service in their local government area designed to support refugees and asylum seekers. In these scenarios, occupational therapists could draw upon their distinctive expertise in the relationship between occupational and health to demonstrate their value. Alternatively, therapists could disseminate their skills to teachers by informing them about the services they can provide for children with special needs in classroom environments. Throughout the profession's history, there have been calls to action for occupational therapists, encouraging them to incorporate professional promotion in their practice. Jacobs (2012) highlighted this point by stating, 'We, as occupational therapy practitioners and students, are the ones best equipped to promote occupational therapy . . . each of us should take responsibility for the promotion of occupational therapy and also learn strategies for promoting occupational therapy from one another' (p. 668). More recently, Pattison et al. (2018) proposed, 'every occupational therapist needs to be an activist in promoting our profession's core values at every opportunity' (p. 241).

Professional associations or collectives, such as Occupational Therapy Australia and Occupational Therapy New Zealand Whakaora Ngangahau Aotearoa, also play a key role in the promotion of occupational therapy. In Australia, Occupational Therapy Australia engages in regular promotional activities targeted at the broader community, federal government, funding bodies, key stakeholders, and potential occupational therapists. At a professional level, they promote the benefits of engaging in the occupational therapy profession as well as the benefits of working with an occupational therapist (Occupational Therapy Australia, 2025).

It is now difficult to imagine occupational therapists being excluded from the opportunity to offer mental health services under a universal health funding scheme (fees); however, that was almost the case. For example, Occupational Therapy Australia promoted occupational therapists to the government for inclusion as health professionals accessible under a mental health care plan. This work resulted in the inclusion of occupational therapists as listed mental health specialists and consequently, people in Australia are now able to access government-funded occupational therapy to support their mental health. In recent times, occupational therapy professional associations, nationally and internationally, have increased their utilisation of social media platforms (including Facebook, X, and LinkedIn). Through these mediums, it has been and is possible to promote individual occupational therapy organisations, promote the profession to a range of local and international audiences, and demonstrate the scope of occupational therapy and current advocacy activities (Hamilton et al., 2016).

40.6 Vignette

A student reads on the student digital notice board that the Occupational Therapy School is looking for third-year occupational therapy students to be on the Student Council. The school considers the council the student leadership group that represents and advocates on behalf of its peers. The student thought nominating for the council would be a good idea, as they have not been happy about several things that have happened in the previous two years of their course, and this would be a forum where they could express their displeasure to the school leadership. They sent an email nominating themselves but did not take the time to read the responsibilities of the role, which included consulting with their peers and representing the third-year occupational therapy year group's interests.

The school accepts their nomination, and they are invited to attend the monthly Student Council meetings. At the first meeting, they say nothing. They decide not to attend the second meeting as they need to complete an assessment task. At the third meeting, they spend ten minutes going over concerns related to their own experiences. Before the fourth meeting, they are approached by several student peers who have only just found out they are on the student council. The student peers want to discuss an issue that is impacting most of the year group and ask that they represent their issues at the next meeting. The student listens to what they have to say and indicates that they will advocate on behalf of the group. At the meeting, the third-year occupational therapy representative raises some issues that they, based on their own experiences, want to support and be an advocate for. However, they do not feel confident in raising their own peer groups' concerns as promised when the chair moves on to a subsequent agenda item. After the meeting, the student reports back to their student peers that there was no time on the agenda to discuss their concerns and that they would do it at the next meeting.

Questions to consider based on the case study.

1. What do you think the student representative should have done before joining the Student Council?
2. How could the student representative have been better prepared to help and advocate for their peers?
3. How did the student representatives' own issues affect their ability to help and advocate for their peers?
4. How might the student representatives' actions affect how their peers see them as a leader?
5. What can the student representative do next time to balance their concerns with their peers' needs?

40.7 Conclusion

This chapter has defined the concepts of leadership, advocacy, and promotion and provided examples of these concepts within occupational therapy practice. Occupational therapists use these skills in daily practice to live our values and advance the participation of our clients at an individual, group, community, and population level. The chapter has highlighted the skills occupational therapy students and new graduates need to develop to enable them to be effective in their professional practice.

40.8 Summary

- Leadership, advocacy, and promotion are all concepts that are part of daily occupational therapy practice.
- Occupational therapists have skill sets that enable them to actively pursue leadership, advocacy, entrepreneurship, and promotion.
- Development of these skills can commence during university training and be enhanced in the workplace.

40.9 Review and reflection questions

- Why does occupational therapy need to have good leaders who exhibit 'Little l' leadership?
- What strategies can student and new graduate occupational therapists employ to develop their own leadership skills?
- Why are advocacy and promotion important for health professions and health professionals?
- What are some examples of advocacy that have recently been shown by the occupational therapy professional association in your country?

References

Alla, X. (2024). Lifelong learning. *Interdisciplinary Journal of Research and Development, 11*(1), 27–27. https://doi.org/10.56345/ijrdv11n105

Amiri, N. A., & Ali, M. (2023). The roles of nurses as marketers: A literature review. *Journal of Health Management, 25*(2), 327–333. https://doi.org/10.1177/09720634231177336

Boop, C., Cahill, S. M., Davis, C., Dorsey, J., Gibbs, V., Herr, B., Kearney, K., Metzger, L., Miller, J., & Owens, A. (2020). Occupational Therapy Practice Framework: Domain and process, 4th edition. *American Journal of Occupational Therapy, 74*(Supp 2), 1–85. https://doi.org/10.5014/ajot.2020.74S2001

Canavesi, A., & Minelli, E. (2022). Servant leadership: A systematic literature review and network analysis. *Employee Responsibilities and Rights Journal, 34*(3), 267–289. https://doi.org/10.1007/s10672-021-09381-3

Duarte, A. P., Ribeiro, N., Semedo, A. S., & Gomes, D. R. (2021). Authentic leadership and improved individual performance: Affective commitment and individual creativity's sequential mediation. *Frontiers in Psychology, 12*, 675749. https://doi.org/10.3389/fpsyg.2021.675749

Errida, A., & Lotfi, B. (2021). The determinants of organizational change management success: Literature review and case study. *International Journal of Engineering Business Management, 13.* https://doi.org/10.1177/18479790211016

Hamilton, A. L., Burwash, S. C., Penman, M., Jacobs, K., Hook, A., Bodell, S., Ledgerd, R., & Pattison, M. (2016). Making connections and promoting the profession: Social media use by World Federation of Occupational Therapists member organisations. *Digital Health, 2*, 1–15. https://doi.org/10.1177/2055207616653844

Hunter, C., & Pride, T. (2021). Critiquing the Canadian Model of Client-Centered Enablement (CMCE) for Indigenous contexts. *Canadian Journal of Occupational Therapy, 88*(4), 329–339. https://doi.org/10.1177/00084174211042960

Jacobs, K. (2012). PromOTing occupational therapy: Words, images, and actions. *American Journal of Occupational Therapy, 66*(6), 652–671. https://doi.org/10.5014/ajot.2012.666001

Jacobs, K. (2024). Marketing and management of occupational therapy services. In *Occupational therapy essentials for clinical competence* (pp. 605–614). Routledge.

King, D., & Curtin, M. (2014). Occupational therapists' use of advocacy in brain injury rehabilitation settings. *Australian Occupational Therapy Journal, 61*(6), 446–457. https://doi.org/10.1111/1440-1630.12149

Kirsh, B. H. (2015). Transforming values into action: Advocacy as a professional imperative. *Canadian Journal of Occupational Therapy, 82*(4), 212–223. https://doi.org/10.1177/0008417415601395

Kotter, J. P. (2008). *Force for change: How leadership differs from management.* Simon and Schuster.

McGuier, E. A., Kolko, D. J., Aarons, G. A., Schachter, A., Klem, M. L., Diabes, M. A., Weingart, L. R., Salas, E., & Wolk, C. B. (2024). Teamwork and implementation of innovations in healthcare and human service settings: A systematic review. *Implementation Science, 19*(1), 49. https://doi.org/10.1186/s13012-024-01381-9

McKinnon, S., Petrone, N., & Tarbet, A. (2024). The role of an occupational therapy practitioner in professional advocacy: A scoping review. *Translational Science in Occupation, 1*(2), 3. https://doi.org/10.32873/unmc.dc.tso.1.2.02

Northouse, P. G. (2015). *Leadership. Theory and practice.* SAGE Publications.

Occupational Therapy Australia. (2025). *Media and advocacy.* https://otaus.com.au/media-and-advocacy/advocacy

Occupational Therapy Board of New Zealand. (2022). *General scope of practice: Kaiwhakaora Ngangahau Occupational Therapist.* Retrieved March 7, 2025, from https://otboard.org.nz/site/ces/scope

Pattison, M., Baptiste, S., McKinstry, C., Sarkies, M. N., White, J., Henderson, K., Haas, R., Bowles, J., Sharber, J., & Silverman, F. (2018). A vision splendid; visioning for the future of occupational therapy. *Australian Occupational Therapy Journal, 65*(3), 238–242. https://doi.org/10.1111/1440-1630.12490

Pinto, H., Sampaio, F., Ferreira, S., & Elston, J. (2024). Academic social entrepreneurship: A contemporary reflection from Schumpeter's economic sociology. *Businesses, 4*(4), 723–737. https://doi.org/10.3390/businesses4040040

Promotion. (2015). *In Oxford dictionaries online.* http://www.oxforddictionaries.com/definition/english/promotion

Reed, B. N., Klutts, A. M., & Mattingly II, T. J. (2019). A systematic review of leadership definitions, competencies, and assessment methods in pharmacy education. *American Journal of Pharmaceutical Education, 83*(9), 7520. https://doi.org/10.5688/ajpe7520

Rodger, S. (2011). *Final report: Building capacity among emerging occupational therapy academic leaders in curriculum renewal and evaluation at UQ and nationally.* https://ltr.edu.au/resources/Rodger_Report_UQ_2011_0.pdf

Rodger, S. (2012). Leadership through an occupational lens: Celebrating our territory. *Australian Occupational Therapy Journal, 59*(3), 172–179. https://doi.org/10.1111/j.1440-1630.2012.00995.x

Rogers, J., & Hartstein, D. (2018). *The value of contemporary professional associations.*

Tan, W.-L., Williams, J., & Tan, T.-M. (2005). Defining the 'social' in 'social entrepreneurship': Altruism and entrepreneurship. *The International Entrepreneurship and Management Journal, 1*(3), 353–365. https://doi.org/10.1007/s11365-005-2600-x

Taylor, J., O'Hara, L., Talbot, L., & Verrinder, G. (2021). *Promoting health: The primary health care approach* (7th ed.). Elsevier Australia.

van Oort, B., van 't Riet, H., Parejo Pagador, A., Lescrauwaet Noboa, R., & Aantjes, C. (2023). Understanding the what, how, and why in advocacy: Assessing the applicability of participatory process evaluation methodology in an advocacy context. *Evaluation, 29*(4), 509–527. https://doi.org/10.1177/13563890231200057

VanPuymbrouck, L., Chun, E. M., Hesse, E. D., Ranneklev, K., & Sanchez, C. (2024). Developing client self-advocacy in occupational therapy: Are we practicing what we preach? *Occupational Therapy International, 2024*(1), 1662671. https://doi.org/10.1155/2024/1662671

Vito, R. (2020). How do social work leaders understand and ideally practice leadership? A synthesis of core leadership practices. *Journal of Social Work Practice, 34*(3), 263–279. https://doi.org/10.1080/02650533.2019.1665002

Yeo, A., Lee, S. S., Lim, V. K., Godsey, J. A., Kuok, K., Gunawan, J., & Liaw, S. Y. (2025). Strategies to elevate the brand image of nursing: A scoping review. *International Nursing Review, 72*(2), e70026. https://doi.org/10.1111/inr.70026

Zahra, S. A., Gedajlovic, E., Neubaum, D. O., & Shulman, J. M. (2009). A typology of social entrepreneurs: Motives, search processes and ethical challenges. *Journal of Business Venturing, 24*(5), 519–532. https://doi.org/10.1016/j.jbusvent.2008.04.007

CHAPTER 41

Moving forward

Occupational therapy in Australia and Aotearoa New Zealand's future

Ema Tokolahi, Yvonne Thomas, Ted Brown, Stephen Isbel, and Louise Gustafsson

Authors' positionality statement
We are Western-educated occupational therapists with postgraduate qualifications working in leadership positions in Australia and Aotearoa New Zealand. We are white, cisgender, able-bodied, English-speaking individuals. We acknowledge our white privilege, our Global North outlook, and the impacts of colonial hegemony on the Aboriginal and Torres Strait Islander peoples of Australia and Māori communities in Aotearoa New Zealand. We support decolonisation, indigenisation, racial equality, queer inclusivity, cultural sensitivity, social and occupational justice, and gender-affirmative and culturally safe and responsive health care and education. We believe in the importance of building respectful relationships with Aboriginal and Torres Strait Islander peoples of Australia and Māori communities in Aotearoa New Zealand underpinned by seeking truth, recognition, and reconciliation. This impacts our world view, how we understand the perspectives of others, and our scholarly writing.

Key terms
- Aotearoa New Zealand
- Australia
- Cultural responsivity
- Future practice
- Occupational therapy

Objectives
Upon completion of this chapter, the reader will be able to:

- Reflect on what active partnership might look like in practice and recognising its value for occupational therapy
- Consider the potential future for occupational therapy in relation to decolonisation, globalisation, and artificial intelligence

DOI: 10.4324/9781003495666-44

- Outline potential future areas of occupational therapy practice
- Reflect and plan your career as a culturally responsive occupational therapist and how you might contribute to strengthen our profession

41.1 Introduction

Australia and Aotearoa New Zealand are vibrant and diverse nations, rich in landscapes and cultural heritage. Their histories extend far beyond the arrival of white settlers, rooted in the enduring presence and knowledge of Indigenous Peoples. Over time, occupational participation has evolved in both countries in response to changing contexts of sovereignty, oppression, colonialism, resistance, and renaissance. The diverse physical, social, cultural, and political environments of Australia and Aotearoa New Zealand profoundly shape the range of occupations people engage in and their access to them. Today, both lands are home to politically active Indigenous Peoples seeking reconciliation and redress for historical and contemporary injustices. These countries sit within a global network, both influencing and being influenced by international movements, which further diversifies the nature and quality of occupational participation and access to culturally meaningful occupations.

41.2 Active partnerships

We, the editors of this book, would like to acknowledge and mihi the many Aboriginal, Torres Strait Islander, and Māori authors who have contributed ideas and writing in the chapters of this book. We also acknowledge the lack of those authors serving as editors with the ability to contribute to strategic decision-making and oversight of the book as a whole. Subsequently, we can see that the book privileges the views of WEIRD (western, education, industrial, rich, and democratic) (Henrich et al., 2010) occupational therapists, and greater inclusion of Aboriginal, Torres Strait Islander, and Māori peoples' perspectives is needed. We recognise that genuine partnership was not fully realised in the production of this book. As editors and as a profession, we are on a journey to achieve more culturally responsive and safe practices – we recognise such journeys take time, commitment, and humility. Yarning and whakawhanaungatanga (relationship building) require patience, energy, and trust – these things cannot (and should not) be rushed.

We are learning when our time is to step up and speak out or step back and make space (Bell, 2024). When stepping up we must identify and call out racism and inequality. This pushes us to critically reflect on our own practices and how these may not be as JEDI-oriented (just, equitable, diverse-affirming, and inclusive) as we had hoped. When stepping back, we must make space for perspectives and practices different to our own to be recognised and respected in their own right. Stepping back requires us to consistently foster culturally safe environments where colleagues, clients and others feel genuinely invited to contribute – without fear of being trapped, ambushed, or tokenised. This parallels how we, as a profession, can approach practice and highlights some of the issues that are equally relevant and present for clinicians on a daily basis.

41.3 Revisiting the paradigm shifts

As discussed in Chapter 1, we are in the midst of change or paradigm shifts, including globalisation, decolonisation, and the rapid advancement in artificial intelligence.

Further planetary health, including pandemics, natural disasters, and environmental pollution are increasingly impacting health and wellbeing and therefore require an occupational response. As a profession we recognise the importance and value of our holistic approach with human flourishing and decentring scientific approaches, without devaluing these, whilst giving greater priority and privilege to our humanity, compassion, relational, justice-oriented, and ancient intelligence. These shifts are expanded on here to consider how these may impact future occupational therapy education, practice, and knowledge generation.

Over recent years, there has been a distinct acceleration towards decolonisation in the occupational therapy profession (Huot & Forwell, 2024), which looks and feels different across Australia and Aotearoa New Zealand. Progress is rarely linear and is halting at times. Some members of the profession actively seek to resist recycling characteristics of colonialism in their knowledge and skills bases and in the structures and systems in which they practice (Ahmed-Landeryou, 2024). Some remain oblivious to the imperial gaze that informs decision-making and action and serves to oppress and reinforce racial disparities. Many are somewhere in between, knowing change is needed but feeling uncertain and paralysed to act (Bell, 2024; Crawford & Langridge, 2022). Future occupational therapy requires continuous, active, and intentional engagement in decolonial praxis to manifest real, sustainable change in occupational therapy education; professional practice; and knowledge generation, translation, and integration (Ahmed-Landeryou, 2024).

Decolonising will include shifting from an individual focus to addressing determinants of health, working with communities and populations at 'social, environmental, and structural levels to modify what people can do in their everyday lives and promote social inclusion' (Hocking & Tokolahi, 2025, p. 552). Such work will require the profession to be vulnerable and present in uncomfortable spaces (Peters et al., 2024), where we may critically reflect on our individual and collective ways of knowing and doing. For ideas and inspiration, we may choose to look globally, outside our local context, and explore how others are approaching decolonising praxis. However, our profession may need to look outwards and inwards to critically interrogate the role of globalisation in our profession's future given tensions to meet local needs (Huot & Forwell, 2024). As a profession, we know where we want to be, but we are not there yet; to achieve this we must accept our responsibility to take steps to advance this paradigm shift and move forward on this journey.

The future of occupational therapy will include greater adoption and integration of artificial intelligence (AI) to increase efficiency and accuracy and improve client outcomes (Kokkotis et al., 2025; Stover & Jacobs, 2025). AI is increasingly utilised to streamline time-consuming administrative tasks, including clinical note taking and report writing (Bracken et al., 2025), and to support evidence-based practice (Ferreira, 2023). Increased efficiencies afforded by using AI hold great potential for increased therapist availability to interact with clients and improve job satisfaction and therapist retention (Stover & Jacobs, 2025). In the future we will see increased adoption of AI in therapy in motor function assessment and recovery; AI will be integrated with assistive devices, the use of robotics, and the expanding application in cognitive assessment and interventions (Kaelin et al., 2021; Kokkotis et al., 2025). While occupational therapy is still in the early stages of adopting artificial intelligence, there is an urgent need for more research into how AI can support occupational participation. Occupational therapists are increasingly called to collaborate with developers and clients in designing and implementing AI solutions that address individual participation needs (Kaelin et al., 2024).

As we look to the future of occupational therapy in Australia and Aotearoa New Zealand, the profession will continue to evolve. With growing populations of older people, and increased prevalence of chronic health conditions, the demand for occupational therapy will continue to grow (Australian Institute of Health and Welfare [AIHW], 2024). Current health systems, primarily focused on individualised hospital-based care, are overwhelmed with long waiting times for both emergency and elective procedures. Primary care access is restricted for many due to a lack of physicians, especially in rural and remote areas, and the cost of general practitioner appointments. Occupational therapy, together with other allied health professions, will be needed to work in extended and advanced roles in primary and preventative health care as well as to facilitate more effective rehabilitation and discharges following hospital care. Occupational therapy will continue to evolve and grow to meet the demands of our communities, as it has since the profession began. The pace and direction of our evolution over the next ten years will be influenced by these changing paradigms.

41.4 Ka mua, ka muri: walking backwards into the future

'Ka mua, ka muri' is a Māori whakatauki (proverb, not attributed to a single author) that signifies the importance of the past for informing the future. We invite you, as a student or a current practicing occupational therapist, to reflect on how far you have come in your own journey and encourage you to look forward to being a part of an ever-changing responsive profession that aims to meet the occupational needs of those they serve. You may find your place in an established practice area or be an innovator who shapes a new area of practice for the benefit of your community and future occupational therapists. You may find your place in research or knowledge generation that keeps the profession growing with the foundations firmly embedded in evidence. You may find yourself in administration, management, and governance roles that directly influence occupational therapy service provision and people who access those services. Wherever you find yourself, make a difference with people, strengthen the profession through gathering and generating evidence to support practice, and be innovative and responsive to change. As evidenced by the past, the future will bring changes to our populations, health, the environment, where and how people live, and what occupations are important to access. The systems that support those who access occupational therapy will change, and occupational therapists need to help lead positive transformations in health, education, social services, and other government-level initiatives.

Take some time to reflect on your future and how you want to contribute to creating a culturally responsive, evidence-based future for the occupational therapy profession. Recording your aspirations and intentions is important because as a lifelong learner it helps you to stay focused and be accountable to your own professional development plan. We present the following six key questions to reflect on when developing your goals and suggest that you record your answers.

41.5 Reflective questions

- Who will benefit from my work as an occupational therapist, and how will I know this?
- How will I align my practice with JEDI principles: justice, equity, diversity, and inclusion?
- What attitudes, knowledge and skills do I need to develop practice that is more culturally safe and responsive?
- How will I initiate opportunities (for me and those I serve) to access resources and supports so that I can deliver more culturally safe and responsive practice?
- Who can I learn from and who can I support and mentor as I develop my professional identity and practices?
- How do I use my knowledge and skills to influence future occupational therapy practice and practitioners by standing up and stepping back?
- Consider reviewing your plan in six months – you may find you are ready to revise your goals and update your responses. Keep developing and progressing your career, and you will keep contributing to the growth of occupational therapy in Australia and Aotearoa New Zealand.

41.6 Conclusion

We would like to conclude with acknowledgements of the leaders from the occupational therapy profession who have generously provided their knowledge and experiences of practice. Contributing authors generously and expertly share their insights – from in-depth discussions of foundational concepts to compelling presentations of professional issues and examples of both innovative and everyday practices – enriching the knowledge of future occupational therapists and enhancing the services they provide.

This book offers a snapshot of occupational therapy practice at a particular moment in time. Local and global contexts will continue to shape and inform the way occupational therapy practice develops and looks in near and distant futures. As both countries work towards reconciliation, decolonisation, and indigenisation of practices, policies, and curricula, occupational therapy practice must also evolve and adapt. Therefore, as a text on occupational therapy practice and professional issues in Australia and Aotearoa New Zealand, this book is imperfect and a work in progress.

There is enormous work to be done within the profession – and beyond – to achieve equity and occupational justice for all peoples but particularly for Aboriginal and Torres Strait Islander Peoples in Australia and Māori in Aotearoa New Zealand. This work cannot, and should not, be the responsibility of Indigenous Peoples only. Non-Indigenous occupational therapists must continue to serve as allies, co-resisters, and accomplices to advance equity and occupational justice. While this book does not claim to have all the answers, we hope it contributes meaningfully to the ongoing dialogue and action required to move the occupational therapy profession forward.

We end this book by presenting you with a wero. Wero is a Māori concept that can be described as a challenge (Te Aka., 2025), one that is not simply accepted; it is taken up with intention and readiness. Our wero to you is this: What actions will you take to ensure your practice is culturally safe, promotes equity, actively resists oppression, and enables access and occupational participation for the people of Australia and/or Aotearoa New Zealand?

References

Ahmed-Landeryou, M. J. (2024). A critical reflection from inside, looking back and forward: Theorising perspectives on decolonising occupational science theory and practice. *Journal of Occupational Science, 31*(1), 32–46. https://doi.org/10.1080/14427591.2023.2246986

Australian Institute of Health and Welfare (AIHW). (2024). *Australia's health 2024: In brief.* AIHW. https://www.aihw.gov.au/reports/australias-health/australias-health-2024-in-brief/summary

Bell, A. (2024). *Becoming Tangata Tiriti: Working with Māori, honouring the Treaty.* Auckland University Press.

Bracken, A., Reilly, C., Feeley, A., Sheehan, E., Merghani, K., & Feeley, I. (2025). Artificial intelligence (AI)–powered documentation systems in healthcare: A systematic review. *Journal of Medical Systems, 49*, 28. https://doi.org/10.1007/s10916-025-02157-4

Crawford, A., & Langridge, F. (2022). Pākehā/Palangi positionality: Disentangling power and paralysis. *New Zealand Medical Journal, 135*(1561), 102–110. https://doi.org/10.26635/6965.5734

Ferreira, R. M. (2023). New evidence-based practice: Artificial intelligence as a barrier breaker. *World Journal of Methodology, 13*(5), 384–389. https://doi.org/10.5662/wjm.v13.i5.384

Henrich, J., Heine, S. J., & Norenzayan, A. (2010). The weirdest people in the world? *The Behavioral and Brain Sciences, 33*(2–3), 61–135. https://doi.org/10.1017/S0140525X0999152X

Hocking, C., & Tokolahi, E. (2025). Occupation and health promotion. In M. N. Ikiugu, S. D. Taff, S. Kantartzis, & N. Pollard (Eds.), *Routledge companion to occupational therapy theories, concepts and models* (pp. 551–564). Routledge.

Huot, S., & Forwell, S. (2024). Special issue: Occupation and society: Global to local perspectives for the future. *Journal of Occupational Science, 31*(1), 3–10. https://doi.org/10.1080/14427591.2024.2308085

Kaelin, V. C., Nilsson, I., & Lindgren, H. (2024). Occupational therapy in the space of artificial intelligence: Ethical considerations and human-centered efforts. *Scandinavian Journal of Occupational Therapy, 31*(1). https://doi.org/10.1080/11038128.2024.2421355

Kaelin, V. C., Valizadeh, M., Salgado, Z., Parde, N., & Khetani, M. A. (2021). Artificial intelligence in rehabilitation targeting the participation of children and youth with disabilities: Scoping review. *Journal of Medical Internet Research, 23*(11), e25745. https://doi.org/10.2196/25745

Kokkotis, C., Kansizoglou, I., Stampoulis, T., Giannakou, E., Siaperas, P., Kallidis, S., Koutra, M., Koutra, C., Beneka, A., & Bebetsos, E. (2025). Artificial intelligence as assessment tool in occupational therapy: A scoping review. *BioMedInformatics, 5*(2), 22. https://doi.org/10.3390/biomedinformatics5020022

Peters, L., Abrahams, K., Francke, M., Rustin, L., & Minen, G. (2024). Towards developing a decolonial transdisciplinary praxis that supports a socially-transformative occupational science: Emergent insights from an educational project in South Africa. *Journal of Occupational Science, 31*(1), 73–87. https://doi.org/10.1080/14427591.2023.2233970

Stover, A. D., & Jacobs, K. (2025). Embracing artificial intelligence (AI) in occupational therapy practice: Bridging workforce gaps and redefining care. *WORK, 80*(3), 1021–1028. https://doi.org/10.1177/10519815241312447

Te Aka. (2025). *Wero.* Māori Dictionary. https://maoridictionary.co.nz/search?idiom=&phrase=&proverb=&loan=&histLoanWords=&keywords=wero

Index

professional practice *see* standards of
practice, professional
professional promotion 542
professional reasoning 106–107, 109,
131, 316–317, 323–324, 385, 406, 464,
481; aspects of 318–321; influences on
321–322; intuition 321; overview of *322,
322–323, 329*; reflection 321–322
professional roles and responsibilities 96–99,
101–102, 106, 254–255, 257
professional socialisation 245
professionalisation (professionalism) 9,
26–28, 34, 74, 191; NDIS 66; Pacific
Peoples 235–236; standards of 32
professional standards and guidelines 251
project 255–256
project placement 255
promotion 538, 541–543
protective factors 503
proxemics (non-verbal communication) 122
proximal determinants 504
psychometrics study, occupational therapy
assessment 396–397; reliability 400;
responsiveness 402; validity 401–402
Psychosocial Impact of Assistive Devices
Scale 472
public health services 50–51, 74, 77
public policy 484
public safety to youth safety 179–180
public space 194
Pussin, J.-B. 18
Puutu Kunti Kurrama and Pinikura Peoples
(PKKP Aboriginal Corporation) 361

qualitative methods 288–289
quality in practice placements 253–254, 259
quantitative methods 288–289
quaternary care in Australia 50
Quebec User Evaluation of Satisfaction with
Assistive Technology (QuEST 2.0) 472
Queensland's OT Futures 252
questioning skills **124**

race-based rules 24
racial equality 11
racism 29, 73, 223, 236, 548–549
racist eugenics 25
rainbow families 155
randomised control trial 288
Rangatira 217–219
Ranger programmes 362
RE-AIM (Reach, Effectiveness, Adoption,
Implementation, and Maintenance)
framework 307
real-time supervision 257
real-world practice scenarios 244
reconciliation 5, 11, 25, 30, 32, 34, 46, 154, 156;
Australian Indigenous Voice referendum 33

reconstruction aides 26
recovery efforts 481
recruitment and retention in rural areas
518, **519**
redress inequities 495
re-evaluation of occupational therapy 384
referendum 30–31; Australian Indigenous
Voice 33
reflection **125**, 254, 256, 258, 379–380
reflective practices 131, 149–150, 505
reflective supervision 149–150
reflexivity 157, 289
regional areas, occupational therapy practice
in 514
Regional University Study Hub (RUSH) 520
Registration Boards 107
regulation/registration authorities 84–86;
facilitators of change 92; knowledge
sharing and professional learning 87–88;
lobbying and advocacy 92; OTBA 86;
OTBNZ 87; OTC 86; professional practice
(*see* standards of practice, professional)
regulatory authorities 106
rehabilitation 10, 26–28, 74, 78–79, 99,
252, 351, 464, 468, 496; American
rehabilitation approaches 26; post-war
28–30; programmes by ACC 75
rehabilitation case manager (RCM) 531,
533–534
reintegration 26
relationality 156
relational practice: kinship, country,
and collaboration 155–156, 158;
whakawhanaungatanga and whānau-
centred practice in 156
relationship-focused practice 142, 144, 149;
characteristics of *144*; *see also* person/
family-centred collaborative relationship-
focused practice
relevance 300–302, 311
religious/spiritual occupations 433
remote areas 482–483; occupational therapy
practice in 514, 517; primary health care
in 550
renaissance 541
repatriation 26; post-war 28–30
research: advocate 287; appraisal 309–311;
collaborators 286–287; consumer 287;
evidence 300; paradigms 287–289, 294;
producers 286–287; translation 304;
utilisation 304
ResearchGate 287
resettlement 26
residential aged care facilities (RACF) 52,
54, 351
Residential Environment Impact Scale 472
resilience 16, 34, 154, 206, 210, 212, 245,
269, 454

For Product Safety Concerns and Information please contact our EU
representative GPSR@taylorandfrancis.com
Taylor & Francis Verlag GmbH, Kaufingerstraße 24, 80331 München, Germany